プラクティカル
医学英語辞典

羽白　清　著

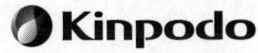

プラクティカル
医学英語辞典

松田 徳一郎 著

Kanehara

序　文

　本書「プラクティカル医学英語辞典」は，あらゆる医療職と医療系学生が医学英語の基礎を身に付けてそれぞれの分野で実際に活用する手引きになることを目標としています．今日，医学を学び，医療に従事する者にとって，英語の知識は必須となっていますが，その必要性の程度は，英語の医学用語を理解したい，最新の医学情報を英語で読みたい，診療に必要なベッドサイドの英語表現を覚えたいなど立場によりいろいろでしょう．

　現在，医学英語に関する書物は世に溢れていますが，基礎的知識から活用表現までを集約した小冊子は見当たりません．本書の背景には，42年前に初版を出版した自著「臨床英文の正しい書き方」があります．この本は英語で診療録を記載するために必要な基本語句と例文を多数列挙して，アメリカの病院で通用する書式と表現を和英対照で示したものです．幸い好評で改訂を重ねてロングセラーとなっていますが，読者からは臨床の現場で利用しやすい「臨床英文」小型版の要望が多く寄せられていました．

　そこで「臨床英文の正しい書き方」を発展させ臨床医学関連の用語数を大幅に増やして応用表現を収載するとともに，医学英語の基礎的語彙を加えて本書を編集しました．基本的な解剖学的用語をはじめ医療関連用語を網羅していますが，単に医学用語を羅列した字引ではなく，英語で診察して診療録を書くことに役立つ実用的な参考書としました．たとえば英文診療録の記載については，実際の診療の過程を踏んで症状，診察所見，検査所見，診断，治療の項目の順に用語を配列しています．

　本書の特色の一つとして，冠名用語に英文の説明文を加えました．医学の分野では人名を冠した疾患，症候群，検査名が多いのですが，主な冠名用語に簡潔な説明を加えて，内容の理解を助けると同時に説明文を読むことにより医学英語の自習にな

ることを期待しています.

　本書一冊で, 和英・英和医学用語辞典, 略語集, 冠名用語集, 診療録記載法, 診療会話・プレゼンテーション・紹介状の英語表現集, 実用医薬品集を兼ねた盛り沢山の内容です. 医師と看護師をはじめいろいろな分野の医療職の方々と, 医療系の学生の皆様の学習書として実用書として活用されることを願っています. 採用した医学用語は, 実際にアメリカの病院で臨床に携わる際にも役に立つレベルであり, 医学生には USMLE Step 2 CS や OSCE の準備にもなるでしょう.

　本書中の会話英語について校閲と助言を戴いた立命館大学講師, John Gorman 先生に謝意を表します. また本書の企画と編集から刊行に至るまで多大のご尽力をいただいた金芳堂社長市井輝和氏と編集部村上裕子氏に心からお礼申し上げます.

　2010年4月1日

　　　　　　　　　　　　　　　　　　　　　　　　　著者

凡　例

1．本書の利用方法

　本書は医師と看護師に限らず，すべての医療関係の学生と専門職が学校や病院で遭遇する英語の医学用語を正しく理解し実地で利用できるように編集した活用辞典である．原則として日本語から出発して対応する英語を検索するという方針で用語を収載したが，医学用語の索引を充実させたので和英・英和辞書としても利用できる．日常手元に置いて英語でどう表現するのか疑問が生じたときに参照し活用していただきたい．

2．本書の構成

- 医学英語の基礎と医療関連用語：医学英語の習得にはまず語彙を豊かにすることが前提となるが，医学用語の成り立ち，語源，接辞，類似語などの解説に加えて医療関連用語を多数示して，興味深く語彙を増やせるように配慮した．臨床医学各分野のテキストブックをはじめ，英字新聞・雑誌の医療記事や英文医学文献の読解に必要な医学用語を網羅し，現代の医療に対応する up-to-date の用語を採用した．
- 英文診療録：英文診療録の構成と記載内容について，POS の診療録を含めて解説し，英文診療録の記載に必要な語句と表現を示した．英文で書かれた診療録や症例報告を読む際の手引きにもなる．
- 診療録用語：診療の流れに沿って，身体の系統ごとに愁訴・症状―診察所見―検査法―疾患名―治療法の順に用語を配列して実際の記録の助けになるように工夫した．いろいろな疾患の症状，徴候，検査項目，治療法を見出し語に列挙してあるので診療のチェックリストにも使える．
- 診療英会話：問診，診察，患者説明に際して必要な英会話表現を列挙し，実際に応用できるように具体的な内容とした．医療者側からだけでなく，受診する立場からも身体と病気の表現ができるように一般英語表現も充実させた．
- 症例プレゼンテーション：回診やカンファレンスで症例のプ

レゼンテーションを要領よく行うために必要な慣用表現を短文で示し，実際の症例を提示した．
- 英文紹介状：通常のビジネスレターの形式に準じるが，医師が書く紹介状の実際について医学的事項を含む短文で例示し，紹介状の実例を示した．
- 略語：略語は各医学用語語末の括弧内に示し，X章に略語集としてまとめた．略語の総数は3,159語である．さらに医薬品略号，元素記号，単位の一覧表をⅧ章に示した．ラテン語以外の略語ではピリオドを省略した．
- 人体解剖図：人体各部の名称を和英対照で列挙し，代表的な用語はイラストで示した．

3．見出し語

　見出し語の配列法は，各テーマの実情に応じて五十音順または項目の内容順とした．医学用語名は，原則として日本医学会医学用語管理委員会編「医学会医学用語辞典―英和―」第3版（南山堂，2007）に基づき，各専門学会の用語集を参照した．見出し語の同義語はコンマで併記した．医学用語には読みの難解なものが多いので，見出し語にはすべてふりがなをつけた．取り上げた見出し語の総数は10,900項目に上る．また診療英会話例文および症例提示と紹介状に関する実用例文の総数は1,154例である．

4．医学用語の英語

　原則として米国式綴りを採用し，単語の不定冠詞，定冠詞は省略した．生物学名の属名はイタリック体で示した．用語は主として名詞で示したが，形容詞，動詞などの派生語を併記して活用の便宜をはかった．

5．冠名用語

　人名を冠した病名，症候群，検査などの冠名用語 eponym には，英語の短文で簡単な説明を加えた．個々の用語の要点を把握できると同時に，医学英語の学習にも役立つことを期待している．すなわち冠名用語の英文説明を読んで医学用語の理解の

凡　例　v

程度を確かめる自習ができる．総計663項目を収載し，巻末に英語の「冠名用語索引」を「英語索引」から独立させて別に設けた．なお人名用語の所有格を表すアポストロフィ s は省略した．

6．医薬品名

　治療法の見出し語として医薬品名は一般名で示したが，対応する英語表記に続いて《　》内に商品名の例を随時示した．抗菌薬と抗癌剤については，略号ごとに系統，用法，商品名などの情報を加えて独立させた．商品名は利用者の便宜を図って例示したが，掲載した商品が唯一のものではなく，またこれを推奨するものでもない．詳細は一般名から各種医薬品集を参照されたい．

7．Tidbits

　医学用語に関連する Tidbits ("small pieces of interesting information" という意味) を息抜きの囲みとして挿入した．

8．索　引

　日本語索引，英語索引，冠名用語索引（英語），薬剤商品名索引があり，それぞれの用語の記載ページを示した．

9．略号，記号

〔英〕：英語　〔独〕：ドイツ語　〔仏〕：フランス語
〔ラ〕：ラテン語　〔名〕：名詞　〔形〕：形容詞　〔動〕：動詞
〔複〕：複数　〔話〕：口語
syn.：同義語　　cf：参照　　＜：派生，由来
（　）：代用，交換，説明
例：父方（母方）の paternal (maternal), on the father's (mother's) side
　　→父方の　paternal, on the father's side
　　　母方の　maternal, on the mother's side

目 次

I章. 医学英語の基礎 …………………………… 1

1. 医学用語 ………………………………… 2
医学用語　2
医学用語の構成要素　2
医学用語造語法　2
医学用語の標準化　3

2. 身体部位・臓器名 ……………………… 5
身体部位・臓器名の語源　5

3. 接　辞 …………………………………… 10
接頭辞　10
連結形　12
接尾辞　17
国際単位系の接頭辞　20

4. ラテン語 ………………………………… 21
常用されるラテン語　21
処方箋に用いられるラテン語　22

5. 術語と日常語 …………………………… 25
術語と日常語の対比　25

6. カタカナ用語 …………………………… 29
カタカナ用語の語源　29

7. 紛らわしい医学用語 …………………… 34
紛らわしい医学用語　34

8. 色彩・形状の表現 ……………………… 39
色　彩　39
形　状　39

II章. 医療関連用語 …………………………… 41

1. 医療行為 ………………………………… 42
医療行為　42
倫理綱領　44

2. 医事法制 ………………………………… 46
法　制　46
医事法　46

3. 医療保険制度 …………………………… 48
医療保険制度　48
英米の医療保険　50

4. 保健医療施設 ……………………………………………… 52
保健医療施設　*52*
医療施設：病院　*52*
病院部門：診療科　*53*
病院部門：診療科以外　*54*
介護施設　*55*

5. 医療従事者 …………………………………………………… 57
医療関係職種　*57*
病院内職掌　*59*
診療医・専門医　*59*
専門看護師　*60*
認定看護師　*60*

6. 医学教育 ……………………………………………………… 62
医療系教育機関　*62*
医科大学職名　*62*
基礎医学　*63*
臨床医学　*63*
看護学　*65*
医学教育用語　*66*

Ⅲ章. 英文診療録 ……………………………………………… 69

1. 診療録 ………………………………………………………… 70
診療録の構成　*70*

2. 診療録の記載 ………………………………………………… 71
患者識別情報　*71*
情報源　*71*
主　訴　*71*
現病歴　*72*
既往歴　*73*
家族歴　*73*
社会歴　*74*
系統別病歴　*75*
身体的検査　*75*
診察用具　*77*
検査法　*78*
画像検査　*79*
測定法　*80*
病理所見　*82*
診　断　*84*
治療法　85
手　術　*86*

看　護　*89*
栄　養　*90*
経過記録　*91*
要　約　*93*

3. 問題志向型システム …………………………………… 95
問題志向型システム　*95*

4. 問題志向型診療録 ……………………………………… 95
問題志向型診療録の構成　*95*

5. POMRの記載 …………………………………………… 96
データベース　*96*
問題リスト　*96*
初期計画　*96*
経過記録　*96*
監　査　*96*

6. 診療録記載に用いられる略語・記号 ………………… 98
略語・記号　*98*

IV章. 診療録用語 …………………………………………… 103

1. 全身状態 ………………………………………………… 104
症状・徴候　*104*
感染症　*107*
膠原病　*110*
難病（特定疾患）　*111*
治療法　*117*
補完代替医療　*118*

2. 疼　痛 …………………………………………………… 120
症状・徴候　*120*
治療法　*122*

3. 眼 ………………………………………………………… 125
愁訴・症状　*125*
診察所見・徴候　*127*
検査法　*131*
疾患名　*133*
治療法　*135*

4. 耳鼻咽喉 ………………………………………………… 139
愁訴・症状　*139*
診察所見・徴候　*140*
検査法　*141*
疾患名　*143*
治療法　*145*

5. 口腔, 歯 147
- 愁訴・症状 *147*
- 診察所見・徴候 *148*
- 検査法 *149*
- 疾患名 *150*
- 治療法 *152*

6. 呼吸器系 154
- 愁訴・症状 *154*
- 診察所見・徴候 *156*
- 検査法 *158*
- 疾患名 *163*
- 治療法 *167*

7. 循環器系 172
- 愁訴・症状 *172*
- 診察所見・徴候 *173*
- 検査法 *178*
- 疾患名 *183*
- 治療法 *188*

8. 消化器系 194
- 愁訴・症状 *194*
- 診察所見・徴候 *197*
- 検査法 *199*
- 疾患名 *204*
- 治療法 *210*

9. 腎・泌尿器系 216
- 愁訴・症状 *216*
- 診察所見・徴候 *217*
- 検査法 *217*
- 疾患名 *221*
- 治療法 *224*

10. 生殖器系 228
- 愁訴・症状 *228*
- 診察所見・徴候 *231*
- 胎位 *233*
- 検査法 *234*
- 疾患名 *236*
- 治療法 *241*

11. 内分泌・代謝系 244
- 愁訴・症状 *244*
- 診察所見・徴候 *245*
- 検査法 *246*
- 疾患名 *251*
- 治療法 *257*

12. 血液・造血器系 261
- 愁訴・症状 *261*
- 診察所見・徴候 *262*
- 検査法 *263*
- 疾患名 *269*
- 治療法 *274*

13. 筋・骨格系 278
- 愁訴・症状 *278*
- 診察所見・徴候 *279*
- 検査法 *283*
- 疾患名 *284*
- 治療法 *288*

14. 精神・神経系 293
- 愁訴・症状 *293*
- 恐怖症 *296*
- 診察所見・徴候 *297*
- 検査法 *303*
- 疾患名 *306*
- 治療法 *314*

15. 皮膚 318

愁訴・症状	*318*	疾患名	*324*
診察所見・徴候	*319*	治療法	*328*
検査法	*321*		

16. 小児科 ……………………………………………………… *330*

愁訴・症状	*330*	疾患名	*334*
診察所見・徴候	*331*	治療法	*343*
検査法	*333*		

V章. 診療英会話 ……………………………………………… *345*

1. 問診の英会話 ……………………………………………… *346*
インタビューを始める　*346*
患者の訴え　*347*
症状につて尋ねる　*350*
全身状態　*352*
疼痛　*353*
眼　*355*
耳鼻咽喉　*356*
呼吸器・循環器系　*357*
消化器系　*359*
泌尿器系　*361*
生殖器系　*362*
内分泌系　*363*
骨・関節・筋肉系　*364*
精神・神経系　*365*
皮膚　*366*
患者像　*367*
既往歴　*370*
家族歴　*371*

2. 診察の英会話 ……………………………………………… *372*
診察前　*372*
バイタルサイン　*372*
頭部　*373*
胸部　*374*
腹部　*375*
四肢　*376*
診察後　*377*

3. 患者説明の英会話 ………………………………………… *378*
病状・診断の説明　*378*
検査の説明　*379*
治療方針の説明　*381*
服薬指導　*385*

VI章. 症例プレゼンテーション……………………… *391*

1. 基本短文例……………………………………… *392*
症例検討　*392*
患者紹介　*392*
患者像　*394*
現病歴　*395*
既往歴　*396*
家族歴　*397*
身体所見　*398*
検査所見　*400*
診　断　*401*
計　画　*403*

2. 実　例……………………………………………… *405*
症例提示　*405*

VII章. 英文紹介状……………………………………… *409*

1. 基本短文例……………………………………… *410*
挨拶文句　*410*
本　文　*410*
結びの句　*416*
署　名　*417*

2. 実　例……………………………………………… *418*
紹介状　*418*
紹介状返答　*419*

VIII章. 略号, 記号……………………………………… *421*

1. 医薬品略号……………………………………… *422*
抗菌薬　*422*
抗癌剤　*429*
分子標的治療薬　*433*

2. 元素記号………………………………………… *434*
3. 単　位…………………………………………… *438*

IX章. 人体解剖図……………………………………… *441*

1. 人　体…………………………………………… *442*
頭　*442*　　　　　　　　　　上　肢　*444*
胴体, 体幹　*444*　　　　　　下　肢　*446*

xii

2. 表面解剖学 ... 448
面　448
方　向　448
部　位　450
体表面線　454
体　腔　455

3. 感覚器 ... 456
眼　456
耳　458
鼻　460
皮　膚　462

4. 口　腔 ... 464
口　464
歯　464
咽　頭　465

5. 呼吸器系 ... 466
気　道　466
気　管　466
肺　466
気管支肺区域　468
胸　膜　468
縦　隔　468

6. 循環器系 ... 470
心　臓　470
動　脈　471
静　脈　476
リンパ系　478

7. 消化器系 ... 480
消化器　480
食　道　480
胃　480
腸　480
肝　臓　484
胆　道　484
膵　臓　484

8. 泌尿器・生殖器系 ... 486
泌尿器系　486
男性生殖器系　488
女性生殖器系　488

9. 内分泌系 ... 490
内分泌臓器　490

10. 骨格系 ... 492
骨　492
関　節　495
軟　骨　495

靱帯 *496*
11. 筋肉系 ... *498*
筋肉 *498*
腱 *501*
12. 神経系 ... *502*
中枢神経系 *502*
末梢神経系 *505*
13. 補遺 ... *508*
細胞 *508*
遺伝子 *508*
組織 *512*
体液 *512*

X章. 略語集 ... *515*

索引
日本語索引 ... *614*
英語索引 ... *701*
冠名用語索引 ... *825*
薬剤商品名索引 ... *833*

Tidbits

gobbledygook	4	perleche	153
lien	9	Sutton's law	171
Occam's razor	19	azygos	193
sesquipedalian words	20	bezoar	209
ラテン語の略語	24	Bristol stool form scale	215
Brevity is the soul of wit.	28	NOTES	227
ムンテラ	33	bariatric surgery	260
homophone	38	six-pack	277
quack	45	regimen	292
oxymoron	47	mnemonic	317
portmanteau word	51	uncountable noun	329
acronym	56	gargoylism	344
"comedical" staff	61	tautology	371
topology	68	data	390
Chief Concern	70	back-formation	407
euthanasia	94	Ich bin ein Berliner.	417
octothorp	97	Leggett's tree	420
OOPS. OOB.	101	extremity	447
homeopathy	119	anatomical position	448
cannabis	124	phlegmatic	479
biopsy	138	double noun	485
red herring	146	funny bone	497

I 章

医学英語の基礎

1. 医学用語

● 医学用語　Medical terminology ●

医学用語 いがくようご	medical terms
専門用語 せんもんようご	technical terminology
術語 じゅつご	technical terms
医学英語 いがくえいご	medical English
医学目的の英語 いがくもくてきのえいご	English for medical purposes (EMP)
日常語 にちじょうご	vernacular
俗語 ぞくご	slang
隠語 いんご	jargon
医師間通用語 いしかんつうようご	medical argot, medical jargon, medicalese
語の原形 ごのげんけい	etymon
語源 ごげん	etymology
派生語 はせいご	derivative
語形変化 ごけいへんか	inflection

● 医学用語の構成要素　Word structure ●

語根 ごこん	root（語の中核となる要素で意味を表す．ギリシャ語，ラテン語由来が多い）
接辞 せつじ	affix（接頭辞，挿入辞，接尾辞の総称）
接頭辞 せっとうじ	prefix（語根の前に付いて修飾する）
接尾辞 せつびじ	suffix（語根の後に付いて修飾する）
連結母音 れんけつぼいん	combining vowel (-o-)（語根と語根，語根と接尾辞をつなぐ）
連結形 れんけつけい	combining form（語根＋連結母音）

● 医学用語造語法　Word-formation ●

肝炎 かんえん	hepatitis: hepat 肝（語根）／ itis 炎（接尾辞）
アミラーゼ	amylase: amyl でんぷん（語根）／ ase 酵素（接尾辞）
血液学 けつえきがく	hematology: hemat 血液（語根）／ o（連結母音）／ logy 学（接尾辞）
眼瞼下垂 がんけんかすい	blepharoptosis: blephar 眼瞼（語根）／ o（連結母音）／ ptosis 下垂（接尾辞）
甲状腺機能亢進症 こうじょうせんきのうこうしんしょう	hyperthyroidism: hyper 過度（接頭辞）／ thyroid 甲状腺（語根）／ ism 状態（接尾辞）
多発関節痛 たはつかんせつつう	polyarthralgia: poly 多発（接頭辞）／ arthr 関節（語根）／ algia 痛（接尾辞）

1. 医学用語

高脂血症 こうしけっしょう	hyperlipidemia: hyper 過度（接頭辞）/ lipid 脂質（語根）/ emia 血症（接尾辞）
下顎半切除術 かがくはんせつじょじゅつ	hemimandibulectomy: hemi 半（接頭辞）/ mendibul 下顎（語根）/ ectomy 切除（接尾辞）
軟骨無形成症 なんこつむけいせいしょう	achondroplasia: a 無（接頭辞）/ chondr 軟骨（語根）/ o（連結母音）/ plasia 形成（接尾辞）
精子形成能低下 せいしけいせいのうていか	hypospermatogenesis: hypo 低下（接頭辞）/ spermat 精子（語根）/ o（連結母音）/ genesis 形成（接尾辞）
総胆管十二指腸吻合 そうたんかんじゅうにしちょうふんごう	choledochoduodenostomy: choledoch 総胆管（語根）/ o（連結母音）/ duoden 十二指腸（語根）/ o（連結母音）/ stomy 開口（接尾辞）
肝脾腫 かんひしゅ	hepatosplenomegaly: hepat 肝（語根）/ o（連結母音）/ splen 脾（語根）/ o（連結母音）/ megaly 腫大（接尾辞）
脳波 のうは	electroencephalogram: electr 電気（語根）/ o（連結母音）/ encephal 脳（語根）/ o（連結母音）/ gram 記録（接尾辞）
膿気心膜症 のうきしんまくしょう	pyopneumopericardium: pyo 膿（連結形）/ pneumo 気（連結形）/ peri 周囲（接頭辞）/ cardi 心臓（語根）/ um 組織（接尾辞）（注：pericardium 心膜）
子宮卵管造影法 しきゅうらんかんぞうえいほう	hysterosalpingography: hystero 子宮（連結形）/ salpingo 卵管（連結形）/ graphy 造影（接尾辞）
耳鼻咽喉科学 じびいんこうかがく	otorhinolaryngology: oto 耳（連結形）/ rhino 鼻（連結形）/ laryngo 喉頭（連結形）/ logy 学（接尾辞）

●医学用語の標準化　Standardization●

統合医学用語システム とうごういがくようご—	Unified Medical Language System (UMLS)
国際医学用語コード こくさいいがくようご—	Systematized Nomenclature of Medicine (SNOMED)
医学件名標目集 いがくけんめいひょうもくしゅう	Medical Subject Headings (MeSH)
疾病及び関連保健問題の国際統計分類第10回修正 しっぺいおよ—かんれんほけんもんだい—こくさいとうけいぶんるいだい—	International Statistical Classification of Diseases and Related Health Problems, Tenth Revision (ICD-10)

国際病理学用語コード Systematized Nomenclature of Pathology (SNOP)
看護実践国際分類 International Classification for Nursing Practice (ICNP)
国際科学用語 International Scientific Vocabulary (ISV)

Tidbits

gobbledygook

本来は回りくどく難解なお役所言葉（officialese）を指す口語でgobble は七面鳥の鳴き声．第二次大戦中の米国下院議員，Maury Maverick（一匹狼 maverick の語源となった Samuel A Maverick とは別人）が官僚の複雑な用語（convoluted language of bureaucrats）は少年時代にテキサスで聞いた果てしない七面鳥の馬鹿げた鳴き声を思い出させるとして名付けたといわれる．医学論文にしばしば見られる冗長な難解表現についても用いられる．E-mail の文字化けも gibberish, gobbledygook, garbled text などという．

2. 身体部位・臓器名

●身体部位・臓器名の語源 Body parts●

臓器名	ラテン語	ギリシャ語	英語	派生語
足 あし	pes	pous	foot	pes planus 扁平足, podagra 足部痛風
頭 あたま	caput	kephalē	head	caput medusae メズサの頭, cephalic 頭部の
胃 い	stomachus	gastēr	stomach	gastric 胃の, gastrolith 胃石
腕 うで	brachium	brachiōn	arm	brachial 腕の, brachioradialis 腕撓骨筋
頤 おとがい	mentum	geneion	chin	mentoplasty 頤形成術, geniohyoid 頤舌骨筋
顔 かお	facies	prosōpon	face	facial 顔面の, prosopoplegia 顔面神経麻痺
体 からだ	corpus	sōma	body	corpus luteum 黄体, somatotype 体型
関節 かんせつ	junctura	arthron	joint	arthritis 関節炎, arthroscope 関節鏡
肝臓 かんぞう	jecur	hēpar	liver	hepatic 肝の, hepatomegaly 肝腫大
気管 きかん	trachea	tracheia	windpipe	tracheal 気管の, tracheostomy 気管切開
気管支 きかんし	bronchus	bronchos	bronchus	bronchial 気管支の, bronchography 気管支造影
胸郭 きょうかく	thorax	thōrax	thorax	thoracic 胸の, thoracoplasty 胸郭形成術
胸骨 きょうこつ	sternum	sternon	breast bone	sternal 胸骨の, sternotomy 胸骨切開
筋 きん	musculus	mys	muscle	muscular 筋の, myoma 筋腫

I章 医学英語の基礎

臓器名	ラテン語	ギリシャ語	英 語	派生語
口 <ruby>く<rt></rt>ち</ruby>	os	stoma	mouth	oral 経口的, stomatitis 口内炎
唇 <ruby>くち<rt></rt>びる</ruby>	labium	cheilos	lip	labial 唇の, cheilitis 口唇炎
毛 <ruby>け<rt></rt></ruby>	pilus	thrix	hair	piloerection 立毛, trichophagia 食毛症
脛骨 <ruby>けい<rt></rt>こつ</ruby>	tibia	knēmē	shinbone	tibial 脛骨の, tibialgia 脛骨痛
血液 <ruby>けつ<rt></rt>えき</ruby>	sanguis	haima	blood	sanguine 多血質の, hemodialysis 血液透析
血管 <ruby>けっ<rt></rt>かん</ruby>	vas	angeion	vessel	vasodilation 血管拡張, angiography 血管造影法
結腸 <ruby>けっ<rt></rt>ちょう</ruby>	colon	kolon	colon	colonic 結腸の, colonoscope 結腸内視鏡
腱 <ruby>けん<rt></rt></ruby>	tendo	tenōn	tendon	tendovaginitis 腱鞘炎, tenodesis 腱固定
喉頭 <ruby>こう<rt></rt>とう</ruby>	larynx	larynx	larynx	laryngeal 喉頭の, laryngoscopy 喉頭鏡検査
骨 <ruby>こ<rt></rt>つ</ruby>	os	osteon	bone	osseous 骨性, ossification 骨化
骨格 <ruby>こっ<rt></rt>かく</ruby>	sceletus	skeleton	skeleton	skeletal 骨格の, exoskeleton 外骨格
骨盤 <ruby>こつ<rt></rt>ばん</ruby>	pelvis	pellis	pelvis	pelvic 骨盤の, pelvimetry 骨盤計測
臍 <ruby>さい<rt></rt></ruby>	umbilicus	omphalos	navel	umbilical 臍の, omphalocele 臍帯ヘルニア
鎖骨 <ruby>さ<rt></rt>こつ</ruby>	clavicula	kleis	collarbone	clavicular 鎖骨の, cleidotomy 鎖骨離断術
子宮 <ruby>し<rt></rt>きゅう</ruby>	uterus	hystera	uterus	uterine 子宮の, hysteropexy 子宮固定術

2. 身体部位・臓器名

臓器名	ラテン語	ギリシャ語	英　語	派生語
膝 _{ひざ}	genu	gony	knee	genicular 膝関節の, gonatocele 膝関節腫
歯肉 _{しにく}	gingiva	oulon	gum	gingival 歯肉の, gingivitis 歯肉炎
舌 _{した}	lingua	glōssa	tongue	lingual 舌の, glossitis 舌炎
小脳 _{しょうのう}	cerebellum	parenkephalida	cerebellum	cerebellar 小脳の, cerebellopontine 小脳橋の
静脈 _{じょうみゃく}	vena	phleps	vein	venous 静脈性, phlebitis 静脈炎
食道 _{しょくどう}	oesophagus	oisophagos	esophagus	esophageal 食道の, esophagitis 食道炎
神経 _{しんけい}	nervus	neuron	nerve	nervous 神経（質）の, neurology 神経学
心臓 _{しんぞう}	cor	kardia	heart	cor pulmonale 肺性心, cardiology 心臓病学
腎臓 _{じんぞう}	ren	nephros	kidney	renal 腎臓の, nephritis 腎炎
膵臓 _{すいぞう}	pancreas	pankreas	pancreas	pancreatic 膵臓の, pancreatitis 膵炎
精神 _{せいしん}	mens	psychē	mind	mental 精神的, psychotherapy 精神療法
精巣 _{せいそう}	testis	orchis	testicle	testicular 精巣の, orchiopexy 精巣固定術
脊椎 _{せきつい}	spina	rhachis	spine	spinal 脊椎の, rachiodynia 脊椎痛
前立腺 _{ぜんりつせん}	prostata	prostatēs	prostate	prostatic 前立腺の, prostatitis 前立腺炎
大腿骨 _{だいたいこつ}	femur	mēros	thighbone	femoral 大腿（骨）の, meralgia 大腿痛
大脳 _{だいのう}	cerebrum	enkephalos	cerebrum	cerebral 大脳の, cerebrospinal 脳脊

I章 医学英語の基礎

臓器名	ラテン語	ギリシャ語	英　語	派生語
				髄の
腸 ちょう	intestinum	enteron	intestine	intestinal 腸管の, enterocolitis 小腸結腸炎
椎骨 ついこつ	vertebra	spondylos	vertebra	vertebral 椎骨の, spondylolisthesis 脊椎すべり症
爪 つめ	unguis	onyx	nail	ungual 爪の, onycholysis 爪剝離症
手 て	manus	cheir	hand	manual 用手の, macrocheiria 巨手症
頭蓋 とうがい	cranium	kranion	skull	cranial 頭蓋の, 頭側の, craniotomy 開頭
動脈 どうみゃく	arteria	artēria	artery	arterial 動脈性, arteriole 細動脈
軟骨 なんこつ	cartilago	chondros	cartilage	catilaginous 軟骨性, chondrosarcoma 軟骨肉腫
乳房 にゅうぼう	mamma	mastos	breast	mammography 乳房X線撮影法, mastectomy 乳房切除術
脳 のう	encephalon	enkephalos	brain	encephalitis 脳炎, encephalocele 脳瘤
歯 は	dens	odous	tooth	dental 歯の, odontogenic 歯原性
肺 はい	pulmonis	pneumōn	lung	pulmonary 肺の, pneumonia 肺炎
鼻 はな	nasus	rhis	nose	nasal 鼻の, rhinitis 鼻炎
腹 はら	abdomen	koilia	belly	abdominal 腹部の, celiac 腹腔の
脾臓 ひぞう	splen, lien	splēn	spleen	splenic, lienal 脾の, splenomegaly 脾腫
皮膚 ひふ	cutis	derma	skin	cutaneous 皮膚の, dermatitis 皮膚炎
膀胱 ぼうこう	vesica	kystis	bladder	vesical 膀胱の, cystoscope 膀胱鏡

2. 身体部位・臓器名

臓器名	ラテン語	ギリシャ語	英 語	派生語
耳 みみ	auris	ous	ear	aural 耳の, otorrhea 耳漏
眼 め	oculus	ophthalmos	eye	ocular 眼の, ophthalmia 眼炎
指 ゆび	digitus	daktylos	finger, toe	digital 指の, arachnodactyly くも指症
卵管 らんかん	tuba uterina	salpinx	salpinx	tubal pregnancy 卵管妊娠, salpingography 卵管造影法
卵巣 らんそう	ovarium	oophoron	ovary	ovarian 卵巣の, oophorectomy 卵巣摘出術
肋骨 ろっこつ	costa	pleura	rib	costal 肋骨の, pleural 胸膜の

---Tidbits---

lien

"The lien remains active." は,「脾臓は活動性を保っている」という意味だろうか? 実は新聞記事の1行なのでこの lien は「留置権, 担保権」のことである. 医学用語では「外転」の abduction は一般には「拉致, 誘拐」であり,「嵌頓」incarceration は一般では「投獄」の意味である.「移植片」graft には「収賄, 不正利得」というよからぬ意味もある.「無痛性」の indolent は, 一般には lazy の意味になるので注意を要する.

3. 接辞

●接頭辞　Prefix●

接頭辞	意味	例
a-, an-	無, 非	anoxia 無酸素症, asymmetry 非対称
ab-	から, 離れて	aberration 迷入, abnormal 異常の
ad-	移動, 付加, 増加	adnerval 神経近傍の, adrenal 副腎の
ambi-	両側	ambidexterity 両手利き, ambivalence 両価性
ana-	上へ, 離れて	analysis 分析, anaplasia 退形成
ante-	前	antegrade 順行性, antepartum 分娩前の
anti-	反, 抗	antibiotic 抗生物質, antibody 抗体
auto-	自身, 同一	autoimmunity 自己免疫, autonomy 自律性
bi-	二, 重	bilateral 両側性, bigeminy 二段脈
bis-	二, 二度	bisacromial 両肩峰の, bisferious 二峰性の
cata-	下方	catabolism 異化作用, cataplexy 情動脱力発作
circum-	周囲	circumference 周径, circumscribed 限局性の, 辺縁明瞭な
con-	共に	concentration 集中, conjoined 結合した
contra-	反対, 逆	contraindication 禁忌, contralateral 反対側性
de-	分離, 否定	decerebration 除脳, dehydration 脱水
di-	二	dimer 二量体, dioxide 二酸化物
dia-	通って	diaphoresis 発汗療法, diathermy ジアテルミー療法
dis-	分離	disarticulation 関節離断術, disinfection 消毒
dys-	困難, 不良	dysmenorrhea 月経困難, dyspepsia 消化不良
ecto-	外側, 表面	ectoderm 外胚葉, ectopic 異所性
en-	中	encapsulated 被包性, enzyme 酵素
endo-	内, 内部	endoderm 内胚葉, endogenous 内因性
ento-	内	entotic 耳内, entozoon 内部寄生動物
epi-	上, 次	epidural 硬膜外, epithelium 上皮
eu-	良好, 正常	euphoria 多幸症, euthyroid 甲状腺機能正常の
ex-	外, 外部	excision 切除, excretion 排泄

接頭辞	意 味	例
exo-	外側	exocrine 外分泌, exotropia 外斜視
extra-	外, 外部	extracellular 細胞外, extravasation 血管外遊出
hemi-	半分	hemicrania 片側頭痛, hemiplegia 半側麻痺
hyper-	過度, 上	hypertension 高血圧, hyperthermia 高体温, 温熱療法
hypo-	低下, 下	hypothyroidism 甲状腺機能低下症, hypoxia 低酸素症
in-	内, 無	inactivation 不活化, incontinence 失禁
infra-	下方	infraorbital 眼窩下の, infrared 赤外線の
inter-	間, 中間	intercostal 肋間の, intermenstrual 月経間の
intra-	内, 内部	intracellular 細胞内, intravenous 静脈内
iso-	等, 同	isotonic 等張の, isotope 同位元素
macro-	巨大	macroglossia 巨大舌, macromolecule 高分子
mal-	不良	malformation 奇形, malnutrition 栄養不良
mega-	巨大	megacolon 巨大結腸, megakaryocyte 巨核球
meso-	中, 中間	mesocolon 結腸間膜, mesothelioma 中皮腫
meta-	後, 変化	metamorphosis 変態, metastasis 転移
micro-	微小	microcirculation 微小循環, microscope 顕微鏡
multi-	多数	multinodular 多結節の, multipara 経産婦
neo-	新	neonatal 新生児の, neoplasm 腫瘍, 新生物
pachy-	厚い	pachydermia 硬性皮膚, pachyglossia 舌肥厚
pan-	全体, すべて	pancytopenia 汎血球減少, panhypopituitarism 汎下垂体機能低下
para-	傍, 対	paraaortic 傍大動脈, paraplegia 対麻痺
per-	通して	percutaneous 経皮, peroral 経口的
peri-	周囲	pericardium 心膜, perivascular 血管周囲性
poly-	多数	polycythemia 多血症, polyneuritis 多発神経炎

12　I章　医学英語の基礎

接頭辞	意　味	例
post-	後	postmortem 死後の, postoperative 術後
pre-	前	precancerous 前癌の, precordial 前胸の
pro-	前	prodrome 前駆症状, prophylaxis 予防法
pseudo-	偽	pseudohypoparathyroidism 偽性副甲状腺機能低下症, pseudomembrane 偽膜
re-	再	reinfection 再感染, reoperation 再手術
retro-	後, 後方	retroflexion 後屈, retroperitoneum 腹膜後腔
semi-	半分	semicoma 半昏睡, semilunar 半月型
sub-	下方	subcostal 肋骨下, subcutaneous 皮下
super-	上, 過度	superinfection 重感染, supersecretion 分泌過多
supra-	上方	supraclavicular 鎖骨上, suprapubic 恥骨上
syn-	共, 結合	syndrome 症候群, synthesis 合成
trans-	通って, 超えて	translocation 転位, transplantation 移植
tri-	三, 三重	tricuspid 三尖弁の, trigeminy 三段脈
ultra-	超	ultrafiltration 限外濾過, ultrasonography 超音波検査法
un-	否定	unconscious 無意識の, undifferentiated 未分化
uni-	単一	unilateral 一側性, unilocular 単房性

● 連結形　Combining form ●

連結形	意　味	例
abdomino-	腹部	abdominocentesis 腹腔穿刺, abdominoperineal 腹会陰式
acro-	先端, 末端, 頂	acrodynia 肢端疼痛症, acromegaly 先端巨大症
adeno-	腺	adenocarcinoma 腺癌, adenomatous 腺腫様
adipo-	脂肪	adipose 脂肪の, adiposity 脂肪過多, 肥満
adreno-	副腎	adrenocortical 副腎皮質の, adrenomyeloneuropathy 副腎脊髄末梢神経障害
andro-	男性	androgen アンドロゲン, android 男性様
angio-	血管	angiography 血管造影法, angioneurotic 血管神経性

連結形	意味	例
antero-	前	anterolateral 前外側の, anteroseptal 前壁中隔の
arterio-	動脈	arteriosclerosis 動脈硬化, arteriovenous 動静脈の
arthro-	関節	arthroplasty 関節形成術, arthroscopy 関節鏡検査
audio-	聴覚	audioanalgesia 聴覚性鎮痛, audiometry 聴覚検査
bio-	生命, 生	biochemistry 生化学, biopsy 生検
brachy-	短	brachycephaly 短頭症, brachydactyly 短指症
brady-	遅	bradycardia 徐脈, bradypnea 緩徐呼吸
broncho-	気管支	bronchodilator 気管支拡張薬, bronchopneumonia 気管支肺炎
carcino-	癌	carcinogen 発癌物質, carcinomatosis 癌腫症
cardio-	心臓	cardiopulmonary 心肺の, cardiovascular 心血管の
cephalo-	頭	cephalohematoma 頭血腫, cephalometry 頭蓋計測
cerebro-	脳	cerebrospinal 脳脊髄の, cerebrovascular 脳血管の
chemo-	化学	chemotaxis 化学走性, chemotherapy 化学療法
chole-	胆汁	cholelithiasis 胆石, cholestasis 胆汁うっ滞
chondro-	軟骨	chondroblastoma 軟骨芽腫, chondronecrosis 軟骨壊死
chromo-	色	chromophobe 色素嫌性, chromosome 染色体
cortico-	皮質	corticospinal 皮質脊髄の, corticotropin 副腎皮質刺激ホルモン
cysto-	嚢胞, 膀胱	cystadenoma 嚢胞腺腫, cystoscopy 膀胱鏡検査
cyto-	細胞	cytoplasm 細胞質, cytotoxic 細胞毒性
derm(at)o-	皮膚	dermatology 皮膚科学, dermography 皮膚描記症
dextro-	右	dextrocardia 右胸心, dextromanual 右利きの
dolicho-	長	dolichocephaly 長頭症, dolichocolon 長結腸症

連結形	意味	例
dorso-	背	dorsal 背側の, dorsoventral 背腹方向の
electro-	電気	electrocoagulation 電気凝固, electromyogram 筋電図
encephalo-	脳	encephalitis 脳炎, encephalomalacia 脳軟化
entero-	腸	enterochromaffin 腸クロム親和性, enterococcus 腸球菌
erythro	赤	erythroblast 赤芽球, erythroderma 紅皮症
fibro-	線維	fibroma 線維腫, fibrosis 線維症
gastro-	胃	gastritis 胃炎, gastrojejunostomy 胃空腸吻合
glyco-	糖	glycogenesis 糖源生成, glycoprotein 糖タンパク質
gyneco-	婦人	gyncology 婦人科学, gynecomastia 女性化乳房
hemo-	血液	hemophilia 血友病, hemothorax 血胸
hepato-	肝	hepatocellular 肝細胞性, hepatomegaly 肝腫大
hetero-	異種	heteroantibody 異種抗体, heterophile 異種親和性
homeo-	同種	homeopathy ホメオパシー, homeostasis 恒常性
hydro-	水	hydrocephalus 水頭症, hydrogen 水素
hystero-	子宮	hysteropexy 子宮固定術, hysteroscope 子宮鏡
iatro-	医師	iatrogenic 医原性
idio-	特殊, 独自	idiopathic 特発性, idiosyncrasy 特異体質
juxta-	近傍	juxta-articular 関節傍の, juxtaglomerular 傍糸球体の
karyo-	核	karyolysis 核融解, karyotyping 核型分類
kerato-	角質, 角膜	keratitis 角膜炎, keratosis 角化症
laparo-	腹	laparoscopy 腹腔鏡, laparotomy 開腹術
lepto-	細, 薄	leptocephalia 狭小頭蓋, leptomeninx 軟膜
leuko-	白	leukocyte 白血球, leukoplakia 白板症
levo-	左	levocardia 左胸心, levoversion 左方視
lipo-	脂肪	lipoma 脂肪腫, lipoprotein リポタンパク質

3. 接辞   15

連結形	意味	例
litho-	石, 結石	lithiasis 結石症, lithotripsy 砕石術
melano-	黒	melanocyte メラニン細胞, melanoma 黒色腫
meningo-	膜, 髄膜	meningococcus 髄膜炎菌, meningorrhagia 髄膜出血
meno-	月経	menopause 閉経期, menoschesis 月経抑制
mono-	単一	monocyte 単球, monopolar 単極性
myelo-	脊髄, 骨髄	myelofibrosis 骨髄線維症, myelopoiesis 骨髄造血
myo-	筋肉	myocarditis 心筋炎, myofibroma 筋線維腫
nephro-	腎	nephropexy 腎固定術, nephrotoxicity 腎毒性
neuro-	神経	neuroblastoma 神経芽腫, neurotropic 向神経性
normo-	正常	normochromic 正色素性, normotensive 正常血圧性
oligo-	欠乏	oligodendroglia 希突起膠細胞, oliguria 乏尿
onco-	腫瘍	oncogenesis 発癌, oncovirus 癌ウイルス
ophthalmo-	眼	ophthalmoplegia 眼筋麻痺, ophthalmoscopy 眼底検査法
ortho-	直, 正常	orthopnea 起座呼吸, orthostatic 起立性
osteo-	骨	osteomalacia 骨軟化症, osteomyelitis 骨髄炎
patho-	病気	pathogenic 病原性, pathophysiology 病態生理学
pedo-	小児	pedodontics 小児歯科学, pedophilia 小児性愛
pedo-	足	pedicure ペディキュア, pedometer 歩数計
phlebo-	静脈	phlebitis 静脈炎, phlebotomy 静脈切開術
pneumo-	肺, 空気	pneumonectomy 肺全摘除術, pneumothorax 気胸
poikilo-	異型, 変形	poikilocyte 異型赤血球, poikiloderma 多形皮膚萎縮
polio-	灰色	polioencephalitis 灰白脳炎, poliomyelitis 灰白髄炎
postero-	後	posterioanterior 後前の, posterolateral

連結形	意味	例
		後外側の
proto-	最初，原始	protodiastolic 拡張初期，protoplasm 原形質
psycho-	精神	psychoanalysis 精神分析，psychosomatic 心身症的
radio-	放射(性，能)	radioactivity 放射能，radiolucency 放射線透過性
radio-	橈骨	radiocarpal 橈骨手根骨の，radioulnar 橈骨尺骨の
reno-	腎	renogram レノグラム，renovascular 腎血管性
rhino-	鼻	rhinophony 鼻声，rhinorrhea 鼻汁
sarco-	肉	sarcoid 類肉腫，サルコイド，sarcoma 肉腫
sclero-	硬，強膜	scleroderma 硬皮症，scleroiritis 強膜虹彩炎
sero-	血清，漿液	seronegative 血清学的陰性，serositis 漿膜炎
somato-	体	somatosensory 体性感覚の，somatotype 体型
spondylo-	脊椎	spondylolisthesis 脊椎すべり症，spondylolysis 脊椎分離症
steato-	脂肪	steatohepatitis 脂肪性肝炎，steatorrhea 脂肪便
tachy-	速	tachycardia 頻脈，tachypnea 頻呼吸
thermo-	熱	thermometer 温度計，thermoregulation 体温調節
thoraco-	胸	thoracoscopy 胸腔鏡検査，thoracotomy 開胸術
thrombo-	血栓	thromboembolism 血栓塞栓，thrombolysis 血栓溶解
uro-	尿	urogenital 尿路性器の，urolithiasis 尿路結石症
vaso-	血管	vasoconstriction 血管収縮，vasomotor 血管運動
ventriculo-	心室，脳室	ventriculography 心室（脳室）造影法，ventriculometry 脳室内圧測定
ventro-	腹	ventral 腹側の，ventrolateral 腹側外側の

● 接尾辞 Suffix ●

接尾辞	意味	例
-algesia	痛	analgesia 痛覚消失, 鎮痛, hyperalgesia 痛覚過敏
-algia	痛	arthralgia 関節痛, neuralgia 神経痛
-ase	酵素	lipase リパーゼ, protease タンパク質分解酵素
-blast	芽細胞	monoblast 単芽球, osteoblast 骨芽細胞
-cele	腫脹, ヘルニア	encephalocele 脳瘤, rectocele 直腸瘤
-centesis	穿刺	paracentesis 穿刺, thoracentesis 胸腔穿刺
-coccus	球菌	pneumococcus 肺炎球菌, staphylococcus ブドウ球菌
-cyte	細胞	erythrocyte 赤血球, granulocyte 顆粒球
-derma	皮膚	erythroderma 紅皮症, scleroderma 硬皮症
-dynia	痛	mastodynia 乳房痛, pleurodynia 胸膜痛
-ectasis	拡張	bronchiectasis 気管支拡張症, telangiectasis 毛細血管拡張症
-ectomy	切除	gastrectomy 胃切除, hysterectomy 子宮摘出
-emia	血液の状態	leukemia 白血病, hypoglycemia 低血糖症
-gen	生ずるもの	allergen アレルゲン, antigen 抗原
-genesis	発生	carcinogenesis 発癌, histogenesis 組織発生
-gram	記録, 図	audiogram 聴力図, electrocardiogram 心電図
-graphy	記録, 造影	angiography 血管造影法, electrocardiography 心電図検査
-ia	状態, 病	arachnodactylia くも状指, hysteria ヒステリー
-ism	状態, 病	alcoholism アルコール依存症, anabolism 同化
-itis	炎	bronchitis 気管支炎, arthritis 関節炎
-logy	学	dermatology 皮膚科学, pathology 病理学
-lysis	溶解	hemolysis 溶血, thrombolysis 血栓溶解
-malacia	軟化 (症)	encephalomalacia 脳軟化, osteomalacia 骨軟化症

接尾辞	意味	例
-mania	狂気	erotomania 色情狂, kleptomania 盗癖
-megaly	肥大, 巨大	splenomegaly 脾腫, acromegaly 先端巨大症
-meter	計測（器）	carorimeter 熱量計, spirometer 肺活量計
-odynia	痛	acrodynia 肢端疼痛症, glossodynia 舌痛
-oid	類似, 様	lymphoid リンパ球様, sarcoid 類肉腫
-oma	腫瘍	carcinoma 癌, leiomyoma 平滑筋腫
-osis	症, 病的増加	leucocytosis 白血球増加, tuberculosis 結核
-pathy	疾患, 症	nephropathy 腎症, retinopathy 網膜症
-penia	欠乏	neutropenia 好中球減少, thrombocytopenia 血小板減少
-pexy	固定	gastropexy 胃固定術, orchiopexy 精巣固定術
-phagia	食う, 嚥下	aerophagia 空気嚥下症, polyphagia 過食
-phasia	言語	aphasia 失語症, dysphasia 発語障害
-philia	傾向, 愛好	eosinophilia 好酸球増加, necrophilia 死体愛
-phobia	恐怖	acrophobia 高所恐怖症, claustrophobia 閉所恐怖症
-phonia	声	aphonia 失声症, rhinophonia 鼻声
-plasia	形成	hyperplasia 過形成, metaplasia 異形成
-plasty	形成術	angioplasty 血管形成術, rhinoplasty 鼻形成術
-plegia	麻痺	hemiplegia 半側麻痺, paraplegia 対麻痺
-pnea	呼吸	dyspnea 呼吸困難, orthopnea 起座呼吸
-poiesis	生産	erythropoiesis 赤血球産生, hematopoiesis 造血
-ptosis	下垂	blepharoptosis 眼瞼下垂, gastroptosis 胃下垂
-rrhaphy	縫合	herniorrhaphy ヘルニア縫合術, perineorrhaphy 会陰縫合
-rrhea	流出, 漏出	leukorrhea 白色帯下, rhinorrhea 鼻汁
-rrhexis	破裂	karyorrhexis 核崩壊, metrorrhexis 子宮破裂
-sclerosis	硬化	arteriosclerosis 動脈硬化, atherosclerosis 粥状硬化
-scope	鏡, 検査器	cystoscope 膀胱鏡, laparoscope 腹腔鏡

接尾辞	意味	例
-stasis	静止, うっ血	cholestasis 胆汁うっ滞, hemostasis 止血
-stomy	開口	colostomy 人工肛門造設, pancreaticojejunostomy 膵管空腸吻合
-tomy	切開	laparotomy 開腹, tracheotomy 気管切開
-tripsy	破砕	lithotripsy 砕石術
-trophy	栄養	atrophy 萎縮, hypertrophy 肥大
-uria	尿	albuminuria アルブミン尿, polyuria 多尿

Tidbits

Occam's razor

「オッカムの剃刀」とは,英国のスコラ哲学者 William of Occam (1285 - 1349) が唱えた唯名論 nominalism の格言,"Entities should not be multiplied unnecessarily." (必要以上に実体を増やしてはならない) のこと.正しい思考を妨げる無用の「ひげ」は剃り落とすべきという比喩で,無用な複雑化を避け最も簡潔な理論をとるべきとする.言い換えれば,「複数の理論があるときには一番単純な理論を用いること」,「同等の仮説がある場合,単純なほうを採用すること」.この節約の原理 the principle of economy, law of parsimony は科学の諸分野に適用されてきたが,医学では診断学で diagnostic parsimony の是非について議論の的となっている.Ockham's razor とも綴る.

●国際単位系の接頭辞　Measurement prefixes●

接頭辞	記号	冪指数	倍量と分量	
exa-	E	10^{18}	1,000,000,000,000,000,000	百京倍
peta-	P	10^{15}	1,000,000,000,000,000	千兆倍
tera-	T	10^{12}	1,000,000,000,000	一兆倍
giga-	G	10^{9}	1,000,000,000	十億倍
mega-	M	10^{6}	1,000,000	百万倍
kilo-	k	10^{3}	1,000	千倍
hecto-	h	10^{2}	100	百倍
deca-	da	10	10	十倍
deci-	d	10^{-1}	0.1	十分の一
centi-	c	10^{-2}	0.01	百分の一
milli-	m	10^{-3}	0.001	千分の一
micro-	μ	10^{-6}	0.000 001	百万分の一
nano-	n	10^{-9}	0.000 000 001	十億分の一
pico-	p	10^{-12}	0.000 000 000 001	一兆分の一
femto-	f	10^{-15}	0.000 000 000 000 001	千兆分の一
atto-	a	10^{-18}	0.000 000 000 000 000 001	百京分の一

---Tidbits---

sesquipedalian words

sesqui- は「一倍半」を意味する連結形で，sesquicentennial は「百五十年祭」である．sesquipedalian は「1 フィート半」の原義から「長い言葉」，「多音節語」の意味になった．Oxford English Dictionary で最長の語ということで floccinaucinihilipilification（無価値とみなすこと）が有名だが，Webster's Third New International Dictionary では pneumonoultramicroscopicsilicovolcanoconiosis が45字で最多とされた．要するに「塵肺」のことで本書の読者は容易に分解して理解できるであろう．このように医学用語は合成して長くなりえるが，acetylseryltyrosil … で始まる1,185字の化学名には及ばない（Dmitri A Borgman, 1967）．しかしこの記録もすぐ267個のアミノ酸を有する酵素名の1,913字に破られた由である．

4. ラテン語

● 常用されるラテン語　Commonly used Latin words ●

ラテン語	略語	英語	意味
a posteriori		from what comes after	帰納的, 経験的, 後天的
a priori		from what is before	演繹的, 先験的, 先天的
ad hoc		for this	この目的に, 特別の〔英〕ad hoc committee 特別委員会
ad libitum	ad lib.	at pleasure	随意に, 適宜〔英〕ad-lib 即興的, アドリブ
circa	ca.	about	およそ（通例年数の前に付ける）
confero	cf.	compare	参照せよ
cum	c̄	with	と共に
de facto		from the fact	事実上
de novo		anew	新規に
ditto	do.	the same	同上, 同前（ラテン語由来のイタリア語）
et alii	et al.	and others	およびその他
et cetera	etc.	and so forth	など, その他
et sequens	et seq.	and the following one	以下参照
exempli gratia	e. g.	for example	たとえば
ibidem	ibid.	in the same place	同じ箇所（章, 節）に
id est	i. e.	that is	すなわち, 換言すれば
idem	id.	the same	同上, 同著者
in situ		in the natural or normal place	自然位で, 正常所在で, 元の位置に（腫瘍では発生部位に限局し隣接組織に侵襲しないもの）
in toto		as a whole	全体で
in utero		inside the uterus	子宮内
in vitro		within a glass	試験管内, 生体外

ラテン語	略 語	英 語	意 味
in vivo		within the living body	生体内
manuscriptum	MS.	manuscript	原稿
nota bene	NB, n. b.	note well	よく注意せよ
opere citato	op. cit.	in the work cited	前掲（引用）書中に
per		for each, by	につき，により〔英〕per hour/day/week/gallon/rail
per annum	p. a.	for each year	1年につき
per capita		for each person	1人当たり
per se		in itself	それ自体，本質的に
post mortem		after death	死後 〔英〕postmortem 死後の，検死の，検死，事後の検討
post operationem	p. o.	after operation	手術後 〔英〕postoperative 術後の
post partum		after childbirth	産後 〔英〕postpartum 産後の
post scriptum	PS	postscript	追伸
quod vide	q. v.	which see	その項を見よ
sine	s̄	without	なしに
versus	vs.	against	対
vide	v.	see	見よ，参照せよ
videlicet	viz.	namely	すなわち

● 処方箋に用いられるラテン語　Latin words in prescriptions ●

ラテン語	略 語	英 語	意 味
ad		to, up to	まで
adde	add.	add	加えよ
ampulla	amp.	ampule	アンプル
ana	aā	of each	各々
ante cibum	a. c.	before meals	食前
ante meridiem	a. m.	before noon	午前
aqua	aq.	water	水
auris dextra	AD	right ear	右耳
auris sinistra	AS	left ear	左耳
aures unitas	AU	both ears together	両耳

ラテン語	略 語	英 語	意 味
auris utreque	AU	each ear	各耳
bis in die	b. i. d.	twice a day	1日2回
capsula	cap.	capsule	カプセル
detur	d., dtr.	let it be given	与えよ
diebus alternis	dieb. alt.	on alternate days	隔日（q. o. d. が慣用される）
diebus tertiis	dieb. tert.	every third day	三日目毎
gutta	gt.	a drop	一滴
guttae	gtt.	drops	滴
hora	h.	hour	時間
hora somni	h. s.	at bedtime	眠前
liquor	Liq.	liquid	液
lotio	lot.	lotion	ローション
misce	M.	mix	混和せよ
nil per os	n. p. o.	nothing by mouth	絶食
oculus dexter	OD	right eye	右眼
oculus sinister	OS	left eye	左眼
oculi unitas	OU	both eyes	両眼
oculus uterque	OU	each eye	各眼
omni mane	o. m.	every morning	毎朝
omni nocte	o. n.	every night	毎晩
per anum		through the anus	経肛門的
per os	p. o.	by mouth	経口的
post cibum	p. c.	after meals	食後
post meridiem	p. m.	afternoon	午後
pro re nata	p. r. n.	as needed	必要時
pulvis	pulv.	powder	散剤
quantum libet	q. l.	as much as desired	所要量
quantum satis	q. s.	sufficient quantity	十分量
quantum sufficit	q. s.	as much as suffices	十分量
quaque	q.	each, every	毎
quaque die	q. d.	every day	毎日
quaque hora	q. h.	every hour	毎時
quaque quarta hora	q. q. h.	every four hours	4時間毎（通常 q. 4h. と記す）
quater in die	q. i. d.	four times a day	1日4回
recipe	Rx	take	服用

ラテン語	略語	英語	意味
repetatur	Rep.	let it be repeated	反復せよ
secundum artem	s. a.	according to art	常法に従って
semis	ss.	half	半分
signetur	Sig.	let it be labeled	表示せよ
si opus sit	s. o. s.	if it is necessary	必要時
statim	stat.	immediately	直ちに
syrupus	syr.	syrup	シロップ
ter in die	t. i. d.	three times a day	1日3回
unguentum	ung.	ointment	軟膏
ut dictum	ut dict.	as directed	指示通り

---Tidbits---

ラテン語の略語

一般に略語のピリオドは省略する傾向にあるが，学会や出版社により方針が異なり，ラテン語の場合も不要 (AMA)，要 (Dorland) と一定しない．b. i. d. あるいは t. i. d. を bid, tid とすると単語と紛らわしくなるので，処方用語では小文字のとき必ずピリオドを付けて，付けない場合は大文字にするという意見もある．

5. 術語と日常語

●術語と日常語の対比　Technical and lay terms●

術　語	意　味	日常語
abdomen	腹部	belly
acne vulgaris	尋常性痤瘡	pimple
acute anterior poliomyelitis	急性脊髄前角炎	polio
allergic rhinitis	アレルギー性鼻炎	hay fever
alopecia	脱毛症	baldness
analgesic	鎮痛薬	painkiller
anemia	貧血	low blood count, thin blood
arteriosclerosis	動脈硬化症	hardening of the arteries
arthralgia in children	成長痛	growing pains
aseptic	無菌性	germ-free
baby produced by artificial insemination	人工授精児	test-tube baby
bronchitis	気管支炎	chest colds
caisson disease	潜函病	bends
calf cramps	腓腹筋痙攣	charley horse
cerebral vascular accident	脳血管障害	stroke
cerumen	耳垢	earwax
clavicle	鎖骨	collarbone
clavus	鶏眼	corn
cocaine	コカイン	snow
comedo	面皰	blackhead
condyloma acuminatum	尖圭コンジローマ	venereal wart
congelation	凍傷	frostbite
congenital vascular nevus	母斑	birthmark
conjunctivitis	結膜炎	pink eye
contusion	挫傷	bruise, black-and-blue
convulsions	痙攣発作	fits
decubitus ulcer	褥瘡性潰瘍	bedsore
delirium tremens	振戦せん妄	horrors
depression	うつ病	blues
diaphragmatic hernia	横隔膜ヘルニア	upside-down stomach
dysmenorrhea	月経困難	cramps, period pains

術 語	意 味	日常語
dyspepsia	消化不良	indigestion
encephalitis	脳炎	brain fever
enuresis	夜尿症	bed-wetting
ephelides	雀卵斑	freckles
epidemic parotitis	流行性耳下腺炎	mumps
epileptic seizures	てんかん発作	fits
epistaxis	鼻出血	nosebleed
eructation	おくび	belching, burping
esophagus	食道	gullet
euthanasia	安楽死	mercy killing
exophthalmos	眼球突出	popeyes
exudate	滲出液	weep
flatulence, flatus	鼓腸, 放屁	gas, wind
furuncle	フルンケル	boil
gastric hyperacidity	胃酸過多	acid stomach
gastrointestinal tract	消化管	guts
genu valgum	外反膝	knock-knees
genu varum	内反膝	bowleg
glomerulonephritis	糸球体腎炎	Bright disease
gonorrhea	淋病	clap
gonorrheal ophthalmia	淋菌性眼炎	babies' sore eyes
halitosis	口臭	bad breath
hemophilia	血友病	bleeder's disease
hemorrhoids	痔核	piles
hepatitis	肝炎	yellow jaundice
hernia	ヘルニア	rupture
herniation of the intervertebral disc	椎間板ヘルニア	slipped disc
herpes simplex	単純ヘルペス	cold sore, fever sore
herpes zoster	帯状疱疹	shingles
hordeolum	麦粒腫	stye
hyperemesis gravidarum	妊娠悪阻	morning sickness
hyperglycemia	高血糖	high blood sugar
icterus	黄疸	jaundice
infectious mononucleosis	伝染性単核球症	glandular fever
influenza	インフルエンザ	flu
inguen	鼠径	groin
injection	注射	shot
inoculation	接種	shot

術 語	意 味	日常語
laxative	緩下薬	physic
leukorrhea	白色帯下	whites
menopause	閉経期	change of life
menstruation	月経	period
microbe	微生物	bug
myocardial infarction	心筋梗塞	coronary, heart attack
narcotic	麻薬	dope
nevus	母斑	mole
nocturnal emission	夜間遺精, 夢精	wet dream
Parkinson disease	パーキンソン病	shaking palsy
patella	膝蓋	kneecap
pectus carinatum	鳩胸	chicken breast
pernio	凍瘡	chilblain
pertussis	百日咳	whooping cough
placenta	胎盤	afterbirth
pollenosis, pollinosis	花粉症	hay fever
pruritus	掻痒	itching
psychiatrist	精神科医	head doctor
psychoneurosis	精神神経症	nervous breakdown
puerperal sepsis	産褥敗血症	childbed fever
pyrosis	胸やけ	heartburn
rubella	風疹	German measles
salpingitis	卵管炎	infection of the tubes
scabies	疥癬	itch
septicemia	敗血症	blood-poisoning
singultus	しゃっくり	hiccup
sinusitis	副鼻腔炎	sinus trouble
stimulant (amphetamine, caffeine)	刺激薬	pep pill
strabismus	斜視	cross-eye, squint
streptococcal pharyngitis	連鎖球菌性咽頭炎	strep throat
sudamina	汗疹	heat rash
sycosis vulgaris	尋常性毛瘡	barbers' itch
syphilis	梅毒	bad blood, the pox
tetanus	破傷風	lockjaw
thrush, moniliasis	口腔カンジダ症	white mouth
tibia	脛骨	shinbone
tinea cruris	股部白癬	jockstrap itch

術　語	意　味	日常語
tinea pedis	足部白癬	athlete's foot
tinnitus	耳鳴	ringing in the ears
tonsillitis, pharyngitis, laryngitis	上気道炎	sore throat
torticollis	斜頸	wryneck
trachea	気管	windpipe
trichophytosis	白癬症	ringworm
tuberculosis	結核	consumption
ulcer	潰瘍	sore
unconsciousness	意識消失	blackout
urticaria	蕁麻疹	hives
uterus	子宮	womb
vaginal bleeding	腟出血	spotting
valvular disease of the heart	心臓弁膜症	leaky heart
varicella	水痘	chickenpox
verruca	疣	wart
vertigo	めまい	dizziness, staggers
vesicle	小水疱	blister
virus	ウイルス	bug
vomit	吐く	throw up

Tidbits

Brevity is the soul of wit.

医療用語が一般の人には難解でしばしば誤解されていることが指摘され対策が検討されている（例えば，膠原病，ショック，誤嚥，予後，寛解など）．咳嗽，吃逆，嘈囃，肺臓などの医学用語が，せき，しゃっくり，むねやけ，たこのことと簡単に分かっては医者の沽券に関わると思っていたかどうかは分からないが，英語でも singultus, pyrosis とラテン語で煙に巻いたり難解な表現で虚勢を張ったりする医師もいる．"near" の代わりに "in close proximity to", "catch a cold easily" の代わりに "have a proclivity for contracting coryza" など．科学論文では，難解語句や冗長表現を避けて簡潔明快に書くことが必須であり，名著 "The Elements of Style" (Strunk & White) に強調されているが，既に Shakespeare が "Brevity is the soul of wit." (Hamlet) （簡潔は機知の精髄）と述べている．

6. カタカナ用語

● カタカナ用語の語源　Katakana terms ●

カタカナ用語	原　語	意　味
アイテル	Eiter〔独〕	膿, 〔英〕pus
アウゲ	Auge, Augenheilkunde〔独〕	眼, 眼科, 〔英〕eye, ophthalmology
アウス	Auskratzung〔独〕	掻爬, 〔英〕curettage
アウフネーメン	aufnehmen〔独〕	受け入れる（入院）, 〔英〕admit
アッペ	Appendicitis〔独〕, appendicitis〔英〕	虫垂炎
アテレク	Atelektase〔独〕, atelectasis〔英〕	無気肺
アナムネ	Anamnese〔独〕	既往歴, 病歴, 〔英〕history
アプラ	aplastische Anämie〔独〕, aplastic anemia〔英〕	再生不良性貧血
アポ	Apoplexie〔独〕, apoplexy〔英〕	脳卒中
アミトロ	amyotrophische Lateralsklerose〔独〕	筋萎縮性側索硬化症
アルフェト	α-fetoprotein〔英〕	αフェトプロテイン
アルホス	alkaline phosphatase〔英〕	アルカリホスファターゼ
アンギオ	Angiographie〔独〕	血管撮影, 〔英〕angiography
アンプタ	Amputation〔独〕	切断, 〔英〕amputation
イクテルス	Ikterus〔独〕	黄疸, 〔英〕icterus, jaundice
イムラッド	IMRAD: Introduction, Methods, Results, and Discussion〔英〕	緒言, 方法, 結果, 考察（科学論文の構成）
インオペ	inoperabel〔独〕	手術不能の, 〔英〕inoperable
ウロ	Urologie〔独〕	泌尿器科, 〔英〕urology
エスエス	SS: Schwangerschaft〔独〕	妊娠, 〔英〕pregnancy
エッセン	Essen〔独〕	食事
エデーム	Ödem〔独〕	浮腫, 〔英〕edema
エピ	epilepsy〔英〕	てんかん
エピ	epidural anesthesia〔英〕	硬膜外麻酔
エピジオ	Episiotomie〔独〕, epis-	会陰切開術

カタカナ用語	原　語	意　味
	iotomy〔英〕	
エムケー	MK: Magenkrebs〔独〕	胃癌
エリトロ	Erythrozyten〔独〕	赤血球，〔英〕erythrocyte
エルケー	LK: Lungenkrebs〔独〕	肺癌，〔英〕lung cancer
エルブレ	erbrechen〔独〕	嘔吐する，〔英〕vomit
エント	Entlassung, entlassen〔独〕	退院，〔英〕discharge
エンボリ	embolization〔英〕	塞栓形成術
オーベー	o. B.: ohne Befund〔独〕	所見なし，〔英〕unremarkable
オーベン	oben〔独〕	上の（上司）
オスキー	OSCE: objective structured clinical examination〔英〕	客観的臨床能力試験
オト	Otorhinolaryngologie〔独〕	耳鼻咽喉科，〔英〕otorhinolaryngology
オペ	Operation〔独〕, operation〔英〕	手術
オルト	Orthopädie〔独〕	整形外科，〔英〕orthopedics
カイザー	Kaiserschnitt〔独〕	帝王切開，〔英〕cesarean section
カテ	Katheter〔独〕	カテーテル，〔英〕catheter
カマ，カマグ	煆製マグネシア magnesia usta〔ラ〕	酸化マグネシウム 〔英〕calcined magnesia = magnesium oxide
カルチ	Karzinom〔独〕	癌，〔英〕carcinoma, cancer
ギネ	Gynäkologie〔独〕	婦人科，〔英〕gynecology
キント	Kind, Kindheilkunde〔独〕	小児，小児科，〔英〕infant, pediatrics
クール	Kurs〔独〕, cours〔仏〕	治療単位
クランケ	Kranke〔独〕	患者，〔英〕patient
グリッペ	Grippe〔独〕	インフルエンザ，〔英〕influenza
クレブス	Krebs〔独〕	癌（発音はクレープス）
ゲブルト	Geburt〔独〕	出産，〔英〕birth
ケモ	chemotherapy〔英〕	化学療法
コアグラ	Koagulum〔独〕, coagulum〔英〕	凝血塊

6. カタカナ用語

カタカナ用語	原 語	意 味
コート	Kot〔独〕	糞便, 〔英〕stool, feces
ゴノ	Gonorrhoe〔独〕, gonorrhea〔英〕	淋病
コンタミ	contamination〔英〕	汚染
コントラ	Kontraindikation〔独〕, contraindication〔英〕	禁忌
ザー	SAH: subarachnoid hemorrhage〔英〕	くも膜下出血
サーズ	SARS: severe acute respiratory syndrome〔英〕	重症急性呼吸器症候群
シゾ	Schizophrenie〔独〕	統合失調症（発音はシツォフレニー）
シーネ	Schiene〔独〕	副子, 〔英〕splint
シャーカステン	Schaukasten〔独〕	ショーケース（フィルムビューアー）〔英〕x-ray viewer
シャッテン	Schatten〔独〕	陰影, 〔英〕shadow
ステト	Stethoskop〔独〕, stethoscope〔英〕	聴診器
ステる	sterben〔独〕	死亡する（発音はシュテルベン）
スパイロ	spirometer〔英〕	肺活量計
ズブアラ	subarachnoideale Blutung〔独〕	くも膜下出血
ズポ	Suppositorium〔独〕	坐剤, 〔英〕suppository
セグ	segmented neutrophil〔英〕	分葉核好中球
ゼク	Sektion〔独〕	剖検, 〔英〕autopsy
ソープ	SOAP: subjective data, objective data, assessment, plan〔英〕	主観的データ, 客観的データ, 評価, 計画
ゾンデ	Sonde〔独〕	消息子, 〔英〕probe
タキ	tachycardia〔英〕	頻脈
ツッカー	Zucker〔独〕	糖（血糖, ブドウ糖液），〔英〕sugar
ツモール	Tumor〔独〕	腫瘍, 〔英〕tumor
ディアベ	Diabetes〔独〕	糖尿病, 〔英〕diabetes
ディスポ	disposable〔英〕	使い捨て
テーベー	TB: Tuberkulose〔独〕	結核, 〔英〕tuberculosis
デルマ	Dermatologie〔独〕	皮膚科, 〔英〕dermatology

32　I章　医学英語の基礎

カタカナ用語	原　語	意　味
トモ	Tomographie〔独〕, tomography〔英〕	断層撮影法
ナート	Naht〔独〕	縫合, 〔英〕suture
ニッシェ	Nische〔独〕	ニッシェ, 壁龕〔英〕niche
ニーレ	Niere〔独〕	腎臓, 〔英〕kidney
ネーベン	Nebenarbeit〔独〕	副業, バイト
ネクる	Nekrose〔独〕, necrosis〔英〕	壊死（をきたす）
ノイトロ	neutrophile Leukozyten〔独〕	好中球, 〔英〕neutrophil leukocyte
ノルアド	noradrenaline〔英〕	ノルアドレナリン
バイタル	vital signs〔英〕	生命徴候
バウフ	Bauch〔独〕	腹, 〔英〕abdomen
ハーツー	HER2: human epidermal growth factor receptor type 2	ヒト上皮増殖因子受容体2型
パト	Pathologie〔独〕	病理学, 〔英〕pathology
ハルン	Harn〔独〕	尿, 〔英〕urine
ピエロ	Pyelographie〔独〕	腎盂造影法, 〔英〕pyelography
ファル	Fall〔独〕	症例, 〔英〕case
プシ	Psychiatrie, psychisch〔独〕	精神医学, 精神科, 精神病の
ブラディ	bradycardia〔英〕	徐脈
プルス	Puls〔独〕	脈拍, 〔英〕pulse
ブルート	Blut〔独〕	血液, 〔英〕blood
プレート	platelet〔英〕	血小板
ブロンコ	bronchoscopy〔英〕	気管支鏡
ベッケン	Becken〔独〕	骨盤, 〔英〕pelvis
ヘマト	Hämatokrit〔独〕	ヘマトクリット, 〔英〕hematocrit
ヘモ	Hämorrhoid〔独〕	痔, 〔英〕hemorrhoid
ヘルツ	Herz〔独〕	心臓, 〔英〕heart
ポリペク	polypectomy〔英〕	ポリープ切除術
マーゲン	Magen〔独〕	胃, 〔英〕stomach
マルク	Knochenmark〔独〕	骨髄（骨髄穿刺）,〔英〕bone marrow
マンマ	Mamma〔独〕	乳房, 〔英〕breast
ミエロ	Myelographie〔独〕	脊髄造影法, 〔英〕myelography

6. カタカナ用語

カタカナ用語	原 語	意 味
ミエロ	Myelozyten〔独〕	骨髄球, 〔英〕myelocyte
ムンテラ	Mundtherapie〔独〕	患者説明
メタ	Metastase〔独〕, metastasis〔英〕	転移
ラパ	Laparotomie〔独〕, laparotomy〔英〕	開腹
ラパコレ	laparoscopic cholecystectomy〔英〕	腹腔鏡下胆嚢摘除術
ラボ	Laboratorium〔独〕, laboratory〔英〕	検査室, 研究室
リコール	Liquor〔独〕	髄液, 〔英〕cerebrospinal fluid
リハ, リハビリ	rehabilitation〔英〕	リハビリテーション
ルンゲ	Lunge〔独〕	肺, 〔英〕lung
ルンバール	Lumbalpunktion〔独〕	腰椎穿刺, 〔英〕lumbar puncture
レーシック	LASIK: laser-assisted in-situ keratomileusis〔英〕	レーザー角膜内切削形成術
レーベル	Leber〔独〕	肝臓, 〔英〕liver
レスピ	respirator〔英〕	人工呼吸器
レセ, レセプト	Rezept〔独〕	診療報酬明細書(本来処方箋の意)
ロイコ	Leukozyten〔独〕	白血球, 〔英〕leukocyte
ロイマ	Rheumatismus〔独〕	リウマチ, 〔英〕rheumatism
ワイセ	weisses Blutkörperchen〔独〕	白血球, 〔英〕white blood cell

Tidbits

ムンテラ

Mund(口)と Therapie(治療)を結びつけた和製語で,以前口先で言いくるめる意味で用いられた.「学問的に昇華し医師と患者とのラポールを作る手段としたい」(間中喜雄:むんてら,創元医学新書, 1963)という意見もあったが,概して後ろめたい隠語として使われた. ムンテラには informed consent の時代にふさわしくないニュアンスがある. なお Mundtherapie は通常のドイツ語辞書には無いが,「正常な飲食と発語のための口腔リハビリ」の意味で用いられている (http://www.heinrich-piepmeyer-haus.de).

7. 紛らわしい医学用語

● 紛らわしい医学用語　Easily confused terms ●

紛らわしい医学用語	日本語	注
abduction / adduction	外転 / 内転	
absorption / adsorption	吸収 / 吸着	
actin / actinic	アクチン / 光線性, 紫外線の	actinic cheilitis 日射性口唇炎
afferent / efferent	求心性 / 遠心性	
alkalosis / ankylosis	アルカローシス / 強直	
ambulance / ambulatory	救急車 / 歩行の, 通院の	ambulation 歩行
ampule / ampulla	アンプル / 膨大部	ampule＜ampulla〔ラ〕
anaplasia / aplasia	退形成 / 無形成	
anatomic / anastomotic	解剖の / 吻合の	
ante- / anti-	前 / 抗	anterior 前の, antibody 抗体
anuresis / enureis	尿閉 / 夜尿症	anuresis = urinary retention
aphagia / aphasia	嚥下不能 / 失語症	
arteriosclerosis / atherosclerosis	動脈硬化 / 粥状硬化	
aseptic / acetic	無菌性 / 酢酸の	
aura / aural	前兆 / 耳の	
aural / oral	耳の / 口の	発音は同じ
axillary / auxiliary	腋窩の / 補助の	
bolus / bullous	丸い塊 / 水疱性	bolus of food 食塊
born / borne	生まれた / 運んだ（過去分詞）	air-borne infection 空気感染
bronchial / branchial	気管支の / 鰓の	branchial cleft 鰓溝
buccal / buckle	頬の / バックル	発音は同じ
caliber / caliper	口径 / 側径器	calipers（通常複数）カリパス
callus / callous	胼胝 / 胼胝性	発音は同じ
calyx / calx	腎杯 / 踵	
cancer / chancre	癌 / 下疳	canker sore 口唇潰瘍
cancerous / cancellous	癌性の / 海綿状の	

7. 紛らわしい医学用語

紛らわしい医学用語	日本語	注
casualty / casuistry	死傷者 / 決疑論	
cecal / thecal	盲腸の / 鞘の	cecum 盲腸, theca 卵胞膜
cerebrum / cerebellum	大脳 / 小脳	
cholic / colic	胆汁の / 結腸の, 仙痛	
choroid / colloid	脈絡膜 / コロイド	
cirrhosis / xerosis	肝硬変 / 乾皮症	xerosis [ziróusəs]
complement / compliment	補体 / 賛辞	発音は同じ
coarse / course	粗大 / 経過, クール	発音は同じ
conscious / conscience	意識のある / 良心	
convulsion / convolution	痙攣 / 脳回	
cord / chord	索 / 索	発音は同じ, chorda に由来し同義
cytology / sitology	細胞学 / 栄養学	発音は同じ, 栄養学 dietetics
demography / dermography	人口学 / 皮膚描記症	
depletion / depilation	喪失 / 抜毛	
diffuse / defuse	びまん性 / 信管を外す, 静める	発音は同じ
discrete / discreet	分離した / 慎重な	発音は同じ
diseased / deceased	病的 / 死去した	
diuresis / diuretics	利尿 / 利尿薬	
dysphagia / dysphasia	嚥下障害 / 発語障害	
dysphonia / dysphoria	発声障害 / 気分変調	
elicit / illicit	引き出す / 違法な	発音は同じ
endemic / pandemic	地方病性 / 汎発流行性	
esotropia / exotropia	内斜視 / 外斜視	
etiology / etymology	病因論 / 語源学	
facial / fascial	顔面の / 筋膜の	
familial / familiar	家族性 / ありふれた	
foci / fossae	病巣 / 窩	単数 focus / fossa
fovea / phobia	窩 / 恐怖症	fovea centralis 中心

36 I章 医学英語の基礎

紛らわしい医学用語	日本語	注
		窩
fungus / fungous	真菌 / 真菌の	発音は同じ，真菌の fungal
generic / genetic	属の / 遺伝の	generic name 属名，一般名（薬）
genus / genu	属 / 膝	
gland / glans	腺 / 亀頭	
hemostasis / homeostasis	止血 / 恒常性	
hemothorax / hemithorax	血胸 / 片側胸部	
heterotopia / heterotropia	異所性 / 斜視	
homogenous / homogeneous	同質性 / 均質性	
hypochondrium / hypochondriac	下肋部 / 心気的	
hysterical / historical	ヒステリー性 / 病歴の	
icterus / ictus	黄疸 / 発作	ictus epilepticus てんかん発作
ileac / iliac	回腸の / 腸骨の	発音は同じ
ileal / ilial	回腸の / 腸骨の	発音は同じ
ileum / ilium	回腸 / 腸骨	発音は同じ
illusion / elusion	錯覚 / 逃避	発音は同じ，〔形〕illusive/elusive
incidence / incidents	発病率 / 出来事	
infancy / infantry	幼年期 / 歩兵	
infra- / intra-	下 / 内	infrared 赤外線の，intracranial 頭蓋内
initiation / institution	開始 / 施設	
innocuous / inoculable	無害の / 接種可能の	inoculation 予防接種（n は 1 個）
keratosis / keratitis	角化症 / 角膜炎	
labile / labial	不安定な / 唇の	
lien / lean	脾臓 / 痩せた	発音は同じ
malaria / miliaria	マラリア / 汗疹	
malleolus / malleus	果・踝 / ツチ骨	
malocclusion / mesioclusion	不正咬合 / 近位咬合	-cc- / -c- に注意
mental / mental	精神の / 頤の	綴りと発音は同じ

7. 紛らわしい医学用語

紛らわしい医学用語	日本語	注
miosis / meiosis	縮瞳 / 減数分裂	発音は同じ
miotic / mitotic	縮瞳の / 核分裂の	
miotic / myopic	縮瞳の / 近視性	
mucus / mucous	粘液 / 粘液性	発音は同じ
navel / naval	臍 / 海軍の	発音は同じ
nocturia / nycturia	夜間頻尿 / 夜間多尿	区別せず夜間尿として同義に用いられる
os / os	口 / 骨	複数は ora / ossa
palpable / palpebral	触知可能の / 眼瞼の	
parameter / parametric	パラメーター / 子宮傍の	parametric は「parameter の」〔形〕でもある
parental / parenteral	親の / 非経口的	
parous / porous	経産の / 多孔性	
pedicle / pediculus	柄・脚 / シラミ	
perennial / perineal	通年性 / 会陰の	
perineal / peritoneal	会陰の / 腹膜の	
perineal / peroneal	会陰の / 腓骨の	
pleural / plural	胸膜の / 複数(の)	発音は同じ
pleuritis / pruritus	胸膜炎 / 掻痒	
podiatrist / pediatrist	足治療医 / 小児科医	小児科医は通常 pediatrician
polypoid / polyploid	ポリープ状 / 多倍数体	
potion / portion	水薬の一服 / 一部	
prescribe / proscribe	処方する / 禁止する	
principle / principal	原理 / 主要な	発音は同じ
prostate / prostrate	前立腺 / 疲憊する	
psychosis / sycosis	精神病 / 毛瘡	発音は同じ
pubic / public	陰部の / 公共の	反意語!
radicle / radical	小根 / 根, 根治的	発音は同じ
rationale / rational	理論的根拠 / 合理的	
renal / lienal	腎臓の / 脾臓の	
scirrhus / scirrhous	硬性癌 / 硬性癌の	発音は同じ
site / sight / cite	部位 / 視覚 / 引用する	発音は同じ
soul / sole	精神 / 足底	発音は同じ
speculum / spectrum	鏡 / スペクトル	vaginal speculum 腟鏡
sprain / strain	捻挫 / 挫傷, 緊張, 系統	

I章 医学英語の基礎

紛らわしい医学用語	日本語	注
stationary / stationery	静止の / 文房具	発音は同じ
stature / statue	身長 / 像	
sulfa / sulfur	サルファ(剤) / イオウ	
super- / supra-	超 / 上	superego 超自我, supranuclear 核上
tarsus / tarsus	足根 / 瞼板	綴りと発音は同じ
tenia / tinea	ひも, 条虫 / 白癬	taenia coli 結腸ひも
tic / tick	チック / ダニ	発音は同じ
topical / tropical	局所性 / 熱帯性	
tortuous / torturous	蛇行性 / 苦痛な	torture 虐待, 拷問
tubercular / tuberculous	結節の / 結核性	
tympanic / tympanitic	鼓室性 / 鼓音性	
ureter / urethra	尿管 / 尿道	
urinary / urinal	尿の / しびん	
vesicle / vesical	小水疱 / 膀胱の	発音は同じ
villus / villous	絨毛 / 絨毛状	発音は同じ
viscous / viscus	粘着性 / 内臓	発音は同じ
waist / waste	腰 / 浪費, 廃棄物	発音は同じ

Tidbits

homophone

異綴同音異義語は homophone, 同綴同音異義語は homonym で, 同綴異音異義語は heteronym である. ラテン語の onymum (名前) に由来する接尾辞 -onym の例は, 他に acronym 頭字語, synonym 同義語, antonym 反意語, eponym 冠名用語, metonym 換喩語など, 接頭辞 onom- の例は onomatopoeia 擬声語.

8．色彩・形状の表現

● 色彩　Color ●

白色 はくしょく	white, whitish
黒色 こくしょく	black, blackish
赤色 せきしょく	red, reddish
桃色 ももいろ	pink, pinkish
緋色 ひいろ，深紅色 しんこうしょく	scarlet
黄色 おうしょく	yellow, yellowish
褐色 かっしょく	brown, brownish
橙色 とうしょく	orange
青色 せいしょく	blue, bluish
空色 そらいろ	azure, sky blue
緑色 りょくしょく	green, greenish
紫色 ししょく	purple, purplish
灰色 かいしょく	gray, grayish
蒼白色 そうはくしょく	pale
肌色 はだいろ	flesh-colored
さび色	rusty
青銅色 せいどうしょく	bronze, bronzy

● 形状　Shape ●

三角形 さんかくけい	triangle, 〔形〕triangular
正三角形 せい―	equilateral triangle
二等辺三角形 にとうへん―	isosceles triangle
不等辺三角形 ふとうへん―	scalene triangle
直角三角形 ちょっかく―	right-angled triangle
鋭角三角形 えいかく―	acute triangle
鈍角三角形 どんかく―	obtuse triangle
四辺形 しへんけい	quadrilateral, 〔形〕quadrilateral
平行四辺形 へいこうしへんけい	parallelogram
正方形 せいほうけい	square, 〔形〕square
長方形 ちょうほうけい	rectangle, 〔形〕rectangular
菱形 りょうけい	rhombus, 〔複〕rhombi, 〔形〕rhomboid
偏菱形 へんりょうけい	rhomboid, 〔形〕rhomboidal
台形 だいけい	trapezoid, 〔形〕trapezoidal
不等辺四辺形 ふとうへんしへんけい	trapezium, 〔形〕trapezial
多角形 たかくけい	polygon, 〔形〕polygonal
正多角形 せいたかくけい	regular polygon
五角形 ごかくけい	pentagon, 〔形〕pentagonal
六角形 ろっかくけい	hexagon, 〔形〕hexagonal

八角形 はっかくけい	octagon, 〔形〕octagonal
円形 えんけい	circle, 〔形〕circular
半円形 はんえんけい	semicircle
楕円形 だえんけい	ellipse, 〔形〕elliptic
卵形 らんけい	oval, 〔形〕oval
三日月形 みかづきけい	crescent, 〔形〕crescent
環 かん	ring, annulus, 〔形〕annular
立方体 りっぽうたい	cube, 〔形〕cubic, cuboid
直方体 ちょくほうたい	rectangular solid
平行六面体 へいこうろくめんたい	parallelepiped
円柱 えんちゅう	cylinder, 〔形〕cylindrical
三角柱 さんかくちゅう	triangular prism
球体 きゅうたい	sphere, 〔形〕spherical
半球体 はんきゅうたい	hemisphere, 〔形〕hemispherical
楕円体 だえんたい	ellipsoid, 〔形〕ellipsoidal
円錐 えんすい	cone, 〔形〕conical
角錐 かくすい	pyramid, 〔形〕pyramidal
紡錘 ぼうすい	spindle, 〔形〕spindle-shaped, fusiform
亜鈴 あれい	dumbbell, 〔形〕dumbbell-shaped
鋸歯 きょし	sawtooth, 〔形〕saw-toothed, serrated
梨 なし	pear, 〔形〕pear-shaped, piriform
星 ほし	star, stella, 〔形〕star-shaped, stellate
蜂巣 ほうそう	honeycomb, 〔形〕honeycombed
分葉 ぶんよう	lobulation, 〔形〕lobulated
クローバー	clover, 〔形〕cloverleaf
茎 けい	peduncle, stalk, 〔形〕pedunculated, stalked
広基 こうき	broad base, 〔形〕sessile, broad based
乳頭 にゅうとう	papilla, 〔形〕papillary
カリフラワー	cauliflower, 〔形〕cauliflower-like
絨毛 じゅうもう	villus, 〔形〕villous, villose
棘 とげ	spine, 〔形〕spinous, spiny
樹状突起 じゅじょうとっき	dendrite, 〔形〕dendritic, dendric
結節 けっせつ	node, 〔形〕nodal
小結節 しょうけっせつ	nodule, 〔形〕nodular
ポリープ	polyp, 〔形〕polypoid
印環 いんかん	signet ring
ドーナツ	doughnut, torus, 〔形〕doughnut-shaped
噴火口 ふんかこう	crater, 〔形〕crater-like, crater-shaped, crateriform
螺旋 らせん	spiral, helix, 〔形〕spiral
蛇行 だこう	tortuosity, 〔形〕tortuous

II章

医療関連用語

1. 医療行為

● 医療行為　Medical practice ●

医業停止処分 いぎょうていししょぶん	suspension of medical practice
医事裁判 いじさいばん	medical trial
医師賠償責任保険 いしばいしょうせきにんほけん	medical professional liability insurance
医事紛争 いじふんそう	medical dispute
医事紛争処理委員会 いじふんそうしょりいいんかい	Malpractice Council
医道審議会 いどうしんぎかい	Medical Ethics Council
医薬食品局 いやくしょくひんきょく	Pharmaceutical and Food Safety Bureau
医薬品医療機器総合機構 いやくひんいりょうききそうごうきこう	Pharmaceuticals and Medical Devices Agency (PMDA)
医薬分業 いやくぶんぎょう	separation of pharmacy from medical practice
医療 いりょう	medical care
医療過誤 ─かご	malpractice, medical malpractice
医療過誤訴訟 ─かごそしょう	malpractice litigation, malpractice suit
医療監査 ─かんさ	medical audit
医療監視 ─かんし	medical inspection
医療機関認定合同委員会（米国） ─きかんにんていごうどういいんかい	Joint Commission on Accreditation of Healthcare Organizations (JCAHO)
医療技術評価 ─ぎじゅつひょうか	medical technology assessment (MTA)
医療機能評価 ─きのうひょうか	evaluation of medical practice
医療行政 ─ぎょうせい	medical administration
医療計画 ─けいかく	medical care plan
医療資源利用群（米国） ─しげんりようぐん	Resource Utilization Groups (RUG)
医療事故 ─じこ	medical accident
医療情報 ─じょうほう	medical information
医療水準 ─すいじゅん	medical care standard, quality of health care
医療制度 ─せいど	medical system, system of medical services
医療訴訟 ─そしょう	medical lawsuit
医療廃棄物 ─はいきぶつ	medical waste
医療費 ─ひ	health care cost
医療費適正化計画 ─ひてきせいかけいかく	health care cost control program
医療扶助 ─ふじょ	medical assistance

1. 医療行為　43

医療法人 いりょうほうじん	medical corporation, medical juridical person
医療倫理 いりょうりんり	medical ethics
医療連携 いりょうれんけい	referral system
遠隔医療 えんかくいりょう	telemedicine
共同介護 きょうどうかいご	shared care
グループ診療 グループしんりょう	group practice
健康管理手帳 けんこうかんりてちょう	personal health record
健康政策局 けんこうせいさくきょく	Health Policy Bureau
公害 こうがい	environmental pollution
公衆衛生行政 こうしゅうえいせいぎょうせい	public health administration
厚生労働省 こうせいろうどうしょう	Ministry of Health, Labour and Welfare
高齢化社会 こうれいかしゃかい	aging society
国家医療 こっかいりょう	state medicine
国際病院評価機構 こくさいびょういんひょうかきこう	Joint Commission International (JCI)
災害派遣医療チーム さいがいはけんいりょうチーム	disaster medical assistance team (DMAT)
在宅医療 ざいたくいりょう	home-based medical care
在宅介護 ざいたくかいご	home care, in-home care, home health care
裁判外紛争解決 さいばんがいふんそうかいけつ	alternative dispute resolution (ADR)
時間外診療 じかんがいしんりょう	after-hours practice
施設内審査委員会 しせつないしんさいいんかい	institutional review board (IRB)
社会医療 しゃかいいりょう	socialized medicine
守秘義務 しゅひぎむ	confidentiality
守秘義務違反 しゅひぎむいはん	breach of confidentiality, breach of confidence
診断書 しんだんしょ	medical certificate
診療ガイドライン しんりょうガイドライン	clinical practice guideline
診療圏 しんりょうけん	catchment area
診療情報開示 しんりょうじょうほうかいじ	medical information disclosure
生命倫理 せいめいりんり	bioethics
説明義務 せつめいぎむ	accountability
代診 だいしん	deputizing service, locum tenens
段階的患者管理 だんかいてきかんじゃかんり	progressive patient care (PPC)
地域医療 ちいきいりょう	community health care, community medicine
注意義務 ちゅういぎむ	attention obligation
電子カルテ でんしカルテ	electronic medical record (EMR)
同僚検討 どうりょうけんとう	peer review

44　II章　医療関連用語

届出義務 とどけできむ	reporting responsibility
トリアージ	triage
トリアージタッグ	triage tag
日本医師会 にほんいしかい	Japan Medical Association (JMA)
日本医療機能評価機構 にほんいりょうきのうひょうかきこう	Japan Council for Quality Health Care (JCQHC)
日本看護協会 にほんかんごきょうかい	Japanese Nursing Association (JNA)
日本生命倫理学会 にほんせいめいりんりがっかい	Japan Association for Bioethics
日本病院薬剤師会 にほんびょういんやくざいしかい	Japanese Society of Hospital Pharmacists (JSHP)
日本薬剤師会 にほんやくざいしかい	Japan Pharmaceutical Association (JPA)
病院情報システム びょういんじょうほう	hospital information system (HIS)
標準化死亡比 ひょうじゅんかしぼうひ	standardized mortality rate (SMR)
へき地診療 へきちしんりょう	medical care in remote site (in less populated area)
包括医療 ほうかついりょう	comprehensive medical care
訪問看護 ほうもんかんご	home-visit nursing care
保健医療システム ほけんいりょう	health care system
無医地区 むいちく	medically underserved area, doctorless area
無資格診療 むしかくしんりょう	unlicenced medical practice
有害薬物反応 ゆうがいやくぶつはんのう	adverse drug reaction (ADR)
有害事象 ゆうがいじしょう	adverse event
利害関係 りがいかんけい	conflict of interest
倫理委員会 りんりいいんかい	ethics committee

● 倫理綱領　Code of ethics ●

国際看護師協会看護師の倫理綱領 こくさいかんごしきょうかいかんごしのりんりこうりょう	ICN Code of Ethics for Nurses (International Council of Nurses)
国際助産師連盟助産師の倫理綱領 こくさいじょさんしれんめいじょさんしのりんりこうりょう	ICM Code of Ethics for Midwives (International Confederation of Midwives)
世界医師会医の国際倫理綱領 せかいいしかいいのこくさいりんりこうりょう	WMA International Code of Medical Ethics (World Medical Association)
世界医師会患者の権利に関するリスボン宣言 せかいいしかいかんじゃのけんりかんするりすぼんせんげん	WMA Declaration of Lisbon on the Rights of the Patient
ナイチンゲール誓詞 ーせいし	Nightingale Pledge

〈*An adaptation of the physician's Hippocratic Oath for nurses, originally composed in 1893 by a committee chaired by Lystra Gretter; it portrays the role and duties of nurses and guides nursing ethics. It was named in honor of the esteemed founder of modern nursing.*⟩

日本医師会医の倫理綱領	JMA Code of Medical Ethics (Japan Medical Association)
ニュルンベルク綱領	Nuremberg Code
ヒポクラテスの誓い	Hippocratic Oath

⟨*An oath of ethical professional behavior taken by physicians as they began medical practice; one of the well-known phrases is, "never do harm to anyone". It has been revised over the centuries; a modern version of the oath written by Louis Lasagna was widely used.*⟩

米国医師会倫理綱領	AMA Code of Ethics (American Medical Association)
米国病院協会患者の権利章典	AHA Patients' Bill of Rights (American Hospital Association)(現在は Patient Care Partnership と改題)
ヘルシンキ宣言	Declaration of Helsinki

Tidbits

quack

quack-quack はアヒルのガーガー鳴く鳴き声であるが，quack には藪医者やにせ医者の意味がある．膏薬売りがその効能をあひるのようにがなり立てるので quacksalver と呼ばれたことに由来すると言われる．いんちき療法を quackery, quack remedies, いかさま薬を quack medicine という．

2. 医事法制

● 法制 Legislation ●

法律 ほうりつ	act (a law that has been officially accepted by the legislature)
政令 せいれい	cabinet order
省令 しょうれい	ordinance of the ministry
規則 きそく	rule
県(市)条例 けん(し)じょうれい	prefectural (municipal) ordinance

● 医事法 Medical law ●

医師法 いしほう	Medical Practitioners Law
医療法 いりょうほう	Medical Service Law
覚せい剤取締法 かくせいざいとりしまりほう	Stimulants Control Law
学校保健法 がっこうほけんほう	School Health Law
環境基本法 かんきょうきほんほう	Environmental Law
感染症予防法 かんせんしょうよぼうほう	Law for the Prevention of Infectious Diseases and the Medical Care of People Suffering from Infectious Diseases
結核予防法 けっかくよぼうほう	Tuberculosis Prevention Law
検疫法 けんえきほう	Quarantine Act
健康増進法 けんこうぞうしんほう	Health Promotion Law
歯科医師法 しかいしほう	Dental Act
死体解剖保存法 したいかいぼうほぞんほう	Law concerning Autopsy and Preservation of Corpse
児童福祉法 じどうふくしほう	Child Welfare Act
食品衛生法 しょくひんえいせいほう	Food Sanitation Act
身体障害者福祉法 しんたいしょうがいしゃふくしほう	Law for the Welfare of the People with Physical Disabilities
精神保健福祉法 せいしんほけんふくしほう	Law on Mental Health and Welfare for People with Mental Disorders
臓器移植法 ぞうきいしょくほう	Organ Transplantation Law
地域保健法 ちいきほけんほう	Community Health Law
知的障害者福祉法 ちてきしょうがいしゃふくしほう	Law for the Welfare of the People with Intellectual Disability
保健師助産師看護師法 ほけんしじょさんしかんごしほう	Public Health Nurse, Midwife and Nurse Law
保健所法 ほけんじょほう	Health Center Act
母子保健法 ぼしほけんほう	Maternal and Child Health Law
母体保護法 ぼたいほごほう	Maternal Protection Law
薬剤師法 やくざいしほう	Pharmacists Law
薬事法 やくじほう	Pharmaceutical Affairs Law

予防接種法 よぼうせつしゅほう	Immunization Law
麻薬及び向神経薬取締法 まやくおよ——こうしんけいやくとりしまりほう	Narcotic and Psychotropic Drugs Control Law
老人福祉法 ろうじんふくしほう	Welfare Law for the Elderly
老人保健法 ろうじんほけんほう	Health and Medical Service Law for the Elderly
労働安全衛生法 ろうどうあんぜんえいせいほう	Industrial Safety and Health Act

Tidbits

oxymoron

oxymoron とは,両立しない言葉を組み合わせて修辞的効果を上げようとする「矛盾語法」であり,open secret, cruel kindness, polite discourtesy などがその例である.この oxymoron 自体が oxymoron であり,ギリシャ語の oxúmōros (pointedly-foolish あるいは sharp-dull) に由来する.医学用語にレトリックは不要であるが,ill health, dry rale, child psychiatrist, differentiated stem cell, feel numb などが oxymoron といえる.

3. 医療保険制度

● 医療保険制度　Medical insurance system ●

医療過誤保険（いりょうかごほけん）	malpractice insurance
医療費控除（いりょうひこうじょ）	medical expenses deduction
医療保険（いりょうほけん）	medical treatment insurance
介護保険（かいごほけん）	long-term care insurance
確定拠出年金（かくていきょしゅつねんきん）	defined contribution pension
がん保険（がんほけん）	cancer insurance
管理医療（かんりいりょう），マネージドケア	managed care
給付金（きゅうふきん）	benefits
共済組合健康保険（きょうさいくみあいけんこうほけん）	mutual aid association health insurance
組合管掌健康保険（くみあいかんしょうけんこうほけん）	society-managed health insurance
健康保険（けんこうほけん）	health insurance
健康保険組合（けんこうほけんくみあい）	health insurance society
健康保険適用（けんこうほけんてきよう）	health care coverage
健康保険による払い戻し（けんこうほけんによるはらいもどし）	health insurance reimbursement
健康保険被保険者証（けんこうほけんひほけんしゃしょう），保険証（ほけんしょう）	health insurance certificate
高額医療（こうがくいりょう）	high-cost medical care, expensive care
高額療養費（こうがくりょうようひ）	high medical expenses
後期高齢者医療制度（こうきこうれいしゃいりょうせいど）	medical insurance system for people aged 75 and older
厚生年金保険（こうせいねんきんほけん）	employees' pension insurance
公的健康保険（こうてきけんこうほけん）	public health insurance
公的年金（こうてきねんきん）	public pension
高度先進医療（こうどせんしんいりょう）	highly-advanced medical technology
国民皆保険（こくみんかいほけん）	universal health insurance
国民健康保険（こくみんけんこうほけん），国保（こくほ）	National Health Insurance
国民年金保険（こくみんねんきんほけん）	national pension insurance
個人健康保険（こじんけんこうほけん）	private health insurance
自己負担額（じこふたんがく）	co-payment
自己負担限度額（じこふたんげんどがく）	out-of-pocket maximum
自己負担率（じこふたんりつ）	co-payment rate
失業保険（しつぎょうほけん）	unemployment insurance
自費診療費（じひしんりょうひ）	out-of-pocket medical expenses
社会保険（しゃかいほけん）	social insurance

3. 医療保険制度

社会保険庁 しゃかいほけんちょう	Social Insurance Agency
社会保障 しゃかいほしょう	social security
障害年金 しょうがいねんきん	disability pension
傷害保険 しょうがいほけん	accident insurance
診断群分類別包括評価 しんだんぐんぶんるいべつほうかつひょうか	diagnosis procedure combination (DPC)
診断別関連群 しんだんべつかんれんぐん	diagnosis-related group (DRG)
診療報酬 しんりょうほうしゅう	fee for medical services
診療報酬点数 しんりょうほうしゅうてんすう	medical fee points
生活保護 せいかつほご	public assistance, welfare
政府管掌健康保険 せいふかんしょうけんこうほけん	government-managed health insurance
生命保険 せいめいほけん	life insurance
船員保険 せんいんほけん	seamen's insurance
相互扶助 そうごふじょ	mutual aid, reciprocal help
損害補償 そんがいほしょう	indemnity
退職者医療制度 たいしょくしゃいりょうせいど	medical care system for retirees
退職年金 たいしょくねんきん	retirement pension
滞納 たいのう	nonpayment
脱退一時金 だったいいちじきん	lump-sum withdrawal payment
中央社会保険医療協議会 ちゅうおうしゃかいほけんいりょうきょうぎかい	Central Social Insurance Medical Council
出来高払い方式 できだかばらいほうしき	fee-for-service plans
日本年金機構 にほんねんきんきこう	Japan Pension Service
年金 ねんきん	pension, annuity
年金受給者 ねんきんじゅきゅうしゃ	pensioner
被扶養者 ひふようしゃ	dependent
被保険者 ひほけんしゃ	insured person, the insured
被用者保険 ひようしゃほけん	employees' health insurance
保険会社 ほけんがいしゃ	insurance company
保険給付 ほけんきゅうふ	insurance benefits
保険金受給者 ほけんきんじゅきゅうしゃ	beneficiary
保険契約者 ほけんけいやくしゃ	policy-holder, the insured
保険証書 ほけんしょうしょ	insurance policy
保険料 ほけんりょう	insurance premium, premium
免責額 めんせきがく	deductible
養老保険 ようろうほけん	endowment insurance
療養費 りょうようひ	medical expenses, health expenditure
老人医療費 ろうじんいりょうひ	medical expenditure for the elderly
老齢基礎年金 ろうれいきそねんきん	old-age basic pension
労働者災害補償保険 ろうどうしゃさいがいほしょうほけん, 労災 ろうさい	workmen's accident compensation insurance

II章

● 英米の医療保険　Medical insurance in UK and the USA. ●

アメリカ健康保険企画（米国）	America's Health Insurance Plans (AHIP)
医療者選択会員制団体健康保険（米国）	preferred providers organization (PPO)
医療保険の通算可能性と説明責任に関する法律（米国）	Health Insurance Portability and Accountability Act (HIPAA)
英国保健省	Department of Health (DOH)
健康維持機構（米国）	health maintenance organization (HMO)
国民保健サービス（英国）	National Health Service (NHS)
国民保健サービス・地域医療法（英国）	National Health Service and Community Care Act
小児健康保険制度（米国）	State Children's Health Insurance Program (SCHIP)
食料切符支給計画（米国）	food stamp program
ブルークロス（米国）	Blue Cross
ブルーシールド（米国）	Blue Shield
米国保健福祉省	Department of Health and Human Services (DHHS)
メディケア（米国）	Medicare
メディケイド（米国）	Medicaid
メディケア・メディケイドセンター（米国）	Centers for Medicare and Medicaid Services (CMS)
老齢・遺族・障害者年金および健康保険（米国）	Old Age, Survivors, Disability, and Health Insurance (OASDHI)

---Tidbits---

portmanteau word

portmanteau は大型の両開きスーツケースで,「二つ以上の用途を兼ねた」という形容詞にもなる. 従って「かばん語」とは2語の音と意味を混ぜて作った合成語のことで, brunch (breakfast+lunch), motel (motor+hotel), smog (smoke+fog) がよく知られている. そのほか bit (binary+digit), pixel (picture+element), infomercial (information+commercial), workaholic (work+alcoholic), Medicaid (medical+aid), medevac (medical+evacuation), などがあるが, MDeity (MD+deity) は過去の言葉としたい.

4. 保健医療施設

● 保健医療施設　Health-care facilities ●

病院 びょういん	hospital
療養所 りょうようじょ	sanatorium
診療所 しんりょうじょ	clinic
助産所 じょさんじょ	maternity home
保健所 ほけんじょ	public health center

● 医療施設：病院　Medical facilities: hospitals ●

医療センター いりょう—	medical center
エイズ治療拠点病院 —ちりょうきょてんびょういん	key hospital for AIDS treatment
開放式病院 かいほうしきびょういん	open hospital
隔離病院 かくりびょういん	isolation hospital
がんセンター	cancer center
関連病院 かんれんびょういん	affiliated hospital
救急病院 きゅうきゅうびょういん	emergency hospital
救命救急センター きゅうめいきゅうきゅう—	emergency and critical care center
教育病院 きょういくびょういん	teaching hospital
県立病院 けんりつびょういん	prefectural hospital
結核病院 けっかくびょういん, 結核療養所 けっかくりょうようじょ	tuberculosis hospital, sanatorium
公立病院 こうりつびょういん	public hospital, government hospital
国立病院 こくりつびょういん	national hospital, state-run hospital
国立病院機構 こくりつびょういんきこう	National Hospital Organization
災害医療センター さいがいいりょう—	disaster medical center
産科病院 さんかびょういん, 産院 さんいん	maternity hospital, lying-in hospital
小児病院 しょうにびょういん	children's hospital
市立病院 しりつびょういん	city hospital, municipal hospital
私立病院 しりつびょういん	private hospital
精神病院 せいしんびょういん	mental hospital
総合病院 そうごうびょういん	general hospital
大学病院 だいがくびょういん	university hospital
地域医療支援病院 ちいきいりょうしえんびょういん	support hospital for regional medical care
特定機能病院 とくていきのうびょういん	specialized function hospital
分娩施設 ぶんべんしせつ	birthing center
閉鎖式病院 へいさしきびょういん	closed hospital
母子保健センター ぼしほけん—	center for maternal and child health
夜間病院 やかんびょういん	night hospital

4. 保健医療施設　53

野戦病院 やせんびょういん　　　field hospital
老人病院 ろうじんびょういん　　geriatric hospital

● 病院部門：診療科　Department / Division (D.) ●

アレルギー科　　　　　D. of Allergy
移植外科 いしょくげか　　D. of Transplant Surgery
一般外科 いっぱんげか　　D. of General Surgery
核医学科 かくいがくか　　D. of Nuclear Medicine
眼科 がんか　　　　　　　D. of Ophthalmology
感染症科 かんせんしょうか　D. of Infectious Disease
肝臓科 かんぞうか　　　　D. of Hepatology
矯正歯科 きょうせいしか　D. of Orthodontics
胸部外科 きょうぶげか　　D. of Thoracic Surgery
形成外科 けいせいげか　　D. of Plastic Surgery
外科 げか　　　　　　　　D. of Surgery
血液科 けつえきか　　　　D. of Hematology
血管外科 けっかんげか　　D. of Vascular Surgery
口腔外科 こうくうげか　　D. of Oral Surgery
呼吸器科 こきゅうきか　　D. of Pulmonary Disease, D. of Respiratory Medicine
産婦人科 さんふじんか　　D. of Obstetrics and Gynecology (Ob-Gyn)
歯科 しか　　　　　　　　D. of Dentistry
耳鼻咽喉科 じびいんこうか　D. of Oto(rhino)laryngology (ENT)
腫瘍科 しゅようか　　　　D. of Oncology
循環器科 じゅんかんきか　D. of Cardiology
消化器科 しょうかきか，胃腸科 いちょうか　D. of Gastroenterology
小児科 しょうにか　　　　D. of Pediatrics
小児外科 しょうにげか　　D. of Pediatric Surgery
神経内科 しんけいないか　D. of Neurology
心血管外科 しんけっかんげか　D. of Cardiovascular Surgery
腎臓科 じんぞうか　　　　D. of Nephrology
心臓外科 しんぞうげか　　D. of Cardiac Surgery
心療内科 しんりょうないか　D. of Psychosomatic Medicine
整形外科 せいけいげか　　D. of Orthopedic Surgery, D. of Orthopedics
精神科 せいしんか　　　　D. of Psychiatry
性病科 せいびょうか　　　D. of Venereology
総合内科 そうごうないか　D. of General Internal Medicine
直腸肛門科 ちょくちょうこうもんか　D. of Proctology
頭頚部外科 とうけいぶげか　D. of Head and Neck Surgery

54　II章　医療関連用語

内科 ないか	D. of Medicine, D. of Internal Medicine
内視鏡部 ないしきょうぶ	D. of Endoscopy, Endoscopy Unit
内分泌科 ないぶんぴか	D. of Endocrinology
脳外科 のうげか	D. of Brain Surgery
脳神経外科 のうしんけいげか	D. of Neurosurgery, D. of Neurological Surgery
泌尿器科 ひにょうきか	D. of Urology
皮膚科 ひふか	D. of Dermatology
病理部 びょうりぶ	D. of Pathology
美容外科 びようげか	D. of Cosmetic Surgery
ペインクリニック	pain clinic
放射線科 ほうしゃせんか	D. of Radiology
麻酔科 ますいか	D. of Anesthesiology
免疫科 めんえきか	D. of Immunology
リウマチ病科 リウマチびょうか	D. of Rheumatology
臨床病理部 りんしょうびょうりぶ	D. of Clinical Pathology
老年科 ろうねんか	D. of Geriatrics

● 病院部門：診療科以外　Other departments ●

受付 うけつけ	reception desk
栄養部 えいようぶ	nutrition and food services
X線検査室 エックスせんけんさしつ	X-ray room
会計 かいけい	cashier
回復室 かいふくしつ	recovery room (RR)
外来 がいらい	outpatient department (OPD)
看護部 かんごぶ	department of nursing
冠疾患集中治療室 かんしっかんしゅうちゅうちりょうしつ	coronary care unit (CCU)
カンファレンス室 カンファレンスしつ	conference room
緩和ケア病棟 かんわケアびょうとう	palliative care unit (PCU)
救急室 きゅうきゅうしつ	emergency room (ER)
救急治療部 きゅうきゅうちりょうぶ	emergency department (ED)
検査室 けんさしつ	laboratory (lab)
産科病棟 さんかびょうとう	maternity ward
事務部 じむぶ	business office
集中治療室 しゅうちゅうちりょうしつ	intensive care unit (ICU)
手術室 しゅじゅつしつ	operating room (OR)
食堂 しょくどう	cafeteria, dining room
処置室 しょちしつ	procedure room, treatment room
診察室 しんさつしつ	doctor's office, examining room, examination room
新生児室 しんせいじしつ	nursery

4．保健医療施設 55

新生児集中治療室	neonatal intensive care unit (NICU)
セルフケア・ユニット	self-care unit (SCU)
全身麻酔後回復室	postanesthesia care unit (PACU)
洗濯室	laundry
中央材料室	central supply room (CSR)
中央滅菌材料部門	central sterile supply department (CSSD)
ナースステーション	nurse's station
病棟	floor, ward, wing
病歴室	medical record library
分娩室	delivery room, birthing room
ホスピス	hospice
待合室	waiting room
薬剤部，薬局	pharmacy
理学療法部	department of physical therapy
霊安室	mortuary, morgue

● 介護施設　Nursing-care facilities ●

介護保険施設	long-term care insurance facility
介護療養型医療施設	medical care facility for the elderly
介護老人保健施設	health care facility for the elderly
軽費老人ホーム，ケアハウス	home for the elderly with a moderate fee, care house
通所介護施設	day services center for the elderly
特別養護老人ホーム，指定介護老人福祉施設	special nursing home for the elderly
認知症高齢者グループホーム	group home for the elderly with dementia
有料老人ホーム	private nursing home
養護老人ホーム	nursing home for the elderly
老人介護支援センター	supportive center for long-term care for the elderly
老人短期入所施設	short-stay facility for the elderly
老人福祉センター	welfare center for the elderly

―――――――――――――――――――――― Tidbits ――

acronym

acronymとは，各語の頭文字を組み合わせて作った語で，NATO，NASA，AIDS，SARSなどのように一語として発音される「頭字語」である．この点で厳密にはMIT，IBM，AST，CKDのように一字ずつ発音するinitialism「頭文字語」とは区別される．医学用語にはユネスコ読みのacronymよりinitialismのほうが圧倒的に多いが，口語ではBUN，NICU，SOAPなどを一語として発音することもある．かつて「キャッツキャン」と言われて戸惑ったことがあるが，CAT scanのことであった．

5. 医療従事者

● 医療関係職種　Medical professionals ●

あん摩マッサージ指圧師	practitioner of amma-massage-acupressure, masseur
医学物理士	medical physicist
医師	doctor, physician
一般医	generalist, general practitioner (GP)
開業医	practitioner
かかりつけ医	primary physician, family doctor, family physician
学校医	school doctor, school physician
家庭医	family doctor, family physician
監察医	medical examiner
勤務医, 病院医	hospitalist, house physician
警察医	police doctor
研究者	researcher
産業医	occupational physician
歯科医	dentist
指導医	clinical teacher, preceptor
獣医	veterinarian
主治医	attending physician
診断医	diagnostician
専門医	specialist
対診医	consultant
当直医	doctor on call, on-call doctor
臨床医	clinician
移植コーディネーター	transplant coordinator
医薬情報担当者	medical representative (MR)
医療ソーシャルワーカー	medical social worker (MSW)
栄養士	dietician, dietitian
音楽療法士	music therapist
介護支援専門員	care manager
介護福祉士	certified care worker
看護師	nurse
看護師, 登録看護師	registered nurse (RN)
准看護師, 実務看護師	licensed practical nurse (LPN)

がん専門薬剤師	board certified oncology pharmacy specialist (BCOPS)
がん薬物療法認定薬剤師	board certified pharmacist in oncology pharmacy (BCPOP)
管理栄養士	registered dietician (dietitian)
義肢装具士	artificial limb fitter, prosthetist and orthotist
救急救命士	emergency medical technician (EMT)
灸師	practitioner of moxibustion, moxibustionist
言語聴覚士	speech and hearing therapist
呼吸療法認定士	certified respiratory therapist
作業療法士	occupational therapist (OT)
歯科衛生士	dental hygienist
歯科技工士	dental technician
視能訓練士	orthoptist (ORT)
社会福祉士	certified social worker
柔道整復師	judo therapist, osteopath (整骨医)
手話通訳士	sign language interpreter
助産師	midwife, maternity nurse, birthing assistant
診療情報管理士	medical record administrator
診療放射線技師	radiological technologist
精神科ソーシャルワーカー	psychiatric social worker (PSW)
精神保健福祉士	certified mental health and welfare worker
専門看護師	certified nurse specialist (CNS)
治験コーディネーター	clinical research coordinator (CRC)
糖尿病療養指導士	certified diabetes educator
ナースプラクティショナー	nurse practitioner (NP)
認定看護師	certified nurse (CN)
鍼師	practitioner of acupuncture, acupuncturist
病院薬剤師	hospital pharmacist
保育士	child care person
保健師	public health nurse (PHN)
薬剤師	pharmacist
理学療法士	physical therapist (PT)
臨床検査技師	medical technologist (MT)

5. 医療従事者 59

| 臨床工学技士 りんしょうこうがくぎし | clinical engineering technologist |
| 臨床心理士 りんしょうしんりし | clinical psychologist |

● 病院内職掌　Hospital staff ●

院長 いんちょう	director
副院長 ふくいんちょう	vice-director
看護部長 かんごぶちょう	director of nursing
事務部長 じむぶちょう	general manager
診療部長 しんりょうぶちょう	department head
薬局長 やっきょくちょう	head pharmacist
技師長 ぎしちょう	head technologist
医員 いいん	staff doctor (physician, surgeon), medical staff
研修医 けんしゅうい	clinical trainee
レジデント	resident, resident physician
看護師長 かんごしちょう	head nurse
主任看護師 しゅにんかんごし	charge nurse
病棟看護師 びょうとうかんごし	floor nurse, staff nurse
手術室看護師 しゅじゅつしつかんごし	operating room nurse, scrub nurse
看護助手 かんごじょしゅ	nurse's aide
事務員 じむいん	clerk
医療補助者 いりょうほじょしゃ	allied health personnel, paramedical staff

● 診療医・専門医　Clinicians / Specialists ●

アレルギー専門医 せんもんい	allergist
一般外科医 いっぱんげかい	general surgeon
眼科医 がんかい	ophthalmologist
肝臓病医 かんぞうびょうい	hepatologist
矯正歯科医 きょうせいしかい	orthodontist
胸部外科医 きょうぶげかい	thoracic surgeon
形成外科医 けいせいげかい	plastic surgeon
外科医 げかい	surgeon
血液病医 けつえきびょうい	hematologist
血管外科医 けっかんげかい	vascular surgeon
口腔外科医 こうくうげかい	oral surgeon
産科医 さんかい	obstetrician
歯科医 しかい	dentist
耳鼻咽喉科医 じびいんこうかい	oto(rhino)laryngologist
腫瘍専門医 しゅようせんもんい	oncologist
循環器病医 じゅんかんきびょうい	cardiologist
消化器病医 しょうかきびょうい	gastroenterologist

II章 医療関連用語

小児科医 しょうにかい	pediatrician
小児外科医 しょうにげかい	pediatric surgeon
神経内科医 しんけいないかい	neurologist
腎臓病医 じんぞうびょうい	nephrologist
心臓外科医 しんぞうげかい	cardiac surgeon
整形外科医 せいけいげかい	orthopedic surgeon, orthopedist
精神科医 せいしんかい	psychiatrist
精神分析専門医 せいしんぶんせきい	psychoanalyst
性病科医 せいびょうかい	venereologist
直腸肛門科医 ちょくちょうこうもんかい	proctologist
内科医 ないかい	internist
内視鏡医 ないしきょうい	endoscopist
内分泌科医 ないぶんぴつかい	endocrinologist
脳外科医 のうげかい	brain surgeon
脳神経外科医 のうしんけいげかい	neurosurgeon
泌尿器科医 ひにょうきかい	urologist
皮膚科医 ひふかい	dermatologist
病理医 びょうりい	pathologist
美容外科医 びようげかい	cosmetic surgeon
婦人科医 ふじんかい	gynecologist
放射線科医 ほうしゃせんかい	radiologist
麻酔科医 ますいかい	anesthesiologist
免疫専門医 めんえきせんもんい	immunologist
リウマチ病医 ーびょうい	rheumatologist
臨床病理医 りんしょうびょうりい	clinical pathologist
老年病専門医 ろうねんびょうせんもんい	geriatrician

● 専門看護師　Certified Nurse Specialist (CNS) ●

がん看護 ーかんご	cancer nursing
精神看護 せいしんかんご	psychiatric mental health nursing
地域看護 ちいきかんご	community health nursing
老人看護 ろうじんかんご	gerontological nursing
小児看護 しょうにかんご	child health nursing
母性看護 ぼせいかんご	women's health nursing
慢性疾患看護 まんせいしっかんかんご	chronic care nursing
急性・重症患者看護 きゅうせい・じゅうしょうかんじゃかんご	critical care nursing
感染症看護 かんせんしょうかんご	infection control nursing
家族支援 かぞくしえん	family health nursing

● 認定看護師　Certified Nurse (CN) ●

救急看護 きゅうきゅうかんご	emergency nursing

5. 医療従事者

皮膚・排泄ケア (ひふ・はいせつ)	wound, ostomy and continence nursing
集中ケア (しゅうちゅう)	intensive care
緩和ケア (かんわ)	palliative care
がん化学療法看護 (かがくりょうほうかんご)	cancer chemotherapy nursing
がん性疼痛看護 (つうかんご)	cancer pain management nursing
訪問看護 (ほうもんかんご)	visiting nursing
感染管理 (かんせんかんり)	infection control
糖尿病看護 (とうにょうびょうかんご)	diabetes nursing
不妊症看護 (ふにんしょうかんご)	infertility nursing
新生児集中ケア (しんせいじししゅう)	neonatal intensive care
透析看護 (とうせきかんご)	dialysis nursing
手術看護 (しゅじゅつかんご)	perioperative nursing
乳がん看護 (にゅう)	breast cancer nursing
摂食・嚥下障害看護 (せっしょく・えんげしょうがいかんご)	dysphagia nursing
小児救急看護 (しょうにきゅうきゅうかんご)	pediatric emergency nursing
認知症看護 (にんちしょうかんご)	dementia nursing
脳卒中リハビリテーション看護 (のうそっちゅう—かんご)	stroke rehabilitation nursing
がん放射線療法看護 (ほうしゃせんりょうほうかんご)	radiation therapy nursing

Tidbits

"comedical" staff

「コメディカルスタッフ」は，病院職員のうち診療補助部門の職員の総称として定着しているが和製英語である．paramedicalの"para-"にある「準」，「補足」，「従属」の含意が嫌われたこと，英語圏ではparamedicといえば「落下傘衛生兵」や「救急救命士」を指すことなどから"co-"（共同，相互，同等）が選ばれたと思われる．なおcomedic(al)は「喜劇的な，滑稽な」を意味することにも要注意．comedical staffと名乗るとPatch Adamsと間違えられるかもしれない．

6. 医学教育

●医療系教育機関　Medical and health-related schools●

医学部 いがくぶ	school of medicine, medical school, faculty of medicine
医科大学 いかだいがく	medical school, medical college, medical university
医療科学大学 いりょうかがくだいがく	university of medical science
医療福祉大学 いりょうふくしだいがく	university of medical welfare
栄養大学 えいようだいがく	nutrition university, college of nutrition
看護学校 かんごがっこう	school of nursing
看護大学 かんごだいがく	college of nursing, nursing university
看護福祉大学 かんごふくしだいがく	university of nursing and welfare
研究機関 けんきゅうきかん	research institute
歯学部 しがくぶ	school of dentistry
歯科大学 しかだいがく	dental college, dental university
社会福祉大学 しゃかいふくしだいがく	university of social welfare
獣医学部 じゅういがくぶ	school of veterinary medicine
総合大学 そうごうだいがく	university
大学院 だいがくいん, 大学院大学	graduate school
単科大学 たんかだいがく	college
短期大学 たんきだいがく	junior college
福祉大学 ふくしだいがく	university of welfare
保健医療大学 ほけんいりょうだいがく	university of health sciences
保健衛生大学 ほけんえいせいだいがく	health university
薬学部 やくがくぶ	school of pharmacy
薬科大学 やっかだいがく	pharmaceutical university, university of pharmacy

●医科大学職名　Medical school staff●

学長 がくちょう	president
副学長 ふくがくちょう	vice president
医学部長 いがくぶちょう	dean of the school of medicine
副学部長 ふくがくぶちょう	associate dean
医学部教授会 いがくぶきょうじゅかい	medical faculty
教授 きょうじゅ	professor
臨床教授 りんしょうきょうじゅ	clinical professor
准教授 じゅんきょうじゅ	associate professor
講師 こうし	lecturer
助教 じょきょう	assistant professor
研究員 けんきゅういん	research personnel
研究助手 けんきゅうじょしゅ	research assistant

● 基礎医学　Basic medicine ●

医学教育学	medical education
医真菌学	medical mycology
遺伝学	genetics
医動物学	medical zoology
衛生学	hygienics
疫学	epidemiology
解剖学	anatomy
環境保健学	environmental health
奇形学	teratology
寄生虫学	parasitology
血清学	serology
公衆衛生学	public health
行動科学	behavioral science
骨学	osteology
細菌学	bacteriology
細胞遺伝学	cytogenetics
実験医学	experimental medicine
実験動物学	laboratory animal science
生化学	biochemistry
生態学	ecology
生理学	physiology
組織学	histology
組織病理学	histopathology
発生学	embryology
微生物学	microbiology
病理学	pathology
分子遺伝学	molecular genetics
分子生物学	molecular biology
法医学	legal medicine, forensic medicine
免疫学	immunology
薬理学	pharmacology

● 臨床医学　Clinical medicine ●

アレルギー学	allergology
移植外科学	transplant surgery
遺伝医学	medical genetics
遺伝子工学	genetic engineering
医用生体工学	medical bioengineering
医療経済学	medical economics
医療社会学	medical sociology
医療情報学	medical informatics

II章 医療関連用語

医療倫理学 いりょうりんりがく	medical ethics
宇宙医学 うちゅういがく	aerospace medicine
栄養学 えいようがく	dietetics
核医学 かくいがく	nuclear medicine
画像診断学 がぞうしんだんがく	diagnostic imaging
家庭医学 かていいがく	family medicine
眼科学 がんかがく	ophthalmology
環境医学 かんきょういがく	environmental medicine
肝臓学 かんぞうがく	hepatology
義肢学 ぎしがく	prosthetics
気象医学 きしょういがく	medical climatology
救急医学 きゅうきゅういがく	emergency medicine
矯正歯科学 きょうせいしかがく	orthodontics
胸部外科学 きょうぶげかがく	thoracic surgery
形成外科学 けいせいげかがく	plastic surgery
外科学 げかがく	surgery
血液学 けつえきがく	hematology
血管外科学 けっかんげかがく	vascular surgery
高圧医学 こうあついがく	hyperbaric medicine
航空医学 こうくういがく	aviation medicine
口腔病学 こうくうびょうがく	stomatology
口腔外科学 こうくうげかがく	oral surgery
呼吸器内科学 こきゅうきないかがく	respiratory medicine
産科学 さんかがく	obstetrics
産業医学 さんぎょういがく	occupational medicine
産婦人科学 さんふじんかがく	obstetrics and gynecology
歯科学 しかがく	dentistry
耳鼻咽喉科学 じびいんこうかがく	otorhinolaryngology
社会医学 しゃかいいがく	social medicine
周産期医学 しゅうさんきいがく	perinatology
腫瘍学 しゅようがく	oncology
消化器病学 しょうかきびょうがく	gastroenterology
小児外科学 しょうにげかがく	pediatric surgery
小児科学 しょうにかがく	pediatrics
神経内科学 しんけいないかがく	neurology
神経耳科学 しんけいじかがく	neurotology
心身医学 しんしんいがく	psychosomatic medicine
心臓病学 しんぞうびょうがく	cardiology
腎臓病学 じんぞうびょうがく	nephrology
心臓外科学 しんぞうげかがく	cardiac surgery
診療情報学 しんりょうじょうほうがく	clinical informatics
スポーツ医学 スポーツいがく	sports medicine

整形外科学 せいけいげかがく	orthopedics
整骨医学 せいこついがく	osteopathic medicine
精神医学 せいしんいがく	psychiatry
生物統計学 せいぶつとうけいがく	biostatistics
地域医療学 ちいきいりょうがく	community medicine
直腸病学 ちょくちょうびょうがく, 肛門病学 こうもんびょうがく	proctology
動物行動学 どうぶつこうどうがく	ethology
内科学 ないかがく	internal medicine
内分泌学 ないぶんぴつがく	endocrinology
熱帯医学 ねったいいがく	tropical medicine
脳神経外科学 のうしんけいげかがく	neurosurgery
肺臓学 はいぞうがく	pulmonology
泌尿器科学 ひにょうきかがく	urology
皮膚科学 ひふかがく	dermatology
病理学 びょうりがく	pathology
美容外科学 びようげかがく	cosmetic surgery
婦人科学 ふじんかがく	gynecology
物理療法学 ぶつりりょうほうがく	physical medicine
放射線医学 ほうしゃせんいがく	radiology
麻酔科学 ますいかがく	anesthesiology
予防医学 よぼういがく	preventive medicine
リウマチ病学 ―びょうがく	rheumatology
リハビリテーション医学 ―いがく	rehabilitation medicine
旅行医学 りょこういがく	travel medicine, emporiatrics
臨床病理学 りんしょうびょうりがく	clinical pathology
臨床免疫学 りんしょうめんえきがく	clinical immunology
老年医学 ろうねんいがく	geriatrics, gerontology

● 看護学 Nursing ●

家族看護学 かぞくかんごがく	family nursing
看護疫学 かんごえきがく	nursing epidemiology
看護管理学 かんごかんりがく	nursing administration
看護教育学 かんごきょういくがく	nursing education
看護倫理 かんごりんり	nursing ethics
基礎看護学 きそかんごがく	basic nursing
クリティカルケア看護学 ―かんごがく	critical care nursing
小児看護学 しょうにかんごがく	pediatric nursing
助産学 じょさんがく	midwifery
成育看護学 せいいくかんごがく	development nursing

66　Ⅱ章　医療関連用語

生活環境看護学 せいかつかんきょうかんごがく	environmental health nursing
精神看護学 せいしんかんごがく	psychiatric nursing
成人看護学 せいじんかんごがく	adult nursing
地域看護学 ちいきかんごがく	community health nursing
母性看護学 ぼせいかんごがく	maternal-child nursing
予防看護学 よぼうかんごがく	preventive nursing
臨床看護学 りんしょうかんごがく	clinical nursing
老年看護学 ろうねんかんごがく	geriatric nursing

●医学教育用語　Terminology of medical education●

医学士 いがくし	Medicinae Doctor, Doctor of Medicine (MD)
医学生涯教育 いがくしょうがいきょういく	continuing medical education (CME)
医学博士 いがくはくし	Philosophiae Doctor, Doctor of Philosophy (PhD)
医学部教育 いがくぶきょういく	undergraduate medical education
医師国家試験 いしこっかしけん	national examination for medical practitioner
医師免許交付 いしめんきょこうふ	medical licensure
一般目標 いっぱんもくひょう	general instructional objective (GIO)
医療面接 いりょうめんせつ	medical interview
外国語としての英語 がいこくご—えいご	English as a foreign language (EFL)
外国語としての英語テスト がいこくご—えいご—	Test of English as a Foreign Language (TOEFL)
外国人医師卒後教育委員会（米国）がいこくじんいしそつごきょういくいいんかい	Educational Commission for Foreign Medical Graduates (ECFMG)
回診 かいしん	rounds,〔動〕make rounds
開放型質問 かいほうがたしつもん	open-ended question
学位 がくい	academic degree
学位論文 がくいろんぶん	dissertation
学際的 がくさいてき	interdisciplinary
学士号 がくしごう	bachelor's degree
学歴社会 がくれきしゃかい	credential society, credentialism
客観的臨床能力試験 きゃっかんてきりんしょうのうりょくしけん	objective structured clinical examination (OSCE)
教育学 きょういくがく	pedagogy
教育目標 きょういくもくひょう	educational objective
教育目標分類体系 きょういくもくひょうぶんるいたいけい	taxonomy of educational objectives
教員能力開発 きょういんのうりょくかいはつ	faculty development (FD)
共用試験 きょうようしけん	common achievement tests

6. 医学教育

健康診断書 けんこうしんだんしょ	health certificate
コア・カリキュラム	core curriculum
講義 こうぎ	lecture
講義時間割 こうぎじかんわり	syllabus
口頭試問 こうとうしもん	oral examination
行動目標 こうどうもくひょう	specific behavioral objective (SBO)
国際コミュニケーション英語能力テスト こくさいコミュニケーションえいごのうりょくテスト	Test of English for International Communication (TOEIC)
根拠に基づく医療 こんきょにもとづくいりょう	evidence-based medicine (EBM)
根拠に基づく看護 こんきょにもとづくかんご	evidence-based nursing (EBN)
コンピュータ処理多岐選択試験 コンピュータしょりたきせんたくしけん	computer-based testing (CBT)
実習 じっしゅう	exercise
質問に基づく学習 しつもんにもとづくがくしゅう	inquiry-based learning (IBL)
修士号 しゅうしごう	master's degree
宿題 しゅくだい	assignment, homework
診療参加型臨床実習 しんりょうさんかがたりんしょうじっしゅう	clinical clerkship
成績 せいせき	academic standing, grade
専門医制度 せんもんいせいど	specialty board system
専門職間教育 せんもんしょくかんきょういく	interprofessional education
早期体験 そうきたいけん	early exposure
早期臨床体験 そうきりんしょうたいけん	clinical early exposure
卒業証書 そつぎょうしょうしょ	diploma
卒業論文 そつぎょうろんぶん	graduation thesis
卒後医学教育 そつごいがくきょういく	postgraduate medical education
卒後医学教育認定協議会(米国) そつごいがくきょういくにんていきょうぎかい	Accreditation Council for Graduate Medical Education (ACGME)
卒後臨床研修 そつごりんしょうけんしゅう	postgraduate clinical training
大学入学許可 だいがくにゅうがくきょか	matriculation
第二言語としての英語 だいにげんごとしてのえいご	English as a second language (ESL)
多肢選択式試問 たしせんたくしきしもん	multiple-choice question (MCQ)
地域立脚型学習 ちいきりっきゃくがたがくしゅう	community-based learning
チューター制 チューターせい	tutorial system
適性検査 てきせいけんさ	aptitude test
日本医学教育学会	Japan Society for Medical Education

認定専門医	certified specialist
標準模擬患者	standardized patient (SP)
米国医師免許試験	United States Medical Licensing Examination (USMLE)
閉鎖型質問	closed question
ポートフォリオ	portfolio
北米看護診断協会	North American Nursing Diagnostic Association (NANDA)
模擬患者	simulated patient (SP)
模擬装置	simulator
問題基盤型学習	problem-based learning (PBL)
問題志向型システム	problem-oriented system (POS)
問題志向型診療録	problem-oriented medical record (POMR)
文部科学省	Ministry of Education, Culture, Sports, Science and Technology
理学士	Bachelor of Science (BS)
理学修士	Master of Science (MS)
履歴書	résumé, curriculum vitae (CV)
臨床学習	bedside learning (BSL)
臨床技能	clinical skills (CS)
臨床知識	clinical knowledge (CK)
臨床病理検討会	clinical-pathological conference (CPC)

Tidbits

topology

医学用語としての topology は，通常局所解剖学 regional anatomy の意味で topography ともいうが，数学者にとっては位相，位相幾何学，地理学者には地形学，コンピュータ分野ではトポロジーなどいろいろ解釈が違う．topological psychology はトポロジー心理学（位相心理学）．topo-（＜topos）は場所を意味する combining form である．紛らわしい綴りの tropology は，比喩の使用ないし比喩的語法を意味する．

Ⅲ章

英文診療録

1. 診療録

●診療録の構成　Components of medical record●

患者識別情報 かんじゃしきべつじょうほう	patient identification, identifying information
情報源 じょうほうげん	source of information
主訴 しゅそ	chief complaint (CC)
現病歴 げんびょうれき	history of present illness (HPI), present illness (PI)
既往歴 きおうれき	past history (PH), past medical history (PMH)
家族歴 かぞくれき	family history (FH)
社会歴 しゃかいれき	social history (SH)
系統別病歴 けいとうべつびょうれき	review of systems (ROS), system review
身体的検査 しんたいてきけんさ，診察 しんさつ	physical examination (PE)
検査所見 けんさしょけん	laboratory findings
診断 しんだん	diagnosis
計画 けいかく	plan
指示 しじ	order
経過記録 けいかきろく	progress notes
要約 ようやく	summary

Tidbits

Chief Concern

初診時の患者の訴えは，診療録では「主訴」として記載され Hauptklage〔独〕，Chief Complaint〔英〕と同様にわが国でも定着しているが，Chief Concern（関心事）とするほうがよいとの提唱がある（AMA Manual of Style, 2007）．Complaintには"pejorative and confrontational"（軽蔑的，対決的）の意味合いがあるという理由であるが，さていかがなものか？

2．診療録の記載

● 患者識別情報　Identification ●

氏名，生年月日，性別，年齢	name, date of birth, sex, age
現住所，電話番号	home address, telephone number
職業，雇用主，住所	occupation, employer's name, address
紹介医	referring physician
緊急時連絡（氏名，住所，電話番号）	notify in case of emergency: name, address, telephone number
健康保険	health insurance
保険証券番号	insurance ID number

● 情報源　Information source ●

情報は〜から得た	Information was obtained from (the patient, his wife, her cousin, the police officer who brought him in).
従前の診療録から補足した	Information was supplemented by old medical records.
信頼性	credibility
情報は信頼できる	Information is reliable.

● 主訴　Chief complaint ●

患者自身の言葉で	in the patient's own words
〜痛	pain in 〜, -ache, -algia, -dynia
〜困難	difficulty in 〜, trouble in 〜, distress, dys-
〜消失	loss of 〜, lack of 〜, a-, an-
〜不能	inability of 〜, disability of 〜, incapacity for 〜
〜減少，縮小	decrease in 〜, reduction in 〜, decline in 〜
〜増加，増大	increase in 〜, enlargement of 〜
過度〜	excessive 〜, hyper-
〜不規則	irregularity in 〜, irregular 〜
〜不快感	discomfort in 〜
〜感	a sensation of 〜, a feeling of 〜
心配事	worries about 〜

入院前 にゅういんまえ	before admission, prior to admission (PTA)
最近〜日間 さいきん〜にちかん	for the last 〜 days
昨日から きのう	since yesterday
〜ヵ月前から 〜まえかげつ	since 〜 months ago
2時間の 2じかん	of 2 hours' duration

● 現病歴 Present illness ●

発生順（年代順）に はっせいじゅん（ねんだいじゅん）に	in chronological order
発病 はつびょう, 発症 はっしょう	onset
発病年齢 はつびょうねんれい	age of onset
突然の発病 とつぜんはつびょう	sudden (abrupt) onset
緩徐な発病 かんじょはつびょう	slow (gradual, insidious) onset
病気 びょうき	illness, sickness, disease, disorder, trouble
罹患する りかん	suffer from (be ill with, be afflicted with, be troubled with) 〜, contract (get, catch) 〜, sustain (an injury, a wound)
病臥する びょうが	be ill (sick) in bed, be bedridden, be confined to bed
症状 しょうじょう	symptom
初期症状 しょきしょうじょう	initial symptom, presenting symptom
症状が出現する しょうじょうしゅつげん	start, begin, appear, develop, occur
症状に気付く しょうじょうきづ	note, notice, recognize, become aware of
発見（指摘）される はっけん（してき）	be found, be discovered, be detected, be pointed out
随伴する ずいはん	accompany
誘因 ゆういん	an inducing cause (factor), a motive, a trigger
引き起こす ひお	cause, induce, bring about, provoke, precipitate
健康診査 けんこうしんさ	health examination, checkup
人間ドック にんげん	complete (comprehensive) physical examination (checkup)
集団検診 しゅうだんけんしん	mass screening, group checkup
来院 らいいん	a visit to a hospital, 〔動〕visit (attend, present to) a hospital
入院 にゅういん	hospitalization, admission to a hospital,

	〔動〕be hospitalized, be admitted
紹介 しょうかい	referral, 〔動〕refer
紹介率 しょうかいりつ	referral rate
退院 たいいん	discharge, 〔動〕be discharged (released), leave a hospital

● 既往歴　Past history ●

既往症 きおうしょう	previous illnesses
小児期疾患 しょうにきしっかん	childhood illnesses
重病 じゅうびょう	serious illness
入院 にゅういん	hospitalization
手術 しゅじゅつ	operation
外傷 がいしょう	injury, wound, trauma
事故 じこ	accident

● 家族歴　Family history ●

家族 かぞく	family, a family member
核家族 かくかぞく	nuclear family
拡大家族 かくだいかぞく	extended family
親 おや	parent,〔複〕parents
父親（母親）ちちおや（ははおや）	father (mother)
父方（母方）の ちちかた（ははかた）の	paternal (maternal), on the father's (mother's) side
父系（母系）の ふけい（ぼけい）の	patrilineal (matrilineal)
兄弟（姉妹）きょうだい（しまい），同胞 どうほう	a brother or sister, sibling
配偶者（夫，妻）はいぐうしゃ（おっと，つま）	spouse (husband, wife)
子供 こども	child,〔複〕children
息子（娘）むすこ（むすめ）	son (daughter)
祖父（祖母）そふ（そぼ）	grandfather (grandmother)
義父（義母）ぎふ（ぎぼ）	father-in-law (mother-in-law)
親族 しんぞく	relation, kin, sib, a relative
親等 しんとう	degrees of relationship (consanguinity)
一（二，四）親等の親族 いっ（に，よん）しんとうのしんぞく	a relation (relative) in the first (second, fourth) degree
血縁 けつえん	blood relative, consanguinity
肉親 にくしん	immediate family
家系図 かけいず	pedigree, family tree, genealogical tree
発端者 ほったんしゃ	proband, propositus, index case
遺伝性疾患 いでんせいしっかん	hereditary disease, inherited disease
常染色体優性遺伝 じょうせんしょくたいゆうせいいでん	autosomal dominant inheritance

III章 英文診療録

常染色体劣性遺伝	autosomal recessive inheritance
伴性遺伝	sex-linked inheritance
X染色体連鎖性遺伝	X-linked inheritance
X染色体連鎖優性	X-linked dominant
X染色体連鎖劣性	X-linked recessive
先天性疾患	congenital disease
体質性疾患	constitutional disease
血族結婚	consanguineous marriage
死亡	death
死因	the cause of one's death
病死する	die of ~ (cancer, hunger), die from ~ (wound, burn)
老衰で死亡する	die of old age
事故死(戦死)する	be killed in an accident (a battle)
自殺	suicide, 〔動〕kill oneself, commit suicide, take one's life

● 社会歴 Social history ●

出生地	birth place
出生証明書	birth certificate
職業	occupation, job
退職	retirement, 〔動〕retire
失業	unemployment
教育	education, schooling
結婚歴	marital status
既婚(未婚)の	married (unmarried)
離婚	divorce, 〔動〕divorce
別居	separation, 〔動〕separate
宗教	religion
信仰	faith, belief
生活状況	living conditions
生活様式	life style
趣味	hobbies
習慣	habits
飲酒	drinking
喫煙	smoking
食習慣	dietary habits
睡眠	sleep

● 系統別病歴　Review of systems ●

全身 ぜんしん	general
頭部 とうぶ	head
眼 め	eyes
耳鼻咽喉 じびいんこう	ears, nose, throat (ENT)
頚部 けいぶ	neck
呼吸器系 こきゅうきけい	respiratory system
循環器系 じゅんかんきけい	cardiovascular system
消化器系 しょうかきけい	gastrointestinal system
泌尿生殖器系 ひにょうせいしょくきけい	urogenital system, genitourinary system
筋骨格系 きんこつかくけい	musculoskeletal system
内分泌系 ないぶんぴけい	endocrine system
造血器系 ぞうけつきけい	hematopoietic system
神経系 しんけいけい	nervous system
皮膚 ひふ	skin, integument

● 身体的検査　Physical examination ●

生命徴候 せいめいちょうこう, バイタル	vital signs (VS)
体温 たいおん, 脈拍 みゃくはく, 呼吸 こきゅう	temperature, pulse, respiration (TPR)
脈拍数 みゃくはくすう, 呼吸数 こきゅうすう, 心拍数 しんぱくすう	pulse rate (PR), respiration rate (RR), heart rate (HR)
口腔温 こうくうおん	oral temperature
腋窩温 えきかおん	axillary temperature
直腸温 ちょくちょうおん	rectal temperature
収縮期血圧 しゅうしゅくきけつあつ, 最大血圧 さいだいけつあつ	systolic blood pressure (SBP), maximal blood pressure
拡張期血圧 かくちょうきけつあつ, 最小血圧 さいしょうけつあつ	diastolic blood pressure (DBP), minimal blood pressure
コロトコフ音 おん	Korotkoff sounds
〈sounds heard over an artery when the cuff pressure is reduced during auscultatory measurement of blood pressure〉	
脈圧 みゃくあつ	pulse pressure
平均動脈圧 へいきんどうみゃくあつ	mean arterial pressure (MAP)
基礎血圧 きそけつあつ	basal blood pressure
外来血圧 がいらいけつあつ	office blood pressure
家庭血圧 かていけつあつ	home blood pressure
自由行動下血圧測定 じゆうこうどうかけつあつそくてい	ambulatory blood pressure monitoring (ABPM)
体重 たいじゅう	weight (wt), body weight (BW)

身長	height (ht)
腹囲	abdominal circumference, abdominal girth
頭囲	head circumference
体格	physique, build
発育良好な	well-developed (WD)
普通(小柄, 大柄)の体格	of average (small, large) build
栄養	nutrition, nourishment
栄養良好な	well-nourished (WN)
栄養不良の	poorly nourished, malnourished, undernourished
悪液質	cachexia, 〔形〕cachectic
見掛けの年齢	apparent age
重態	serious condition
危篤状態	critical condition
瀕死の	moribund
ヒポクラテス顔貌	hippocratic face 〈a livid face with hollow eyes, concave cheeks, and collapsed temples, indicating close to death〉
外傷重症度スコア	injury severity score (ISS)
一般健康状態	general state of health
意識レベル	level of consciousness
意識明瞭な	conscious, alert, aware
意識不明の	unconscious
昏睡	coma, 〔形〕comatose
見当識	orientation
見当識のある(ない)	oriented (disoriented)
気分	mood
体位	posture, position, 〔形〕postural, positional
立位	standing posture, erect position, upright position
臥位	recumbent posture, lying position
背臥位	supine position, dorsal decubitus, face-up position, lying on the back
腹臥位	prone position, ventral decubitus, face-down position, lying on the stomach
側臥位	lateral decubitus, lying on the side
右側臥位	right lateral decubitus, lying on the right side

左側臥位 ひだりそくがい	left lateral decubitus, lying on the left side
膝胸位 しつきょうい	knee-chest position, genupectoral position
砕石位 さいせきい	lithotomy position, dorsosacral position
ファウラー体位 ──たいい	Fowler position

⟨*an inclined position obtained by raising the head of the bed about 50 cm*⟩

トレンデレンブルク体位 ──たいい	Trendelenburg position

⟨*a supine position with the head lower than the pelvis*⟩

シムズ体位 ──たいい	Sims position

⟨*left lateral decubitus with the left arm behind the back and the right leg flexed*⟩

歩行 ほこう	gait
個人衛生 こじんえいせい	personal hygiene
視診 ししん	inspection, 〔動〕inspect
触診 しょくしん	palpation, 〔動〕palpate, 〔形〕palpatory
打診 だしん	percussion, 〔動〕percuss
聴診 ちょうしん	auscultation, 〔動〕auscultate, 〔形〕auscultatory
双手触診 そうしゅしょくしん	bimanual palpation
直腸指診 ちょくちょうししん	digital rectal examination (DRE)

● 診察用具 Instruments ●

聴診器 ちょうしんき	stethoscope
血圧計 けつあつけい	sphygmomanometer, blood pressure manometer, blood pressure cuff
体温計 たいおんけい	thermometer, clinical thermometer
懐中電灯 かいちゅうでんとう	flashlight, penlight
眼底鏡 がんていきょう	ophthalmoscope
耳鏡 じきょう	otoscope, ear speculum
鼻鏡 びきょう	nasal speculum
額帯鏡 がくたいきょう	head mirror
舌圧子 ぜつあつし	tongue depressor, tongue blade, wooden spatula
ハンマー	hammer, percussion hammer, reflex hammer, patellar hammer
ストップウォッチ	stopwatch
ゴム手袋 ──てぶくろ	rubber gloves
使い捨て手袋 つかいすてぶくろ	disposable gloves
指嚢 しのう	finger cot

潤滑剤	lubricant
腟鏡	vaginal speculum
巻尺	tape measure
物差し	scale, ruler
拡大鏡	loupe, magnifying glass, hand lens
音叉	tuning fork
安全ピン	safety pin

● 検査法　Examination ●

臨床検査	clinical test
臨床現場即時検査	point-of-care testing (POCT)
検尿	urinalysis (UA), examination of urine
検便	examination of feces
血液検査	blood test
血液学的検査	hematologic test
血液化学検査	blood chemistry test
血清学的検査	serologic test
免疫学的検査	immunological test
細菌学的検査	bacteriological examination
生理機能検査	physiological function test
X線検査	x-ray examination, radiologic examination, roentgen examination
内視鏡検査	endoscopy, endoscopic examination
経口内視鏡検査	peroral endoscopy
内視鏡下生検	endoscopic biopsy
直視下生検	direct-vision biopsy
針生検	needle biopsy
細針生検	fine-needle biopsy
吸引生検	aspiration biopsy
パンチ生検	punch biopsy
円錐切除診	cone biopsy
細胞診	cytology, cytological examination
剥離細胞診	exfoliative cytology
吸引細胞診	aspiration cytology
吸引生検細胞診	aspiration biopsy cytology (ABC)
細針吸引	fine needle aspiration (FNA)
組織学的検査	histological examination
病理学的検査	pathological examination
剖検	autopsy, postmortem examination
光学顕微鏡	light microscope

位相差顕微鏡	phase microscope
蛍光顕微鏡	fluorescence microscope
電子顕微鏡	electron microscope (EM)
走査型電子顕微鏡	scanning electron microscope (SEM)

● 画像検査　Imaging examinations ●

X線写真	radiograph, x-ray film
単純X線撮影法	plain radiography
断層撮影法	laminography, tomography
造影X線撮影法	contrast radiography
X線造影剤	contrast medium, contrast material
血管造影法	angiography
ディジタル差分血管造影法	digital subtraction angiography (DSA)
コンピュータ断層撮影法	computed tomography (CT), computerized axial tomography (CAT)
動的コンピュータ断層撮影法	dynamic computed tomography
高分解能コンピュータ断層撮影法	high-resolution computed tomography (HRCT)
ヘリカルコンピュータ断層撮影法	helical computed tomography, spiral CT
多列検出器型コンピュータ断層撮影法	multidetector-row computed tomography (MDCT)
マルチスライスコンピュータ断層撮影法	multislice computed tomography (MSCT)
三次元コンピュータ断層撮影法	3 dimensional computed tomography
CT血管造影法	CT angiography (CTA)
ハンスフィールド単位	Hounsfield unit (HU)

⟨a unit of x-ray attenuatim used for CT scans; air is −1000, water 0, and bone +100⟩

磁気共鳴画像検査	magnetic resonance imaging (MRI)
磁気共鳴血管撮影法	magnetic resonance angiography (MRA)
ガドリニウム	gadolinium
核医学検査	radionuclide study
放射性医薬品	radiopharmaceutical

放射線核種 radionuclide
放射性同位元素 radioisotope (RI)
シンチグラフィー scintigraphy
シンチスキャン scintiscan
陽電子放出断層撮影法 positron emission tomography (PET)
¹⁸F 標識フルオロデオキシグルコース ¹⁸F-fluorodeoxyglucose (FDG)
単光子放出コンピュータ断層撮影法 single-photon emission computed tomography (SPECT)
超音波検査法 ultrasonography (US), ultrasonographic examination
B モード超音波法 B-mode ultrasonography
ドプラ超音波法 Doppler ultrasonography
⟨*a basic method of ultrasound diagnosis using frequency-shift between emitted waves and their echoes, based on the principle of the Doppler effect; measures the direction and velocity of the blood flow*⟩

● 測定法 Assays ●

一元放射免疫拡散法 single radial immunodiffusion (SRID)
受身赤血球凝集反応 passive hemagglutination (PHA)
化学発光酵素免疫測定法 chemiluminescent enzyme immunoassay (CLEIA)
化学発光免疫測定法 chemiluminescent immunoassay (CLIA)
核酸増幅法 nucleic acid amplification technique (NAT)
ガス液体クロマトグラフィー gas-liquid chromatography (GLC)
ガスクロマトグラフィー gas chromatography (GC)
ガス固体クロマトグラフィー gas-solid chromatography (GSC)
ガスクロマトグラフィー・質量分析法 gas chromatography-mass spectrometry (GC-MS)
間接蛍光抗体法 indirect fluorescent antibody technique (IFA)
間接赤血球凝集法 indirect hemagglutination (IHA)

2. 診療録の記載

逆受身赤血球凝集反応	reversed passive hemagglutination (RPHA)
逆転写酵素・ポリメラーゼ連鎖反応	reverse transcriptase-polymerase chain reaction (RT-PCR)
競合的タンパク結合分析法	competitive protein binding analysis (CPBA)
蛍光インサイチュー・ハイブリダイゼーション	fluorescence in situ hybridization (FISH)
蛍光酵素免疫測定法	fluorescent enzyme immunoassay (FEIA)
蛍光抗体法	fluorescent antibody technique (FA)
蛍光偏光免疫検定法	fluorescence polarization immunoassay (FPIA)
蛍光免疫測定法	fluorescent immunoassay (FIA)
高速液体クロマトグラフィー	high-performance liquid chromatography (HPLC)
酵素免疫吸着法	enzyme-linked immunosorbent assay (ELISA)
酵素免疫測定法	enzyme immunoassay (EIA)
混合受身赤血球凝集反応	mixed passive hemagglutination (MPHA)
紫外線分光光度法	ultraviolet spectrophotometry
赤血球凝集反応	hemagglutination (HA)
赤血球凝集抑制反応	hemagglutination inhibition (HI)
対向流免疫電気泳動法	counterimmunoelectrophoresis
多元酵素免疫測定法	enzyme multiplied immunoassay technique (EMIT)
中和試験	neutralization test (NT)
直接蛍光抗体法	direct fluorescent antibody technique (DFA)
電気化学発光免疫測定法	electrochemiluminescent immunoassay (ECLIA)
二重免疫拡散法	double immunodiffusion (DID)
薄層クロマトグラフィー	thin-layer chromatography (TLC)

Ⅲ章

比較ゲノムハイブリダイゼーション ひかく	comparative genomic hybridization (CGH)
微粒子計数免疫凝集測定法 びりゅうしけいすうめんえきぎょうしゅうそくていほう	particle counting immunoassay (PCIA)
放射酵素測定法 ほうしゃこうそそくていほう	radioenzymatic assay (REA)
放射性免疫吸着試験 ほうしゃせいめんえききゅうちゃくしけん	radioimmunosorbent test (RIST)
放射免疫測定法 ほうしゃめんえきそくていほう	radioimmunoassay (RIA)
補体結合反応 ほたいけつごう	complement fixation (CF)
ポリアクリルアミド・ゲル電気泳動法 でんいどうでん	polyacrylamide gel electrophoresis (PAGE)
ポリメラーゼ連鎖反応 れんさはんのう	polymerase chain reaction (PCR)
免疫電気泳動法 めんえきでんきえいどうほう	immunoelectrophoresis (IEP)
免疫粘着赤血球凝集反応 めんえきねんちゃくせっけつきゅうぎょうはんのう	immune adherence hemagglutination (IAHA)
免疫比濁法 めんえきひだくほう	turbidimetric immunoassay (TIA)
免疫放射定量測定 めんえきほうしゃていりょうそくてい	immunoradiometric assay (IRMA)
誘導結合プラズママススペクトロメトリー ゆうどうけつごう	inductively coupled plasma mass spectrometry (ICP-MS)
ラテックス凝集反応 ぎょうしゅうはんのう	latex agglutination (LA)
リガーゼ連鎖反応 れんさはんのう	ligase chain reaction (LCR)
粒子凝集反応 りゅうしぎょうしゅうはんのう	particle agglutination (PA)
レーザー免疫測定法 めんえきそくていほう	laser immunoassay (LIA)

●病理所見　Pathological findings●

悪性 あくせい	malignancy, 〔形〕malignant
アポトーシス	apoptosis
異型 いけい	atypia, 〔形〕atypical
萎縮 いしゅく	atrophy, 〔形〕atrophic
異所性 いしょせい	heterotopia, 〔形〕heterotopic
印環細胞 いんかんさいぼう	signet ring cell
うっ血 けつ	congestion, 〔形〕congestive
壊死 えし	necrosis, 〔形〕necrotic
遠隔転移 えんかくてんい	distant metastasis
炎症 えんしょう	inflammation, 〔形〕inflammatory
炎症細胞 えんしょう	inflammatory cells
過形成 かけいせい	hyperplasia, 〔形〕hyperplastic

過誤腫 かごしゅ	hamartoma, 〔形〕hamartomatous
化生 かせい	metaplasia, 〔形〕metaplastic
顆粒 かりゅう	granule, 〔形〕granular
癌 がん	cancer, carcinoma, 〔形〕cancerous, carcinomatous
奇形 きけい	anomaly, malformation, 〔形〕anomalous, malformed
奇形腫 きけいしゅ	teratoma, 〔形〕teratomatous
虚血 きょけつ	ischemia, 〔形〕ischemic
筋腫 きんしゅ	myoma, 〔形〕myomatous
血管腫 けっかんしゅ	hemangioma, 〔形〕hemangiomatous
結節 けっせつ	node, 〔形〕nodal
梗塞 こうそく	infarction, 〔形〕infarcted
骨腫 こつしゅ	osteoma, 〔形〕osteomatous
再生 さいせい	regeneration, 〔形〕regenerative
自己融解 じこゆうかい	autolysis, 〔形〕autolytic
脂肪腫 しぼうしゅ	lipoma, 〔形〕lipomatous
充血 じゅうけつ	hyperemia, 〔形〕hyperemic
出血 しゅっけつ	bleeding, hemorrhage, 〔形〕hemorrhagic
腫瘍 しゅよう	tumor, 〔形〕tumorous
小結節 しょうけっせつ	nodule, 〔形〕nodular
神経腫 しんけいしゅ	neuroma, 〔形〕neuromatous
滲出 しんしゅつ	exudation, 〔形〕exudative
浸潤 しんじゅん	infiltration, 〔形〕infiltrative
線維腫 せんいしゅ	fibroma, 〔形〕fibromatous
線維症 せんいしょう	fibrosis, 〔形〕fibrotic
腺癌 せんがん	adenocarcinoma
腺腫 せんしゅ	adenoma, 〔形〕adenomatous
腺様嚢胞癌 せんようのうほうがん	adenoid cystic carcinoma (ACC)
増殖 ぞうしょく	proliferation, 〔形〕proliferative
退形成 たいけいせい	anaplasia, 〔形〕anaplastic
低形成 ていけいせい	hypoplasia, 〔形〕hypoplastic
転移 てんい	metastasis, 〔形〕metastatic
肉芽 にくげ	granulation
肉芽腫 にくげしゅ	granuloma, 〔形〕granulomatous
肉腫 にくしゅ	sarcoma, 〔形〕sarcomatous
嚢胞 のうほう	cyst, 〔形〕cystic
膿瘍 のうよう	abscess, 〔形〕abscessed
播種 はしゅ	dissemination, 〔形〕disseminated
瘢痕 はんこん	scar, cicatrix, 〔形〕cicatricial
肥大 ひだい	hypertrophy, 〔形〕hypertrophic
浮腫 ふしゅ	edema, 〔形〕edematous

分化 ぶんか	differentiation, 〔形〕differentiated
変性 へんせい	degeneration, 〔形〕degenerative
扁平上皮癌 へんぺいじょうひがん	squamous cell carcinoma (SCC)
未分化 みぶんか	undifferentiation, 〔形〕undifferentiated
無形成 むけいせい	aplasia, 〔形〕aplastic
良性 りょうせい	benignancy, 〔形〕benign
濾出 ろしゅつ	transudation, 〔形〕transudative

● 診断 Diagnosis ●

診断 しんだん	diagnosis, 〔動〕diagnose, make a diagnosis of, diagnosticate, 〔形〕diagnostic
対診 たいしん	consultation
症候診断学 しょうこうしんだんがく	pathognomy
疾病特徴的 しっぺいとくちょうてき	pathognomonic
診断基準 しんだんきじゅん	diagnostic criteria
診断印象 しんだんいんしょう	diagnostic impression
暫定診断 ざんていしんだん, 仮診断 かりしんだん	provisional diagnosis, tentative diagnosis
推定診断 すいていしんだん	presumptive diagnosis, suspected diagnosis
予備的診断 よびてきしんだん	preliminary diagnosis
臨床診断 りんしょうしんだん	clinical diagnosis
診察的診断 しんさつてきしんだん, 身体的診断 しんたいてきしんだん	physical diagnosis
術前診断 じゅつぜんしんだん	preoperative diagnosis
看護診断 かんごしんだん	nursing diagnosis
検査室診断 けんさしつしんだん	laboratory diagnosis
血清診断 けっせいしんだん	serum diagnosis
X線診断 エックスせんしんだん	x-ray diagnosis, roentgen diagnosis
画像診断 がぞうしんだん	imaging diagnosis
顕微鏡的診断 けんびきょうてきしんだん	microscopic diagnosis
細胞学的診断 さいぼうがくてきしんだん	cytologic diagnosis
生物学的診断 せいぶつがくてきしんだん	biological diagnosis
病理診断 びょうりしんだん	pathological diagnosis
解剖学的診断 かいぼうがくてきしんだん	anatomical diagnosis
病因診断 びょういんしんだん	etiologic diagnosis
確定診断 かくていしんだん	definite diagnosis, established diagnosis
最終診断 さいしゅうしんだん	final diagnosis
主要診断 しゅようしんだん	principal diagnosis
死亡前診断 しぼうぜんしんだん	antemortem diagnosis
死亡診断書 しぼうしんだんしょ	death certificate
早期診断 そうきしんだん	early diagnosis

出生前診断 しゅっせいぜん──	prenatal diagnosis
着床前診断 ちゃくしょうぜんしょ──	preimplantation diagnosis
着床前遺伝子診断 ちゃくしょうぜんいでんし──	preimplantation genetic diagnosis (PGD)
部位診断（脊髄）ぶい──（せきずい）	niveau diagnosis, segmental diagnosis
治療的診断 ちりょうてき──	diagnosis ex juvantibus, therapeutic diagnosis
鑑別診断 かんべつ──	differential diagnosis (DD)
鑑別する かんべつ──	differentiate, distinguish, discriminate
除外診断 じょがい──	diagnosis by exclusion
除外する じょがい──	exclude, rule out
疑診 ぎしん	suspected diagnosis
疑わしい（ありそうでない）うたが	doubtful, unlikely, 〔動〕doubt, 〔名〕doubt
疑わしい（疑いをかける）うたが	suspicious, likely, 〔動〕suspect, 〔名〕suspicion
誤診 ごしん	misdiagnosis, diagnostic error, wrong diagnosis, 〔動〕make a wrong diagnosis, misdiagnose
予後 よご	prognosis (forecast of the outcome, prospect of recovery)
予後を判定する よご──はんてい──	prognose, prognosticate
国際疾病分類 こくさいしっぺいぶんるい	International Classification of Diseases (ICD)
悪性腫瘍臨床国際分類 あくせいしゅようりんしょうこくさいぶんるい	TNM Classification of Malignant Tumors

● 治療法　Treatment ●（Ⅳ章　診療録用語の各系統治療法参照）

投薬 とうやく	medication, administration of a medicine, 〔動〕give (administer) a medicine
投与径路 とうよけいろ	route of administration
処方箋薬 しょほうせんやく	prescription drug
日本薬局方 にほんやっきょくほう	Japanese Pharmacopoeia (JP)
国際薬局方 こくさいやっきょくほう	International Pharmacopeia (IP)
米国薬局方 べいこくやっきょくほう	United States Pharmacopeia (USP)
一般用医薬品 いっぱんよういやくひん	over-the-counter drug (OTC), non-prescription drug
後発医薬品 こうはついやくひん	generic drug
治験薬 ちけんやく	investigational new drug (IND)
偽薬 ぎやく, プラセボ	placebo
希用薬 きようやく	orphan drug
処方薬 しょほうやく	prescribed drug

86　III章　英文診療録

一般名 いっぱんめい	generic name
商標名 しょうひょうめい	brand name
添付文書 てんぷぶんしょ	patient package insert (PPI)
服薬遵守 ふくやくじゅんしゅ	compliance
服薬不履行 ふくやくふりこう	noncompliance
アドヒアランス	adherence
錠剤 じょうざい	tablet
カプセル剤 ざい	capsule
圧迫包装 あっぱくほうそう	press through package (PTP)
散剤 さんざい	powder
顆粒剤 かりゅうざい	granule
水薬 すいやく	liquid medicine
シロップ剤 ざい	syrup
エリキシル剤 ざい	elixir
トローチ	lozenge, troche
舌下錠 ぜっかじょう	sublingual (SL) tablet
含嗽剤 がんそうざい	gargle, mouthwash
エアゾール剤 ざい	aerosol
坐剤 ざざい	suppository
注射器 ちゅうしゃき	syringe
注射針 ちゅうしゃしん	needle
皮下注射 ひかちゅうしゃ	subcutaneous (sc) injection, hypodermic injection
皮内注射 ひないちゅうしゃ	intradermal injection, intradermic injection
筋肉内注射 きんにくないちゅうしゃ	intramuscular (IM) injection
静脈内注射 じょうみゃくないちゅうしゃ	intravenous (IV) injection
心内注射 しんないちゅうしゃ	intracardiac injection
腹腔内注射 ふくくうないちゅうしゃ	intraperitoneal (IP) injection
髄腔内注射 ずいくうないちゅうしゃ	intrathecal (IT) injection
関節内注射 かんせつないちゅうしゃ	intra-articular injection
点滴注入 てんてきちゅうにゅう	drip infusion
軟膏剤 なんこうざい	ointment
硬膏剤 こうこうざい	plaster
クリーム剤 ざい	cream
ローション剤 ざい	lotion
貼布剤 ちょうふざい	patch
治療薬濃度測定 ちりょうやくのうどそくてい	therapeutic drug monitoring (TDM)

● 手術　Operation ●

手術 しゅじゅつ	operation, surgery, 〔形〕operative, operating

手術記録 しゅじゅつきろく	operative note
無菌操作 むきんそうさ	sterile technique
手洗い てあらい	surgical hand scrub
麻酔 ますい	anesthesia
全身麻酔 ぜんしんますい	general anesthesia
吸入麻酔 きゅうにゅうますい	inhalation anesthesia
笑気・酸素・エーテル麻酔 しょうき・さんそ・——ますい	gas-oxygen-ether (GOE) anesthesia
笑気・酸素・フローセン麻酔 しょうき・さんそ・——ますい	gas-oxygen-fluothane (GOF) anesthesia
笑気・酸素・イソフルレン麻酔 しょうき・さんそ・——ますい	gas-oxygen-isoflurane (GOI) anesthesia
静脈麻酔 じょうみゃくますい	intravenous anesthesia
局所麻酔 きょくしょますい	local anesthesia
腰椎麻酔 ようついますい	lumbar anesthesia
脊髄くも膜下麻酔 せきずいまくかますい	spinal anesthesia, subarachnoid anesthesia
仙骨麻酔 せんこつますい	sacral anesthesia
硬膜外麻酔 こうまくがいますい	epidural anesthesia
表面麻酔 ひょうめんますい	surface anesthesia
浸潤麻酔 しんじゅんますい	infiltration anesthesia
ニューロレプト麻酔 ますい	neuroleptanesthesia (NLA)
温存 おんぞん	preservation
開窓 かいそう	fenestration, 〔動〕fenestrate
核出 かくしゅつ	enucleation, 〔動〕enucleate
郭清 かくせい	dissection, 〔動〕dissect
拡張 かくちょう	dilation, 〔動〕dilate
間置 かんち	interposition, 〔動〕interpose
貫通 かんつう	transfixion, 〔動〕transfix
結紮 けっさつ	ligation, 〔動〕ligate
減圧 げんあつ	decompression, 〔動〕decompress
牽引 けんいん	traction
固定 こてい	fixation, 〔動〕fix
再建 さいけん	reconstruction, 〔動〕reconstruct
止血 しけつ	hemostasis
試験切開 しけんせっかい	exploration, 〔動〕explore
充填 じゅうてん	filling, 〔動〕fill
修復 しゅうふく	repair, 〔動〕repair
授動 じゅどう	mobilization, 〔動〕mobilize
焼灼 しょうしゃく	cauterization, 〔動〕cauterize
整復 せいふく	replacement
切開 せっかい	incision, 〔動〕incise, make an incision

正中切開 せいちゅうせっかい	median incision, midline incision
正中傍切開 せいちゅうぼうせっかい	paramedian incision
横切開 おうせっかい	transverse incision
交互切開 こうごせっかい	gridiron incision
コッヘル切開 ―せっかい	Kocher incision

⟨a subcostal incision, for the biliary tract on the right and for the spleen on the left⟩

ファンネンスチール切開	Pfannenstiel incision

⟨a curved transverse incision above the symphysis, mainly for the access to the uterus⟩

マクバーニー切開	McBurney incision

⟨an incision parallel to the right external oblique muscle, above the anterior superior iliac spine, for appendectomy⟩

切除 せつじょ	resection, excision, 〔動〕resect, excise
切断 せつだん	amputation, 〔動〕amputate
穿孔術 せんこうじゅつ	trephination, trepanation
創傷離開 そうしょうりかい	wound dehiscence
掻爬 そうは	curettage
断端 だんたん	stump
摘出 てきしゅつ	extirpation, 〔動〕extirpate
デブリードマン	debridement
排液 はいえき	drainage
剥離 はくり	abrasion
吻合 ふんごう	anastomosis, 〔動〕anastomose
閉鎖 へいさ	closure, 〔動〕close
縫合 ほうごう	suture, 〔動〕suture
アルバート縫合 ―ほうごう	Albert suture

⟨the first row of stitches is passed through all layers of the intestinal wall⟩

一次縫合 いちじほうごう	primary suture
巾着縫合 きんちゃくほうごう	purse-string suture
結節縫合 けっせつほうごう	interrupted suture, knotted suture
マットレス縫合 ―ほうごう	mattress suture
ランベール縫合 ―ほうごう	Lembert suture

⟨inverting suture used in intestinal anastomosis, producing serosal apposition but not entering the intestinal lumen⟩

連続縫合 れんぞくほうごう	continuous suture
接合縫合 せつごうほうごう	coaptation suture, apposition suture
離断 りだん	transection, 〔動〕transect
手術用器具 しゅじゅつようきぐ	surgical instruments
メス	scalpel
鋏 はさみ	scissors
鉗子 かんし	forceps, clamp

有鉤鑷子 ゆうこうせっし	toothed forceps
無鉤鑷子 なこうせっし	non-toothed forceps
把持鉗子 はじかんし	grasping forceps
止血鉗子 しけつかんし	hemostatic forceps, hemostat
モスキート鉗子 かんし	mosquito clamp, mosquito forceps
コッヘル鉗子 かんし	Kocher forceps
⟨a toothed hemostatic forceps with transverse serrations⟩	
腸鉗子 ちょうかんし	intestinal clamps
分娩鉗子 ぶんべんかんし	obstetrical forceps
ピンセット	thumb forceps
開創鉤 かいそうこう	retractor
持針器 じしんき	needle holder
吻合器 ふんごうき	stapler
消息子 しょうそくし, ゾンデ	probe
排膿管 はいのうかん, ドレイン	drain
ガーゼ	gauze

● 看護 Nursing ●

看護 かんご	nursing
看護基準 きじゅん	nursing standard
看護記録 きろく	nursing record
看護業務 ぎょうむ	nursing service
看護ケア	nursing care
看護手順 てじゅん	nursing procedure
看護技術 ぎじゅつ	nursing art, nursing skill
看護過程 かてい	nursing process
看護介入 かいにゅう	nursing intervention
看護介入分類 かいにゅうぶんるい	Nursing Interventions Classification (NIC)
看護成果分類 せいかぶんるい	Nursing Outcomes Classification (NOC)
看護計画 けいかく	nursing care plan
看護監査 かんさ	nursing audit
クリニカルパス	clinical pathway (CP)
フォーカスチャーティング	focus charting
チーム看護 かんご	team nursing
プライマリーナーシング	primary nursing
床上安静 しょうじょうあんせい	bed rest
絶対安静 ぜったいあんせい	complete bed rest
食事介助 しょくじかいじょ	feeding
清拭 せいしき	bed bath, sponge bath
座浴 ざよく	sitz bath, hip bath
足浴 そくよく	foot bath

浣腸 かんちょう	enema, 〔動〕give an enema
グリセリン浣腸 ―ちょう	glycerin enema (GE)
石鹸浣腸 せっけんかんちょう	soapsuds enema (SSE)
浣腸器 かんちょうき	enema syringe
便器 べんき	bedpan
室内便器 しつないべんき	commode
摘便 てきべん	stool extraction
尿器 にょうき, しびん	urinal
導尿 どうにょう	catheterization, 〔動〕catheterize
留置カテーテル りゅう―	indwelling catheter
彎曲カテーテル わんきょく―	elbowed catheter, catheter coudé
体位変換 たいいへんかん	positional change, postural change
体位性排液法 たいいせいはいえきほう	postural drainage
包帯交換 ほうたいこうかん	dressing changes
膿盆 のうぼん	emesis basin
抑制帯 よくせいたい	restraint
離被架 りひか	cradle
担架 たんか	stretcher
車輪付き担架 しゃりんつきたんか	gurney
車椅子 くるまいす	wheelchair
歩行器 ほこうき	walker

● 栄養 Nutrition ●

食事 しょくじ	meal, diet, 〔形〕dietary
普通食 ふつうしょく	regular diet
流動食 りゅうどうしょく	liquid diet
軟食 なんしょく	soft diet
固形食 こけいしょく	solid diet
無刺激食 むしげきしょく	bland diet
基礎食 きそしょく	basal diet
均衡食 きんこうしょく	balanced diet
除外食 じょがいしょく	elimination diet
成分栄養 せいぶんえいよう	elemental diet (ED)
高(低)カロリー食 こう(てい)しょく	high (low) calorie diet
超低カロリー食 ちょうていしょく	very low calorie diet (VLCD)
高タンパク食 こう―しょく	high protein diet
低脂肪食 ていしぼうしょく	low fat diet
低残渣食 ていざんさしょく	low residue diet
高繊維食 こうせんいしょく	high fiber diet
無塩食 むえんしょく	salt-free diet
減塩食 げんえんしょく	low salt diet, low sodium diet

2. 診療録の記載 91

糖尿病食 とうにょうびょうしょく	diabetic diet
減量食 げんりょうしょく	reducing diet
適法食品（ユダヤ教）てきほうしょくひん（——きょう）	kosher food
経腸栄養 けいちょうえいよう	enteral nutrition
非経口栄養 ひけいこうえいよう	parenteral nutrition (PN)
完全静脈栄養 かんぜんじょうみゃくえいよう	total parenteral nutrition (TPN)
経静脈高カロリー輸液 けいじょうみゃくこう——ゆえき	intravenous hyperalimentation (IVH)
在宅経腸栄養法 ざいたくけいちょうえいようほう	home enteral nutrition (HEN)
在宅中心静脈栄養法 ざいたくちゅうしんじょうみゃくえいようほう	home parenteral nutrition (HPN)

● 経過記録　Progress notes ●

経過 けいか	course, progress
進行 しんこう	progression, 〔形〕progressive
急性 きゅうせい	acute
亜急性 あきゅうせい	subacute
慢性 まんせい	chronic
陳旧性 ちんきゅうせい	old
潜在性 せんざいせい	latent
前駆期 ぜんくき	prodromal stage
初期 しょき	initial stage
早期 そうき	early stage
移行期 いこうき	transitional stage
進行期 しんこうき	advanced stage
末期 まっき	terminal stage
悪化 あっか	worsening, aggravation, deterioration, 〔動〕get worse, be aggravated
再発 さいはつ	relapse, recurrence, 〔形〕recurrent, 〔動〕relapse, recur
軽減 けいげん	relief, remission, 〔動〕relieve, lessen
改善 かいぜん	improvement, amelioration, 〔動〕improve, ameliorate
不変 ふへん	no change, 〔形〕unchanged, unimproved, stationary
不可逆性 ふかぎゃくせい	irreversibility, 〔形〕irreversible
最低点 さいていてん	nadir
治癒 ちゆ	cure, recovery, healing, 〔動〕recover, heal, be cured

回復	recovery, recuperation, 〔動〕recover, recuperate
回復期	convalescence
完全寛解	complete remission (CR)
部分寛解	partial remission (PR)
限定された経過をとる	self-limited
全生存期間	overall survival (OS)
無病生存期間	disease-free survival (DFS)
無増悪生存期間	progression-free survival (PFS)
無再発生存期間	relapse-free survival (RFS)
無症候期間	disease-free interval
生存率	survival rate
5年生存率	5-year survival rate
平均余命	life expectancy
延命	life prolongation
生命維持装置	life support system
生活の質	quality of life (QOL)
日常生活動作	activities of daily living (ADL)
日常生活関連動作	activities parallel to daily living (APDL)
手段的日常生活動作	instrumental activities of daily living (IADL)
行動状況	performance status (PS)
機能的自立度評価法	functional independence measure (FIM)
バーセル指数	Barthel index (BI)

⟨a method used to evaluate ADL on long-range basis⟩

カルノフスキースケール	Karnofsky scale

⟨a performance scale to evaluate a patient's progress after a therapeutic procedure⟩

グラスゴー転帰尺度	Glasgow Outcome Scale (GOS)
包括的機能評価スケール	Global Assessment of Functioning (GAF) scale
急性生理慢性健康評価	acute physiology and chronic health evaluation (APACHE)
国際生活機能分類	International Classification of Functioning, Disability, and Health (ICF)
カプラン・マイヤー生存曲線	Kaplan-Meier survival curve

⟨commonly used life table that estimates percent survival at the *time of each endpoint*⟩

死亡率 しぼうりつ	mortality rate
標準化死亡比 ひょうじゅんかしぼうひ	standardized mortality rate (SMR)
特定死因死亡比 とくていしいんしぼうひ	proportionate mortality rate (PMR)
自然死 しぜんし	natural death
突然死 とつぜんし	sudden death
異状死 いじょうし	unnatural death
脳死 のうし	brain death
安楽死 あんらくし	euthanasia
尊厳死 そんげんし	death with dignity

● 要約 Summary ●

退院時要約 たいいんじようやく	discharge summary
入院時診断 にゅういんじしんだん	admitting diagnosis
退院時診断 たいいんじしんだん	discharge diagnosis
転帰 てんき	outcome
合併症 がっぺいしょう	complications
手術名 しゅじゅつめい	operation
組織診断 そしきしんだん	histological diagnosis
入院経過抄録 にゅういんけいかしょうろく	summary of the hospital course
在院日数 ざいいんにっすう	length of the hospital stay
退院時病状 たいいんじびょうじょう	condition at discharge
退院時指示 たいいんじしじ	discharge orders
退院時指導 たいいんじしどう	discharge instructions
外来受診日 がいらいじゅしんび	clinic return date
食事指導 しょくじしどう	diet instructions
退院時投薬 たいいんじとうやく	discharge medication

---- Tidbits ----

euthanasia

euthanasiaは,接頭辞eu-(good, well)と死を意味するギリシャ語のthanatosから成り,文字通りにはgood death,具体的にはquiet, painless deathのことである.積極的安楽死active euthanasia, mercy killing,消極的安楽死passive euthanasia,患者の意思による安楽死voluntary euthanasiaなどを区別する.

オランダではeuthanasiaといえばvoluntary euthanasiaを意味し,"A deliberate termination of an individual's life at that individual's request, by another. Or, in medical practice, the active and deliberate termination of a patient's life, on that patient's request, by a doctor." と定義される (Dutch Government Commission of Euthanasia).

関連する表現には, living will, physician-assisted suicide, lethal injection, Oregon Death with Dignity Act, Washington Initiative 1000などがある.

Thanatosはギリシャ神話で死の擬人神であるが,死を意味する接頭辞thanato-から, thanatosis 壊死, thanatology 死亡学, thanatophobia 死恐怖症, thanatopsis 死観などの語が作られた.

3. 問題志向型システム

● 問題志向型システム　Problem-oriented system (POS) ●

患者の問題	patient's problems
患者中心の医療	patient-centered medicine
問題解決	problem-solving
オーディット，監査	audit
インフォームドコンセント	informed consent (IC)
医療チーム	health-care team
問題志向型診療録	problem-oriented medical record (POMR)
問題志向型看護記録	problem-oriented nursing record (PONR)
問題志向型医療情報システム	Problem-oriented Medical Information System (PROMIS)
問題・知見カプラー	Problem-Knowledge Coupler (PKC)
情報源別診療録	source-oriented medical record (SOMR)

4. 問題志向型診療録

● 問題志向型診療録の構成　Components of POMR ●

問題リスト	problem list
データベース	data base
患者像	patient profile
主訴	chief complaint
現病歴	present illness
既往歴	past history
家族歴	family history
系統別病歴	system review
身体的所見	physical findings
検査所見	laboratory findings
初期計画	initial plan
経過記録	progress notes

5. POMRの記載（「診療録の記載」(p.71) 参照）

● データベース Data base ●

限定基礎データ	defined data base
個人歴	personal history
平均一日の過ごし方	how to spend the typical day (one's routine day, an average day)
一連の出来事	sequence of events

● 問題リスト Problem list ●

問題番号	problem number (#)
活動性問題	active problem
未解決問題	unresolved problem
非活動性問題	inactive problem
解決済み問題	resolved problem
一時的問題	temporary problem
医学的問題	medical problems
潜在的問題	potential problems
心理的問題	psychological problems
家庭的問題	family problems

● 初期計画 Initial plan ●

診断的計画	diagnostic plan
治療的計画	therapeutic plan
教育的計画	educational plan

● 経過記録 Progress notes ●

叙述式記録	narrative notes
SOAP形式	SOAP format
主観的データ	subjective data (S)
客観的データ	objective data (O)
評価	assessment (A)
計画	plan (P)
SOAPIE形式	SOAPIE format (SOAP + Intervention, Evaluation)
フローシート	flow sheet

● 監査 Audit ●

徹底的	thoroughness
信頼性	reliability
分析的	analytical sense
効率性	efficiency (TRASE)

5. POMRの記載   97

―Tidbits―

octothorp

POMRに欠くことのできない問題番号にはNo.（＜numero）の代わりにナンバー記号（#）を使うことが多い．#は，poundの記号にも用いられるが，しばしばsharp嬰記号（♯）と混同されている．このnumber signはまたhash mark, crosshatch, octothorpなどという．octothorpの謂れとして，呼び名の無いまま通用していた#記号には8個の突起があるのでまず"octo"と名付け，当初意味の無い"therp"を付けて造語したが，その後"thorp"（村の意味がある）に変わったという話が伝わっている．

6. 診療録記載に用いられる略語・記号（「ラテン語」(p. 21)参照）

● 略語・記号　Abbreviations and symbols ●

略語・記号	原　語	意　味
ab	abortion	流産
abd	abdomen	腹部
adm	admission	入院
AJ	ankle jerk	アキレス腱反射
ASAP	as soon as possible	できるだけ早く
BP	blood pressure	血圧
BRP	bathroom privileges	トイレ許可
BS	bowel sounds	腸音
BS	breath sounds	呼吸音
Bx	biopsy	生検
c/o	complains of	を訴える
c̄	cum (with)	と共に
CC	chief complaint	主訴
CNS	central nervous system	中枢神経系
CV	cardiovascular	心血管の
CXR	chest x-ray	胸部 X 線写真
D/C	discontinue, or discharge	中止または退院
DOB	date of birth	生年月日
DTR	deep tendon reflex	深部腱反射
Dx	diagnosis	診断
EENT	eyes, ear, nose, and throat	眼耳鼻咽頭
ENT	ear, nose, and throat	耳鼻咽頭
EOM	extraocular muscles	外眼筋
EOM	extraocular movements	外眼運動
EtOH	ethyl alcohol	アルコール
EUA	examination under anesthesia	麻酔下診察
FH	family history	家族歴
GI	gastrointestinal	消化器の
GU	genitourinary	泌尿生殖器の
H&P	history and physical examination	病歴と身体的検査
Hct	hematocrit	ヘマトクリット
HEENT	head, eyes, ears, nose, and throat	頭，眼，耳，鼻，咽頭
HPI	history of present illness	現病歴
HR	heart rate	心拍数
hr	hour	時，時間

6. 診療録記載に用いられる略語・記号   99

略語・記号	原 語	意 味
ht	height	身長
HTN	hypertension	高血圧
Hx	history	病歴
JVD	jugular venous distention	頚静脈拡張
KJ	knee jerk	膝蓋腱反射
L	left	左
L&W	living and well	生存・健康
LKS	liver, spleen, and kidneys	肝臓, 脾臓, 腎臓
LLQ	left lower quadrant	左下腹部
LOC	level of consciousness	意識レベル
LSB	left sternal border	胸骨左縁
LUQ	left upper quadrant	左上腹部
LVH	left ventricular hypertrophy	左室肥大
Ⓜ	murmur	心雑音
mo	month	月
N/V	nausea and vomiting	悪心・嘔吐
neg	negative	陰性, なし
NKA	no known allergy	アレルギーなし
NKDA	no known drug allergy	薬剤アレルギーなし
NSR	normal sinus rhythm	正常洞調律
P	pulse	脈拍
P&A	percussion and auscultation	打聴診
p̄	after	の後
Pap	Papanicolaou smear	パパニコロースミア
PE	physical examination	身体的検査
PERLA	pupils equal and reactive to light and accommodation	瞳孔同大, 対光・調節反射あり
PERRLA	pupils equal, round, reactive to light and accommodation	瞳孔同大, 整円, 対光・調節反射あり
PH	past history	既往歴
PI	present illness	現病歴
PMI	point of maximal impulse	最強拍動点
PR	pulse rate	脈拍数
pt	patient	患者
PTA	prior to admission	入院前
R	right	右
R	respiration	呼吸
R/O	rule out	除外せよ
RLQ	right lower quadrant	右下腹部
ROS	review of systems	系統別病歴

III 章

略語・記号	原　語	意　味
RR	respiratory rate	呼吸数
RTC	return to clinic	外来再診
RUQ	right upper quadrant	右上腹部
Rx	treatment, prescription	治療，処方
s̄	sine (without)	なしに
SH	social history	社会歴
Sx	symptoms	症状
T	temperature	体温
UA	urinalysis	検尿
UCHD	usual childhood diseases	通常の小児期疾患
VO	verbal order	口頭指示
VS	vital signs	生命徴候
WD	well-developed	発育良好な
wk	week	週
WN	well-nourished	栄養良好な
WNL	within normal limits	正常範囲
wt	weight	体重
yo	year(s) old	歳
yr	year	年
#	number	数
(−)	absent	なし
(+)	present	あり
?	questionable	疑わしい
@	at	において
<	less than	より小
>	greater than	より大
×	times	回，倍
↑	increase, increased, elevated	増加，上昇
↓	decrease, decreased, diminished	減少，下降
△	change	変化
ō	none	無し
♂	male	男性
♀	female	女性
□	male, living	男性，生存
○	female, living	女性，生存
■	male, deceased	男性，死亡
●	female, deceased	女性，死亡

＊一般に認められている略語・記号もあるが内輪で慣用されているだけのものもあり要注意．

―― Tidbits ――

OOPS. OOB.

医学論文では略語の初出時に必ず何の略であるかを明記するが、診療録ではしばしば自明のこととして用いられて分かりにくいことがある。特に誤解を招いてはならないのが指示であるが、TPR, NPO, BRP, RICE などは問題ないとしても、TLC とあれば total lung capacity でも thin-layer chromatography でもなくて、tender loving care である。OOB は out of bed, HOB は head of bed であり、KVO は keep vein open のこと、TKO (to keep open) ともいう。

IV章

診療録用語

1. 全身状態

●症状・徴候　Symptoms / Signs●

健康状態 けんこうじょうたい	the condition of one's health, health
健康な けんこう	healthy, well
健康である けんこう	be well, be in good health
健康を保つ けんこうをたもつ	stay healthy, keep fit
疲労 ひろう	fatigue, weariness, tiredness, lassitude, exhaustion
疲れる つかれる	become (get) tired (wearied, weary, fatigued, exhausted)
疲れを覚える つかれをおぼえる	feel tired, feel fatigued
易疲労感 いひろうかん	fatigability, 〔形〕fatigable, easily fatigued
違和感 いわかん	malaise (=a vague feeling of bodily discomfort and fatigue)
脱力 だつりょく	weakness, feebleness, lack of strength
衰弱 すいじゃく	debility, prostration
虚弱な きょじゃく	weak, feeble, frail, sickly, infirm
衰弱する すいじゃく	weaken, become weak, be debilitated, be worn out
無力 むりょく	asthenia, 〔形〕asthenic
慢性疲労症候群 まんせいひろうしょうこうぐん	chronic fatigue syndrome (CFS)
不定愁訴 ふていしゅうそ	unidentified complaint
不定愁訴症候群 ふていしゅうそしょうこうぐん	unidentified clinical syndrome
不定症状 ふていしょうじょう	equivocal symptom, nonspecific symptom
医学的に説明困難な症状 いがくてきにせつめいこんなんなしょうじょう	medically unexplained symptoms (MUS)
睡眠 すいみん	sleep
不眠(症) ふみん(しょう)	insomnia, sleeplessness, 〔形〕insomnious, insomniac, sleepless
不眠症の人 ふみんしょうのひと	insomniac
睡眠相後退症候群 すいみんそうこうたいしょうこうぐん	delayed sleep phase syndrome (DSPS)
睡眠時随伴症 すいみんじずいはんしょう	parasomnia
居眠り いねむり	doze, nap, 〔動〕doze, take a nap
昼間過眠 ひるまかみん	excessive daytime sleepiness (EDS)
寝言 ねごと	sleeptalking, somniloquism
夢 ゆめ	dream, 〔動〕dream
悪夢 あくむ	nightmare
夢遊症 むゆうしょう	sleepwalking, somnambulism
夢遊症者 むゆうしょうしゃ	sleepwalker, somnambulist

1. 全身状態

体重 たいじゅう	weight, body weight
体重増加 たいじゅうぞうか	weight gain, increase in weight, 〔動〕gain weight, put on weight
体重減少 たいじゅうげんしょう	weight loss, loss of weight, 〔動〕lose weight
肥満 ひまん	obesity, fatness, 〔形〕obese, fat, corpulent
太りすぎの ふと	overweight, too heavy, too fat
るいそう	emaciation, excessive leanness, 〔形〕emaciated
痩せた や	thin, lean, slim
発熱 はつねつ	fever, pyrexia, 〔動〕become feverish, have (run) a fever
熱のある ねつ	feverish, febrile, pyrexial
無熱の むねつ	afebrile, feverless
高熱 こうねつ	high fever
弛張熱 しちょうねつ	remittent fever
間欠熱 かんけつねつ	intermittent fever
稽留熱 けいりゅうねつ, 持続熱 じぞくねつ	continued fever, continuous fever
脱水熱 だっすいねつ	dehydration fever, thirsty fever
不明熱 ふめいねつ	fever of unknown origin (FUO), essential fever
食事性熱産生 しょくじせいねつさんせい	diet-induced thermogenesis (DIT)
特異動的作用 とくいどうてきさよう	specific dynamic action (SDA)
悪性高体温症 あくせいこうたいおんしょう	malignant hyperthermia
熱射病 ねっしゃびょう	heat stroke
熱疲労 ねつひろう	heat exhaustion
日射病 にっしゃびょう	sunstroke
悪寒 おかん	chill, rigor
悪寒戦慄 おかんせんりつ	shaking chills, shivering with chills
発汗 はっかん	sweating, perspiration, diaphoresis, 〔動〕sweat, perspire, 〔形〕diaphoretic
寝汗 ねあせ	night sweat
脱水 だっすい	dehydration, 〔形〕dehydrated, 〔動〕dehydrate
感染 かんせん	infection
市中感染 しちゅうかんせん	community-acquired infection
院内感染 いんないかんせん	nosocomial infection, hospital-acquired infection
空気感染 くうきかんせん	airborne infection
飛沫感染 ひまつかんせん	droplet infection

IV章 診療録用語

日和見感染 ひよりみかんせん	opportunistic infection
感染経路 かんせんけいろ	route of infection
細菌感染 さいきんかんせん	bacterial infection
不顕性感染 ふけんせいかんせん	latent infection, subclinical infection, asymptomatic infection
ウイルス感染 —かんせん	viral infection
垂直感染 すいちょくかんせん	vertical infection
水平感染 すいへいかんせん	horizontal infection
病巣感染 びょうそうかんせん	focal infection
二次感染 にじかんせん	secondary infection
感染症 かんせんしょう	infectious disease
新興感染症 しんこうかんせんしょう	emerging infectious disease
再興感染症 さいこうかんせんしょう	re-emerging infectious disease
人畜共通感染症 じんちくきょうつうかんせんしょう	zoonosis
伝染病 でんせんびょう	communicable disease, contagious disease
流行病 りゅうこうびょう	epidemic disease, epidemic
地方病 ちほうびょう, 風土病 ふうどびょう	endemic disease, endemic
汎発性流行病 はんぱつせいりゅうこうびょう	pandemic disease, pandemic
届出疾患 とどけでしっかん	notifiable disease, reportable disease
全身病 ぜんしんびょう	systemic disease
職業病 しょくぎょうびょう	occupational disease
先天性疾患 せんてんせいしっかん	congenital disease
遺伝性疾患 いでんせいしっかん	hereditary disease, inborn genetic disease
チャネル病 —びょう	channelopathy, channel disease
家族病 かぞくびょう	familial disease
医原病 いげんびょう	iatrogenic disease, diseases of medical practice (DOMP)
共存疾患 きょうぞんしっかん	comorbidity
器質性疾患 きしつせいしっかん	organic disease
機能性疾患 きのうせいしっかん	functional disease
代謝性疾患 たいしゃせいしっかん	metabolic disease
欠乏性疾患 けつぼうせいしっかん	deficiency disease
変性疾患 へんせいしっかん	degenerative disease
膠原病 こうげんびょう	collagen disease
自己免疫疾患 じこめんえきしっかん	autoimmune disease
悪性疾患 あくせいしっかん	malignant disease
悪性腫瘍 あくせいしゅよう	malignant tumor, malignant neoplasm
分子病 ぶんしびょう	molecular disease
難病 なんびょう	intractable disease

1. 全身状態　107

不治の病 ふじのやまい	incurable disease
敗血症 はいけつしょう	sepsis
多臓器不全 たぞうきふぜん	multiple organ failure (MOF)
多臓器不全症候群 たぞうきふぜんしょうこうぐん	multiple-organ dysfunction syndrome (MODS)
全身性炎症反応症候群 ぜんしんせいえんしょうはんのうしょうこうぐん	systemic inflammatory response syndrome (SIRS)

● 感染症　Infectious Diseases ●

1. 全数把握の対象　Notify all cases

一類感染症 (診断後直ちに届出)	Category I (notify promptly)

エボラ出血熱 けつねつ	Ebola hemorrhagic fever
クリミア・コンゴ出血熱 しゅつけつねつ	Crimean-Congo hemorrhagic fever
痘瘡 とうそう	smallpox
南米出血熱 なんべいしゅつけつねつ	South American hemorrhagic fever
ペスト	plague
マールブルグ熱 ねつ	Marburg fever
ラッサ熱 ねつ	Lassa fever

二類感染症 (診断後直ちに届出)	Category II (notify promptly)

急性灰白髄炎 きゅうせいはいはくずいえん	acute poliomyelitis
結核 けっかく	tuberculosis
ジフテリア	diphtheria
重症急性呼吸器症候群 じゅうしょうきゅうせいこきゅうきしょうこうぐん	severe acute respiratory syndrome (SARS)

三類感染症 (診断後直ちに届出)	Category III (notify promptly)

コレラ	cholera
細菌性赤痢 さいきんせいせきり	bacillary dysentery
腸管出血性大腸菌感染症 ちょうかんしゅっけつせいだいちょうきんかんせんしょう	enterohemorrhagic Escherichia coli infection
腸チフス ちょう	typhoid fever
パラチフス	paratyphoid fever

四類感染症 (診断後直ちに届出)	Category IV (notify promptly)

| E 型肝炎 がたかんえん | hepatitis E |
| A 型肝炎 がたかんえん | hepatitis A |

IV 章

黄熱（おうねつ）	yellow fever
Q熱（ねつ）	Q fever
狂犬病（きょうけんびょう）	rabies, hydrophobia
炭疽（たんそ）	anthrax
トリインフルエンザ（とり）	avian influenza
ボツリヌス症（しょう）	botulism
マラリア	malaria
野兎病（やとびょう）	tularemia, rabbit fever
ウエストナイル熱（ねつ）	West Nile fever
エキノコックス症（しょう）	echinococcosis
オウム病（びょう）	psittacosis, parrot fever
オムスク出血熱（しゅっけつねつ）	Omsk hemorrhagic fever
回帰熱（かいきねつ）	relapsing fever
キャサヌル森林病（しんりんびょう）	Kyasanur forest disease
コクシジオイデス症（しょう）	coccidioidomycosis
サル痘（とう）	monkeypox
腎症候性出血熱（じんしょうこうせいしゅっけつねつ）	hemorrhagic fever with renal syndrome
西部ウマ脳炎（せいぶのうえん）	Western equine encephalitis (WEE)
ダニ媒介脳炎（ばいかいのうえん）	tick-borne encephalitis
つつが虫病（むしびょう）	tsutsugamushi disease, scrub typhus
デング熱（ねつ）	dengue fever, dengue
東部ウマ脳炎（とうぶのうえん）	Eastern equine encephalitis
ニパウイルス感染症（かんせんしょう）	Nipah virus infection
日本紅斑熱（にほんこうはんねつ）	Japanese spotted fever
日本脳炎（にほんのうえん）	Japanese encephalitis
ハンタウイルス肺症候群（はいしょうこうぐん）	hantavirus pulmonary syndrome
Bウイルス病（びょう）	B virus disease
鼻疽（びそ）	equinia, farcy, malleus
ブルセラ症（しょう）	brucellosis, Malta fever
ベネズエラウマ脳炎（のうえん）	Venezuelan equine encephalitis (VEE)
ヘンドラウイルス感染症（かんせんしょう）	Hendra virus infection
発疹チフス（ほっしん）	typhus
ライム病（びょう）	Lyme disease
リッサウイルス感染症（かんせんしょう）	Lyssavirus infection
リフトバレー熱（ねつ）	Rift Valley fever
類鼻疽（るいびそ）	melioidosis, Whitmore disease
レジオネラ症（しょう）	legionellosis, legionnaires disease

レプトスピラ症	leptospirosis
ロッキー山紅斑熱	Rocky Mountain spotted fever (RMSF)

五類感染症 (7日以内に届出)	Category V (notify within 7days)
ウイルス性肝炎（E型, A型を除く）	viral hepatitis (excluding hepatitis A and E)
クリプトスポリジウム症	cryptosporidiosis
後天性免疫不全症候群	acquired immunodeficiency syndrome
梅毒	syphilis
アメーバ赤痢	amebic dysentery
急性脳炎	acute encephalitis
クロイツフェルト・ヤコブ病	Creutzfeldt-Jakob disease
劇症型溶血性連鎖球菌感染症	fulminant hemolytic streptococcus infection
ジアルジア症	giardiasis
髄膜炎菌性髄膜炎	meningococcal meningitis
先天性風疹症候群	congenital rubella syndrome
破傷風	tetanus
バンコマイシン耐性黄色ブドウ球菌感染症	vancomycin-resistant staphylococcus aureus infection
バンコマイシン耐性腸球菌感染症	vancomycin-resistant enterococcus infection
風疹	rubella, German measles
麻疹	rubeola, measles

2. 定点把握の対象　To be reported by sentinel clinics and hospitals

五類感染症	Category V
インフルエンザ定点 (週単位報告)	Influenza (weekly report)
インフルエンザ	influenza
小児科定点 (週単位報告)	Pediatric diseases (weekly report)
RS ウイルス感染症	RS (respiratory syncytial) virus infection
咽頭結膜熱	pharyngoconjunctival fever
A群溶血性連鎖球菌咽頭	α-hemolytic streptococcal pharyngitis

IV章 診療録用語

炎 (ぐんようけっせいれん/さきゅうきんいんとうえん)	
感染性胃腸炎 (かんせんせいいちょうえん)	infectious gastroenteritis
水痘 (すいとう)	varicella
手足口病 (てあしくちびょう)	hand-foot-and-mouth disease
伝染性紅斑 (でんせんせいこうはん)	infectious erythema
突発性発疹 (とっぱつせいほっしん)	exanthema subitum, roseola
百日咳 (ひゃくにちぜき)	pertussis
ヘルパンギーナ	herpangina
流行性耳下腺炎 (りゅうこうせいじかせんえん)	epidemic parotitis, mumps
眼科定点 (週単位報告)	Eye diseases (weekly report)
急性出血性結膜炎 (きゅうせいしゅっけつせいけつまくえん)	acute hemorrhagic conjunctivitis (AHC)
流行性角結膜炎 (りゅうこうせいかくけつまくえん)	epidemic keratoconjunctivitis (EKC)
性感染症定点 (月単位報告)	STD (monthly report)
性器クラミジア感染症 (せいき—かんせんしょう)	genital chlamydial infection
性器ヘルペスウイルス感染症 (せいき—かんせんしょう)	genital herpesvirus infection
尖圭コンジローマ (せんけい)	condyloma acuminatum
淋菌感染症 (りんきんかんせんしょう)	gonococcal infection
基幹定点 (月単位報告)	Sentinel hospitals (monthly report)
クラミジア肺炎 (いえん)	chlamydial pneumonia
細菌性髄膜炎 (さいきんせいずいまくえん)	bacterial meningitis
マイコプラズマ肺炎 (いえん)	mycoplasmal pneumonia
無菌性髄膜炎 (むきんせいずいまくえん)	aseptic meningitis
基幹定点 (週単位報告)	Sentinel hospitals (weekly report)
ペニシリン耐性肺炎球菌感染症 (—たいせいはいえんきゅうきんかんせんしょう)	penicillin-resistant pneumococcal infection
メチシリン耐性黄色ブドウ球菌感染症 (—たいせいおうしょく—きゅうきんかんせんしょう)	methicillin-resistant staphylococcus aureus infection
薬剤耐性緑膿菌感染症 (やくざいたいせいりょくのうきんかんせんしょう)	drug-resistant pseudomonas infection

(感染症法：2008年1月1日改正施行 Infectious Diseases Control Law: revised 1/1/2008)

● 膠原病　Collagen diseases ●

リウマチ熱 (ねつ)	rheumatic fever
関節リウマチ (かんせつ)	rheumatoid arthritis (RA)
全身性エリテマトーデス	systemic lupus erythematosus (SLE)

1. 全身状態

強皮症	scleroderma
多発性筋炎,皮膚筋炎	polymyositis (PM), dermatomyositis (DM)
結節性多発動脈炎	polyarteritis nodosa (PN)
混合性結合組織病	mixed connective tissue disease (MCTD)
シェーグレン症候群	Sjögren syndrome (SjS)
抗リン脂質抗体症候群	antiphospholipid antibody syndrome (APS)
ベーチェット病	Behçet disease
フェルティー症候群	Felty syndrome
スティル病	Still disease
側頭動脈炎	temporal arteritis
高安動脈炎	Takayasu arteritis
川崎病	Kawasaki disease
アレルギー性肉芽腫性血管炎	allergic granulomatous angiitis
顕微鏡的多発血管炎	microscopic polyangiitis (MPA)
白血球破砕皮膚血管炎	cutaneous leukocytoclastic vasculitis
ウェゲナー肉芽腫症	Wegener granulomatosis
大動脈症候群	aortitis syndrome
CREST症候群	CREST syndrome

● 難病(特定疾患) Intractable diseases ●

*印は医療費助成のある特定疾患治療研究事業対象疾患を示す.

*脊髄小脳変性症	spinocerebellar degeneration
*シャイ・ドレーガー症候群	Shy-Drager syndrome
もやもや病,ウィリス動脈輪閉塞症	moyamoya disease, occlusion of the circle of Willis
正常圧水頭症	normal-pressure hydrocephalus
*多発性硬化症	multiple sclerosis
*重症筋無力症	myasthenia gravis

IV章 診療録用語

ギラン・バレー症候群	Guillain-Barré syndrome (GBS)
フィッシャー症候群	Fisher syndrome
*慢性炎症性脱髄性多発神経炎	chronic inflammatory demyelinating polyneuropathy (CIDP)
多巣性運動ニューロパチー	multifocal motor neuropathy
クロウ・深瀬症候群	Crow-Fukase syndrome
*筋萎縮性側索硬化症	amyotrophic lateral sclerosis (ALS)
*脊髄性進行性筋萎縮症	progressive spinal muscular atrophy (PSMA)
*球脊髄性筋萎縮症	spinobulbar muscular atrophy (SBMA)
脊髄空洞症	syringomyelia
*パーキンソン病	Parkinson disease
*ハンチントン病	Huntington disease
*進行性核上性麻痺	progressive supranuclear palsy
線条体黒質変性症	striatonigral degeneration
ペルオキシソーム病	peroxisomal disorder
*ライソゾーム病	lysosomal storage diseases
*クロイツフェルト・ヤコブ病	Creutzfeldt-Jakob disease (CJD)
*ゲルストマン・ストロイスラー・シャインカー病	Gerstmann-Sträussler-Scheinker disease (GSS)
*致死性家族性不眠症	fatal familial insomnia
*亜急性硬化性全脳炎	subacute sclerosing panencephalitis (SSPE)
進行性多巣性白質脳症	progressive multifocal leukoencephalopathy (PML)
*後縦靱帯骨化症	ossification of posterior longitudinal ligament (OPLL)
*黄色靱帯骨化症	ossification of yellow ligament (OYL)
前縦靱帯骨化症	ossification of anterior longitudinal ligament (OALL)
*広範脊柱管狭窄症	disseminated spinal canal stenosis

1. 全身状態

*特発性大腿骨頭壊死症	idiopathic necrosis of the femoral head
特発性ステロイド性骨壊死症	idiopathic osteonecrosis due to corticosteroid
*網膜色素変性症	retinitis pigmentosa
加齢黄斑変性	age-related macular degeneration (AMD, ARMD)
難治性視神経症	intractable optic neuropathy
突発性難聴	sudden deafness
特発性両側性感音性難聴	idiopathic bilateral sensorineural hearing loss
メニエール病	Meniere disease
遅発性内リンパ水腫	delayed endolymhatic hydrops
*プロラクチン分泌異常症	abnormal secretion of prolactin
*ゴナドトロピン分泌異常症	abnormal secretion of gonadotropin
*拘束型心筋症	restrictive cardiomyopathy (RCM)
*ミトコンドリア病	mitochondrial disease
*ファブリー病	Fabry disease
家族性突然死症候群, QT延長症候群	familial sudden death syndrome, long QT syndrome
原発性高脂血症	primary hyperlipidemia
*特発性間質性肺炎	idiopathic interstitial pneumonia
*サルコイドーシス	sarcoidosis
びまん性汎細気管支炎	diffuse panbronchiolitis (DPB)
*潰瘍性大腸炎	ulcerative colitis
*クローン病	Crohn disease
自己免疫性肝炎	autoimmune hepatitis (AIH)
*原発性胆汁性肝硬変	primary biliary cirrhosis
*劇症肝炎	fulminant hepatitis
特発性門脈圧亢進症	idiopathic portal hypertension (IPH)
肝外門脈閉塞症	extrahepatic portal obstruction (EHO)
*バッド・キアリ症候群	Budd-Chiari syndrome

肝内結石症	intrahepatic cholelithiasis
原発性硬化性胆管炎	primary sclerosing cholangitis (PSC)
膵嚢胞線維症	cystic fibrosis of pancreas
*重症急性膵炎	severe acute pancreatitis
慢性膵炎	chronic pancreatitis
*アミロイドーシス	amyloidosis
*ベーチェット病	Behçet disease
*全身性エリテマトーデス	systemic lupus erythematosus (SLE)
*多発性筋炎・皮膚筋炎	polymyositis, dermatomyositis
シェーグレン症候群	Sjögren syndrome
成人スティル病	adult Still disease
*高安病, 大動脈炎症候群	Takayasu disease, aortitis syndrome
*バージャー病	thromboangiitis obliterans, Buerger disease
*結節性多発動脈炎	polyarteritis nodosa
*ウェゲナー肉芽腫症	Wegener granulomatosis
アレルギー性肉芽腫性血管炎	allergic granulomatous angiitis (AGA)
*悪性関節リウマチ	malignant rheumatoid arthritis, rheumatoid vasculitis
側頭動脈炎	temporal arteritis (TA)
抗リン脂質抗体症候群	antiphospholipid antibody syndrome
*強皮症	scleroderma
好酸球性筋膜炎	eosinophilic fasciitis
硬化性萎縮性苔癬	lichen sclerosus et atrophicus (LSA)
*原発性免疫不全症候群	primary immunodeficiency syndrome
若年性肺気腫	juvenile emphysema
ランゲルハンス細胞組織球症	Langerhans cell histiocytosis (LCH)
*ADH 分泌異常症	abnormal secretion of ADH

1. 全身状態

中枢性摂食異常症	central eating disorder
原発性アルドステロン症	primary aldosteronism
偽性低アルドステロン症	pseudohypoaldosteronism
グルココルチコイド抵抗症	glucocorticoid receptor anomaly
副腎酵素欠損症	adrenal enzyme deficiency
副腎低形成，アジソン病	hypoadrenocorticism, Addison disease
偽性副甲状腺機能低下症	pseudohypoparathyroidism
ビタミンD受容機構異常症	vitamin D receptor anomaly
甲状腺刺激ホルモン受容体異常症	TSH receptor anomaly
甲状腺ホルモン不応症	thyroid hormone resistance
*再生不良性貧血	aplastic anemia
溶血性貧血	hemolytic anemia
不応性貧血，骨髄異形成症候群	refractory anemia, myelodysplastic syndrome
骨髄線維症	myelofibrosis
特発性血栓症	idiopathic thrombosis
血栓性血小板減少性紫斑病	thrombotic thrombocytopenic purpura (TTP)
*特発性血小板減少性紫斑病	idiopathic thrombocytopenic purpura (ITP)
IgA腎症	IgA nephropathy
急速進行性糸球体腎炎	rapidly progressive glomerulonephritis (RPGN)
難治性ネフローゼ症候群	intractable nephrotic syndrome
多発性嚢胞腎	polycystic kidney
*肥大型心筋症	hypertrophic cardiomyopathy (HCM)
*拡張型心筋症	dilated cardiomyopathy (DCM)
肥満低換気症候群	obesity-hypoventilation syndrome

IV章 診療録用語

肺胞低換気症候群	alveolar hypoventilation syndrome
＊原発性肺高血圧症	primary pulmonary hypertension
＊慢性肺血栓塞栓症	chronic pulmonary thromboembolism
＊混合性結合組織病	mixed connective tissue disease
＊神経線維腫症Ⅰ型，レックリングハウゼン病	neurofibromatosis type 1, Recklinghausen disease
＊神経線維腫症Ⅱ型	neurofibromatosis type 2
結節性硬化症，プリングル病	tuberous sclerosis, Pringle disease
＊表皮水疱症	epidermolysis bullosa
＊膿疱性乾癬	pustular psoriasis
＊天疱瘡	pemphigus
＊大脳皮質基底核変性症	corticobasal degeneration
＊重症多形滲出性紅斑（急性期）	severe erythema exudativum multiforme (EEM)
＊肺リンパ脈管筋腫症	pulmonary lymphangioleiomyomatosis (LAM)
進行性骨化性線維異形成症	fibrodysplasia ossificans progressiva (FOP)
色素性乾皮症	xeroderma pigmentosum (XP)
＊スモン	subacute myelo-optico-neuropathy (SMON)
＊下垂体機能低下症	hypopituitarism
＊クッシング病	Cushing disease
＊先端巨大症	acromegaly
原発性側索硬化症	primary lateral sclerosis (PLS)
有棘赤血球を伴う舞踏病	chorea with acanthocytes
HTLV-1関連脊髄障害	HTLV-1-associated myelopathy (HAM)
先天性魚鱗癬様紅皮症	congenital ichthyosiform erythroderma

● 治療法　Treatment ●

原因療法（げんいんりょうほう）	causal therapy
保存的療法（ほぞんてきりょうほう）	conservative therapy
薬物療法（やくぶつりょうほう）	drug therapy, pharmacotherapy, medicinal treatment
催眠薬（さいみんやく）	hypnotic
解熱処置（げねつしょち）	antipyresis
解熱薬（げねつやく）	antipyretic
抗生物質療法（こうせいぶっしつりょうほう）	antibiotic therapy
抗生物質（こうせいぶっしつ）	antibiotics
抗菌物質（こうきんぶっしつ）	antibacterial agent (substance)
抗結核薬（こうけっかくやく）	antitubercular (antituberculous) agent
抗真菌薬（こうしんきんやく）	antifungal agent
抗ウイルス薬（こう―やく）	antiviral agent
生物学的製剤（せいぶつがくてきせいざい）	biological product, biological drug
補充療法（ほじゅうりょうほう）	replacement therapy, substitution therapy
ホルモン療法（―りょうほう）	hormone therapy, hormonal therapy, endocrine therapy
放射線治療（ほうしゃせんちりょう）	radiation therapy (RT), radiotherapy
術中放射線治療（じゅっちゅうほうしゃせんちりょう）	intraoperative radiotherapy (IORT)
体外放射線照射療法（たいがいほうしゃせんしょうしゃりょうほう）	external-beam radiation therapy (EBRT)
定位放射線治療（ていいほうしゃせんちりょう）	stereotactic radiotherapy (SRT)
三次元原体放射線治療（さんじげんげんたいほうしゃせんちりょう）	three-dimensional conformal radiotherapy (3D-CRT)
強度変調放射線治療（きょうどへんちょうほうしゃせんちりょう）	intensity-modulated radiation therapy (IMRT)
密封小線源治療（みっぷうしょうせんげんちりょう）	brachytherapy
陽子線治療（ようしせんちりょう）	proton beam therapy
重粒子線治療（じゅうりゅうしせんちりょう）	heavy ion therapy
インターベンショナルラジオロジー	interventional radiology (IVR)
遺伝子治療（いでんしちりょう）	gene therapy
分子標的療法（ぶんしひょうてきりょうほう）	molecularly targeted therapy
免疫抑制療法（めんえきよくせいりょうほう）	immunosuppressive therapy
食事療法（しょくじりょうほう）	diet therapy, dietary therapy
経口補液療法（けいこうほえきりょうほう）	oral rehydration therapy (ORT)
運動療法（うんどうりょうほう）	exercise therapy, kinesitherapy
作業療法（さぎょうりょうほう）	occupational therapy

理学療法 りがくりょうほう	physical therapy (PT), physiotherapy
姑息的療法 こそくてきりょうほう	palliative therapy
支持療法 しじりょうほう	supportive therapy
維持療法 いじりょうほう	maintenance therapy
治癒的治療 ちゆてきちりょう	curative treatment
対症療法 たいしょうりょうほう	symptomatic therapy, expectant treatment
経験的治療 けいけんてきちりょう	empiric therapy
予防的治療 よぼうてきちりょう	preventive treatment, prophylactic treatment, prophylaxis
化学療法 かがくりょうほう	chemotherapy
外科療法 げかりょうほう	surgical treatment, operative treatment
集学的治療 しゅうがくてきちりょう	multidisciplinary therapy
再生医療 さいせいいりょう	regenerative medicine
補完代替医療 ほかんだいたいいりょう	complementary and alternative medicine (CAM)
個別化医療 こべつかいりょう	personalized health care, tailor-made medicine
根治療法 こんちりょうほう	radical treatment
民間療法 みんかんりょうほう	folk remedies
家庭療法 かていりょうほう	home remedies
末期医療 まっきいりょう	terminal care

● 補完代替医療　Complementary and alternative medicine ●

アーユルヴェーダ	Ayurveda
アロマセラピー，芳香療法 ほうこうりょうほう	aromatherapy
温泉療法 おんせんりょうほう	balneotherapy
カイロプラクティック	chiropractic
漢方 かんぽう	Chinese herbal medicine
灸療法 きゅうりょうほう	moxibustion
キレート療法 ─りょうほう	chelation therapy
クナイプ式療法 ─しきりょうほう	kneippism
クリスチャンサイエンス	Christian Science
虹彩学 こうさいがく	iridology
催眠療法 さいみんりょうほう	hypnotherapy
サウナ	sauna
指圧療法 しあつりょうほう	acupressure
自然療法 しぜんりょうほう	naturopathy
整骨療法 せいこつりょうほう	osteopathy
禅式長寿法 ぜんしきちょうじゅほう	macrobiotics
太極拳 たいきょくけん	tai chi

1. 全身状態

大量ビタミン療法 (たいりょう—りょうほう)	megavitamin therapy
中国伝統医学 (ちゅうごくでんとういがく)	traditional Chinese medicine
バイオフィードバック(ほう)	biofeedback (BF)
鍼療法 (はりりょうほう)	acupuncture
ホメオパシー	homeopathy
マッサージ療法 (—りょうほう)	massage therapy
水治療法 (みずちりょうほう)	hydrotherapy
黙想法 (もくそうほう)	meditation
薬草療法 (やくそうりょうほう)	herbal medicine, herbalism
ヨガ	yoga
ロルフィング	Rolfing

Tidbits

homeopathy

ドイツ人医師 Samuel Hahnemann (1755-1843) が提唱した治療体系. 健康人に投与すると似たような症状を引き起こす極微量の薬を病人に少しずつ投与して治癒力を高めようとする. このことから日常の臨床で投与量が非常に少ないとき "homeopathic dose" ということがある. homeopathy (同種療法) の逆は allopathy (逆症療法).

2. 疼 痛

● 症状・徴候　Symptoms / Signs ●

疼痛 とうつう	pain, ache, soreness, 〔形〕painful, aching, achy, sore
〜が痛む いた	〜 aches, 〜 hurts, have a pain in 〜
体性痛 たいせいつう	somatic pain
表在痛 ひょうざいつう	superficial pain
深部痛 しんぶつう	deep pain
内臓痛 ないぞうつう	visceral pain
異痛 いつう	allodynia
頭痛 ずつう	headache, cephalalgia
前頭部（後頭部，側頭部）痛 ぜんとうぶ（こうとうぶ，そくとうぶ）つう	frontal (occipital, temporal) pain
片頭痛 へんずつう	migraine
片側頭痛 へんそくずつう	hemicrania
緊張性頭痛 きんちょうせいずつう	tension headache
群発頭痛 ぐんぱつずつう	cluster headache
顔面痛 がんめんつう	facial pain
眼痛 がんつう	sore eyes, ophthalmalgia
耳痛 じつう	earache, sore ears, otalgia
咽頭痛 いんとうつう	sore throat, pharyngalgia
歯痛 しつう	toothache, odontalgia, odontodynia
胸痛 きょうつう	chest pain, pectoralgia
前胸部痛 ぜんきょうぶつう	precordial pain
胸骨下痛 きょうこつかつう	substernal pain
胸膜痛 きょうまくつう	pleuritic pain, pleurodynia, pleuralgia, costalgia
腹痛 ふくつう	abdominal pain
心窩部痛 しんかぶつう	epigastric pain, epigastralgia
上（下）腹部痛 じょう（か）ふくぶつう	upper (lower) abdominal pain
右（左）上腹部痛 みぎ（ひだり）じょうふくぶつう	right (left) upper quadrant pain
右（左）下腹部痛 みぎ（ひだり）かふくぶつう	right (left) lower quadrant pain
側腹部痛 そくふくぶつう	flank pain
背痛 はいつう	backache, back pain
腰痛 ようつう	low back pain, lumbago, lumbar pain
関節痛 かんせつつう	joint pain, arthralgia
筋肉痛 きんにくつう	muscle pain, muscular pain, myalgia
骨痛 こつつう	bone pain, ostalgia
神経痛 しんけいつう	neuralgia

2. 疼痛

三叉神経痛 さんさしんけいつう	trigeminal neuralgia, tic douloureux
肋間神経痛 ろっかんしんけいつう	intercostal neuralgia
坐骨神経痛 ざこつしんけいつう	sciatic pain, sciatica, ischiatic neuralgia
帯状疱疹後神経痛 たいじょうほうしんごしんけいつう	postherpetic neuralgia (PHN)
求心路遮断性疼痛 きゅうしんろしゃだんせいとうつう	deafferentation pain
複合性局所疼痛症候群 ふくごうせいきょくしょとうつうしょうこうぐん	complex regional pain syndrome (CRPS)
灼熱痛 しゃくねつつう	causalgia
月経痛 げっけいつう	menstrual pain, cramps, menorrhalgia
陣痛 じんつう	labor pains
共圧陣痛 きょうあつじんつう	bearing-down pains
偽陣痛 ぎじんつう	false pains
成長痛 せいちょうつう	growing pains
幻肢痛 げんしつう	phantom limb pain, phantom pain
神経根痛 しんけいこんつう	root pain
関連痛 かんれんつう	referred pain
放散痛 ほうさんつう	radiating pain
帯状痛 たいじょうつう	girdle pain
仙痛 せんつう	colic, colicky pain
圧痛 あつつう	tenderness, 〔形〕tender
突発痛 とっぱつつう	breakthrough pain
疼痛の性質 とうつうのせいしつ―	character of a pain
鋭い するど	sharp
鈍い にぶ	dull
刺すような さ―	lancinating, piercing, stabbing, darting, terebrating
裂くような さ―	tearing, rending
割れるような わ―	splitting
焼けるような や―	burning
ずきずきする	throbbing
がんがんする	pounding
しくしくする	gnawing, nagging
ちくちくする	pricking, prickling
ひりひりする	smarting, stinging
きりきりする	griping
激しい はげ―	severe, intense, violent; excruciating, tormenting, agonizing
難治性の なんちせい―	intractable
痛覚閾値 つうかくいきち	pain threshold
疼痛許容レベル とうつうきょよう―	pain tolerance level

IV章 診療録用語

| 視覚的評価尺度 しかくてきひょうかしゃくど | visual analog scale (VAS) |
| フェイススケール | face scale |

● 治療法 Treatment ●

疼痛管理 とうつうかんり	pain control
疼痛緩和 とうつうかんわ	pain relief
鎮痛 ちんつう	analgesia, 〔形〕analgesic
鎮痛薬 ちんつうやく	analgesic, anodyne, painkiller, pain reliever
WHO 疼痛緩和ラダー とうつうかんわ	WHO's pain relief ladder
アセトアミノフェン	acetaminophen《カロナール》
アセチルサリチル酸 さん	acetylsalicylic acid (ASA)《アスピリン》
麦角誘導体 ばっかくゆうどうたい	ergot derivatives
酒石酸エルゴタミン しゅせきさん	ergotamine tartrate《カフェルゴット》
セロトニン受容体作動薬 じゅようたいさどうやく	serotonin receptor agonist
スマトリプタンコハク酸塩	sumatriptan succinate《イミグラン》
ナラトリプタン塩酸塩	naratriptan hydrochloride《アマージ》
非ステロイド系抗炎症薬 ひけいこうえんしょうやく	nonsteroidal anti-inflammatory drug (NSAID)
シクロオキシゲナーゼ抑制薬 よくせいやく	cyclooxygenase (COX)-2 inhibitor
ジクロフェナクナトリウム	diclofenac sodium《ボルタレン》
インドメタシン	indomethacin《インダシン》
イブプロフェン	ibuprofen《ブルフェン》
ナプロキセン	naproxen《ナイキサン》
ナブメトン	nabumetone《レリフェン》
メロキシカム	meloxicam《モービック》
麻薬 まやく	narcotic
アヘン	opium
アヘンアルカロイド塩酸塩	opium alkaloid hydrochlorides《オピアル》
モルヒネ塩酸塩	morphine hydrochloride《塩酸モルヒネ》
モルヒネ硫酸塩水和物	morphine sulfate hydrate《MSコンチン》
オキシコドン塩酸塩	oxycodone hydrochloride《オキシコンチン》
コデインリン酸塩	codeine phosphate《リン酸コデイン》
コカイン塩酸塩	cocaine hydrochloride《塩酸コカイン》
フェンタニルクエン酸塩	fentanyl citrate《フェンタニル》
フェンタニル	fentanyl《デュロテップMTパッチ》
ペチジン塩酸塩	pethidine hydrochloride《オピスタン》

2. 疼痛

メサドン塩酸塩	methadone hydrochloride 《USP》
オピオイド	opioid
ペンタゾシン	pentazocine 《ソセゴン》
ブプレノルフィン塩酸塩	buprenorphine hydrochloride 《レペタン》
臨時追加投与	rescue dose, breakthrough dose
局所麻酔薬	local anesthetic
リドカイン	lidocaine 《キシロカイン》
ニューロレプト鎮痛	neuroleptanalgesia
自己調節鎮痛法	patient controlled analgesia (PCA)
自己調節硬膜外鎮痛法	patient controlled epidural analgesia
神経ブロック	nerve block
発痛点注射	injection of trigger points
硬膜外ブロック	epidural block
交感神経ブロック	sympathetic block
星状神経節ブロック	stellate ganglion block
腹腔神経叢ブロック	celiac plexus block
腕神経叢ブロック	brachial plexus block
くも膜下ブロック	subarachnoid block
末梢神経ブロック	peripheral nerve block
下垂体ブロック	pituitary neuroadenolysis
硬膜外腔鏡	epiduroscopy
経皮的電気神経刺激法	transcutaneous electrical nerve stimulation (TENS)
脊髄電気刺激法	spinal cord stimulation (SCS)
交感神経切除術	sympathectomy

―― Tidbits ――

cannabis

cannabis とは大麻のことで,大麻草 Cannabis sativa の葉や花弁から抽出されるテトラヒドロカンナビノール tetrahydrocannabinol (THC) に陶酔・催幻覚作用がある.cannabis と同義に用いられるマリファナ marijuana は乾燥大麻,ハシッシュ hashish は大麻樹脂であり,液体大麻を hash oil という.大麻草は衣服や紐用の線維の原料にもなる植物で hemp と総称する.嗜好品としての大麻は,わが国では大麻取締法 Cannabis Control Law により厳しく規制されているが,gateway drug (cocaine や heroin などのより強力な麻薬を常用するきっかけになる「入り口」薬物),cannabis dependence (依存性),medical marijuana (医療用マリファナ:癌,エイズ,多発性硬化症,緑内障など) の観点から種々議論があり,外国の一部ではマリファナ合法化の動きもある.

3. 眼

● 愁訴・症状　Complaints / Symptoms ●

視覚 しかく	vision, sight, visual sense
視覚障害 しかくしょうがい	visual impairment
視力 しりょく	visual acuity (VA), eyesight, vision
視力減退 しりょくげんたい	impairment of visual acuity, impaired vision, fogginess (dimness) of vision, poor (defective) vision, blurring of vision
視力が弱い しりょく―よわ―	have poor eyesight, be weak-sighted, be weak in sight
弱視 じゃくし	lazy eye, amblyopia
低視力 ていしりょく	low vision
視力を失う しりょく―うしな―	lose one's sight (eyesight), become blind
失明 しつめい	loss of vision, blindness
一過性視力障害 いっかせいしりょくしょうがい	fleeting blindness
黒そこひ くろ―, 黒内障 こくないしょう	amaurosis
点字 てんじ	braille
⟨＜Louis Braille; a form of printing with raised dots on the paper, allowing a blind person to read by touching⟩	
眼痛 がんつう	pain in the eye, sore eyes, ocular ache, ophthalmalgia, ophthalmodynia
屈折異常 くっせついじょう	refractive error, ametropia
近視 きんし, 近眼 きんがん	near-sightedness, myopia, 〔形〕near-sighted, myopic
近眼の人 きんがん―ひと	myope
遠視 えんし	far-sightedness, hypermetropia, hyperopia, 〔形〕far-sighted, hyper(metr)opic
遠視の人 えんし―ひと	hypermetrope, hyperope
乱視 らんし	astigmatism, 〔形〕astigmatic
斜視 しゃし	squint, strabismus, heterotropia, 〔形〕squint, cross-eyed, wall-eyed
老視 ろうし	presbyopia, 〔形〕presbyopic
老視者 ろうししゃ	presbyope
色覚 しきかく	color vision
色覚異常 しきかくいじょう	color vision defect, color anomaly, dyschromatopsia
複視 ふくし	double vision, diplopia
物が二重に見える	see double, have double vision

IV章　診療録用語

矯正視力 (きょうせいしりょく)	corrected vision, corrected visual acuity
眼鏡 (めがね)	glasses, spectacles
読書用眼鏡 (どくしょようめがね)	reading glasses
遠用眼鏡 (えんようめがね)	farsighted glasses
遠近両用眼鏡 (えんきんりょうようめがね)	bifocal glasses, bifocals
度の強い(弱い)眼鏡	strong (weak) glasses
眼鏡をかけている	wear glasses
眼鏡で屈折異常を矯正する (めがねーくっせついじょうーきょうせい―)	correct a refractive error with glasses
コンタクトレンズ	contact lens (CL)
サングラス	sunglasses, dark glasses
義眼 (ぎがん)	artificial eye, false eye
鳥目 (とりめ), 夜盲症 (やもうしょう)	night-blindness, nyctalopia, 〔形〕night-blind
疲れ目 (つかれめ), 眼精疲労 (がんせいひろう)	eyestrain, asthenopia
端末表示装置 (たんまつひょうじそうち)	visual display terminal (VDT), video display terminal
飛蚊症 (ひぶんしょう)	flying flies, myiodesopsia, myodesopsia, muscae volitantes
浮遊物 (ふゆうぶつ)	floaters
光輪視 (こうりんし)	halo vision, rainbow vision
光視症 (こうしょう), 閃光視 (せんこうし)	photopsia, photopsy, sparks or lightning flashes
閃輝暗点 (せんきあんてん)	scintillating scotoma
動揺視 (どうようし)	oscillopsia, oscillating vision
涙 (なみだ)	tears
涙が出る (なみだ―)	tears fall (flow), tears come into (well up in) one's eyes
流涙 (異常に多い) (りゅうるい (いじょう―おお―))	lacrimation, overflow of tears, epiphora
眼内異物感 (がんないいぶつかん)	foreign-body sensation, a feeling of something in the eye, grittiness, sandiness
目やに (め―)	discharge from the eye, eye mucus, gum
眼脂で目がくっついている (がんし―め―)	one's eyes are gummed up
まぶた, 眼瞼 (がんけん)	eyelid
二重瞼 (にじゅうまぶた)	double eyelid

3. 眼　127

まばたき	blink, blinking, 〔動〕blink
垂れ下がる瞼 たれさがるまぶた, 伏し目 ふしめ	drooping eyelids
瞼のけいれん まぶた	twitching of the eyelid, 〔動〕one's eyelid flickers
睫毛 まつげ	eyelashes, cilia
さかまつげ	ingrowing eyelashes
付けまつげ つけ	false eyelashes
羞明 しゅうめい	photophobia, abnormal intolerance of light, inability to stand light
まぶしい	dazzling, glaring, blinding
ものもらい	sty, stye
目薬 めぐすり, 点眼薬 てんがんやく	eye drops

● 診察所見・徴候　Physical findings / Signs ●

指数弁 しすうべん	counting fingers (CF), numerus digitorum (n. d.)
手動弁 しゅどうべん	hand movement (HM), motus manus (m. m.)
光覚弁 こうかくべん	light perception (LP), sensus luminis (s. l.)
眼窩縁 がんかえん	orbital margin
眼瞼下垂 がんけんかすい	blepharoptosis
眼瞼遅滞 がんけんちたい	lid lag
眼瞼痙攣 がんけんけいれん	blepharospasm, cillosis, spasmodic quivering of the eyelid
眼瞼後退 がんけんこうたい	lid retraction
眼瞼縮小 がんけんしゅくしょう	blepharophimosis
兎眼 とがん	lagophthalmos, hare's eye
眼瞼反転 がんけんはんてん	eversion of the eyelids
眼瞼内反 がんけんないはん	entropion, entropium
眼瞼外反 がんけんがいはん	ectropion, ectropium
眼瞼結膜露出 がんけんけつまくろしゅつ	exposure of the palpebral conjunctiva
眼瞼皮膚弛緩症 がんけんひふしかんしょう	blepharochalasis
眼脂 がんし	sebum palpebrale, lema
睫毛乱生 しょうもうらんせい	trichiasis
異物 いぶつ	foreign body
瞼裂斑 けんれつはん	pinguecula
翼状片 よくじょうへん	pterygium
内眼角贅皮 ないがんかくぜいひ	epicanthus, epicanthal folds
結膜浮腫 けつまくふしゅ	chemosis, conjunctival edema
結膜充血 けつまくじゅうけつ	conjunctival injection

IV章

| 結膜下出血 | subconjunctival hemorrhage |
| ビトー斑 | Bitot spots |

⟨*superficial white flecks on the conjunctiva, seen in vitamin A deficiency*⟩

フリクテン	phlyctenule (small vesicles on the cornea or conjunctiva)
角膜知覚	corneal sensitivity
角膜異物	corneal foreign body
角膜混濁	corneal opacity
角膜白斑	corneal leukoma
角膜剥離	corneal abrasion
角膜びらん	corneal erosion
角膜潰瘍	corneal ulcer
円錐角膜	keratoconus, conical cornea
角膜血管増殖, パンヌス	pannus (neovascularization of the cornea with proliferation of granulation tissue)
角膜後面沈着物	keratic precipitates (KP)
老人環	arcus senilis, gerontoxon
虹彩異色症	heterochromia iridis
ブラッシュフィールド斑	Brushfield spots

⟨*white spots on the periphery of the iris in newborns; suggestive of Down syndrome*⟩

眼球突出	proptosis, exophthalmos
眼球陥凹	enophthalmos
眼球斜位	heterophoria
内斜位	esophoria (EP)
外斜位	exophoria (XP)
内斜視	esotropia (ET), internal strabismus, convergent strabismus
外斜視	exotropia (XT), external strabismus, divergent strabismus
眼位不同	anisophoria
網膜異常対応	anomalous retinal correspondence (ARC)
遮閉試験	cover test (CT)
遮閉－遮閉除去試験	cover-uncover test (CUT)
交代遮閉試験	alternating cover test
シルマー試験	Schirmer test

⟨*a measurement of tear production using filter paper strips*⟩

涙液層破壊時間 るいえきそうはかいじかん	tear film breakup time (BUT)
眼圧 がんあつ	intraocular pressure (IOP)
外眼運動 がいがんうんどう	extraocular movement (EOM)
眼振 がんしん	nystagmus
視運動性眼振 しうんどうせいがんしん	optokinetic nystagmus (OKN)
律動性眼振 りつどうせいがんしん	jerk nystagmus, rhythmical nystagmus
振子様眼振 ふりこようがんしん	pendular nystagmus, oscillating nystagmus
瞳孔径 どうこうけい	pupil diameter
瞳孔不同 どうこうふどう	anisocoria
瞳孔間距離 どうこうかんきょり	interpupillary distance (IPD)
瞳孔反射 どうこうはんしゃ	pupillary reflex
対光反射 たいこうはんしゃ	light reflex
共感性対光反射 きょうかんせいたいこうはんしゃ	consensual light reflex
調節反射 ちょうせつはんしゃ	accommodation reflex
縮瞳 しゅくどう	miosis, pupillary constriction, 〔形〕miotic
散瞳 さんどう	mydriasis, pupillary dilatation, 〔形〕mydriatic
アーガイルロバートソン瞳孔 どうこう	Argyll Robertson pupil

⟨*miotic irregular pupils responsive to accommodation but nonresponsive to light stimulation; seen in neurosyphilis*⟩

| アディー症候群 しょうこうぐん | Adie syndrome |

⟨*tonic pupil, unilateral slowness in pupillary accommodation and convergence, and reduced deep tendon reflexes; caused by postsynaptic parasympathetic denervation probably due to ciliary ganglionic lesion*⟩

| 相対的瞳孔求心路障害 そうたいてきどうこうきゅうしんろしょうがい | relative afferent pupillary defect (RAPD) |
| マーカスガン瞳孔 どうこう | Marcus Gunn pupil |

⟨*different light reflex with unilateral optic nerve disease*⟩

虹彩血管新生 こうさいけっかんしんせい	rubeosis iridis
周辺紅彩部癒着 しゅうへんこうさいぶゆちゃく	peripheral anterior synechia (PAS)
前房出血 ぜんぼうしゅっけつ	hyphema
前房蓄膿 ぜんぼうちくのう	hypopyon
無水晶体眼 むすいしょうたいがん	aphakia, aphakic eye
水晶体混濁 すいしょうたいこんだく	lenticular opacity, lens opacity
硝子体混濁 しょうしたいこんだく	vitreous opacity, vitreous clouding, opacitas corporis vitrei (OCV)
硝子体浮遊物 しょうしたいふゆうぶつ	vitreous floater
硝子体出血 しょうしたいしゅっけつ	vitreous hemorrhage

IV章　診療録用語

テルソン症候群 こうぐん	Terson syndrome

⟨*vitreous and retinal hemorrhage associated with subarachnoid hemorrhage*⟩

視神経乳頭 ししんけいにゅうとう	optic disk, optic disc, discus nervi optici
乳頭浮腫 にゅうとうふしゅ	papilledema
うっ血乳頭 うっけつにゅうとう	choked disk
乳頭陥凹 にゅうとうかんおう	cupping of the disk
陥凹乳頭比 かんおうにゅうとうひ	cup-disk (C/D) ratio
視神経萎縮 ししんけいいしゅく	optic atrophy
乳頭出血 にゅうとうしゅっけつ	disc hemorrhage
フォスターケネディー症候群 こうぐん	Foster Kennedy syndrome

⟨*ipsilateral optic atrophy with central scotoma and contralateral papilledema, caused by optic nerve meningioma or frontal lobe tumor*⟩

中心窩 ちゅうしんか	fovea centralis, central fovea
黄斑 おうはん	macula, macula lutea
黄斑円孔 おうはんえんこう	macular hole
黄斑上膜 おうはんじょうまく	epimacular membrane
黄斑浮腫 おうはんふしゅ	macular edema
嚢胞様黄斑浮腫 のうほうようおうはんふしゅ	cystoid macular edema (CME)
網膜上膜 もうまくじょうまく	epiretinal membrane (ERM)
網膜出血 もうまくしゅっけつ	retinal hemorrhage
ロート斑 はん	Roth spots

⟨*white-centered retinal hemorrhage seen in leukemia, subacute bacterial endocarditis, or capillary fragility*⟩

動静脈交差部 どうじょうみゃくこうさぶ	arteriovenous crossing
銅線動脈 どうせんどうみゃく	copper-wire artery
小動脈瘤 しょうどうみゃくりゅう	microaneurysm (MA)
ドルーゼン	drusen
新生血管 しんせいけっかん	neovascularization
脈絡膜新生血管 みゃくらくまくしんせいけっかん	choroidal neovascularization (CNV)
網膜新生血管 もうまくしんせいけっかん	retinal neovascularization
網膜内細小血管異常 もうまくないさいしょうけっかんいじょう	intraretinal microvascular abnormality (IRMA)
綿花様白斑 めんかようはくはん	cotton-wool spots, cotton-wool patches (CWP)
軟性白斑 なんせいはくはん	soft exudate
硬性白斑 こうせいはくはん	hard exudate
梨子地眼底 なしじがんてい	peau d'orange fundus, mottled fundus

キース・ワグナー分類　　　Keith-Wagener classification

⟨a classification of hypertensive retinopathy based on arteriolar constriction, cotton-wool patches, hemorrhages, and papilledema⟩

コロボーマ　　　　　　　　coloboma (a defect of ocular tissue)

● 検査法　Examination ●

検眼法	optometry
視力検査	eyesight test
視力検査表	eye chart, eyesight test chart
ランドルト環	Landolt ring

⟨broken rings used in testing of visual acuity⟩

スネレン表　　　　　　　　Snellen chart

⟨a chart imprinted with capital letters in decreasing sizes to test the acuity of distant vision⟩

イェーガー視力検査文字　　Jaeger test type

⟨ordinary printer's type of seven different sizes to test visual acuity⟩

色覚検査	color vision test
屈折検査	refractometry
裸眼視力	uncorrected visual acuity
正視	emmetropia
非正視	ametropia
限界フリッカー値	critical flicker frequency (CFF)
眼底検査法	ophthalmoscopy, funduscopy
倒像眼底検査	indirect ophthalmoscopy
走査レーザー検眼鏡	scanning laser ophthalmoscope (SLO)
検影法	retinoscopy, skiascopy
隅角検査	gonioscopy
細隙灯顕微鏡検査	slit-lamp biomicroscopy
超音波生体顕微鏡	ultrasound biomicroscopy (UBM)
ヘルテル眼球突出計	Hertel exophthalmometer

⟨a handheld device to assess exophthalmos⟩

眼圧測定法	tonometry
圧平眼圧計	applanation tonometer
シェッツ眼圧計	Schiötz tonometer

⟨a tonometer directly applied to the cornea⟩

非接触眼圧計　　　　　　　noncontact tonometer (NCT)

フレンツェル眼鏡　Frenzel glasses
⟨*glasses with 10-diopter lenses; useful for screening nystagmus*⟩
電気眼振検査法　electronystagmography (ENG)
視野計測法　perimetry
平面視野計　tangent screen
ゴールドマン視野計　Goldmann perimeter
⟨*a projection perimeter*⟩
自動視野計　automated perimeter
アムスラーチャート　Amsler chart
⟨*diagram of grids and parallel lines, used to detect defects in central visual fields*⟩
眼底血圧測定法　ophthalmodynamometry (ODN)
網膜動脈圧　retinal arterial pressure (RAP)
網膜中心動脈圧　central arterial pressure of retina (CAP)
硝子体蛍光測定法　vitreous fluorophotometry (VFP)
蛍光眼底撮影法　fluorescein angiography (FAG)
光学的干渉断層検査　optical coherence tomography (OCT)
網膜電図　electroretinogram (ERG)
眼電図　electro-oculogram (EOG)
視野　visual field (VF), field of vision
視野欠損　visual field defect
視野狭窄　contraction of visual field
中心視　central vision
周辺視　peripheral vision
網膜正常対応　normal retinal correspondence (NRC)
半盲　hemianopia, hemianopsia
両鼻側半盲　binasal hemianopia
両耳側半盲　bitemporal hemianopia
同側半盲　homonymous hemianopia
異側半盲　heteronymous hemianopia
水平半盲　altitudinal hemianopia
盲点, マリオット盲点　blind spot, Mariotte spot
⟨*the area of blindness in the visual field corresponding to the optic disk*⟩
暗点　scotoma, 〔複〕scotomata
単眼視　monocular vision
両眼視　binocular vision (BV)
立体視　stereopsis
同時視　simultaneous perception (SP)

3. 眼 *133*

| 融像 ゆうぞう | fusion |
| 視覚誘発電位 しかくゆうはつでんい | visual evoked potential (VEP) |

● 疾患名 Diseases ●

眼瞼炎 がんけんえん	blepharitis
霰粒腫 さんりゅうしゅ	chalazion, 〔複〕chalazia
麦粒腫 ばくりゅうしゅ	hordeolum, 〔複〕hordeola
トラコーマ	trachoma
涙嚢炎 るいのうえん	dacryocystitis
流涙症 りゅうるいしょう	epiphora, illacrimation
鼻涙管狭窄症 びるいかんきょうさくしょう	nasolacrimal duct stenosis
涙嚢鼻腔狭窄症 るいのうびくうきょうさくしょう	dacryocystorhinostenosis
急性出血性結膜炎 きゅうせいしゅっけつせいけつまくえん	acute hemorrhagic conjunctivitis (AHC)
アレルギー性結膜炎 ―せいけつまくえん	allergic conjunctivitis
春季カタル しゅんき―	vernal conjunctivitis
巨大乳頭結膜炎 きょだいにゅうとうけつまくえん	giant papillary conjunctivitis (GPC)
流行性角結膜炎 りゅうこうせいかくけつまくえん	epidemic keratoconjunctivitis (EKC)
上輪部角結膜炎 じょうりんぶかくけつまくえん	superior limbic keratoconjunctivitis (SLK)
トラコーマ封入体結膜炎 ―ふうにゅうたいけつまくえん	trachoma-inclusion conjunctivitis (TRIC)
結膜弛緩症 けつまくしかんしょう	conjunctivochalasis
紫外線角膜炎 しがいせんかくまくえん	ultraviolet keratitis, actinic keratitis
点状表層角膜炎 てんじょうひょうそうかくまくえん	superficial punctate keratitis (SPK)
感染性眼内炎 かんせんせいがんないえん	infectious endophthalmitis
強膜炎 きょうまくえん	scleritis
上強膜炎 じょうきょうまくえん	episcleritis
眼乾燥症 がんかんそうしょう, ドライアイ	dry eye
乾性角結膜炎 かんせいかくけつまくえん	keratoconjunctivitis sicca (KCS)
高眼圧症 こうがんあつしょう	ocular hypertension (OH)
緑内障 りょくないしょう	glaucoma
原発閉塞隅角緑内障 げんぱつへいそくぐうかくりょくないしょう	primary angle-closure glaucoma (PACG)
原発開放隅角緑内障 げんぱつかいほうぐうかくりょくないしょう	primary open-angle glaucoma (POAG)
正常眼圧緑内障	normal-tension glaucoma (NTG)

発達緑内障	developmental glaucoma
隅角後退緑内障	angle-recession glaucoma
続発緑内障	secondary glaucoma
白内障	cataract
前嚢下白内障	anterior subcapsular cataract (ASC)
後嚢下白内障	posterior subcapsular cataract (PSC)
後発白内障	aftercataract
後水晶体線維増殖症	retrolental fibroplasia (RLF)
一過性黒内障	amaurosis fugax
虹彩炎	iritis
虹彩毛様体炎	iridocyclitis
ぶどう膜炎	uveitis
フォークト・小柳・原田症候群	Vogt-Koyanagi-Harada syndrome

⟨bilateral uveitis with meningism, alopecia, poliosis, vitiligo, deafness, and glaucoma; likely autoimmune⟩

眼型白皮症	ocular albinism (OA)
後部硝子体剝離	posterior vitreous detachment (PVD)
脈絡膜剝離	choroidal detachment (CD)
中心性漿液性脈絡網膜症	central serous chorioretinopathy (CSCR)
網膜炎	retinitis
滲出性網膜炎, コーツ病	exudative retinitis, Coats disease

⟨retinal telangiectasia and accumulation of exudate leading to retinal detachment⟩

網膜中心静脈閉塞症	central retinal vein occlusion (CRVO)
網膜中心動脈閉塞症	central retinal artery occlusion (CRAO)
網膜静脈分枝閉塞症	branch retinal vein occlusion (BRVO)
網膜動脈分枝閉塞症	branch retinal artery occlusion (BRAO)
視神経炎	optic neuritis
虚血性視神経障害	ischemic optic neuropathy (ION)
前部虚血性視神経症	anterior ischemic optic neuropathy (AION)

レーバー遺伝性視神経症	Leber hereditary optic neuropathy

⟨*degeneration of the optic nerve in young men, resulting in central visual loss; caused by point mutation of a mitochondrial gene for NADH*⟩

未熟児網膜症	retinopathy of prematurity (ROP)
糖尿病網膜症	diabetic retinopathy (DR)
増殖糖尿病網膜症	proliferative diabetic retinopathy (PDR)
高血圧網膜症	hypertensive retinopathy
急性網膜壊死	acute retinal necrosis (ARN)
網膜色素変性症	retinitis pigmentosa (RP), retinal pigmentary degeneration
急性後部多発性斑状色素上皮症	acute posterior multifocal placoid pigment epitheliopathy (APMPPE)
網膜剥離	retinal detachment (RD)
増殖硝子体網膜症	proliferative vitreoretinopathy (PVR)
加齢黄斑変性	age-related macular degeneration (AMD, ARMD)
小口病	Oguchi disease

⟨*congenital night blindness with gray to yellow fundus; autosomal recessive*⟩

ポリープ状脈絡膜血管症	polypoidal choroidal vasuculopathy (PCV)
網膜芽細胞腫	retinoblastoma
脈絡膜黒色腫	choroidal melanoma
眼筋麻痺	ophthalmoplegia
進行性外眼筋麻痺	progressive external ophthalmoplegia (PEO), ocular myopathy
慢性進行性外眼筋麻痺	chronic progressive external ophthalmoplegia (CPEO)
眼球突出性眼筋麻痺	exophthalmic ophthalmoplegia
眼窩底吹き抜け骨折	orbital floor blow-out fracture (BOF)

● 治療法 Treatment ●

保護眼鏡	protective glasses, safety glasses
二重焦点眼鏡	bifocal glasses
三重焦点眼鏡	trifocal glasses
多焦点レンズ	multifocal lens

ハードコンタクトレンズ	hard contact lens, hydrophobic contact lens
ソフトコンタクトレンズ	soft contact lens, hydrophilic contact lens
使い捨てコンタクトレンズ	disposable contact lens
眼帯	eyepatch
洗眼薬	collyrium, eyewash
散瞳薬	mydriatics
トロピカミド	tropicamide《ミドリン》
縮瞳薬	miotics
塩酸ピロカルピン	pilocarpine hydrochloride《サンピロ》
局所用ベータ遮断薬	topical beta blocker
カルテオロール塩酸塩	carteolol hydrochloride《ミケラン》
炭酸脱水素酵素阻害薬	carbonic anhydrase inhibitor
浸透圧性利尿薬	osmotic diuretics
アセタゾラミド	acetazolamide《ダイアモックス》
ペガプタニブナトリウム	pegaptanib sodium《マクジェン》
ラニビズマブ	ranibizumab《ルセンティス》
人工涙液	artificial tears
視能訓練	orthoptics
弱視視能矯正	pleoptics
レーザー光凝固術	laser photocoagulation
汎網膜光凝固術	panretinal photocoagulation (PRP)
光線力学療法	photodynamic therapy (PDT)
ヘマトポルフィリン誘導体	hematoporphyrin derivative
ベルテポルフィン	verteporfin《ビスダイン》
経瞳孔温熱療法	transpupillary thermotherapy
涙囊鼻腔吻合術	dacryocystorhinostomy (DCR)
ケルマン水晶体乳化術	Kelman phacoemulsification (KPE)

⟨a surgical method of cataract extraction developed in 1967; the lens is emulsified by ultrasonic vibration, irrigated and aspirated through a small incision⟩

水晶体超音波乳化吸引術	phacoemulsification and aspiration (PEA)

白内障嚢内摘出術	intracapsular cataract extraction (ICCE)
白内障嚢外摘出術	extracapsular cataract extraction (ECCE)
眼内レンズ	intraocular lens (IOL)
眼内レンズ挿入眼	pseudophakia
有水晶体眼内レンズ	phakic intraocular lens
レーザー虹彩切開術	laser iridotomy (LI)
レーザー線維柱帯形成術	laser trabeculoplasty (LTP)
レーザー隅角形成術	laser gonioplasty (LGP)
周辺虹彩切除術	peripheral iridectomy
線維柱帯切除術	trabeculectomy
線維柱帯切開術	trabeculotomy
隅角癒着解離術	goniosynechiolysis (GSL)
硝子体手術	vitreous surgery
硝子体切除術	vitrectomy
角膜矯正術	orthokeratology
乱視矯正角膜切開術	astigmatic keratectomy (AK)
放射状角膜切開術	radial keratotomy (RK)
治療的レーザー角膜切除術	phototherapeutic keratectomy (PTK)
レーザー屈折矯正角膜切除術	photorefractive keratectomy (PRK)
レーザー角膜内切削形成術	laser-assisted in-situ keratomileusis (LASIK)
強膜内陥術	scleral buckling
眼球摘出術	enucleation, ophthalmectomy
眼球内容除去術	orbital evisceration
網膜復位術	retinopexy
角膜移植術	keratoplasty, corneal transplantation
層状角膜移植術	lamellar keratoplasty

IV章 診療録用語

全層角膜移植術 (そうじょうかくまくいしょくじゅつ / ぜんそうかくまくいしょくじゅつ)　　penetrating keratoplasty (PKP)

アイバンク　　eye bank

― Tidbits ―

biopsy

生検 biopsy は "removal and examination of tissue from the living body" という意味の名詞であり動詞に用いるのは正しくないが,実際には "The mass was biopsied." のような動詞としての用法をしばしば認めるようになり,許容する意見も増えている.

4. 耳鼻咽喉

● 愁訴・症状 Complaints / Symptoms ●

聴覚 ちょうかく	hearing, the sense of hearing, auditory sense, 〔形〕auditory
聴力 ちょうりょく	hearing, hearing acuity
難聴 なんちょう	impaired hearing, decreased hearing, loss of hearing
耳が遠い みみとお—	be hard of hearing
聾 ろう	deafness, 〔形〕deaf
聴覚過敏 ちょうかくかびん	excessive sensitivity to sound, hyperacusis
耳鳴 じめい	ringing of the ears, tinnitus
耳鳴りがする みみな—	have a ringing in the ears, one's ears ring
耳閉感 じへいかん	feeling of fullness in the ear
耳だれ みみ—, 耳漏 じろう	ear discharge, discharges from ears, otorrhea
耳だれがある	have running ears, have a discharge from the ear
耳痛 じつう	earache, otalgia
耳が痛む みみいた—	have a pain in one's ear, one's ear hurts
耳垢 じこう	earwax, wax in the ear, cerumen
綿棒で耳垢を取る めんぼう—じこう—と—	clean one's ears with a cotton swab
鼓膜 こまく	eardrum, tympanic membrane, 〔形〕tympanic
鼓膜が破れる こまくやぶ—	have one's eardrum ruptured (perforated)
中耳炎 ちゅうじえん	inflammation of the middle ear, otitis media
自声強調 じせいきょうちょう	autophony, autophonia
めまい	dizziness, giddiness, vertigo, 〔形〕dizzy, giddy, vertiginous
平衡障害 へいこうしょうがい	disequilibrium
鼻水 はなみず, 鼻漏 びろう	nasal discharge, snivel, rhinorrhea
後鼻漏 こうびろう	postnasal drip (PND)
鼻水が出る はなみずで—	snivel, run at the nose, have a running nose
鼻をかむ はな—	blow the nose
くしゃみ	sneezing, sneeze, 〔動〕sneeze, have a

140　IV章　診療録用語

	sneezing fit
鼻づまり はな，鼻閉 びへい	nasal obstruction, nasal stuffiness, nasal blockage, nasal congestion
口呼吸 こうこきゅう	mouth breathing
鼻声 はなごえ	nasal voice, nasal tone, twang
鼻出血 びしゅっけつ	nosebleed, bleeding from the nose, nasal hemorrhage, epistaxis
鼻血が出る はなぢ— で—	have a nosebleed
花粉症 かふんしょう	hay fever, pollen allergy
嗅覚 きゅうかく	smell, the sense of smell, olfaction, 〔形〕olfactory
無嗅覚 むきゅうかく	anosmia
嗅覚減退 きゅうかくげんたい	hyposmia
嗅覚異常 きゅうかくいじょう	dysosmia
いびき	snoring, snore,〔動〕snore
睡眠時無呼吸 すいみんじむこきゅう	sleep apnea
咽頭痛 いんとうつう	sore throat
咽頭異物感 いんとういぶっかん	foreign-body sensation in the throat
低い（大きい，太い）声で ひく—（おおき—，ふと—）こえ—	in a low (loud, deep) voice
失声症 しっせいしょう	aphonia
発声障害 はっせいしょうがい	dysphonia, voice disturbance
声が出なくなる こえ— で—	lose one's voice
歌手結節 かしゅけっせつ	singer's nodes
嗄声 させい	hoarseness, a hoarse (husky, harsh, raucous) voice
しわがれ声で —ごえ—	hoarsely, in a hoarse (husky) voice
声がかれる こえ—	get (become) hoarse
扁桃腺が腫れている へんとうせん— は—	have swollen tonsils

● 診察所見・徴候　Physical findings / Signs ●

耳介変形 じかいへんけい	auricular deformity
耳介結節 じかいけっせつ	auricular tubercle, Darwin tubercle

⟨a nodule on the edge of the helix, congenital and harmless; should not be mistaken for a tophus⟩

痛風結節 つうふうけっせつ	tophus
耳輪結節性軟骨皮膚炎 じりんけっせつせいなんこつひふえん	chondrodermatitis noduralis helicis
耳垢栓塞 じこうせんそく	impacted cerumen, impaction of earwax
鼓膜穿孔 こまくせんこう	tympanic membrane perforation

聴覚反射 ちょうかくはんしゃ	acoustic reflex, stapedial reflex
ホールパイク法 ほう	Hallpike maneuver

⟨a test for BPPV; positive if rapid lying from a sitting to a supine position with the head hanging over the edge of the bed causes nystagmus⟩

鼻瘤 びりゅう	rhinophyma
酒皶鼻 しゅさび	rosacea, acne rosacea
鞍鼻 あんび	saddle nose, saddle-back nose, sway-back nose
キーセルバッハ部位 ぶい	Kiesselbach area

⟨the anterior part of the nasal septum rich in capillaries; a common site of epistaxis⟩

鼻中隔彎曲 びちゅうかくわんきょく	septal deviation
鼻中隔穿孔 びちゅうかくせんこう	perforation of the nasal septum
鼻茸 はなたけ	nasal polyp
咽頭反射 いんとうはんしゃ	pharyngeal reflex, gag reflex
咽頭充血 いんとうじゅうけつ	pharyngeal injection
偽膜 ぎまく	pseudomembrane
扁桃腫大 へんとうしゅだい	tonsillar swelling
声門浮腫 せいもんふしゅ	glottis edema
声帯麻痺 せいたいまひ	vocal cord paralysis
ラインケ浮腫 ―ふしゅ	Reinke edema

⟨fluid accumulation in Reinke space of vocal cord; associated with smoking, vocal abuse, and chemical irritants⟩

バトル徴候 ―ちょうこう	Battle sign

⟨postauricular ecchymosis due to basilar skull fracture⟩

コステン症候群 ―しょうこうぐん	Costen syndrome

⟨otalgia, tinnitus, decreased hearing, dizziness, and burning sensation of the tongue and throat; temporomandibular joint dysfunction implicated but not convincing⟩

コーガン症候群 ―しょうこうぐん	Cogan syndrome

⟨oculovestibulo-auditory syndrome, marked by interstitial keratitis, vertigo, tinnitus, hearing loss, and visual loss; often associated with polyarteritis nodosa⟩

● 検査法　Examination ●

耳鏡検査 じきょうけんさ	otoscopy
聴覚検査 ちょうかくけんさ	hearing test, audiometry
オージオメータ	audiometer
皮膚電気反応聴力検査 ひふでんきはんのうちょうりょくけんさ	electric response audiometry (ERA), electrodermal audiometry
聴力図 ちょうりょくず	audiogram
最小可聴域 さいしょうかちょういき	minimum audible field

IV章 診療録用語

最小可聴閾値	minimum audible threshold
一過性閾値減衰試験	temporary threshold decay test (TTD)
一過性閾値変動	temporary threshold shift (TTS)
永久閾値上昇	permanent threshold shift (PTS)
純音聴力検査	pure tone audiometry
語音聴力検査	speech audiometry
語音弁別検査	speech discrimination test
語音聴取閾値検査	speech reception threshold test (SRT)
伝音性難聴	conductive hearing loss, conductive deafness
感音性難聴	sensorineural hearing loss, perceptive deafness
耳鳴検査	tinnitus test
音叉検査	tuning fork test
ウェーバー試験	Weber test

⟨a test for differentiating sensorineural from conductive hearing loss using a vibrating tuning fork placed on the midline of the head⟩

リンネ試験	Rinne test

⟨a vibrating tuning fork is placed on the mastoid process for bone conduction and held next to ear canal for air conduction⟩

骨伝導	bone conduction (BC)
空気伝導	air conduction (AC)
ベツォルト三徴	Bezold triad

⟨prolonged bone conduction, decreased perception of low tones, and negative Rinne test, indicating otosclerosis⟩

両耳音の大きさバランス検査	alternate binaural loudness balance test (ABLB)
短時間増強感覚指数	short increment sensitivity index (SISI)
補充現象	recruitment
蝸電図法	electrocochleography
蝸牛マイクロホン電位	cochlear microphonic potential, cochlear microphonics
蝸牛内直流電位	endocochlear potential
耳音響放射	otoacoustic emission (OAE)
ティンパノメトリー	tympanometry
聴覚誘発電位	auditory evoked potential (AEP)
聴性脳幹反応	auditory brainstem response (ABR), brainstem auditory evoked potential

(BAEP)

耳管通気法 じかんつうきほう	tympanic insufflation
平衡機能検査 へいこうきのうけんさ	equilibrium test
回転試験 かいてんしけん	rotation test
温度眼振試験 おんどがんしんしけん, バラニー検査 ——けんさ	caloric test, Bárány test

〈vestibular function test; warm-water irrigation of the normal ear causes rotatory nystagmus toward the irrigated ear, cold-water irrigation away from that side〉

バラニー指示試験 ——しじしけん	Bárány pointing test

〈positive for a brain lesion if the patient makes a constant error with the eyes closed; the patient is asked to point at an object alternately with the eyes open and closed〉

嗅覚検査 きゅうかくけんさ	olfactometry
嗅電図 きゅうでんず	electro-olfactogram (EOG)
嗅覚認知域のにおい きゅうかくにんちいき——	minimal identifiable odor
耳管鏡検査 じかんきょうけんさ	salpingoscopy
鼻咽腔検査 びいんくうけんさ	nasopharyngoscopy
後鼻鏡検査 こうびきょうけんさ	posterior rhinoscopy
喉頭鏡検査 こうとうきょうけんさ	laryngoscopy
喉頭ストロボスコープ こうとう——	laryngostroboscope

● 疾患名　Diseases ●

老人性難聴 ろうじんせいなんちょう	presbyacusis, presbyacusia
突発性難聴 とっぱつせいなんちょう	sudden deafness
後迷路性難聴 こうめいろせいなんちょう	retrocochlear hearing loss
外耳炎 がいじえん	external otitis, otitis externa
鼓膜炎 こまくえん	myringitis
外傷性鼓膜穿孔 がいしょうせいこまくせんこう	traumatic perforation of the tympanic membrane
急性中耳炎 きゅうせいちゅうじえん	acute otitis media (AOM)
滲出性中耳炎 しんしゅつせいちゅうじえん	otitis media with effusion (OME)
グラデニゴー症候群	Gradenigo syndrome

〈suppurative otitis media with abducens paralysis and trigeminal neuralgia〉

コレステリン腫 ——しゅ, 真珠腫 しんじゅしゅ	cholesteatoma
鼓膜硬化 こまくこうか	tympanosclerosis
耳管炎 じかんえん	salpingitis, eustachian salpingitis

〈Bartolommeo Eustachio; inflammation of the auditory tube〉

耳管狭窄 じかんきょうさく	tubal stenosis

耳管閉塞 じかんへいそく	tubal obstruction
耳管開放症 じかんかいほうしょう	patulous eustachian tube
耳真菌症 じしんきんしょう	otomycosis
内耳炎 ないじえん	labyrinthitis
耳硬化症 じこうかしょう	otosclerosis
聴神経炎 ちょうしんけいえん	acoustic neuritis
聴神経鞘腫 ちょうしんけいしょうしゅ	acoustic neurinoma
メニエール病 ─びょう	Meniere disease

⟨*labyrinthine hydrops or endolymphatic hydrops characterized by vertigo, nausea, tinnitus, and progressive hearing loss*⟩

良性発作性頭位性めまい りょうせいほっさせいとういせい──	benign paroxysmal positional vertigo (BPPV)
前庭神経炎 ぜんていしんけいえん	vestibular neuronitis
乳様突起炎 にゅうようとっきえん	mastoiditis
再発性多発軟骨炎 さいはつせいたはつなんこつえん	relapsing polychondritis (RP)
アレルギー性鼻炎 ──せいびえん	allergic rhinitis
花粉症 かふんしょう	pollinosis, pollenosis
枯草熱 こそうねつ	hay fever
アレルギー性通年性鼻炎 ──せいつうねんせいびえん	perennial allergic rhinitis, nonseasonal allergic rhinitis
萎縮性鼻炎 いしゅくせいびえん	atrophic rhinitis
臭鼻症 しゅうびしょう	ozena
咽頭炎 いんとうえん	pharyngitis
扁桃炎 へんとうえん	tonsillitis
扁桃周囲炎 へんとうしゅういえん	peritonsillitis
扁桃周囲膿瘍 へんとうしゅういのうよう	peritonsillar abscess (PTA)
深頚部膿瘍 しんけいぶのうよう	deep neck abscess
喉頭炎 こうとうえん	laryngitis
喉頭蓋炎 こうとうがいえん	epiglottitis
声門下喉頭炎 せいもんかこうとうえん	subglottic laryngitis, chorditis vocalis inferior
喉頭痙攣 こうとうけいれん	laryngospasm, laryngismus
声帯炎 せいたいえん	chorditis, chorditis vocalis
声帯ポリープ せいたい──	vocal cord polyp
反回神経麻痺 はんかいしんけいまひ	recurrent laryngeal nerve paralysis
副鼻腔炎 ふくびくうえん	sinusitis
上顎洞炎 じょうがくどうえん	maxillary sinusitis
篩骨洞炎 しこつどうえん	ethmoid sinusitis, ethmoiditis
蝶形骨洞炎 ちょうけいこつどうえん	sphenoid sinusitis, sphenoiditis
前頭洞炎 ぜんとうどうえん	frontal sinusitis
上顎洞癌 じょうがくどうがん	maxillary sinus cancer

鼻咽頭癌 びいんとうがん | nasopharyngeal cancer
中咽頭癌 ちゅういんとうがん | oropharyngeal cancer
下咽頭癌 かいんとうがん | hypopharyngeal cancer
喉頭癌 こうとうがん | laryngeal cancer
頭頚部腫瘍 とうけいぶしゅよう | head and neck tumor

● 治療法　Treatment ●

充血除去薬 じゅうけつじょきょやく | decongestant
抗ヒスタミン薬 こう――やく | antihistamine
ジフェンヒドラミン塩酸塩 ――えんさんえん | diphenhydramine hydrochloride《レスタミン》
クロルフェニラミンマレイン酸塩 ――さんえん | chlorpheniramine maleate《ポララミン》
H$_1$受容体拮抗薬 ――じゅようたいきっこうやく | H$_1$-receptor antagonist
ケトチフェンフマル酸塩 ――さんえん | ketotifen fumarate《ザジテン》
エバスチン | ebastine《エバステル》
点鼻液 てんびえき | nasal drop
フルチカゾンプロピオン酸エステル ――さん―― | fluticasone propionate《フルナーゼ》
鼻洗浄 びせんじょう | nasal irrigation, nasal douche
耳管通気法 じかんつうきほう | air douche
エプリー法 ――ほう | Epley maneuver
　〈canal repositioning maneuver to treat benign paroxysmal positional vertigo〉
補聴器 ほちょうき | hearing aid
発声訓練 はっせいくんれん | voice training
食道発声 しょくどうはっせい | esophageal speech
言語療法 げんごりょうほう | speech therapy
耳鳴再訓練療法 じめいさいくんれんりょうほう | tinnitus retraining therapy (TRT)
鼓膜切開術 こまくせっかいじゅつ | tympanostomy, myringotomy
鼓膜形成術 こまくけいせいじゅつ | myringoplasty
鼓室形成術 こしつけいせいじゅつ | tympanoplasty
乳様突起切除術 にゅうようとっきせつじょじゅつ | mastoidectomy
耳小骨摘出術 じしょうこつてきしゅつじゅつ | ossiculectomy
耳小骨形成術 じしょうこつけいせいじゅつ | ossiculoplasty
あぶみ骨摘除術 ――こつてきじょじゅつ | stapedectomy
あぶみ骨形成術 ――こつけいせいじゅつ | stapedioplasty
あぶみ骨板開窓術 ――こつばんかいそうじゅつ | stapes fenestration
迷路摘出術 めいろてきしゅつじゅつ | labyrinthectomy

146　Ⅳ章　診療録用語

人工内耳 じんこうないじ	cochlear implant
鼻出血焼灼 びしゅっけつしょうしゃく	cauterization of nosebleeds
鼻形成術 びけいせいじゅつ	rhinoplasty
鼻中隔矯正術 びちゅうかくきょうせいじゅつ	submucous resection of nasal septum
粘膜下下鼻甲介切除術 ねんまくかかびこうかいせつじょじゅつ	submucous resection of inferior nasal concha
鼻甲介切除術 びこうかいせつじょじゅつ	turbinectomy
扁桃摘出術 へんとうてきしゅつじゅつ	tonsillectomy
アデノイド切除術 ―せつじょ	adenoidectomy
扁桃アデノイド手術 へんとう―しゅじゅつ	tonsillectomy and adenoidectomy (T & A)
咽頭切除術 いんとうせつじょじゅつ	pharyngectomy
喉頭切開術 こうとうせっかいじゅつ	laryngotomy
喉頭摘出術 こうとうてきしゅつじゅつ	laryngectomy
喉頭形成術 こうとうけいせいじゅつ	laryngoplasty
キリアン手術 ―しゅじゅつ	Killian operation

⟨*an operation for frontal sinusitis; excision of the anterior wall, curettage, and communication with the nasal cavity*⟩

口蓋垂軟口蓋咽頭形成術 こうがいすいなんこうがいいんとうけいせいじゅつ	uvulopalatopharyngoplasty (UPPP)
頭蓋顔面合併切除術 とうがいがんめんがっぺいせつじょじゅつ	craniofacial resection
頭頸部再建 とうけいぶさいけん	head and neck reconstruction
根治的頸部リンパ節郭清術 こんちてきけいぶ―せっかくせいじゅつ	radical neck dissection (RND)
機能的頸部リンパ節郭清術 きのうてきけいぶ―せっかくせいじゅつ	functional neck dissection (FND)

Tidbits

red herring

臭いの強い燻製ニシンは若い bloodhound を猟犬として訓練する際に用いられたが，これを悪用して17世紀に犯罪者がニシンを引きずって追っ手の bloodhound をごまかそうとしたという．このことから「巧妙な罠にはまって目的を外される」，「人の注意をほかへそらせるもの」という比喩が生まれ，政争や推理小説の話題となったが，回診やカンファレンスでも鑑別診断の議論の中で聞くことがある．ある症状や所見に惑わされて脇道に入り肝心の診断を見失うのが diagnostic red herring である．

5. 口腔，歯

● 愁訴・症状 Complaints / Symptoms ●

味覚 みかく	taste, the sense of taste, gustation, 〔形〕gustatory
食物の味が分からない	be unable to taste
味覚減退 みかくげんたい	gustatory hypesthesia
味覚異常 みかくいじょう	bad taste in the mouth, dysgeusia
錯味覚 さくみかく	parageusia
唾液 だえき	saliva
唾液分泌 だえきぶんぴ	salivation, salivary secretion
よだれをたらす	drool, drivel
アフタ	aphtha
舌痛 ぜっつう	sore tongue, glossalgia, glossodynia
舌灼熱感 ぜっしゃくねつかん	burning tongue, glossopyrosis
みつくち	harelip
口臭 こうしゅう	bad breath, foul breath
口腔衛生 こうくうえいせい	oral hygiene, dental hygiene
歯を磨く はをみがく	brush (clean) one's teeth
歯ブラシ は	toothbrush
デンタルフロス	dental floss
歯間ブラシ しかん	interdental brush
うがい	gargling, 〔動〕gargle, rinse one's mouth
うがい薬 やく	gargle, mouthwash
歯並び はならび	set of teeth
歯茎 はぐき，歯肉 しにく	gums, gingiva, 〔形〕gingival
前歯 まえば	front teeth
奥歯 おくば	back teeth, molars
歯痛 しつう	toothache, 〔動〕have a toothache, one's tooth aches
歯ぎしり は	grinding of teeth, bruxism
虫歯 むしば	decayed (carious, bad) tooth, dental caries, tooth cavity
乳歯 にゅうし	baby teeth, milk teeth
親知らず おやしらず，智歯 ちし	wisdom tooth, third molar tooth
永久歯 えいきゅうし	permanent teeth
出っ歯 でっぱ	buck teeth, protruding teeth
歯石 しせき	tartar, dental calculus
歯垢 しこう	plaque
抜歯 ばっし	extraction of a tooth, 〔動〕extract a tooth, pull out a tooth

歯が抜ける	lose a tooth, a tooth comes out
歯のない	toothless, edentulous, edentate
歯がぐらぐらする	one's tooth feels loose
歯冠をかぶせる	crown
充塡する	fill up, plug
入れ歯, 義歯	artificial (false) tooth, denture, plate, dental prosthesis
総入れ歯	full denture, complete denture
部分入れ歯	partial denture, clasp denture
入れ歯をしている	wear false teeth, wear a denture
入れ歯をはめる（はずす）	put in (take out) one's denture

● 診察所見・徴候　Physical findings / Signs ●

呼気悪臭	halitosis, foetor ex ore, stomatodysodia
尿臭	urine odor, urinous odor
肝性口臭	hepatic fetor
アセトン臭	acetone odor
開口障害	trismus, lockjaw
唾液分泌減少	hypoptyalism
舌偏倚	tongue deviated (to the right / left)
舌肥厚	pachyglossia
巨大舌	macroglossia
舌乳頭	lingual papillae
苔舌	coated tongue, coating of the tongue, furred tongue
いちご舌	strawberry tongue
黒色舌	black tongue, melanoglossia
毛舌	hairy tongue
黒毛舌	black hairy tongue, glossophytia
亀裂舌	fissured tongue, furrowed tongue, scrotal tongue, crocodile tongue
地図状舌	geographic tongue, benign migratory glossitis
舌痙攣	glossospasm
粘液囊胞	mucous cyst
がま腫	ranula, sublingual cyst
歯牙腫	odontoma
エナメル上皮腫	ameloblastoma
白板症	leukoplakia
唾石	sialolith, salivary calculus, salivary stone
コプリック斑	Koplik spots

⟨small red spots on the buccal mucosa seen early in measles⟩

フォーダイス斑 はん	Fordyce spots

⟨ectopic sebaceous glands in labial and buccal areas⟩

歯肉出血 しにくしゅっけつ	gingival hemorrhage
フェニトイン歯肉増殖症 しにくぞうしょくしょう	phenytoin-induced gingival hyperplasia
エプーリス	epulis, localized gingival enlargement
歯式 しき	dental formula
歯列 しれつ	dentition
歯周ポケット ししゅう	periodontal pocket
う歯 うし	dental caries
有歯の ゆうし	dentulous
無歯の むし	edentulous, toothless
歯牙動揺 しがどうよう	tooth mobility
咬耗症 こうもうしょう	attrition
う食窩 うしょくか	dental cavity
斑状歯 はんじょうし	mottled tooth, dental fluorosis
脱落歯 だつらくし	deciduous tooth
未萌出歯 みほうしゅつし	unerupted tooth
埋没歯 まいぼつし	embedded tooth
沈下歯 ちんかし	submerged tooth
弛緩歯 しかんし	loose tooth
裂離歯 れつりし	avulsed tooth, knocked-out tooth
過剰歯 かじょうし	supernumerary tooth
欠損歯 けっそんし	missing tooth
ハッチンソン歯 し	Hutchinson teeth

⟨notched incisors seen in congenital syphilis⟩

間隙 かんげき	diastema, interdental space
不正咬合 ふせいこうごう	malocclusion, uneven bite
遠心咬合 えんしんこうごう	distoclusion
近位咬合 きんいこうごう	mesioclusion
反対咬合 はんたいこうごう	reversed occlusion
小顎症 しょうがくしょう	micrognathia, micrognathism
顎前突症 がくぜんとつしょう	prognathism
下顎前突症 かがくぜんとつしょう	mandibular protrusion
上顎前突症 じょうがくぜんとつしょう	maxillary protrusion
顎後退症 がくこうたいしょう	retrognathism
下顎後退症 かがくこうたいしょう	mandibular retrusion
上顎後退症 じょうがくこうたいしょう	maxillary retrusion

● 検査法　Examination ●

抗 SS-A/Ro 抗体 こうたい	anti-Sjögren syndrome-A/Ro (SS-A/Ro)

	antibody
抗SS-B/La抗体 こうたい	anti-Sjögren syndrome-B/La (SS-B/La) antibody
プラークコントロールレコード	plaque control record
味覚試験 みかくしけん	gustation test
唾液腺造影法 だえきせんぞうえいほう	sialography
唾液腺シンチグラフィー だえきせん	salivary gland scintigraphy, radionuclide sialography
MR唾液腺造影法 だえきせんぞうえいほう	MR sialography
頭部X線規格撮影法 とうぶせんきかくさつえいほう	cephalometric radiography
ウォーターズ撮影法 さつえいほう	Waters projection

〈*occipitomental projection used for viewing the orbits and maxillary sinuses*〉

X線パノラマ撮影法 せんさつえいほう	panoramic radiography, pantomography
咬翼撮影法 こうよくさつえいほう	bite-wing radiography
唾液腺電図 だえきせんでんず	electrosalivogram
電気歯髄診断器 でんきしずいしんだんき	electric pulp tester

● 疾患名　Diseases ●

口唇炎 こうしんえん	cheilitis
口角炎 こうかくえん	angular cheilitis
口角びらん こうかく	perleche, angular stomatitis
口唇ヘルペス こうしん	herpes labialis, cold sore
口唇裂 こうしんれつ	cleft lip, cheiloschisis
アッシャー症候群 しょうこうぐん	Ascher syndrome

〈*congenital double lip with blepharochalasis and nontoxic goiter*〉

口蓋隆起 こうがいりゅうき	torus palatinus, palatal torus
口蓋披裂 こうがいひれつ	cleft palate
唇顎口蓋披裂 しんがくこうがいひれつ	cheilognathouranoschisis
口蓋垂炎 こうがいすいえん	staphylitis, uvulitis
口内炎 こうないえん	stomatitis
アフタ性口内炎 せいこうないえん	aphthous stomatitis
ベーチェット病 びょう	Behçet disease

〈*multisystem vasculitis characterized by recurrent oral aphthous ulceration, genital ulceration, uveitis with hypopyon, and skin lesions*〉

鵞口瘡 がこうそう	thrush, oral candidiasis

5. 口腔，歯

水癌，壊疽性口内炎	noma, gangrenous stomatitis
舌炎	glossitis
ハンター舌炎	Hunter glossitis

⟨atrophic glossitis seen in pernicious anemia⟩

ルードウィッヒアンギーナ，口底蜂巣炎	Ludwig angina

⟨severe cellulitis of the submaxillary, sublingual, and submental spaces from infected molars or penetrating injury of the floor of the mouth⟩

舌癌	lingual cancer, carcinoma of the tongue
流行性耳下腺炎	mumps, epidemic parotitis
唾液腺炎	sialadenitis, sialoadenitis
唾石症	sialolithiasis, ptyalolithiasis
口内乾燥症	xerostomia
シェーグレン症候群	Sjögren syndrome

⟨keratoconjunctivitis sicca, xerostomia, and lacrimal gland enlargement, seen in menopausal women; often associated with rheumatoid arthritis or other connective tissue diseases⟩

ミクリッツ症候群	Mikulicz syndrome

⟨unilateral or bilateral enlargement of the lacrimal, parotid, and salivary glands with xerostomia; associated with sarcoidosis, leukemia, lymphoma, and SLE⟩

フライ症候群	Frey syndrome

⟨auriculotemporal syndrome; localized flushing and sweating of the earlobe and cheek, elicited by eating chocolate or spicy foods; due to injury to the parotid gland or auriculotemporal nerve⟩

歯肉炎	gingivitis
急性壊死性潰瘍性歯肉炎	acute necrotizing ulcerative gingivitis (ANUG)
塹壕口内炎，ヴァンサン口峡炎	trench mouth, Vincent angina

⟨ulceromembranous pharyngitis as spread of ANUG; caused by fusiform and spirochetal organisms⟩

歯冠周囲炎	pericoronitis
歯髄炎	pulpitis
歯原性嚢胞	odontogenic cyst
石灰化歯原性嚢胞	calcifying odontogenic cyst (COC)
歯根嚢胞	radicular cyst
歯槽膿漏	alveolar pyorrhea
歯槽膿瘍	alveolar abscess
歯周炎	periodontitis

IV章 診療録用語

歯周症 (ししゅうしょう)	periodontosis
歯性上顎洞炎 (しせいじょうがくとうえん)	odontogenic maxillary sinusitis
顎関節症 (がくかんせつしょう)	temporomandibular joint disorder

● 治療法　Treatment ●

含嗽薬 (がんそうやく)	gargle
アズレンスルホン酸ナトリウム	azulene sulfonate sodium《アズノール》
ポビドンヨード	povidone-iodine (PVP-I)《イソジンガーグル》
唇形成術 (くちびるけいせいじゅつ)	cheiloplasty
口蓋形成術 (こうがいけいせいじゅつ)	palatoplasty
唾石摘除術 (だせきてきじょじゅつ)	sialolithotomy
舌切除術 (ぜつせつじょじゅつ)	glossectomy
フッ素 (そ)	fluoride
歯石除去 (しせきじょきょ)	scaling
機械的歯面清掃 (きかいてきしめんせいそう)	professional mechanical tooth cleaning
抜歯 (ばっし)	tooth extraction
歯列矯正 (しれつきょうせい)	orthodontics
歯科補綴術 (しかほてつじゅつ)	prosthodontics
橋義歯術 (きょうぎししじゅつ)	bridge prosthodontics
部分床義歯 (ぶぶんしょうぎし)	partial denture
全部床義歯 (ぜんぶしょうぎし)	complete denture, full denture
固定橋義歯 (こていきょうぎし)	fixed bridge, fixed partial denture
美容歯科学 (びようしかがく)	esthetic dentistry, cosmetic dentistry
歯内療法 (しないりょうほう)	endodontics
シーラント, 密閉剤 (みっぺいざい)	sealant
歯冠修復 (しかんしゅうふく)	crown restoration
陶歯冠 (とうしかん)	porcelain crown
根管治療 (こんかんちりょう)	root canal treatment (RCT)
根管充塡 (こんかんじゅうてん)	root canal filling (RCF)
インレー修復 (しゅうふく)	inlay restoration
陶材インレー (とうざい)	porcelain inlay
複合樹脂インレー (ふくごうじゅし)	composite resin inlay
アマルガム修復 (しゅうふく)	amalgam restoration, silver filling
インプラント義歯 (ぎし)	implant denture
抜髄 (ばつずい)	pulp removal
ルートプレーニング	root planing
歯肉皮弁術 (しにくひべんじゅつ)	flap operation
歯根尖切除術 (しこんせんせつじょじゅつ)	apicoectomy
歯周組織再生誘導手術 (ししゅうそしきさいせいゆうどうしゅじゅつ)	guided tissue regeneration (GTR)

骨再生誘導手術 _{こつさいせいゆうどうしゅじゅつ}	guided bone regeneration (GBR)
歯牙移植 _{しがいしょく}	tooth transplantation
歯牙再植 _{しがさいしょく}	tooth replantation

Tidbits

perleche

「ペルレシュ」と読むフランス語である．もっとも本来の perlèche のアクサン・グラーブはしばしば脱落している．口角びらんないし口角炎のことでカンジダや細菌の感染が原因のこともある．相当する英語は angular cheilitis, angular stomatitis, angular cheilosis, intertrigo labialis など．

英語の医学用語の中にはフランス語からの借用語がかなりありドイツ語よりも多い．馴染み深いものに bruit, rale, malaise, cul-de-sac, tamponade, ballottement などがあり，café-au-lait spots (neurofibromatosis と Albright disease のとき) もよく知られている．診断に際しては coeur en sabot, grand mal, petit mal, chancre, tic douloureux が思い浮かぶ．治療に massage, lavage, bougie, douche, débridement は欠かせない．そのほか en bloc, peau d'orange, fourchette, boutonnière deformity, rouleau formation など．最後は morgue.

6. 呼吸器系

● 愁訴・症状 Complaints / Symptoms ●

呼吸器症状 こきゅうきしょうじょう	respiratory symptoms
上気道症状 じょうきどうしょうじょう	symptoms of the upper respiratory tract
呼吸 こきゅう	breathing, respiration, 〔形〕respiratory
吸気 きゅうき	inspiration, 〔形〕inspiratory
呼気 こき	expiration, 〔形〕expiratory
呼吸する こきゅう, 息をする いき	breathe, respire
深呼吸する しんこきゅう	breathe deeply, take a deep breath, draw a deep breath
鼻で(口で)呼吸する はな(くち)こきゅう	breathe through the nose (the mouth)
腹式呼吸 ふくしきこきゅう	abdominal respiration, diaphragmatic respiration
胸式呼吸 きょうしきこきゅう	thoracic respiration, costal respiration
無呼吸 むこきゅう	apnea
息切れ いきぎれ	shortness of breath
息切れがする いきぎれ	be short of breath, be breathless, be short-winded, be out of breath, lose one's breath
呼吸困難 こきゅうこんなん	difficult in breathing, difficult breathing, dyspnea, 〔形〕dyspneic
運動(労作)性呼吸困難 うんどう(ろうさ)せいこきゅうこんなん	exertional dyspnea, dyspnea on exertion (DOE), difficulty in breathing on exertion (exercise, physical activity, effort)
安静時呼吸困難 あんせいじこきゅうこんなん	dyspnea at rest
夜間呼吸困難 やかんこきゅうこんなん	nocturnal dyspnea
頻呼吸 ひんこきゅう	rapid breathing, tachypnea
起座呼吸 きざこきゅう	orthopnea, 〔形〕orthopneic
あえぎ	panting, a pant, a gasp, 〔動〕pant, gasp
ため息 ためいき	sigh, 〔動〕sigh, give a sigh, draw a long breath
喘息 ぜんそく	asthma
喘鳴 ぜんめい, ぜいぜい	wheeze, wheezing, stridor
ぜいぜい息をする いき	wheeze
喘息発作 ぜんそくほっさ	asthmatic attack
くしゃみ	sneezing, 〔動〕sneeze, give a sneeze
窒息 ちっそく	suffocation, asphyxia

6. 呼吸器系　155

息の詰まる感じ いきつかん	choking sensation
窒息する ちっそく	be suffocated, be choked
しゃっくり	hiccups, singultus, 〔動〕hiccup, have the hiccups
咳 せき	cough, coughing, 〔動〕cough, have a cough
咳き込む せきこ	have a fit of coughing, have a paroxysmal cough
咳払いする せきばら	clear the throat
空咳が出る からせきで	have a dry cough, have a nonproductive cough
痰の出る咳 たんせき	productive cough, cough with sputum
痰の切れない苦しい咳 たんくるせき	hacking cough
痰 たん, 喀痰 かくたん	sputum, phlegm, expectoration
痰を喀出する たんかくしゅつ	cough up phlegm, bring up phlegm, expectorate
(痰が)のどにからむ	stick in the throat
粘い (薄い, 濃い, 泡沫状の) 痰 ねばうすこ ほうまつじょう たん	viscid or tenacious (thin, thick, frothy) sputum
粘液状 (膿性, 漿液性) 痰 ねんえきじょう のうせい しょうえきせい たん	mucoid (purulent, serous) sputum
緑色の (黄色の, さび色の) 痰 りょくしょく きいろ さびいろ たん	greenish (yellow, rusty) sputum
血痰 けったん	bloody sputum
血線の混じった痰 けっせんまたん	blood-streaked sputum, bloodstained sputum
血の色をした痰 ちいろたん	blood-tinged sputum
喀血 かっけつ	hemoptysis, bloody expectoration, 〔動〕cough up (expectorate) blood
かぜ	a cold, common cold
鼻かぜ はな	sniffles, snuffles, head cold, coryza
流感 りゅうかん, インフルエンザ	influenza, the flu, grippe
季節性インフルエンザ きせつせい	seasonal influenza
かぜを引く ひ	catch a cold, have a cold
かぜ気味である ぎみ	have a slight (a touch of) cold
かぜを引いて休んでいる	be in bed with a cold
かぜをこじらせる	aggravate one's cold
胸痛 きょうつう (cf. 疼痛)	chest pain

156　IV章　診療録用語

吸気時痛 きゅうきじつう	pain on inspiration
胸膜痛 きょうまくつう	pleuritic pain, pleurodynia
昼間過眠 ちゅうかんかみん	excessive daytime sleepiness (EDS)
ブリンクマン指数 しすう, 喫煙指数 きつえんしすう	Brinkman index (BI)

　〈average amount of tobacco smoked per day × length of time in years〉

| ピクウィック症候群 しょうこうぐん, 肥満低換気症候群 ひまんていかんきしょうこうぐん | pickwickian syndrome |

　〈<Dickens' Pickwick Papers; obesity-hypoventilation syndrome; obesity, daytime somnolence, hypoventilation and erythrocytosis〉

| アスベスト曝露 ばくろ | asbestos exposure |

● 診察所見・徴候　Physical findings / Signs ●

胸郭 きょうかく	thorax,〔形〕thoracic
樽状胸 たるじょうきょう	barrel chest
鳩胸 はとむね	pectus carinatum, chicken breast, pigeon chest
漏斗胸 ろうときょう	pectus excavatum, funnel chest, foveated chest
ハリソン溝 こう	Harrison groove

　〈a horizontal furrow along the lower border of the chest corresponding to the costal insertion of the diaphragm; seen in chronic respiratory diseases and in children with rickets〉

| くる病じゅず じゅず | rachitic rosary |
| ティーツェ症候群 しょうこうぐん | Tietze syndrome |

　〈painful nonsuppurative swelling of costochondral junctions〉

| 正常呼吸 せいじょうこきゅう | eupnea, normal respiration |
| ボルグ指数 しすう | Borg scale |

　〈a measuring system for dyspnea on scale of 0-10, none to maximal〉

呼吸性移動 こきゅうせいいどう	respiratory excursions, breathing movements
気管偏位 きかんへんい	tracheal deviation
気道閉塞 きどうへいそく	airway obstruction
触覚振盪音 しょっかくしんとうおん	tactile fremitus
皮下気腫 ひかきしゅ	subcutaneous emphysema
打診音 だしんおん	percussion sound
共鳴音 きょうめいおん, 清音 せいおん	resonance,〔形〕resonant
濁音 だくおん	dullness,〔形〕dull
破壺共鳴 はこきょうめい	cracked-pot resonance
空洞音性共鳴 くうどうおんせいきょうめい	amphoric resonance

6. 呼吸器系

グロッコ三角 （さんかく）	Grocco triangle

⟨a triangular area of dullness at the base of the chest, on the opposite side to a pleural effusion⟩

ガーランド三角 （さんかく）　Garland triangle

⟨a triangular area of relative resonance in the lower back near the spine, on the same side of a pleural effusion⟩

スコダ共鳴音 （めいおん）　skodaic resonance

⟨<Josef Skoda; increased percussion resonance at the upper part of the chest, above the level of a large pleural effusion⟩

トラウベ半月部 （はんげつぶ）　Traube semilunar space

⟨a tympanitic area bounded by the left costal arch, heart and liver due to the underlying stomach; dull by a pleural effusion⟩

呼吸音 （こきゅうおん）	breath sounds (BS)
肺胞呼吸音 （はいほうこきゅうおん）	vesicular sounds
気管支肺胞呼吸音 （きかんしはいほうこきゅうおん）	bronchovesicular sounds
気管支呼吸音 （きかんしこきゅうおん）	bronchial sounds
気管呼吸音 （きかんこきゅうおん）	tracheal sounds
空洞音 （くうどうおん）	cavernous breath sounds
呼吸音減弱 （こきゅうおんげんじゃく）	decreased breath sounds
喘鳴 （ぜんめい）	stridor
気管支声 （きかんしせい）	bronchophony
胸声 （きょうせい）	pectoriloquy
囁語胸声 （じょごきょうせい）	whispered pectoriloquy, whispered bronchophony
ヤギ声 （せい）	egophony
小児呼吸 （しょうにこきゅう）	puerile breathing
呼気延長 （こきえんちょう）	prolonged expiration
喘息性呼吸 （ぜんそくせいこきゅう）	asthmatic breathing
断続性（歯車様）呼吸 （だんぞくせい（はぐるまよう）こきゅう）	interrupted (cogwheel) breathing
チェーン・ストークス呼吸 （きこう）	Cheyne-Stokes respiration

⟨alternating periods of deep breathing and apnea; seen in coma from affection of nervous centers⟩

ビオー呼吸 （きゅう）　Biot respiration

⟨ataxic breathing characterized by completely irregular pattern, apneic periods alternating with several identical breaths; occurs with increased intracranial pressure⟩

副雑音 （ふくざつおん）	adventitious sounds
ラ音 （おん）	rale
断続性ラ音 （だんぞくせいおん）	discontinuous sounds
水泡音 （すいほうおん）（粗い断続性	coarse crackles

捻髪音 ねんぱつおん（細かい断続性ラ音） fine crackles
連続性ラ音 れんぞくせいらーおん continuous sounds
笛声音 てきせいおん（高音性連続性ラ音） wheezes
類軋音 るいあつおん（低音性連続性ラ音） rhonchi
声音振盪 せいおんしんとう vocal fremitus
胸膜摩擦音 きょうまくまさつおん pleural friction rub
胸水 きょうすい pleural effusion
ハマン徴候 ―ちょうこう Hamman sign
〈*precordial crunching sound synchronous with each heart beat indicating pneumothorax, pneumomediastinum, or mediastinitis*〉
チアノーゼ cyanosis,〔形〕cyanotic
ばち指 ―ゆび clubbed finger, clubbing of digits
肺性肥厚性骨関節症 はいせいひこうせいこつかんせつしょう hypertrophic pulmonary osteoarthropathy（HPO）
MRC 息切れスケール ―いきぎれ― MRC dyspnea scale（British Medical Research Council）
ウィリアムソン徴候 Williamson sign
〈*much lower BP in the leg as opposed to the arm on the same side; seen in pneumothorax or pleural effusion*〉
ホルネル症候群 ―しょうこうぐん Horner syndrome
〈*unilateral ptosis, miosis, and anhidrosis due to destruction of ipsilateral cervical sympathetic nerve supply, often from lung cancer*〉
パンコースト症候群 Pancoast syndrome
〈*weakness and pain of the arm, and Horner syndrome due to neoplastic involvement of brachial plexus and sympathetic ganglia*〉
ランバート・イートン筋無力症候群 ―きんむりょくしょうこうぐん Lambert-Eaton myasthenic syndrome（LEMS）
〈*an autoimmune myasthenic syndrome with weakness in pelvic and thigh muscles, dry mouth, impotence, and decreased DTRs; often associated with small-cell lung carcinoma*〉

● 検査法　Examination ●

ツベルクリン試験 ―けんし，マントー反応 ―のうはんのう tuberculin test, Mantoux test, tine test, PPD（purified protein derivative）test
動脈血ガス どうみゃくけつ― arterial blood gas（ABG）
パルスオキシメトリー pulse oximetry
水素イオン濃度 すいそ―のうど hydrogen ion concentration（pH）
重炭酸イオン濃度 bicarbonate concentration

動脈血酸素分圧	arterial oxygen tension (PaO$_2$)
動脈血炭酸ガス分圧	arterial carbon dioxide tension (PaCO$_2$)
動脈血酸素飽和度	arterial oxygen saturation (SaO$_2$)
経皮的動脈血酸素飽和度	oxygen saturation by pulse oximetry (SpO$_2$)
肺胞気−動脈血ガス分圧較差	alveolar-arterial gas tension difference
肺胞気−動脈血酸素分圧較差	alveolar-arterial oxygen difference (AaDO$_2$)
肺胞気−動脈血二酸化炭素分圧較差	alveolar-arterial carbon dioxide difference (AaDCO$_2$)
肺胞気−動脈血窒素分圧較差	alveolar-arterial nitrogen difference (AaDN$_2$)
塩基過剰	base excess (BE)
陰イオンギャップ	anion gap (AG)
低酸素症	hypoxia
低酸素血症	hypoxemia
高炭酸ガス血症	hypercapnia
二酸化炭素ナルコーシス	carbon dioxide narcosis, CO$_2$ narcosis
呼吸性アシドーシス	respiratory acidosis
Dダイマー	D dimer
ロイコトリエン	leukotriene (LT)
遅反応性アナフィラキシー物質	slow reacting substance of anaphylaxis (SRS-A)
クレオラ体	creola body
サーファクタントプロテインA	surfactant protein A
サーファクタントプロテインD	surfactant protein D
好酸球塩基性タンパク	eosinophilic cationic proteins (ECP)
クルシュマンらせん体	Curschmann spiral
	⟨*corkscrew-shaped mucinous fibrils found in the sputum in asthma*⟩
喀痰培養	sputum culture
インフルエンザ菌	*Haemophilus influenzae*

肺炎桿菌	*Klebsiella pneumoniae*
肺炎球菌	*Streptococcus pneumoniae, Pneumococcus*
ペニシリン耐性肺炎球菌	penicillin-resistant *Streptococcus pneumoniae* (PRSP)
モラクセラ・カタラーリス	*Moraxella catarrhalis*
レジオネラ・ニューモフィーラ	*Legionella pneumophila*
肺炎マイコプラズマ	*Mycoplasma pneumoniae*
肺炎クラミジア	*Chlamydophila pneumoniae*
結核菌	*Mycobacterium tuberculosis*
非結核性抗酸菌	nontuberculous mycobacterium (NTM)
トリ型結核菌複合体	mycobacterium avium complex (MAC)
カンサシー抗酸菌	*Mycobacterium kansasii*
ニューモシスチス・イロベチ	*Pneumocystis jiroveci*
アデノウイルス	*Adenovirus*
ライノウイルス	*Rhinovirus*
インフルエンザウイルスA型	*Influenza A virus*
インフルエンザウイルスB型	*Influenza B virus*
コロナウイルス	*Coronavirus*
トリインフルエンザウイルス	avian influenza virus
ブタ由来インフルエンザウイルスA型	swine-origin influenza A virus (S-OIV)
パラインフルエンザウイルス	parainfluenza virus
ガフキー号数	Gaffky scale
	⟨*a scale based on the number of tubercle bacilli in the sputum*⟩
インターフェロンγ放出アッセイ	interferon-gamma release assay (IGRA)
クオンティフェロンTB試験	QuantiFERON-TB (QFT) test
抗インフルエンザウイルス抗体	anti-influenza virus antibody
インフルエンザウイルス抗原	influenza virus antigen
赤血球吸着ウイルス	hemadsorption virus

6. 呼吸器系

赤血球吸着試験	hemadsorption test
胸部単純撮影法	plain chest radiography
胸部X線写真	chest roentgenogram, chest x-ray (CXR)
放射線不透過性	radiopacity, 〔形〕radiopaque
放射線透過性	radiolucency, 〔形〕radiolucent
肺紋理	pulmonary markings, lung markings
肺門陰影	hilar shadow
気管支含気像	air bronchogram
スワイヤ・ジェームス症候群	Swyer-James syndrome

〈*unilateral hyperlucent lung; caused by obliterating bronchiolitis in childhood*〉

両側肺門リンパ節腫大	bilateral hilar lymphadenopathy (BHL)
レフグレン症候群	Löfgren syndrome

〈*bilateral hilar lymphadenopathy with erythema nodosum, indicating sarcoidosis*〉

円形陰影	coin lesion
浸潤像	infiltrate
硬化像	consolidation
石灰化	calcification
肺胸膜嚢胞	bleb
空洞	cavity, cavitation
肺尖帽	apical cap
スリガラス様陰影	ground glass appearance
粟粒陰影	miliary shadow
蜂巣状肺	honeycomb lung
板状無気肺	platelike atelectasis, subsegmental atelectasis
肋骨横隔膜角鈍化	blunting of the costophrenic angle
断層撮影法	tomography, laminography, laminagraphy
気管支造影法	bronchography
肺血管造影法	pulmonary angiography
気管支動脈造影法	bronchial arteriography (BAG)
気体縦隔造影法	pneumomediastinography
換気血流スキャン	ventilation-perfusion scan

IV章 診療録用語

血管外肺水分量	extravascular lung water (EVLW)
肺機能検査	pulmonary function test (PFT)
肺活量計	spirometer
肺活量測定	spirometry
全肺気量	total lung capacity (TLC)
肺活量	vital capacity (VC)
最大吸気量	inspiratory capacity (IC)
1回換気量	tidal volume (TV)
予備吸気量	inspiratory reserve volume (IRV)
機能的残気量	functional residual capacity (FRC)
残気量	residual volume (RV)
呼気予備量	expiratory reserve volume (ERV)
努力呼気曲線	maximal expiratory flow-volume curve
努力肺活量	forced expiratory volume (FEV)
1秒量	forced expiratory volume in one second ($FEV_{1.0}$)
1秒率	percent of one second forced expiratory volume ($FEV_{1.0\%}$)
最大呼気流量	peak expiratory flow (PEF)
最大呼気流量計	peak flow meter (PFM)
最大呼気速度	peak expiratory flow rate (PEFR)
最大中間呼気流量率	maximal mid-expiratory flow rate (MMEFR)
一酸化炭素肺拡散能	diffusing capacity of the lung for carbon monoxide (DL_{CO})
吸入酸素濃度	fraction of inspired oxygen (FIO_2)
呼気分析	expired-air analysis
呼気炭酸ガス分圧	expired carbon dioxide tension
呼気中一酸化炭素濃度	expired carbon monoxide concentration
呼気中一酸化窒素濃度	expired nitric oxide concentration
フローボリューム曲線	flow-volume curve
気道可逆性試験	airway reversibility test
気道過敏性試験	bronchial hyperreactivity test
肺換気受容体	ventilatory receptor
プレチスモグラフィー	plethysmography
ポリソムノグラフィー	polysomnography (PSG)
無呼吸指数	apnea index (AI)

6. 呼吸器系　163

無呼吸低換気指数	apnea-hypopnea index (AHI)
睡眠潜時反復検査	multiple sleep latency test (MSLT)
気管支内超音波断層法	endobronchial ultrasonography (EBUS)
気管支鏡検査	bronchoscopy
気管支肺胞洗浄	bronchoalveolar lavage (BAL)
気管支肺胞洗浄液	bronchoalveolar lavage fluid (BALF)
経気管支生検	transbronchial biopsy (TBB)
経気管支吸引生検	transbronchial aspiration biopsy (TBAB)
経気管支肺生検	transbronchial lung biopsy (TBLB)
経気管吸引生検	transtracheal aspiration biopsy (TTAB)
胸腔鏡検査	thoracoscopy
胸腔鏡下生検	thoracoscopic biopsy
胸腔穿刺	thoracentesis, thoracocentesis
縦隔鏡検査	mediastinoscopy

● 疾患名　Diseases ●

上気道感染症	upper respiratory tract infection (URI)
かぜ症候群	common cold syndrome
閉塞性肺疾患	obstructive lung disease
拘束性肺疾患	restrictive lung disease
気管支炎	bronchitis
喘息性気管支炎	asthmatic bronchitis
気管支喘息	bronchial asthma (BA)
運動誘発喘息	exercise-induced asthma (EIA)
副鼻腔気管支症候群	sinobronchial syndrome (SBS)
肺炎	pneumonia
市中肺炎	community-acquired pneumonia
院内肺炎	hospital-acquired pneumonia (HAP), nosocomial pneumonia
誤嚥性肺炎	aspiration pneumonia
メンデルソン症候群	Mendelson syndrome

⟨pulmonary acid aspiration syndrome; aspiration of gastric contents causes chemical pneumonitis and subsequent ARDS⟩

| 原発性異型肺炎 | primary atypical pneumonia (PAP) |
| 過敏性肺炎 | hypersensitivity pneumonia |

IV章 診療録用語

急性好酸球性肺炎	acute eosinophilic pneumonia (AEP)
慢性好酸球性肺炎	chronic eosinophilic pneumonia (CEP)
肺好酸球浸潤	pulmonary infiltration with eosinophilia (PIE)
レフレル症候群	Löffler syndrome ⟨*transient pulmonary infiltrates with eosinophilia; possible parasitic infestation*⟩
人工呼吸器関連肺炎	ventilator-associated pneumonia (VAP)
放射線肺炎	radiation pneumonitis
間質性肺炎	interstitial pneumonia
特発性間質性肺炎	idiopathic interstitial pneumonia (IIP)
特発性肺線維症, ハマン・リッチ症候群	idiopathic pulmonary fibrosis (IPF), Hamman-Rich syndrome
通常型間質性肺炎	usual interstitial pneumonia (UIP)
呼吸細気管支炎関連間質性肺疾患	respiratory bronchiolitis-associated interstitial lung disease (RB-ILD)
急性間質性肺炎	acute interstitial pneumonia (AIP)
非特異性間質性肺炎	nonspecific interstitial pneumonia (NSIP)
リンパ球性間質性肺炎	lymphocytic interstitial pneumonia (LIP)
器質化肺炎を伴う閉塞性細気管支炎	bronchiolitis obliterans with organizing pneumonia (BOOP)
特発性器質化肺炎	cryptogenic organizing pneumonitis (COP)
剝離性間質性肺炎	desquamative interstitial pneumonia (DIP)
びまん性汎細気管支炎	diffuse panbronchiolitis (DPB)
間質性肺疾患	interstitial lung disease (ILD)
気管支拡張症	bronchiectasis
原発性線毛機能不全	primary ciliary dyskinesia (PCD)
慢性閉塞性肺疾患	chronic obstructive pulmonary disease

6. 呼吸器系

慢性閉塞性肺疾患	(COPD)
慢性気管支炎	chronic bronchitis
肺気腫	pulmonary emphysema
先天性肺嚢胞性腺腫様奇形	congenital cystic adenomatoid malformation of lung (CCAM)
在郷軍人病	legionnaires disease
肺結核	pulmonary tuberculosis (TB)
多剤耐性結核	multidrug-resistant tuberculosis (MDR-TB)
非結核性抗酸菌症	nontuberculous mycobacteriosis
真菌性肺疾患	fungal lung disease
肺アスペルギルス症	pulmonary aspergillosis
肺アスペルギローム	pulmonary aspergilloma
アレルギー性気管支肺アスペルギルス症	allergic bronchopulmonary aspergillosis (ABPA)
肺クリプトコックス症	pulmonary cryptococcosis
肺カンジダ症	pulmonary candidiasis
ニューモシスチス肺炎	pneumocystis pneumonia (PCP)
無気肺	atelectasis, 〔形〕atelectatic
嚢胞性線維症	cystic fibrosis (CF)
塵肺	pneumoconiosis
カプラン症候群	Caplan syndrome

〈*pneumoconiosis with rheumatoid arthritis; multiple nodular infiltrates in both lungs*〉

珪肺症	silicosis
石綿肺	asbestosis
肺胞タンパク症	pulmonary alveolar proteinosis (PAP)
サルコイドーシス	sarcoidosis
ヘールフォルト症候群	Heerfoldt syndrome

〈*uveoparotid fever; a form of sarcoidosis with parotid enlargement, uveitis, and Bell palsy*〉

ウェゲナー肉芽腫症	Wegener granulomatosis

〈*necrotizing granulomas of the respiratory tract and glomerulonephritis; the underlying condition is systemic vasculitis*〉

チャーグ・ストラウス症候群	Churg-Strauss syndrome

⟨allergic granulomatous angiitis, i.e. AGA; characterized by asthma, fever, eosinophilia, and granulomatous reactions⟩

肺塞栓症 はいそくせんしょう	pulmonary embolism (PE)
肺塞栓血栓症 はいそくせんけっせんしょう	pulmonary thromboembolism (PTE)
肺梗塞 はいこうそく	pulmonary infarction
肺水腫 はいすいしゅ	pulmonary edema
高地肺水腫 こうちはいすいしゅ	high-altitude pulmonary edema (HAPE)
肺癌 はいがん	lung cancer (LC), bronchogenic carcinoma
小細胞肺癌 しょうさいぼうはいがん	small cell lung carcinoma (SCLC)
非小細胞肺癌 ひしょうさいぼうはいがん	non-small cell lung carcinoma (NSCLC)
大細胞肺癌 だいさいぼうはいがん	large cell lung carcinoma
扁平上皮癌 へんぺいじょうひがん	squamous cell carcinoma (SCC)
肺腺癌 はいせんがん	adenocarcinoma of lung
細気管支肺胞上皮癌 さいきかんしはいほうじょうひがん	bronchioloalveolar cell carcinoma (BAC)
非定型的腺腫様過形成 ひていけいてきせんしゅようかけいせい	atypical adenomatous hyperplasia
肺リンパ脈管筋腫症 はい—みゃくかんきんしゅしょう	pulmonary lymphangioleiomyomatosis (LAM)
上大静脈症候群 じょうだいじょうみゃくしょうこうぐん	superior vena cava syndrome (SVCS)
肺高血圧症 はいこうけつあつしょう	pulmonary hypertension (PH)
原発性肺高血圧症 げんぱつせいはいこうけつあつしょう	primary pulmonary hypertension (PPH)
慢性血栓塞栓性肺高血圧症 まんせいけっせんそくせんせいはいこうけつあつしょう	chronic thromboembolic pulmonary hypertension (CTEPH)
中葉症候群 ちゅうようしょうこうぐん	middle lobe syndrome
急性肺損傷 きゅうせいはいそんしょう	acute lung injury (ALI)
急性呼吸促迫症候群 きゅうせいこきゅうそくはくしょうこうぐん	acute respiratory distress syndrome (ARDS)
びまん性肺胞傷害 —せいはいほうしょうがい	diffuse alveolar damage (DAD)
重症急性呼吸器症候群 じゅうしょうきゅうせいこきゅうきしょうこうぐん	severe acute respiratory syndrome (SARS)
急性呼吸不全 きゅうせいこきゅうふぜん	acute respiratory failure (ARF)
輸血関連急性肺傷害 ゆけつかんれんきゅうせいはいしょうがい	transfusion-related acute lung injury (TRALI)
慢性呼吸不全 まんせいこきゅうふぜん	chronic respiratory failure (CRF)
過換気症候群 かかんきしょうこうぐん	hyperventilation syndrome (HVS)
低換気症候群 ていかんきしょうこうぐん	hypoventilation syndrome
肺胞低換気症候群	alveolar hypoventilation syndrome

6. 呼吸器系

中枢性肺胞低換気症候群	central alveolar hypoventilation syndrome (CAHS)
睡眠時呼吸障害	sleep-disordered breathing (SDB)
睡眠時無呼吸症候群	sleep apnea syndrome (SAS)
閉塞性睡眠時無呼吸症候群	obstructive sleep apnea syndrome (OSAS)
胸膜炎	pleuritis, pleurisy, [形]pleuritic
気胸	pneumothorax
水胸	hydrothorax
血胸	hemothorax
膿胸	pyothorax, pleural empyema
悪性胸膜中皮腫	pleural malignant mesothelioma
縦隔炎	mediastinitis
縦隔気腫	mediastinal emphysema, pneumomediastinum
縦隔腫瘍	mediastinal tumor

● 治療法 Treatment ●

呼吸療法	respiratory therapy, respiratory care
鎮咳薬	antitussive, cough medicine
リン酸コデイン	codeine phosphate
デキストロメトルファン臭化水素酸塩	dextromethorphan hydrobromide hydrate《メジコン》
去痰薬	expectorant
アセチルシステイン	acetylcysteine《ムコフィリン》
気管支拡張薬	bronchodilator
呼吸促進薬	respiratory stimulant
キサンチン誘導体	xanthine derivatives
アミノフィリン	aminophylline《ネオフィリン》
ロイコトリエン拮抗薬	leukotriene antagonist
プランルカスト水和物	pranlukast hydrate《オノン》
メディエーター抑制薬	mediator inhibitor
クロモグリク酸ナトリウム	disodium cromoglycate (DSCG)《インタール》
オマリズマブ	omalizumab《ゾレア》
ノイラミニダーゼ阻害薬	neuraminidase inhibitor

オセルタミビルリン酸塩 そがいやく	oseltamivir phosphate 《タミフル》
ザナミビル水和物 すいわぶつ	zanamivir hydrate 《リレンザ》
ペラミビル	peramivir 《ラピアクタ》
アマンタジン塩酸塩	amantadine hydrochloride 《シンメトレル》
ピルフェニドン	pirfenidone 《ピレスパ》
イソニアジド	isoniazid, isonicotinic acid hydrazide (INH) 《イスコチン》
リファンピシン	rifampicin (RFP) 《リマクタン》
ピラジナミド	pyrazinamide (PZA) 《ピラマイド》
エタンブトール塩酸塩	ethambutol hydrochloride (EB) 《エブトール》
硫酸ストレプトマイシン りゅうさん	streptomycin sulfate (SM) 《硫酸ストレプトマイシン》
エチオナミド	ethionamide (ETH) 《ツベルミン》
サイクロセリン	cycloserine (CS) 《サイクロセリン》
ゲムシタビン塩酸塩	gemsitabine hydrochloride 《ジェムザール》
ゲフィチニブ	gefitinib 《イレッサ》
エルロチニブ	erlotinib 《タルセバ》
ペメトレキセドナトリウム水和物	pemetrexed sodium hydrate 《アリムタ》
肺炎球菌ワクチン はいえんきゅうきん	pneumococcal vaccine 《ニューモバックス NP》
ハイムリック法 ほう	Heimlich maneuver

⟨*forcible pressure to the epigastrium with a quick upward thrust to dislodge an obstructing material from the throat*⟩

口腔内装具 こうくうないそうぐ	oral appliance
気管内挿管 きかんないそうかん	endotracheal intubation
気管チューブ きかん	tracheal tube, endotracheal tube (ETT)
気管内吸引 きかんないきゅういん	tracheal suctioning
酸素療法 さんそりょうほう	oxygen therapy, oxygen inhalation therapy
酸素マスク さんそ	oxygen mask
部分再呼吸マスク ぶぶんさいこきゅう	partial rebreathing mask
非再呼吸式マスク ひさいこきゅうしき	nonrebreathing mask
ベンチュリマスク	Venturi mask

⟨*a face mask enabling a controlled mixture of oxygen and air*⟩

鼻カニューレ び	nasal cannula, nasal prongs

6. 呼吸器系

酸素テント さんそ	oxygen tent
在宅酸素療法 ざいたくさんそりょうほう	home oxygen therapy (HOT)
肺清掃 はいせいそう	pulmonary toilet, bronchopulmonary hygiene
吸入療法 きゅうにゅうりょうほう	inhalation therapy
吸入器 きゅうにゅうき	inhaler, inhalator
定量吸入器 ていりょうきゅうにゅうき	metered-dose inhaler (MDI)
ネブライザー	nebulizer
エアゾール	aerosol
短時間作用型吸入 β_2 刺激薬 たんじかんさようがたきゅうにゅう——しげきやく	short-acting inhaled β_2-agonist (SABA)
長時間作用型吸入 β_2 刺激薬 ちょうじかんさようがたきゅうにゅう——しげきやく	long-acting inhaled β_2-agonist (LABA)
サルメテロール	salmeterol《セレベント》
吸入ステロイド薬 きゅうにゅう——やく	inhaled corticosteroids
ベクロメタゾンプロピオン酸エステル ——さん——	beclomethasone dipropionate (BDP)《キュバール》
フルチカゾンプロピオン酸エステル ——さん——	fluticasone propionate (FP)《フルタイド》
ブデソニド	budesonide (BUD)《パルミコート》
吸入ステロイド・長時間作用型吸入 β_2 刺激薬合剤 きゅうにゅう————・ちょうじかんさようがたきゅうにゅう——しげきやくごうざい	combination inhaled corticosteroid and long-acting inhaled β_2-agonist《アドエア》
呼吸リハビリテーション こきゅう——	pulmonary rehabilitation
胸部理学療法 きょうぶりがくりょうほう	chest physiotherapy
呼吸訓練 こきゅうくんれん	breathing exercise
スパイロメータ呼吸訓練 ——こきゅうくんれん	incentive spirometry
呼吸筋トレーニング こきゅうきん——	respiratory muscles training
体位性排液法 たいいせいはいえきほう	postural drainage
経鼻気管吸引 けいびきかんきゅういん	nasotracheal suctioning
気管支肺洗浄 きかんしはいせんじょう	bronchopulmonary lavage
胸腔洗浄 きょうくうせんじょう	pleural lavage
胸腔ドレーン きょうくう——	thoracostomy tube
禁煙外来 きんえんがいらい	smoking cessation clinic
ニコチン貼付剤 ——ちょうふざい	nicotine patches
人工呼吸 じんこうこきゅう	artificial respiration, assisted ventilation
人工呼吸器 じんこうこきゅうき	respirator, mechanical ventilator
機械的換気 きかいてきかんき	mechanical ventilation

IV章 診療録用語

調節呼吸 ちょうせつこきゅう	controlled mechanical ventilation (CMV)
圧補助換気 あつほじょかんき	pressure support ventilation
非侵襲的陽圧換気 ひしんしゅうてきようあつかんき	noninvasive positive pressure ventilation (NIPPV)
持続陽圧換気 じぞくようあつかんき	continuous positive pressure ventilation (CPPV)
持続陽圧呼吸 じぞくようあつこきゅう	continuous positive pressure breathing (CPPB)
持続気道陽圧呼吸 じぞくきどうようあつこきゅう	continuous positive airway pressure (CPAP)
間欠陽圧呼吸 かんけつようあつこきゅう	intermittent positive pressure breathing (IPPB)
経鼻的持続気道陽圧呼吸 けいびてきじぞくきどうようあつこきゅう	nasal continuous positive airway pressure (NCPAP)
間欠的強制換気 かんけつてきょうせいかんき	intermittent mandatory ventilation (IMV)
同期式間欠的強制換気 どうきしきかんけつてききょうせいかんき	synchronized intermittent mandatory ventilation (SIMV)
二相性陽性気道内圧 にそうせいようせいきどうないあつ	biphasic positive airway pressure (BiPAP)
呼気終末陽圧呼吸 こきしゅうまつようあつこきゅう	positive end-expiratory pressure (PEEP)
陽陰圧換気 よういんあつかんき	positive negative pressure ventilation (PNPV)
高頻度人工換気 こうひんどじんこうかんき	high-frequency oscillation (HFO)
気管支動脈塞栓術 きかんしどうみゃくそくせんじゅつ	bronchial arterial embolization (BAE)
気管支動脈注入 きかんしどうみゃくちゅうにゅう	bronchial arterial infusion (BAI)
光線力学療法 こうせんりきがくりょうほう	photodynamic therapy (PDT)
ポルフィマーナトリウム	porfimer sodium《フォトフリン》
タラポルフィンナトリウム	talaporfirin sodium《レザフィリン》
ビデオ下胸腔鏡手術 ―かきょうくうきょうしゅじゅつ	video-assisted thoracoscopic surgery (VATS)
胸腔鏡下肺嚢胞切除 きょうくうきょうかはいのうほうせつじょ	thoracoscopic bullectomy
胸腔鏡下肺全摘 きょうくうきょうかはいぜんてき	thoracoscopic pneumonectomy
気管切開 きかんせっかい	tracheostomy, tracheotomy
開胸術 かいきょうじゅつ	thoracotomy
胸郭形成術 きょうかくけいせいじゅつ	thoracoplasty
胸膜癒着術 きょうまくゆちゃくじゅつ	pleurodesis

胸膜剝離術 きょうまくはくりじゅつ	pleurolysis
肺塞栓除去術 はいそくせんじょきょじゅつ	pulmonary embolectomy
肺全摘除術 はいぜんてきじょじゅつ	total pneumonectomy
肺葉切除術 はいようせつじょじゅつ	pulmonary lobectomy
肺容量減少術 はいようりょうげんしょうじゅつ	lung volume reduction surgery (LVRS)
肺移植 はいいしょく	lung transplantation
人工肺 じんこうはい	artificial lung

Tidbits

Sutton's law

医学生や研修医が稀有の診断名を並べる傾向を戒める「法則」. 有名な銀行強盗 Willie Sutton は, 何故銀行ばかり狙うのかと尋ねられて, "Cause that's where the money is, you idiot!" と答えたという. ありふれた当然の診断をまず考えなさいという教訓. 同様の意味で, "When you hear hoofbeats in Texas, think horses, not zebras." も cliché となっている.

7. 循環器系

● 愁訴・症状　Complaints / Symptoms ●

心臓の症状 しんぞうのしょうじょう	cardiac symptoms, heart problems, heart trouble
心臓が悪い しんぞうがわるい	have heart trouble, have a weak heart
心臓発作 しんぞうほっさ	heart attack
狭心症発作 きょうしんしょうほっさ	anginal attack
心臓麻痺 しんぞうまひ	heart failure, cardiac arrest
脈 みゃく	pulse, pulsation
脈を打つ みゃくをうつ	pulsate, pulse, throb
頻脈 ひんみゃく	rapid pulse, rapid heartbeat, tachycardia
徐脈 じょみゃく	slow pulse, slow heartbeat, bradycardia
不整脈 ふせいみゃく	irregular pulse, arrhythmia
結滞 けったい	pause in the pulse, skipped pulse, skipped heartbeat
心臓の鼓動 しんぞうのこどう, 心拍 しんぱく	heartbeat
動悸 どうき, 心悸亢進 しんきこうしん	palpitation
動悸がする どうきがする	palpitate, throb
めまい	dizziness, light-headedness, vertigo, 〔形〕dizzy, light-headed, vertiginous
体位性失神 たいいせいしっしん	postural syncope
血圧 けつあつ	blood pressure
血圧を計る けつあつをはかる	take one's blood pressure, measure one's blood pressure
血圧が高い(低い) けつあつがたかい(ひくい)	have high (low) blood pressure
息切れ いきぎれ, 呼吸困難 こきゅうこんなん (cf. 呼吸器系)	shortness of breath, dyspnea
発作性夜間呼吸困難 ほっさせいやかんこきゅうこんなん	paroxysmal nocturnal dyspnea (PND)
胸痛 きょうつう (cf. 疼痛)	chest pain
息が詰まる痛み いきがつまるいたみ	choking pain, suffocative pain
絞扼痛 こうやくつう	tight pain, constricting pain, band-like (vise-like) pain
圧迫痛 あっぱくつう	pressing (squeezing) pain
腕と頚に放散する うでとくびにほうさんする	radiate to arms and neck
胸部不快感 きょうぶふかいかん	discomfort in the chest
前胸部圧迫感 ぜんきょうぶあっぱくかん	precordial oppression

締めつけられる感じ	tightness in the chest, constriction
心臓の雑音	heart murmur, cardiac murmur
循環	circulation
血液の循環が良い(悪い)	have a good (poor) circulation of blood
間欠性跛行	intermittent claudication
浮腫, むくみ	edema, swelling
足首のむくみ	ankle swelling

● 診察所見・徴候　Physical findings / Signs ●

血圧 (左腕, 臥位)	blood pressure (left arm, supine)
血圧 (右腕, 座位)	blood pressure (right arm, sitting)
白衣高血圧	white-coat hypertension
仮面高血圧	masked hypertension
足関節上腕血圧比	ankle-brachial index (ABI)
ヒル徴候	Hill sign

⟨*disproportionate femoral systolic hypertension, 60-100 mmHg higher than brachial, in aortic regurgitation*⟩

脈, 脈拍	pulse
硬脈	hard pulse, pulsus durus
軟脈	soft pulse, pulsus mollis
実脈	full pulse, strong pulse, pulsus plenus
虚脈	weak pulse, pulsus vacuus
速脈	quick pulse, pulsus celer
遅脈	prolonged pulse, pulsus tardus
交互脈	alternating pulse, pulsus alternans
奇脈	paradoxic pulse, pulsus paradoxus
虚脱脈	collapsing pulse, water-hammer pulse, cannonball pulse
コリガン脈	Corrigan pulse

⟨*a full, hard pulse followed by a sudden collapse in aortic regurgitation*⟩

二峰性脈	bisferious pulse, pulsus bisferiens
二段脈	bigeminal pulse, pulsus bigeminus, bigeminy
三段脈	trigeminy
二重脈	pulsus duplex, dicrotic pulse
脈拍欠損	pulse deficit
洞調律	sinus rhythm

IV章 診療録用語

不整脈 ふせいみゃく	arrhythmia
洞不整脈 どうふせいみゃく	sinus arrhythmia
洞頻脈 どうひんみゃく	sinus tachycardia
洞徐脈 どうじょみゃく	sinus bradycardia
呼吸性洞不整脈 こきゅうせいどうふせいみゃく	respiratory sinus arrhythmia
体位性起立性頻拍症候群 たいいせいきりつせいひんぱくしょうこうぐん	postural orthostatic tachycardia syndrome (POTS)
発作性心房頻拍 ほっさせいしんぼうひんぱく	paroxysmal atrial tachycardia (PAT)
異所性心房頻拍, 自動能性心房頻拍 いしょせいしんぼうひんぱく, じどうのうせいしんぼうひんぱく	ectopic atrial tachycardia (EAT), automatic atrial tachycardia (AAT)
多源性心房頻拍 たげんせいしんぼうひんぱく	multifocal atrial tachycardia (MAT), chaotic atrial tachycardia
上室性頻拍 じょうしつせいひんぱく	supraventricular tachycardia (SVT)
房室回帰頻拍 ぼうしつかいきひんぱく	atrioventricular reciprocating tachycardia (AVRT)
洞結節リエントリー頻拍 どうけっせつ——ひんぱく	sinus nodal reentry tachycardia, sinus nodal reentrant tachycardia (SNRT)
房室結節リエントリー頻拍 ぼうしつけっせつ——ひんぱく	atrioventricular nodal reentry tachycardia, atrioventricular nodal reentrant tachycardia (AVNRT)
心室性頻拍 しんしつせいひんぱく	ventricular tachycardia (VT)
促進心室固有調律 そくしんしんしつこゆうちょうりつ	accelerated idioventricular rhythm (AIVR)
心房細動 しんぼうさいどう	atrial fibrillation (AF)
非弁膜症性心房細動 ひべんまくしょうせいしんぼうさいどう	non-valvular atrial fibrillation (NVAF)
心房粗動 しんぼうそどう	atrial flutter (AF)
徐脈頻脈症候群 じょみゃくひんみゃくしょうこうぐん	bradycardia-tachycardia syndrome, brady-tachy syndrome
心室細動 しんしつさいどう	ventricular fibrillation (VF)
ブルガダ症候群 こうぐん	Brugada syndrome
	⟨*sudden VF in a healthy person resulting in sudden death; a channellopathy, autosomal dominant*⟩
心房期外収縮 しんぼうきがいしゅうしゅく	atrial premature complex (contraction) (APC), premature atrial contraction (PAC), atrial extrasystole
心室期外収縮 しんしつせいきがいしゅうしゅく	ventricular premature complex (contraction) (VPC), premature ventricular contraction (PVC), ventricular extrasystole
頸静脈怒張 けいじょうみゃくどちょう	jugular venous distention (JVD)

7. 循環器系

肝頸静脈逆流 かんけいじょうみゃくぎゃくりゅう	hepatojugular reflux (HJR)
心濁音界 しんだくおんかい	area of cardiac dullness
心尖拍動 しんせんはくどう	apex beat
最強拍動点 さいきょうはくどうてん	point of maximal impulse (PMI)
肋間腔 ろっかんくう	intercostal space (ICS)
胸骨左縁 きょうこつさえん	left sternal border (LSB)
胸骨右縁 きょうこつうえん	right sternal border (RSB)
心肥大 しんひだい	cardiomegaly, cardiac enlargement
左室肥大 さしつひだい	left ventricular hypertrophy (LVH)
右室肥大 うしつひだい	right ventricular hypertrophy (RVH)
振戦 しんせん	thrill
心音 しんおん	heart sounds, cardiac sounds
第1（2，3，4）心音 だい1（2，3，4）しんおん	first (second, third, fourth) heart sound (S1, S2, S3, S4)
大動脈（肺動脈）第2音 だいどうみゃく（はいどうみゃく）だい2おん	aortic (pulmonic) second sound (A2, P2)
クリック	click
駆出音 くしゅつおん	ejection sound
開放音 かいほうおん	opening snap (OS)
奔馬調律 ほんばちょうりつ	gallop rhythm
心音の分裂 しんおん―ぶんれつ	splitting of heart sounds
心雑音 しんざつおん	cardiac murmurs, heart murmurs
器質性雑音 きしつせいざつおん	organic murmur
非器質性雑音 ひきしつせいざつおん，機能性雑音 きのうせいざつおん，無害性雑音 むがいせいざつおん	inorganic murmur, functional murmur, innocent murmur
収縮期雑音 しゅうしゅくきざつおん	systolic murmur
拡張期雑音 かくちょうきざつおん	diastolic murmur
収縮早期雑音 しゅうしゅくそうきざつおん	early systolic murmur
拡張早期雑音 かくちょうそうきざつおん	early diastolic murmur, prediastolic murmur
収縮中期雑音 しゅうしゅくちゅうきざつおん	midsystolic murmur
拡張中期雑音 かくちょうちゅうきざつおん	mid-diastolic murmur
前収縮期雑音 ぜんしゅうしゅくきざつおん	presystolic murmur
全収縮期雑音 ぜんしゅうしゅくきざつおん	pansystolic murmur, holosystolic murmur
漸強性雑音 ぜんきょうせいざつおん	crescendo murmur
漸弱性雑音 ぜんじゃくせいざつおん	decrescendo murmur
連続性雑音 れんぞくせいざつおん	continuous murmur
駆出性雑音 くしゅつせいざつおん	ejection murmur
往復雑音 おうふくざつおん	to-and-fro murmur
オースティン・フリント	Austin Flint murmur

176 Ⅳ章 診療録用語

雑音 ざつおん
　〈*a presystolic murmur heard at the apex in aortic regurgitation*〉
グレアム・スティール雑音 　Graham Steell murmur
　〈*a high-pitched diastolic murmur heard in pulmonary regurgitation due to severe pulmonary hypertension*〉

心膜摩擦音 しんまくまさつおん	pericardial friction rub
エワート徴候 ちょうこう	Ewart sign

　〈*dullness to percussion and bronchial breathing at the lower left scapular angle, seen in pericardial effusion*〉

ブロードベント徴候　Broadbent sign
　〈*retraction of the left posterior chest wall between 11th and 12th rib, synchronous with cardiac systole, seen in pericardial adhesion*〉

ベック三主徴 さんしゅちょう　Beck triad
　〈*hypotension, high venous pressure, and diminished heart sounds seen in pericardial tamponade*〉

疣贅 ゆうぜい	vegetation（clots adherent to cardiac valves）
肺うっ血 はいけつ	pulmonary congestion
肺水腫 はいすいしゅ	pulmonary edema
心原性ショック しんげんせい	cardiogenic shock
心停止 しんてい	cardiac arrest（CA）
心原性突然死 しんげんせいとつぜんし	sudden cardiac death（SCD）
心肺停止 しんぱいてい	cardiopulmonary arrest（CPA）
原因不明突然死 げんいんふめいとつぜんし	sudden unexplained death（SUD）
院外心停止 いんがいしんていし	out-of-hospital cardiac arrest（OHCA）
アダムス・ストークス症候群 しょうこうぐん	Adams-Stokes syndrome

　〈*bradycardia, syncope, and convulsions, as a result of AV block or rapid arrhythmias such as ventricular fibrillation*〉

電導収縮解離 でんどうしゅうしゅくかいり	pulseless electrical activity（PEA）
血管迷走神経反射 けっかんめいそうしんけいはんしゃ	vasovagal reflex（VVR）
頸動脈雑音 けいどうみゃくざつおん	carotid bruit
静脈雑音 じょうみゃくざつおん	venous hum, humming-top murmur, bruit de diable
橈骨動脈脈拍 とうこつどうみゃくみゃくはく	radial pulse
アレン試験 けん	Allen test

　〈*radial compression test to assess patency of the ulnar artery*〉

大腿動脈拍動 だいたいどうみゃくはくどう	femoral pulse
膝窩動脈拍動 しっかどうみゃくはくどう	popliteal pulse
後脛骨動脈拍動 こうけいこつどうみゃくはくどう	posterior tibial pulse

足背動脈拍動 そくはいどうみゃくはくどう	dorsalis pedis pulse
デュロジェ徴候 ちょうこう	Duroziez sign

⟨to-and-fro murmur over the femoral artery in aortic regurgitation⟩

ルリーシュ症候群 しょうこうぐん	Leriche syndrome

⟨aortic bifurcation syndrome; thigh and buttock claudication, impotence, absent femoral pulses, and pallor of the legs due to aotoiliac obstruction⟩

下肢浮腫 かしふしゅ	dependent edema
末梢浮腫 まっしょうふしゅ	peripheral edema
圧痕浮腫 あっこんふしゅ	pitting edema
指圧痕 しあつこん	pitting
指圧痕のない	nonpitting
リンパ浮腫 ふしゅ	lymphedema
ミルロイ病 びょう	Milroy disease

⟨congenital lymphedema, autosomal dominant⟩

ウィルヒョウ三徴 さんちょう	Virchow triad

⟨risk factors for vascular thrombosis; stasis, hypercoagulability, and endothelial injury⟩

深部静脈血栓 しんぶじょうみゃくけっせん	deep vein thrombosis (DVT)
ホーマンズ徴候 ちょうこう	Homans sign

⟨calf pain with dorsiflexion of foot; a sign of thrombosis of deep calf veins⟩

レーベンベルク徴候	Löwenberg sign

⟨calf pain by inflation of blood-pressure cuff to 80 mmHg; a sign of DVT⟩

モンドール病 びょう	Mondor disease

⟨thrombophlebitis of the thoracoepigastric vein which crosses the breast and lateral chest wall from the epigastrium to the axilla⟩

トルソー症候群 しょうこうぐん	Trousseau syndrome

⟨migratory superficial thrombophlebitis associated with visceral cancer, especially pancreatic⟩

ベインブリッジ反射 はんしゃ	Bainbridge reflex

⟨increased heart rate caused by increased right atrial pressure⟩

ドミュセー徴候 ちょうこう	de Musset sign

⟨rhythmical jerking of the head in aortic insufficiency and aneurysm⟩

オリバー徴候 ちょうこう	Oliver sign

⟨tracheal tugging; a pulling sensation in the trachea due to aortic aneurysm⟩

オスラー結節 けっせつ	Osler node

⟨painful bluish nodes in the pads of fingers or toes; pathognomonic of subacute bacterial endocarditis⟩

キリップ分類 ぶんるい	Killip classification

⟨a classification for patients with heart failure based on physical *examination, no failure, basal crackles, pulmonary edema, and cardiogenic shock*⟩

ニューヨーク心臓協会分類 — New York Heart Association (NYHA) classification

● 検査法　Examination ●

クレアチンキナーゼ — creatine kinase (CK)
クレアチンリン酸酵素 — creatine phosphokinase (CPK)
クレアチンキナーゼアイソザイム MB — creatine kinase isoenzyme MB (CK-MB)
乳酸デヒドロゲナーゼ — lactate dehydrogenase (LDH), lactic acid dehydrogenase
心筋トロポニン T — cardiac troponin T (cTnT)
心筋トロポニン I — cardiac troponin I (cTnI)
ミオグロビン — myoglobin
ヒト心臓由来脂肪酸結合タンパク — heart-type fatty acid-binding protein (H-FABP)
ミオシン軽鎖 — myosin light chain
心房性ナトリウム利尿ペプチド — atrial natriuretic peptide (ANP)
脳性ナトリウム利尿ペプチド — brain natriuretic peptide (BNP)
脳性ナトリウム利尿ペプチド前駆体 N 端フラグメント — N-terminal pro-brain natriuretic peptide (NT-proBNP)
サイクリックグアノシン一リン酸 — cyclic guanosine monophosphate (cGMP)
脈波伝播速度 — pulse wave velocity
心電図検査 — electrocardiography
心電図 — electrocardiogram (ECG)
胸部誘導 — precordial leads, chest leads
四肢誘導 — limb lead
左（右）軸偏位 — left (right) axis deviation (LAD, RAD)
時計方向回転 — clockwise rotation (CWR)
反時計方向回転 — counterclockwise rotation (CCW)
等電位線 — isoelectric line
PR（PQ）時間延長（短縮） — prolonged (short) PR (PQ) interval
ラウン・ギャノン・レバイン症候群 — Lown-Ganong-Levine (LGL) syndrome

⟨*a short PR interval with a normal QRS complex, frequently associated with atrial tachycardia*⟩

ウォルフ・パーキンソン・ホワイト症候群   Wolff-Parkinson-White (WPW) syndrome
⟨*a short PR interval and a wide QRS complex with a delta wave, associated with paroxysmal tachycardia*⟩

ケント束   Kent bundle
⟨*a muscular bundle running directly between the atrial and ventricular walls; an anatomic basis of WPW syndrome*⟩

ST上昇（下降）	ST elevation (depression)
陰性（逆転，冠性）T波	negative (inverted, coronary) T wave
肺性（僧帽弁性）P波	pulmonary (mitral) P wave, P pulmonale (mitrale)
右房肥大	right atrial enlargement (RAE)
左房肥大	left atrial enlargement (LAE)
QRS群	QRS complex
トルサードドポアンツ，倒錯型心室頻拍	torsade de pointes (TDP)
低電位	low voltage
房室ブロック	atrioventricular (AV) block
1度（2度，3度）房室ブロック	first degree (second degree, third degree) AV block
ウェンケバッハ型ブロック	Wenckebach block

⟨*a type of second degree AV block; there is progressive elongation of PR intervals until the beat is dropped*⟩

左脚ブロック	left bundle branch block (LBBB)
右脚ブロック	right bundle branch block (RBBB)
両脚ブロック	bilateral bundle branch block (BBBB)
不完全脚ブロック	incomplete bundle branch block (IBBB)
完全左脚ブロック	complete left bundle branch block (CLBBB)
完全右脚ブロック	complete right bundle branch block (CRBBB)
左脚前枝ブロック	left anterior hemiblock (LAH), left anterior fascicular block
左脚後枝ブロック	left posterior hemiblock (LPH), left posterior fascicular block
二枝ブロック	bifascicular block
三枝ブロック	trifascicular block
移動性ペースメーカー	wandering pacemaker

ホルター心電計　―しん でんけい　　　Holter electrocardiograph, Holter monitor
〈a portable continuous ECG recorder〉

心イベント記録計　しん―き ろくけい　　cardiac event recorder

運動負荷試験　うんどう かしけんふ　　exercise test, exercise stress test

マスター2階段試験　―2かい だんしけん　　Master two-step test
〈an exercise test to identify coronary insufficiency using a pair of 9-inch steps; the number of trips standardized for age, sex and weight〉

段階的運動負荷試験　だんかいてきうん どうふかしけん　　graded exercise test

トレッドミル試験　―けんし　treadmill test, treadmill stress test

自転車エルゴメーター　じてんしゃ―　bicycle ergometer

ベクトル心電図　―でんず しん　vectorcardiogram (VCG)

ヒス束心電図　―んでんず そくし　His bundle electrogram (HBE)
〈intracardiac electrogram of the lower right atrium, AV node, and His-Purkinje system〉

高右心房心電図　こううしんぼう しんでんず　high right atrial (HRA) electrogram

心音図検査　しんおん ずけんさ　phonocardiography (PCG)

心機図　しん きず　mechanocardiogram

心尖拍動図　しんせん くどうず　apex cardiogram (ACG)

頚動脈波　けいどう みゃくは　carotid pulse wave

頚静脈波　けいじょう みゃくは　jugular pulse wave

胸部X線写真　きょうぶ せんしゃしん―　chest roentgenogram, chest x-ray (CXR)

心臓足首血管指数　しんぞうあしくび けっかんしすう　cardio-ankle vascular index (CAVI)

心胸郭比　しん きょう うかくひ　cardiothoracic ratio (CTR)

大動脈隆起　だいどうみゃ くりゅうき　aortic knob

カーリーB線　―せん　Kerley B lines
〈costophrenic septal lines representing widened interlobular septa in pulmonary edema, usually at the base of the lungs; Kerley A lines are more central than the Kerley B lines〉

ウェスターマーク徴候　Westermark sign
〈loss of lung markings distal to a pulmonary embolus in chest radiography〉

木靴心　きぐつ しん　coeur en sabot, sabot heart, wooden-shoe heart

電気生理学的検査　でんきせいりが くてきけんさ　electrophysiologic study (EPS)

7. 循環器系

洞結節機能回復時間	sinus node recovery time (SNRT)
洞房伝導時間	sinoatrial conduction time (SACT)
心弾道図	ballistocardiogram (BCG)
心エコー検査	echocardiography
心エコー図	echocardiogram
Mモード心エコー法	M-mode echocardiography
ドプラー心エコー図法	Doppler echocardiography

⟨*ultrasonic cardiography; records the flow of RBCs through the cardiovascular system by Doppler ultrasonography techniques*⟩

三次元心エコー法	three-dimensional echocardiography
心筋コントラストエコー法	myocardial contrast echocardiography (MCE)
ストレス心エコー法	stress echocardiography
経食道心エコー検査	transesophageal echocardiography (TEE)
僧帽弁前尖弁後退速度	diastolic descent rate (DDR)
収縮期前方運動	systolic anterior motion (SAM)
タリウムトレッドミル試験	thallium treadmill stress test
タリウム心筋血流スキャン	thallium-201 myocardial perfusion scanning
心筋血流イメージング	myocardial perfusion imaging (MPI)
多関門集積スキャン	multiple-gated acquisition scan (MUGA)
スワン・ガンツカテーテル	Swan-Ganz (SG) catheter

⟨*a balloon-tipped pulmonary artery catheter*⟩

心係数	cardiac index (CI)
心拍出量	cardiac output (CO)
1回心拍出量	stroke volume (SV)
右室圧	right ventricular pressure (RVP)
肺動脈圧	pulmonary artery pressure (PAP)
肺動脈楔入圧	pulmonary wedge pressure (PWP), pulmonary capillary wedge pressure

	(PCWP)
肺血管抵抗 はいけっかんていこう	pulmonary vascular resistance (PVR)
混合静脈血酸素分圧 こんごうじょうみゃくけつさんそぶんあつ	mixed venous oxygen tension
心臓カテーテル法 しんぞう―ほう	cardiac catheterization, heart catheterization
拡張末期圧 かくちょうまっきあつ	end-diastolic pressure (EDP)
拡張末期容量 かくちょうまっきようりょう	end-diastolic volume (EDV)
収縮末期圧 しゅうしゅくまっきあつ	end-systolic pressure (ESP)
収縮末期容量 しゅうしゅくまっきようりょう	end-systolic volume (ESV)
左室拡張終末期圧 さしつかくちょうしゅうまつきあつ	left ventricular end-diastolic pressure (LVEDP)
左室拡張終末期容積 さしつかくちょうしゅうまつきようせき	left ventricular end-diastolic volume (LVEDV)
左室収縮終末期圧 さしつしゅうしゅくしゅうまつきあつ	left ventricular end-systolic pressure (LVESP)
左室収縮終末期容積 さしつしゅうしゅくしゅうまつきようせき	left ventricular end-systolic volume (LVESV)
圧容積関係 あつようせききかんけい	pressure-volume relation (PVR)
駆出率 くしゅつりつ	ejection fraction (EF)
左室駆出率 さしつくしゅつりつ	left ventricular ejection fraction (LVEF)
収縮時間 しゅうしゅくじかん	systolic time intervals
中心静脈圧 ちゅうしんじょうみゃくあつ	central venous pressure (CVP)
全末梢血管抵抗 ぜんまっしょうけっかんていこう	total peripheral resistance (TPR)
フォレスター分類 ―ぶんるい	Forrester classification

⟨*classifies heart failure after right heart catheterization into four subsets according to cardiac index and PCWP; no pulmonary congestion or peripheral hypotension in Class I and both present in Class IV*⟩

心血管造影法 しんけっかんぞうえいほう	angiocardiography (ACG)
心血管動画撮影法 しんけっかんどうがさつえいほう	cineangiocardiography
冠血管造影法 かんけっかんぞうえいほう	coronary angiography (CAG)
左室造影法 さしつぞうえいほう	left ventriculography (LVG)
血管内超音波検査法 けっかんないちょうおんぱけんさほう	intravascular ultrasonography (IVUS)
サーモグラフィー	thermography
ドベーキー分類 ―ぶんるい	DeBakey classification

⟨*a classification of aortic dissection by its location and extent*⟩

●疾患名　Diseases●

洞不全症候群	sick sinus syndrome (SSS)
先天性心疾患	congenital heart disease (CHD)
大動脈縮窄症	coarctation of the aorta
心房中隔欠損	atrial septal defect (ASD)
部分的肺静脈還流異常	partial anomalous pulmonary venous return (PAPVR)
全肺静脈還流異常	total anomalous pulmonary venous return (TAPVR)
心室中隔欠損	ventricular septal defect (VSD)
心内膜床欠損	endocardial cushion defect (ECD)
動脈管開存症	patent ductus arteriosus (PDA), patent Botallo duct
卵円孔開存	patent foramen ovale (PFO)
三尖弁閉鎖症	tricuspid atresia (TA)
ファロー四徴症	tetralogy of Fallot (TOF)

⟨a set of congenital cardiac defects including pulmonary stenosis, ventricular septal defect, dextroposition of the aorta, and right ventricular hypertrophy⟩

主要大動脈肺動脈側副血行路	major aortopulmonary collateral artery (MAPCA)
アイゼンメンゲル複合	Eisenmenger complex

⟨ventricular septal defect with pulmonary hypertension and consequent right-to-left shunt⟩

エプスタイン奇形	Ebstein anomaly

⟨congenital inferior displacement of the tricuspid valve into the right ventricle; often associated with ASD or PFO⟩

大血管転位症	transposition of great vessels
動静脈奇形	arteriovenous malformation (AVM)
肺動静脈瘻	pulmonary arteriovenous fistula (PAVF)
右胸心	dextrocardia
カルタゲナー症候群	Kartagener syndrome

⟨situs inversus associated with bronchiectasis, sinusitis, and ciliary dysmotility; autosomal recessive inheritance⟩

QT延長症候群	long QT syndrome (LQTS)
ロマノ・ワード症候群	Romano-Ward syndrome

⟨hereditary long QT syndrome, characterized by syncope and sometimes VF and sudden death; autosomal dominant⟩

心臓弁膜症	valvular heart disease
大動脈弁閉鎖不全	aortic valve insufficiency, aortic regurgitation (AR)
大動脈輪拡張	annuloaortic ectasia (AAE)

IV章 診療録用語

大動脈弁狭窄 （だいどうみゃくべんきょうさく）	aortic valve stenosis, aortic stenosis (AS)
僧帽弁閉鎖不全 （そうぼうべんへいさふぜん）	mitral valve insufficiency, mitral regurgitation (MR)
僧帽弁狭窄 （そうぼうべんきょうさく）	mitral valve stenosis, mitral stenosis (MS)
僧帽弁逸脱症 （そうぼうべんいつだつしょう）	mitral valve prolapse (MVP)
三尖弁閉鎖不全 （さんせんべんへいさふぜん）	tricuspid valve insufficiency, tricuspid regurgitation (TR)
三尖弁狭窄 （さんせんべんきょうさく）	tricuspid valve stenosis, tricuspid stenosis (TS)
肺動脈弁閉鎖不全 （はいどうみゃくべんへいさふぜん）	pulmonary valve insufficiency, pulmonic regurgitation (PR)
肺動脈弁狭窄 （はいどうみゃくべんきょうさく）	pulmonary valve stenosis, pulmonary stenosis (PS)
連合弁膜症 （れんごうべんまくしょう）	combined valvular disease (CVD)
高血圧症 （こうけつあつしょう）	hypertension (HTN)
本態性高血圧 （ほんたいせいこうけつあつ）	essential hypertension
二次性高血圧 （にじせいこうけつあつ）	secondary hypertension
腎血管性高血圧 （じんけっかんせいこうけつあつ）	renovascular hypertension (RVH)
副腎性高血圧 （ふくじんせいこうけつあつ）	adrenal hypertension
線維筋異形成症 （せんいきんいけいせいしょう）	fibromuscular dysplasia (FMD)
境界域高血圧 （きょうかいいきこうけつあつ）	borderline hypertension, labile hypertension
起立性低血圧 （きりつせいていけつあつ）	orthostatic hypotension
神経調節性失神 （しんけいちょうせつせいしっしん）	neurally mediated syncope (NMS)
頸動脈洞症候群 （けいどうみゃくどうしょうこうぐん）	carotid sinus syndrome
心血管疾患 （しんけっかんしっかん）	cardiovascular disease (CVD)
リウマチ性心疾患 （―せいしんしっかん）	rheumatic heart disease (RHD)
高血圧性心疾患 （こうけつあつせいしんしっかん）	hypertensive heart disease (HHD)
動脈硬化性心疾患 （どうみゃくこうかせいしんしっかん）	arteriosclerotic heart disease (ASHD)
動脈硬化性心血管疾患 （どうみゃくこうかせいしんけっかんしっかん）	arteriosclerotic cardiovascular disease (ASCVD)
冠動脈疾患 （かんどうみゃくしっかん）	coronary artery disease (CAD)
冠動脈性心疾患 （かんどうみゃくせいしんしっかん）	coronary heart disease (CHD)
冠動脈硬化症 （かんどうみゃくこうかしょう）	coronary arteriosclerosis
虚血性心疾患 （きょけつせいしんしっかん）	ischemic heart disease (IHD)
急性冠動脈症候群	acute coronary syndrome (ACS)

狭心症（きょうしんしょう）	angina pectoris (AP)
安定狭心症（あんていきょうしんしょう）	stable angina
不安定狭心症（ふあんていきょうしんしょう）	unstable angina
異型狭心症（いけいきょうしんしょう），プリンツメタル型狭心症（—がたきょうしんしょう）	variant angina pectoris (VAP), Prinzmetal angina

⟨*chest pain occurring at rest and associated with ST segment elevation*⟩

労作性狭心症（ろうさせいきょうしんしょう）	effort angina (EA), angina of effort
安静時狭心症（あんせいじきょうしんしょう）	angina at rest
血管攣縮性狭心症（けっかんれんしゅくせいきょうしんしょう）	vasospastic angina (VSA)
無症候性心筋虚血（むしょうこうせいしんきんきょけつ）	silent myocardial ischemia (SMI)
中間冠状症候群（ちゅうかんかんじょうしょうこうぐん）	intermediate coronary syndrome
心筋梗塞（しんきんこうそく）	myocardial infarction (MI)
急性心筋梗塞（きゅうせいしんきんこうそく）	acute myocardial infarction (AMI)
陳旧性心筋梗塞（ちんきゅうせいしんきんこうそく）	old myocardial infarction (OMI)
前壁（後壁，側壁）心筋梗塞（ぜんぺき（こうへき，そくへき）しんきんこうそく）	anterior (posterior, lateral) myocardial infarction
前壁中隔心筋梗塞（ぜんぺきちゅうかくしんきんこうそく）	anteroseptal myocardial infarction
下壁心筋梗塞（かへきしんきんこうそく）	inferior myocardial infarction, diaphragmatic myocardial infarction
貫壁性心筋梗塞（かんぺきせいしんきんこうそく）	transmural myocardial infarction
心内膜下心筋梗塞（しんないまくかしんきんこうそく）	subendocardial myocardial infarction
ST上昇型心筋梗塞（—じょうしょうがたしんきんこうそく）	ST-elevation myocardial infarction (STEMI)
非ST上昇型心筋梗塞（ひ—じょうしょうがたしんきんこうそく）	non-ST-elevation myocardial infarction (NSTEMI)
心室瘤（しんしつりゅう）	ventricular aneurysm
低心拍出量症候群（ていしんぱくしゅつりょうしょうこうぐん）	low output syndrome (LOS)
心不全（しんふぜん）	heart failure, cardiac failure, cardiac insufficiency
うっ血性心不全（—けっせいしんふぜん）	congestive heart failure (CHF)
左心不全（さしんふぜん）	left-sided heart failure, left ventricular failure

右心不全 うしんふぜん	right-sided heart failure, right ventricular failure
高拍出性心不全 こうはくしゅつせいしんふぜん	high-output heart failure
低拍出性心不全 ていはくしゅつせいしんふぜん	low-output heart failure
駆出率正常心不全 くしゅつりつせいじょうしんふぜん	heart failure with normal left ventricular ejection fraction
拡張期心不全 かくちょうきしんふぜん, 拡張不全 かくちょうふぜん	diastolic heart failure (DHF)
肺性心 はいせいしん	cor pulmonale (CP)
アイエルザ症候群 しょうこうぐん	Ayerza syndrome

〈*polycythemia vera with cor pulmonale, seen with sclerosis of the pulmonary artery*〉

心内膜炎 しんないまくえん	endocarditis
感染性心内膜炎 かんせんせいしんないまくえん	infectious endocarditis, infective endocarditis (IE)
急性細菌性心内膜炎 きゅうせいさいきんせいしんないまくえん	acute bacterial endocarditis (ABE)
急性感染性心内膜炎 きゅうせいかんせんせいしんないまくえん	acute infectious endocarditis (AIE)
亜急性細菌性心内膜炎 あきゅうせいさいきんせいしんないまくえん	subacute bacterial endocarditis (SBE)
非細菌性血栓性心内膜炎 ひさいきんせいけっせんせいしんないまくえん	nonbacterial thrombotic endocarditis (NBTE)
リブマン・サックス心内膜炎 しんないまくえん	Libman-Sacks endocarditis

〈*nonbacterial verrucous endocarditis associated with SLE; vegetations found on the atrioventricular valves and chordae tendineae*〉

レフレル心内膜炎 しんないまくえん	Löffler endocarditis

〈*constrictive endocarditis; fibrotic thickening of the endocardium with eosinophilia, resulting in congestive heart failure, pleural effusion, hepatosplenomegaly, and dependent edema*〉

自己弁心内膜炎 じこべんしんないまくえん	native valve endocarditis (NVE)
人工弁心内膜炎 じんこうべんしんないまくえん	prosthetic valve endocarditis (PVE)
心膜炎 しんまくえん	pericarditis
収縮性心膜炎 しゅうしゅくせいしんまくえん	constrictive pericarditis
心膜滲出液 しんまくしんしゅつえき	pericardial effusion
心膜タンポナーデ しんまく	pericardial tamponade
ドレスラー症候群 しょうこうぐん	Dressler syndrome

〈*post-myocardial infarction syndrome; pericarditis, pleurisy, pneumonia, fever, and leukocytosis after myocardial infarction; possible development of autoantibodies*〉

心筋炎 しんきんえん	myocarditis
心筋症 しんきんしょう	cardiomyopathy (CMP)

特発性心筋症	idiopathic cardiomyopathy (ICM), primary cardiomyopathy
拡張型心筋症	dilated cardiomyopathy (DCM)
うっ血性心筋症	congestive cardiomyopathy (CCM)
肥大型心筋症	hypertrophic cardiomyopathy (HCM)
肥大型閉塞性心筋症	hypertrophic obstructive cardiomyopathy (HOCM)
肥大型非閉塞性心筋症	hypertrophic nonobstructive cardiomyopathy (HNCM)
拘束型心筋症	restrictive cardiomyopathy (RCM)
心内膜心筋線維症	endomyocardial fibrosis (EMF)
不整脈原性右室異形成	arrythmogenic right ventricular dysplasia (ARVD)
特発性肥大型大動脈弁下狭窄症	idiopathic hypertrophic subaortic stenosis (IHSS)
大動脈解離	aortic dissection
動脈瘤	aneurysm
胸部大動脈瘤	thoracic aortic aneurysm (TAA)
腹部大動脈瘤	abdominal aortic aneurysm (AAA)
解離性動脈瘤	dissecting aneurysm
末梢血管疾患	peripheral vascular disease (PVD)
末梢動脈疾患	peripheral arterial disease (PAD)
閉塞性動脈硬化症	arteriosclerosis obliterans (ASO)
閉塞性血栓血管炎, バージャー病	thromboangiitis obliterans (TAO), Buerger disease
急性動脈閉塞疾患	acute arterial occlusive disease
筋・腎障害性代謝異常症候群	myonephropathic metabolic syndrome (MNMS)
高安病, 高安動脈炎	Takayasu disease, Takayasu arteritis

⟨*pulseless disease; progressive obliteration of the aortic arch and branches, manifested by syncope, visual defects, and loss of pulses*⟩

巨細胞動脈炎	giant cell arteritis (GCA)
側頭動脈炎	temporal arteritis (TA)
血栓性静脈炎	thrombophlebitis
下肢静脈瘤	varicose veins of lower extremities
神経循環無力症	neurocirculatory asthenia (NCA), Da

心因性無力症候群, ダコスタ症候群 Costa syndrome
心房粘液腫 atrial myxoma
カーニー複合 Carney complex
〈NAME syndrome; nevi, atrial myxoma, myxoid neurofibromas, and ephelids; adrenal and pituitary tumors may occur〉

● 治療法 Treatment ●

降圧薬	antihypertensive
利尿薬	diuretic
サイアザイド	thiazides
トリクロルメチアジド	trichlormethiazide《フルイトラン》
ループ利尿薬	loop diuretic
フロセミド	furosemide《ラシックス》
スピロノラクトン	spironolactone《アルダクトンA》
アセタゾラミド	acetazolamide《ダイアモックス》
β遮断薬	β-blocker, β-adrenergic blocking agent
プロプラノロール塩酸塩	propranolol hydrochloride《インデラル》
カルシウム拮抗薬	calcium antagonist
カルシウムチャネル遮断薬	calcium channel blocker (CCB)
ニフェジピン	nifedipine《アダラート》
アムロジピンベシル酸塩	amlodipine besilate《アムロジン》
アンギオテンシン変換酵素阻害薬	angiotensin-converting enzyme inhibitor (ACEI)
カプトプリル	captopril《カプトリル》
I型アンギオテンシンII受容体拮抗薬	angiotensin II type I receptor blocker (ARB)
カンデサルタンシレキセチル	candesartan cilexetil《ブロプレス》
イルベサルタン	irbesartan《アバプロ》
選択的アルドステロンブロッカー	selective aldosterone blocker (SAB)
エプレレノン	eplerenone《セララ》
α受容体遮断薬	α-adrenergic antagonist, α-adrenergic blocking agent, α-adrenoreceptor antagonist
プラゾシン塩酸塩	prazosin hydrochloride《ミニプレス》
中枢性交感神経抑制薬	central sympatholytic
メチルドパ	methyldopa《アルドメット》

7. 循環器系

昇圧薬	vasopressor
血管収縮薬	vasoconstrictor
カテコールアミン	catecholamine
アドレナリン，エピネフリン	adrenaline, epinephrine《ボスミン》
ドパミン塩酸塩	dopamine hydrochloride《イノバン》
血管拡張薬	vasodilator
プロスタグランジン	prostaglandin《プロスタンディン》
亜硝酸アミル	amyl nitrite
ヒドララジン塩酸塩	hydralazine hydrochloride《アプレゾリン》
ニトロプルシドナトリウム	sodium nitroprusside (SNP)《ニトプロ》
ニトログリセリン	nitroglycerin (NTG)《ニトログリセリン》
硝酸イソソルビド	isosorbide dinitrate (ISDN)《ニトロール》
一硝酸イソソルビド	isosorbide mononitrate (ISMN)《アイトロール》
皮膚貼布剤	transdermal patch
強心薬	cardiotonic, cardiac stimulant
ジギタリス	digitalis《ジゴキシン，ジギトキシン》
ジギタリス投与，ジギタリス飽和	digitalization
抗不整脈薬	antiarrhythmic
ナトリウムチャネル遮断薬	sodium channel blocker
硫酸キニジン	quinidine sulfate《硫酸キニジン》
プロカインアミド塩酸塩	procainamide hydrochloride《アミサリン》
リドカイン	lidocaine《キシロカイン》
メキシレチン塩酸塩	mexiletine hydrochloride《メキシチール》
アミオダロン塩酸塩	amiodarone hydrochloride《アンカロン》
ニフェカラント塩酸塩	nifekalant hydrochloride《シンビット》
ホスホジエステラーゼ阻害薬	phosphodiesterase inhibitor (PDEI)《レバチオ》
抗凝固療法	anticoagulant therapy (ACT)
抗凝固薬	anticoagulant
血栓溶解薬	thrombolytic agent
ヘパリン	heparin
ワルファリンカリウム	warfarin potassium《ワーファリン》
ウロキナーゼ	urokinase (UK)《ウロキナーゼ》
組織プラスミノーゲン活性化因子	tissue plasminogen activator (t-PA)
アルテプラーゼ	alteplase《アクチバシン》
血小板凝集抑制薬	antiplatelet agent, platelet inhibitor

アスピリン	aspirin《バイアスピリン》
チクロピジン塩酸塩	ticlopidine hydrochloride《パナルジン》
バルサルバ法	Valsalva method
	⟨*forced expiratory effort against a closed glottis; high intrathoracic pressure interferes with venous return to the right atrium*⟩
星状神経節ブロック	stellate ganglion block (SGB)
心臓リハビリテーション	cardiac rehabilitation
心肺蘇生法	cardiopulmonary resuscitation (CPR)
口対口人工呼吸	mouth-to-mouth breathing
アンビュー	Ambu bag
体外心マッサージ	closed chest cardiac massage, external cardiac massage (ECM)
心臓除細動	cardioversion
除細動器	cardioverter, defibrillator
自動体外式除細動器	automated external defibrillator (AED)
植え込み型除細動器	implantable cardioverter-defibrillator (ICD)
植え込み型自動除細動器	automatic implantable cardioverter-defibrillator (AICD)
心臓ペーシング	cardiac pacing
経皮的ペーシング	transcutaneous pacing (TCP)
心臓ペースメーカー	cardiac pacemaker
植え込み型ペースメーカー	implantable (implanted, internal) pacemaker
心臓再同期療法	cardiac resynchronization therapy (CRT)
経皮的冠動脈インターベンション	percutaneous coronary intervention (PCI)
経皮経管的冠動脈形成術	percutaneous transluminal coronary angioplasty (PTCA)
経皮経管的冠動脈再開通術	percutaneous transluminal coronary recanalization (PTCR)
冠動脈内注入血栓溶解療法	intracoronary thrombolysis (ICT)
バルーン血管形成術	balloon angioplasty
レーザー血管形成術	laser angioplasty
エキシマレーザー冠動脈形成術	excimer laser coronary angioplasty (ELCA)

カテーテル焼灼術	catheter ablation
バルーン拡張式血管内ステント	balloon-expandable intravascular stent (BEIS)
薬剤溶出性ステント	drug-eluting stent (DES)
血栓除去術	thrombectomy
フォガティー・カテーテル	Fogarty catheter

⟨*a balloon-tip catheter used to remove emboli and thrombi from blood vessels*⟩

回転性粥腫切除術	rotational atherectomy, rotablation
方向性冠動脈粥腫切除術	directional coronary atherectomy (DCA)
バルーン心房中隔裂開	balloon atrial septostomy (BAS)
冠動脈バイパス移植片	coronary artery bypass graft (CABG)
冠動脈バイパス	coronary artery bypass grafting
大動脈冠動脈バイパス	aortocoronary (AC) bypass
低侵襲心臓外科手術	minimally invasive cardiac surgery (MICS)
血栓内膜切除術	thromboendarterectomy (TEA)
ブラロック・トーシグ手術	Blalock-Taussig operation

⟨*anastomosis of the left or right subclavian artery to the left or right pulmonary artery for TOF or other congenital anomalies*⟩

フォンタン手術	Fontan operation

⟨*surgical correction of single ventricle and tricuspid atresia by anastomosis of the right atrium and the pulmonary artery with closure of ASD*⟩

開心術	open heart surgery
大動脈弁置換術	aortic valve replacement (AVR)
僧帽弁置換術	mitral valve replacement (MVR)
僧帽弁交連切開術	mitral commissurotomy
経皮経静脈的僧帽弁交連切開術	percutaneous transvenous mitral commissurotomy (PTMC)

バルーン弁形成術	balloon valvuloplasty
経皮的バルーン大動脈弁形成術	percutaneous balloon aortic valvuloplasty
大動脈内バルーン・パンピング	intra-aortic balloon pumping (IABP)
経皮的心肺補助装置	percutaneous cardiopulmonay support (PCPS)
静動脈バイパス	veno-arterial bypass (VAB)
補助人工心臓システム	ventricular assist system (VAS)
心室補助装置	ventricular assist device (VAD)
左室補助装置	left ventricular assist device (LVAD)
右室補助装置	right ventricular assist device (RVAD)
両心室補助装置	biventricular assist device (BVAD)
血管内治療	endovascular treatment (EVT)
人工血管	synthetic graft, artificial blood vessel
ポリエチレンテレフタレート	polyethylene terephthalate (PET)
胸部大動脈瘤ステントグラフト内挿術	thoracic endovascular aortic repair (TEVAR)
人工心臓	artificial heart
完全置換型人工心臓	total artificial heart (TAH)
体外循環	extracorporeal circulation (ECC)
人工心肺	artificial heart-lung (AHL), cardiopulmonary bypass (CPB), heart-lung machine
心臓移植	heart transplantation
静脈瘤抜去	stripping of varicose veins
静脈瘤抜去兼筋膜下交通枝結紮	stripping of varicose veins and subfascial ligation of perforator

―― Tidbits ――

azygos

奇静脈 azygos vein の「奇」は,「奇異, 奇特」の「奇」ではなく「奇数」の「奇」である. azygos (発音は ǽzəgəs, eizáigəs) は, ギリシャ語の azygon に由来し, zygon は yoke, すなわち一対の牛馬をつなぐ「くびき (軛)」のことであるから, unpaired「対になっていない, 不対の」を意味する. 生体には一対の臓器が多く, azygos の付いた用語は奇静脈と関係する右肺の奇静脈裂 azygos fissure, 奇静脈葉 azygos lobe くらいである.

8. 消化器系

●愁訴・症状　Complaints / Symptoms●

消化器症状 しょうかきしょうじょう	gastrointestinal symptoms, symptoms of the digestive tract, symptoms of the alimentary canal
胃症状 いしょう	stomach trouble, upset stomach
消化 しょうか	digestion
消化不良 しょうかふりょう	indigestion, dyspepsia
食欲 しょくよく	appetite, desire for food
食欲増進 しょくよくぞうしん	increase (improvement) of appetite
食欲がある	have a good appetite
食欲がない	have no (little, a poor) appetite
食欲が旺盛である しょくよくおうせい―	have a strong (voracious) appetite
食欲不振 しょくよくふしん	poor (bad, weak) appetite, no (little) appetite, loss (lack, decrease) of appetite, anorexia, 〔形〕anorectic, anorexic, anoretic
食欲を失う しょくよくうしな―	lose one's appetite
過食 かしょく	overeating, hyperphagia
空腹 くうふく	hunger, 〔動〕be (feel) hungry
空き腹 すきばら	an empty stomach
食事 しょくじ	meal, diet, 〔動〕have (take, eat) a meal
日に3度食事する ひ―3ど―しょくじ―	eat three meals a day
食事を抜かす しょくじぬ―	skip (miss) a meal
間食する かんしょく	eat between meals
軽い(こってりした)食事 かる―しょくじ	light (heavy) meal
バランスの取れた食事	balanced diet, well-balanced diet
偏った食事 かたよ―しょくじ	unbalanced diet
食物 しょくもつ	food
流動(固形)物 りゅうどう(こけい)ぶつ	liquid (solid) food
油っこい食品 あぶら―しょくひん	fatty food, oily food, greasy food
香辛料に富んだ食品 こうしんりょう―と―しょくひん	spicy food
健康食品 けんこうしょくひん	health food
自然食品 しぜんしょくひん	organic food
食物の好み しょくもつこの―	food preference, likes and dislikes
食事療法 しょくじりょうほう	diet
食事療法をしている	be on a diet, be put on a diet

8. 消化器系

咀嚼 そしゃく	chewing, mastication, 〔動〕chew
嚥下 えんげ	swallowing, 〔動〕swallow, gulp
嚥下困難 えんげこんなん	difficulty in swallowing, dysphagia
食物がのどにつかえる	stick (get caught, get stuck) in one's throat
（茶，ビールで）むせぶ	choke on (be choked by) (tea, beer)
のどに塊を感じる かたまり	feel a lump in the throat
悪心 おしん，吐き気 はきけ	nausea, retch, heaving, nauseous (nauseated) feeling, sickly feeling
吐き気を催す，むかつく	feel nausea (nauseous, nauseated, sick, queasy), heave, feel like vomiting
嘔吐 おうと	vomiting, emesis, 〔動〕vomit, throw up, 〔話〕puke
空えずき からえずき	retching, 〔動〕retch
吐物 とぶつ	vomit, vomitus, vomited matter
コーヒー残渣様の物を吐く ざんさ	vomit coffee-ground materials
吐血 とけつ	hematemesis, 〔動〕vomit blood
下血 げけつ	bloody bowel discharge, passage of bloody stool
黒色便 こくしょくべん	melena, black-colored stool, tarry stool
鮮血便 せんけつべん，顕血便 けんけつべん	hematochezia, grossly bloody stool
肛門出血 こうもんしゅっけつ	anal bleeding
胸やけ むね	heartburn, pyrosis, water brash, 〔動〕have heartburn
胃酸過多 いさんかた	hyperacidity, acid stomach, acid dyspepsia
おくび，げっぷ	belching, eructation, 〔動〕belch, eruct, 〔話〕burp
酸いげっぷ す	sour eructation, brash
逆流 ぎゃくりゅう	regurgitation, 〔動〕regurgitate
二日酔い ふつかよい	hangover, 〔話〕morning after, 〔動〕have a hangover
腹痛 ふくつう (cf. 疼痛)	abdominal pain
空腹痛 くうふくつう	hunger pain
食後痛 しょくごつう	postprandial pain
夜間痛 やかんつう	nocturnal pain
胆石仙痛 たんせきせんつう	biliary colic
膨満痛 ぼうまんつう	gas pains
心窩部痛症候群 しんかぶつうしょうこうぐん	epigastric pain syndrome
食後愁訴症候群 しょくごしゅうそしょうこうぐん	postprandial distress syndrome

慢性機能性腹痛	chronic functional abdominal pain (CFAP)
腹囲, 胴回り	abdominal girth
腹部膨満	abdominal distention, bloating
鼓腸	meteorism, flatulence, gassiness, gaseous distention
腹が張る	be bloated with gas
腹鳴, グル音	borborygmus, gurgling, growling, rumbling
腹がぐうぐう鳴る	have stomach rumbles
腹水	ascites
黄疸	jaundice, icterus
シャルコー三主徴	Charcot triad
	〈*jaundice, fever, and RUQ pain; diagnostic for cholangitis*〉
レイノルズ五徴	Reynolds pentad
	〈*jaundice, fever, RUQ pain, shock, and mental confusion seen in acute obstructive cholangitis*〉
離脱症候群	withdrawal syndrome
便通, 排便	bowel movement (BM), bowel habit
便通がある, 排便する	have a bowel movement, pass stools, defecate, evacuate the bowels
便通がない	be constipated, one's bowels do not move
排便痛	pain on defecation
下痢	diarrhea, loose bowels
抗生物質関連下痢	antibiotic-associated diarrhea (AAD)
便秘	constipation, obstipation (=obstinate constipation)
しぶり腹, 裏急後重	tenesmus, straining at stool
便失禁	fecal incontinence, 〔形〕incontinent of feces
食中毒	food poisoning
便, 糞便	stool, feces, excrement
水様(血, テール)便	watery (bloody, tarry) stool
軟(硬, 固形, 半固形)便	loose or soft (hard, formed, semi-formed) stool or feces
灰白色(粘土色)便	grayish (clay-colored) stool
泥状便	mushy stool

8. 消化器系　197

| 脂肪便 しぼうべん | steatorrhea |
| 放屁 ほうひ | flatus,〔動〕pass gas（wind, flatus）|

●診察所見・徴候　Physical findings / Signs●

肝性口臭 かんせいこうしゅう	fetor hepaticus, liver breath
手掌紅斑 しゅしょうこうはん	palmar erythema
黄疸 おうだん	jaundice, icterus,〔形〕icteric
女性化乳房 じょせいかにゅうぼう	gynecomastia
くも状血管腫 —じょうけっかんしゅ	vascular spider, spider telangiectasia, spider angioma
羽ばたき振戦 はーしんせん	asterixis, liver flap, flapping tremor
カイザー・フライシャー輪 —りん	Kayser-Fleischer ring

⟨a greenish ring encircling the cornea in Wilson disease⟩

| メズサの頭 —あたま | caput medusae, Medusa head |

⟨dilated cutaneous veins around the umbilicus⟩

腹部膨隆 ふくぶぼうりゅう	distention of the abdomen
膨隆した ぼうりゅう—	distended, protuberant, protruding
陥凹した かんぼう—	concave, retracted, scaphoid
平坦な へいたん—	flat
鼓腸 こちょう	meteorism, tympanites,〔形〕tympanitic
呑気症 どんきしょう	aerophagy, aerophagia
蠕動不穏 ぜんどうふおん	visible peristalsis
腹水 ふくすい	ascites,〔形〕ascitic
波動 はどう	fluid wave, fluctuation
濁音移動 だくおんいどう	shifting dullness
圧痛 あっつう	tenderness, pain on pressure,〔形〕tender, painful on pressure
マーフィー徴候 —ちょうこう	Murphy sign

⟨pain on palpation beneath the right costal arch during inspiration, indicating acute cholecystitis⟩

| マクバーニー徴候 —ちょうこう | McBurney sign |

⟨tenderness at two-thirds of the way from the umbilicus to the anterior superior spine, indicating acute appendicitis⟩

| ロブシング徴候 —ちょうこう | Rovsing sign |

⟨palpation in the LLQ induces pain at McBurney point, indicating appendicitis⟩

| コープ徴候 —ちょうこう | Cope sign |

⟨psoas sign; pain induced by hyperextension of the right thigh while lying on the left side; indicative of appendicitis⟩

| 反跳痛 はんちょうつう, ブルンベルグ徴候 —ちょうこう | rebound tenderness, Blumberg sign |

⟨pain on sudden release of steady pressure on the anterior abdomi-

nal wall; indicative of peritonitis⟩

筋性防御 (きんせいぼうぎょ)	muscular defense, guarding
筋硬直 (きんこうちょく)	muscular rigidity
穿孔 (せんこう)	perforation
穿通 (せんつう)	penetration
破裂 (はれつ)	rupture
狭窄 (きょうさく)	stenosis, narrowing
閉塞 (へいそく)	obstruction, blockage
肝濁音界 (かんだくおんかい)	liver dullness
肝腫大 (かんしゅだい)	hepatomegaly
脾腫 (ひしゅ)	splenomegaly
腫瘤触知 (しゅりゅうしょくち)	palpable mass
還納性ヘルニア (かんのう―)	reducible hernia
嵌頓ヘルニア (かんとん―)	incarcerated hernia
腹部浮球感 (ふくぶふきゅうかん)	abdominal ballottement
腸雑音 (ちょうざつおん)	bowel sounds
腹鳴 (ふくめい)	borborygmus
振水音 (しんすいおん)	splashing sound, succussion sound, succussion splash
血管雑音 (けっかんざつおん)	bruit, vascular murmur
クリュヴェイエ・バウムガルテン症候群 (―しょうこうぐん)	Cruveilhier-Baumgarten syndrome

⟨*venous hum in caput medusae caused by portal hypertension due to cirrhosis*⟩

大動脈雑音 (だいどうみゃくざつおん)	aortic bruit
肛門括約筋緊張 (こうもんかつやくきんきんちょう)	anal sphincter tone
ウィルヒョウリンパ節 (―せつ)	Virchow node

⟨*left supraclavicular node metastasis; often first sign of a GI tumor*⟩

| クールボアジエ徴候 | Courvoisier sign |

⟨*severe jaundice with a palpable, nontender gallbladder indicative of biliary obstruction due to a tumor*⟩

| カレン徴候 (―ちょうこう) | Cullen sign |

⟨*periumbilical discoloration of the skin, indicating intraperitoneal hemorrhage in acute hemorrhagic pancreatitis or ruptured ectopic pregnancy*⟩

| グレイターナー徴候 | Grey Turner sign |

⟨*discoloration of the skin in the lumbar region, indicative of retroperitoneal hemorrhage due to acute hemorrhagic pancreatitis*⟩

| ミリッツィ症候群 (―しょうこうぐん) | Mirizzi syndrome |

⟨*cystic duct stone that compresses the bile duct and causes jaundice and acute cholangitis*⟩

8. 消化器系　199

オギルヴィー症候群	Ogilvie syndrome
	⟨*acute colonic pseudo-obstruction due to motility disturbance*⟩
腹部コンパートメント症候群	abdominal compartment syndrome (ACS)
チャイルド分類	Child classification
	⟨*a classification of severity of cirrhosis, A, B and C, based on 5 parameters: total bilirubin, albumin, prothrombin time, ascites, and encephalopathy*⟩
ボールマン分類	Borrmann classification
	⟨*a classification of gastric carcinoma; polypoid, ulcerated, ulcerating-infiltrating, and diffusely infiltrating*⟩
デュークス分類	Dukes classification
	⟨*a staging system of colorectal carcinoma based on the extent of invasion; A, confined to the bowel wall, B, penetrated, and C, with lymph node involvement*⟩

● 検査法　Examination ●

便潜血	fecal occult blood (FOB)
寄生虫卵	ova of parasites
線虫	nematode
回虫	*Ascaris*, roundworm
鞭虫	*Trichuris*, whipworm
鉤虫	*Ancylostoma*, hookworm
蟯虫	*Enterobius vermicularis*, pinworm
アニサキス	*Anisakis*
無鉤条虫	*Taenia saginata*, beef tapeworm
有鉤条虫	*Taenia solium*, pork tapeworm
住血吸虫	*Schistosoma*
肺吸虫	*Paragonimus*, lung fluke
肝吸虫	*Clonorchis sinensis*, liver fluke
肥大吸虫	*Fasciolopsis*
エキノコックス	*Echinococcus*
肝機能検査	liver function test (LFT)
総(直接, 間接)ビリルビン	total (direct, indirect) bilirubin
抱合型(非抱合型)ビリルビン	conjugated (unconjugated) bilirubin
アスパラギン酸アミノトランスフェラーゼ	aspartate aminotransferase (AST)
アラニンアミノトランスフェラーゼ	alanine aminotransferase (ALT)
アルカリホスファターゼ	alkaline phosphatase (ALP)
γグルタミルトランスフ	γ-glutamyltransferase (γ-GT)

IV 章

ェラーゼ	
コリンエステラーゼ	cholinesterase (ChE)
ロイシンアミノペプチダーゼ	leucine aminopeptidase (LAP)
アルブミン・グロブリン比	albumin-globulin ratio (A/G)
総胆汁酸	total bile acid (TBA)
インドシアニングリーン試験	indocyanine green (ICG) test
ヒアルロン酸	hyaluronic acid
プロコラーゲンIIIペプチドIII	procollagen-3-peptide (PIIIP)
アンモニア	ammonia
動脈血中ケトン体比	arterial keton body ratio (AKBR)
ペプシノーゲンI	pepsinogen I (PG I)
ペプシノーゲンII	pepsinogen II (PG II)
分枝鎖アミノ酸	branched-chain amino acid (BCAA)
分枝鎖アミノ酸・チロシンモル比	branched-chain amino acid-tyrosine molar ratio
セルロプラスミン	ceruloplasmin
肝細胞増殖因子	hepatocyte growth factor (HGF)
肝炎ウイルスマーカー	hepatitis virus marker
肝炎関連抗原	hepatitis-associated antigen (HAA)
A型肝炎ウイルス	hepatitis A virus (HAV)
B型肝炎ウイルス	hepatitis B virus (HBV)
C型肝炎ウイルス	hepatitis C virus (HCV)
D型肝炎ウイルス	hepatitis D virus (HDV)
E型肝炎ウイルス	hepatitis E virus (HEV)
G型肝炎ウイルス	hepatitis G virus (HGV)
A型肝炎ウイルス抗体	anti-HAV antibody (HA-Ab)
B型肝炎表面抗原	hepatitis B surface antigen (HBsAg)
HBs抗体	anti-HBs antibody
B型肝炎コア抗原	hepatitis B core antigen (HBcAg)
HBc抗体	anti-HBc antibody
B型肝炎e抗原	hepatitis B envelope antigen (HBeAg)
HBe抗体	anti-HBe antibody

8. 消化器系

C 型肝炎ウイルス抗体	anti-HCV antibody (HC-Ab)
IgM 型 HA 抗体	IgM class antibody to hepatitis A virus
IgM 型 HBc 抗体	IgM class antibody to hepatitis B core antigen
B 型肝炎ウイルス DNA 定量	hepatitis B virus DNA quantification (HBV-DNA)
C 型肝炎ウイルス群別判定	hepatitis C virus serotype
C 型肝炎ウイルス核酸増幅定性	hepatitis C virus RNA detection by amplification with RT-PCR (HCV-RNA)
インターフェロン感受性領域	interferon sensitivity determining region (ISDR)
持続性ウイルス陰性化	sustained virological response (SVR)
抗ミトコンドリア抗体	antimitochondrial antibody (AMA)
腫瘍マーカー	tumor marker
癌胎児性抗原	carcinoembryonic antigen (CEA)
糖鎖抗原19-9	carbohydrate antigen 19-9 (CA19-9)
α フェトプロテイン	α-fetoprotein (AFP)
PIVKA-II, デスγカルボキシプロトロンビン	protein induced by vitamin K absence-II (PIVKA-II), des-γ-carboxy prothrombin (DCP)
塩基性胎児タンパク	basic fetoprotein (BFP)
膵癌胎児抗原	pancreatic oncofetal antigen (POA)
肝血流量	hepatic blood flow (HBF)
食道内圧	esophageal intraluminal pressure
下部食道括約筋圧	lower esophageal sphincter pressure (LESP)
胃液検査	gastric analysis
基礎酸分泌量	basal acid output (BAO)
最高酸分泌量	maximal acid output (MAO)
最大刺激時酸分泌量	peak acid output (PAO)
ヘリコバクター・ピロリ	*Helicobacter pylori* (HP)
迅速ウレアーゼ試験	rapid urease test (RUT)
尿素呼気試験	urea breath test (UBT)
抗ヘリコバクター・ピロリ抗体	anti-Helicobacter pylori antibody

糞便中ヘリコバクター・ピロリ抗原	fecal Helicobacter pylori antigen
腸内細菌叢	intestinal flora
腸内細菌科	Enterobacteriaceae
グラム陰性桿菌	gram-negative bacillus (GNB)
サルモネラ	*Salmonella*

〈<*Daniel Elmer Salmon; a genus of gram-negative bacteria of Enterobacteriaceae*〉

腸炎ビブリオ	*Vibrio parahaemolyticus*
カンピロバクター・ジェジュニ	*Campylobacter jejuni*
黄色ブドウ球菌	*Staphylococcus aureus*
腸管病原性大腸菌	enteropathogenic *Escherichia coli* (EPEC)
腸管付着性大腸菌	enteroadherent *Escherichia coli* (EAEC)
腸管組織侵入性大腸菌	enteroinvasive *Escherichia coli* (EIEC)
腸毒素産生性大腸菌	enterotoxigenic *Escherichia coli* (ETEC)
腸管出血性大腸菌	enterohemorrhagic *Escherichia coli* (EHEC)
コレラ菌	*Vibrio cholerae*
非コレラビブリオ	noncholera vibrios (NCV)
ノロウイルス	*Norovirus*
膵機能検査	pancreatic function test
アミラーゼ	amylase
アミラーゼアイソザイム	amylase isozyme
リパーゼ	lipase
膵分泌性トリプシンインヒビター	pancreatic secretory trypsin inhibitor (PSTI)
エラスターゼ1	elastase 1
アミラーゼクレアチニンクリアランス比	amylase creatinine clearance ratio (ACCR)
セクレチン試験	secretin test
BT-PABA 試験	N-benzoyl-L-tyrosyl-paraaminobenzoic acid (BT-PABA) test
膵機能診断薬	pancreatic function diagnostant (PFD)
食道内圧検査	esophageal manometry
腹部超音波検査	abdominal ultrasonography
腹部単純撮影	plain abdominal radiograph, KUB (kidney, ureter, bladder) film, flat plate

8. 消化器系

空気液面 くうきえきめん	air-fluid level
上部消化管造影法 じょうぶしょうかかんぞうえいほう	upper gastrointestinal series (UGIS)
シャツキー輪 りん	Schatzki ring

⟨*lower esophageal ring; a fibrous constriction or web, usually associated with hiatal hernia*⟩

ニッシェ	niche
ひだ集中 しゅうちゅう	convergence of the folds
陰影欠損 いんえいけっそん, 充満欠損 じゅうまんけっそん	filling defect
二重造影法 にじゅうぞうえいほう	double-contrast radiography
粘膜レリーフ造影法 ねんまくぞうえいほう	mucosal relief radiography
低緊張性十二指腸造影 ていきんちょうせいじゅうにしちょうぞうえい	hypotonic duodenography (HDG)
注腸検査 ちゅうちょうけんさ, バリウム注腸造影	barium enema (BE)
胆嚢造影法 たんのうぞうえいほう	cholecystography
胆管造影法 たんかんぞうえいほう	cholangiography
点滴静注胆管造影法 てんてきじょうちゅうたんかんぞうえいほう	drip infusion cholangiography (DIC)
経皮経肝胆管造影法 けいひけいかんたんかんぞうえいほう	percutaneous transhepatic cholangiography (PTC)
術中胆管造影法 じゅつちゅうたんかんぞうえいほう	operative cholangiography
内視鏡的逆行性胆道膵管造影法 ないしきょうてきぎゃっこうせいたんどうすいかんぞうえいほう	endoscopic retrograde cholangiopancreatography (ERCP)
磁気共鳴胆道膵管造影法 じききょうめいたんどうすいかんぞうえいほう	magnetic resonance cholangiopancreatography (MRCP)
選択的腹腔動脈造影法 せんたくてきふくくうどうみゃくぞうえいほう	selective celiac angiography (SCA)
消化管内視鏡検査 しょうかかんないしきょうけんさ	gastrointestinal endocopy
食道胃十二指腸内視鏡検査 しょくどういじゅうにしちょうないしきょうけんさ	esophagogastroduodenoscopy (EGD)
胃内視鏡検査 いないしきょうけんさ	gastroscopy, 〔形〕gastroscopic
十二指腸内視鏡検査 じゅうにしちょうないしきょうけんさ	duodenoscopy, 〔形〕duodenoscopic
大腸内視鏡検査 だいちょうないしきょうけんさ	colonoscopy, 〔形〕colonoscopic
小腸内視鏡検査 しょうちょうないしきょうけんさ	enteroscopy

IV章 診療録用語

S状結腸内視鏡検査	sigmoidoscopy
直腸鏡検査	proctoscopy
経皮経肝胆道鏡検査	percutaneous transhepatic cholangioscopy (PTCS)
カプセル内視鏡検査	capsule endoscopy
超音波内視鏡検査	endoscopic ultrasonography (EUS)
管腔内超音波検査法	intraductal ultrasonography (IDUS)
腹腔鏡検査	laparoscopy, 〔形〕laparoscopic
胃生検	gastric biopsy
腹腔鏡下生検	laparoscopic biopsy
肝生検	liver biopsy
腹腔穿刺	paracentesis, abdominal paracentesis
診断的腹腔洗浄	diagnostic peritoneal lavage (DPL)
マロリー体	Mallory body

〈*hyaline cytoplasmic inclusions in hepatocytes, seen in alcoholic liver disease*〉

ランソン判定基準　Ranson criteria

〈*five signs at admission and six signs at 48 hours to assess severity of acute pancreatitis*〉

● 疾患名　Diseases ●

上部消化管出血	upper gastrointestinal bleeding
機能性ディスペプシア	functional dyspepsia (FD)
食道憩室	esophageal diverticulum
ツェンカー憩室	Zenker diverticulum

〈*pharyngoesophageal diverticulum; pulsion type*〉

食道静脈瘤	esophageal varix
裂孔ヘルニア	hiatal hernia, hiatus hernia
横隔膜ヘルニア	diaphragmatic hernia
逆流性食道炎	reflux esophagitis
胃食道逆流症	gastroesophageal reflux disease (GERD)
非びらん性胃食道逆流症	non-erosive reflux disease (NERD)
マロリー・ワイス症候群	Mallory-Weiss syndrome

〈*UGI bleeding from lacerations of the mucosa at the gastroesopha-*

geal junction induced by vomiting or retching⟩

ボエルハーヴェ症候群　　Boerhaave syndrome
⟨*esophageal rupture caused by retching or vomiting*⟩

バレット食道　　Barrett esophagus
⟨*metaplasia of the lower esophageal mucosa to columnar-lined epithelium*⟩

アカラシア　　achalasia
食道癌　　esophageal cancer
急性（慢性）胃炎　　acute (chronic) gastritis
急性胃粘膜病変　　acute gastric mucosal lesion (AGML)
消化性潰瘍　　peptic ulcer, peptic ulcer disease (PUD)
胃潰瘍　　gastric ulcer (GU), ulcus ventriculi
クッシング潰瘍　　Cushing ulcer
⟨*small peptic ulcers associated with CNS lesions or after brain surgery*⟩

デュラフォア潰瘍　　Dieulafoy ulcer
⟨*a pinpoint arterial bleeding near the cardia; a submucosal artery causes pressure erosion of the mucosa and ruptures into the lumen*⟩

胃前庭部毛細血管拡張症　　gastric antral vascular ectasia (GAVE)
胃下垂　　gastroptosis
胃腺腫　　gastric adenoma
胃ポリープ　　gastric polyp
異型上皮　　atypical epithelium (ATP)
メネトリエ病　　Ménétrier disease
⟨*hypertrophic gastropathy with thickened gastric folds*⟩

胃粘膜下腫瘍　　gastric submucosal tumor
消化管間質腫瘍　　gastrointestinal stromal tumor (GIST)
胃癌　　gastric cancer
早期胃癌　　early gastric cancer (EGC)
スキルス胃癌　　scirrhous gastric carcinoma
幽門狭窄　　pyloric stenosis
十二指腸炎　　duodenitis
十二指腸潰瘍　　duodenal ulcer (DU), ulcus duodeni
カーリング潰瘍　　Curling ulcer
⟨*duodenal ulcer in burn patients; causes significant bleeding*⟩

十二指腸憩室　　duodenal diverticulum
吻合部潰瘍　　stomal ulcer
腸炎　　enteritis
憩室炎　　diverticulitis
虫垂炎　　appendicitis

メッケル憩室 （けいしつ）	Meckel diverticulum

⟨congenital ileal diverticulum derived from unobliterated omphalomesenteric duct; may be attached to the umbilicus; heterotopic gastric tissue can cause peptic ulceration and bleeding⟩

腸閉塞（ちょうへいそく），イレウス	ileus, intestinal obstruction
感染性腸炎（かんせんせいちょうえん）	infectious enterocolitis
サルモネラ症（しょう）	salmonellosis

⟨Salmonella infections commonly manifested as food poisoning; typhoid fever and paratyphoid fever included⟩

炎症性腸疾患（えんしょうせいちょうしっかん）	inflammatory bowel disease (IBD)
クローン病（びょう）	Crohn disease (CD)

⟨regional enteritis; chronic granulomatous disease of the GI tract, most often in the terminal ileum⟩

潰瘍性大腸炎（かいようせいだいちょうえん）	ulcerative colitis (UC)
中毒性巨大結腸（ちゅうどくせいきょだいけっちょう）	toxic megacolon
虚血性大腸炎（きょけつせいだいちょうえん）	ischemic colitis
非閉塞性腸管虚血症（ひへいそくせいちょうかんきょけつしょう）	nonocclusive mesenteric ischemia (NOMI)
抗生物質関連大腸炎（こうせいぶっしつかんれんだいちょうえん）	antibiotic-associated colitis (AAC)
急性出血性大腸炎（きゅうせいしゅっけつせいだいちょうえん）	acute hemorrhagic colitis (AHC)
偽膜性大腸炎（ぎまくせいだいちょうえん）	pseudomembranous colitis (PMC)
放射線直腸炎（ほうしゃせんちょくちょうえん）	radiation proctitis
過敏性腸症候群（かびんせいちょうしょうこうぐん）	irritable bowel syndrome (IBS)
吸収不良症候群（きゅうしゅうふりょうしょうこうぐん）	malabsorption syndrome
ウィップル病（びょう）	Whipple disease

⟨malabsorption syndrome caused by Tropheryma whippelii, characterized by steatorrhea, lymphadenopathy, arthritis, hyperpigmentation, uveitis, and CNS involvement⟩

胃切除後症候群（いせつじょごしょうこうぐん）	postgastrectomy syndrome
ダンピング症候群（しょうこうぐん）	dumping syndrome
輸入脚症候群（ゆにゅうきゃくしょうこうぐん）	afferent loop syndrome
盲係蹄症候群（もうけいていしょうこうぐん）	blind loop syndrome
タンパク漏出性腸症（ろうしゅっせいちょうしょう）	protein-losing enteropathy
セリアック病（びょう）	celiac disease
腸偽閉塞（ちょうぎへいそく）	intestinal pseudo-obstruction
大腸ポリープ（だいちょう）	colonic polyp

家族性腺腫性ポリポーシス	familial adenomatous polyposis (FAP)
家族性大腸ポリポーシス	familial polyposis coli (FPC)
遺伝性非ポリポーシス大腸癌	hereditary nonpolyposis colorectal cancer (HNPCC), Lynch syndrome
ガードナー症候群	Gardner syndrome

⟨*FAP with extracolonic lesions like osteomas, epidermoid cysts, fibromas, and tooth impactions; autosomal dominant*⟩

ポイツ・ジェガース症候群	Peutz-Jeghers syndrome

⟨*numerous hamartomas in the intestine and melanin spots of the lips, buccal mucosa, and fingers; autosomal dominant*⟩

クロンカイト・カナダ症候群	Cronkhite-Canada syndrome

⟨*hamartomatous polyposis with malabsorption, alopecia, and nail dystrophy*⟩

カウデン病	Cowden disease

⟨*multiple hamartoma syndrome; hamartomas in the stomach, colon, mouth, skin, breast, and thyroid*⟩

ミュア・トレ症候群	Muir-Torre syndrome

⟨*multiple colorectal carcinomas with sebaceous tumors*⟩

大腸憩室症	colonic diverticulosis
結腸癌	colonic cancer
直腸癌	rectal cancer
痔核	hemorrhoid
痔瘻	anal fistula
裂肛	anal fissure, fissure in ano
脂肪肝	fatty liver
急性妊娠脂肪肝	acute fatty liver in pregnancy (AFLP)
急性(慢性, 亜急性)肝炎	acute (chronic, subacute) hepatitis
ウイルス性肝炎	viral hepatitis
A (B, C, D, E) 型肝炎	hepatitis A (B, C, D, E)
輸血後肝炎	post-transfusion hepatitis (PTH)
劇症肝炎	fulminant hepatitis
慢性活動性肝炎	chronic active hepatitis (CAH)
自己免疫性肝炎	autoimmune hepatitis (AIH)
アルコール性肝疾患	alcoholic liver disease (ALD)
非アルコール性脂肪性肝疾患	nonalcoholic fatty liver disease (NAFLD)

IV章 診療録用語

非アルコール性脂肪性肝炎	nonalcoholic steatohepatitis (NASH)
ジーヴ症候群	Zieve syndrome ⟨jaundice, hemolytic anemia, and hyperlipidemia associated with alcoholic fatty liver and cirrhosis⟩
ワイル病	Weil disease ⟨icterohemorrhagic leptospirosis characterized by fever, jaundice, azotemia, bleeding tendency, and myalgia⟩
肝内胆汁うっ滞	intrahepatic cholestasis
体質性高ビリルビン血症	constitutional hyperbilirubinemia
ジルベール症候群	Gilbert syndrome ⟨familial nonhemolytic jaundice due to an inborn error of bilirubin metabolism; elevated unconjugated bilirubin without liver damage⟩
デュビン・ジョンソン症候群	Dubin-Johnson syndrome ⟨familial nonhemolytic jaundice due to a defect of hepatic excretion of conjugated bilirubin; retention of a brown pigment in the hepatic cells characteristic⟩
バイラー病	Byler disease ⟨progressive familial intrahepatic cholestasis; cirrhosis and death in early childhood; autosomal recessive⟩
肝硬変症	cirrhosis of the liver, liver cirrhosis (LC)
非代償性肝硬変	decompensated liver cirrhosis
肝細胞癌	hepatocellular carcinoma (HCC), hepatoma
肝膿瘍	liver abscess, hepatic abscess
肝不全	hepatic failure
肝性脳症	hepatic encephalopathy
原発性硬化性胆管炎	primary sclerosing cholangitis (PSC)
原発性胆汁性肝硬変	primary biliary cirrhosis (PBC)
慢性非化膿性破壊性胆管炎	chronic nonsuppurative destructive cholangitis (CNSDC)
特発性門脈圧亢進症	idiopathic portal hypertension (IPH)
肝外門脈閉塞症	extrahepatic portal obstruction (EHO)
バッド・キアリ症候群	Budd-Chiari syndrome ⟨hepatic vein obstruction⟩
肝静脈閉塞性疾患	veno-occlusive disease (VOD)

8. 消化器系

ヘモクロマトーシス (かんじょうみゃくへいそくせいしっかん)	hemochromatosis
肝レンズ核変性症,ウィルソン病 (かん―かくへんせいしょう)	hepatolenticular degeneration, Wilson disease

⟨*liver cirrhosis, neurological manifestations, and Kayser-Fleischer ring, caused by accumulation of copper in the liver, basal ganglia, and cornea due to abnormal copper transport; autosomal recessive*⟩

胆嚢炎 (たんのうえん)	cholecystitis
胆石症 (たんせきしょう)	cholelithiasis
肝内結石症 (かんないけっせきしょう)	intrahepatic cholelithiasis
胆嚢ポリープ (たんのう―)	gallbladder polyp
胆嚢腺筋腫症 (たんのうせんきんしゅしょう)	gallbladder adenomyomatosis
胆嚢切除後症候群 (たんのうせつじょごしょうこうぐん)	postcholecystectomy syndrome
胆管炎 (たんかんえん)	cholangitis
急性閉塞性化膿性胆管炎 (きゅうせいへいそくせいかのうせいたんかんえん)	acute obstructive suppurative cholangitis (AOSC)
総胆管嚢腫 (そうたんかんのうしゅ)	choledochal cyst
カロリ病 (―びょう)	Caroli disease

⟨*congenital dilatation of the intrahepatic bile ducts*⟩

胆嚢癌 (たんのうがん)	gallbladder cancer
胆管癌 (たんかんがん)	bile duct cancer, cholangiocarcinoma
胆管細胞癌 (たんかんさいぼうがん)	cholangiocellular carcinoma (CCC)
クラッツキン腫瘍 (―しゅよう)	Klatskin tumor

⟨*cholangiocarcinoma at the bifurcation of the common hepatic duct*⟩

急性 (慢性) 膵炎	acute (chronic) pancreatitis
急性出血性膵炎 (きゅうせいしゅっけつせいすいえん)	acute hemorrhagic pancreatitis (AHP)

Tidbits

bezoar

英語では「ビーゾー」と発音するが,日常は「胃石」あるいはドイツ語読みで「ベツォアール」と呼んでいる.胃に限らず人や動物の消化管内結石のことで,ペルシャ語の pādzahr (pād: protector, zahr: stone) に由来し,ウシやヒツジの胃腸内から取り出して解毒に用いられていたことから「解毒薬」を意味していた.成分により,phytobezoar (植物), trichobezoar (毛髪), diosopyrobezoar (柿), pharmacobezoar (薬物) などと呼ぶ.なお胃石は gastrolith という.

210　IV章　診療録用語

急性壊死性膵炎 きゅうせいえしせいすいえん	acute necrotizing pancreatitis (ANP)
慢性石灰化膵炎 まんせいせっかいかすいえん	chronic calcifying pancreatitis, chronic calcific pancreatitis
膵石症 すいせきしょう	pancreatolithiasis
自己免疫性膵炎 じこめんえきせいすいえん	autoimmune pancreatitis (AIP)
膵嚢胞 すいのうほう	pancreatic cyst
膵偽性嚢胞 すいぎせいのうほう	pancreatic pseudocyst
異所性膵 いしょせい	heterotopic pancreas
輪状膵 りんじょうすい	annular pancreas
膵嚢胞線維症 すいのうほうせんいしょう	cystic fibrosis of pancreas
膵島細胞腫瘍 すいとうさいぼうしゅよう	islet cell tumor
膵癌 すいがん	pancreatic cancer
急性腹症 きゅうせいふくしょう	acute abdomen
腹膜炎 ふくまくえん	peritonitis
特発性細菌性腹膜炎 とくはつせいさいきんせいふくまくえん	spontaneous bacterial peritonitis (SBP)
腹膜偽粘液腫 ふくまくぎねんえきしゅ	pseudomyxoma peritonei
鼠径ヘルニア そけい	inguinal hernia
直接鼠径ヘルニア ちょくせつそけい	direct inguinal hernia
間接鼠径ヘルニア かんせつそけい	indirect inguinal hernia
大腿ヘルニア だいたい	femoral hernia, crural hernia
腹壁ヘルニア ふくへき	ventral hernia, abdominal hernia
臍ヘルニア へそ	umbilical hernia
腸壁ヘルニア ちょうへき, リヒターヘルニア	parietal hernia, Richter hernia

⟨*an incarcerated femoral or inguinal hernia in which only the antimesenteric border of the bowel is involved*⟩

● 治療法　Treatment ●

鎮痙薬 ちんけいやく	antispasmodic
抗コリン薬 こう―やく	anticholinergic
制酸薬 せいさんやく	antacid
粘膜保護薬 ねんまくほごやく	mucosal protective agent
スクラルファート水和物 ―すいわぶつ	sucralfate hydrate《アルサルミン》
プロスタグランジンアナログ	prostaglandin analog
ミソプロストール	misoprostol《サイトテック》
H_2受容体拮抗薬 ―じゅようたいきっこうやく	H_2-receptor antagonist, H_2 blocker
シメチジン	cimetidine《タガメット》
プロトンポンプ阻害薬	proton pump inhibitor (PPI)

オメプラゾール	omeprazole《オメプラゾン》
ヘリコバクター・ピロリ除菌療法	Helicobacter pylori eradication therapy
制吐薬	antiemetic
ドンペリドン	domperidone《ナウゼリン》
プロクロルペラジン	prochlorperazine《ノバミン》
グラニセトロン塩酸塩	granisetron hydrochloride《カイトリル》
ニューロキニン1受容体拮抗薬	neurokinin-1 receptor antagonist
下剤	cathartic, purgative, laxative
ピコスルファートナトリウム	sodium picosulfate《ラキソベロン》
センノシド	sennoside《プルゼニド》
止瀉薬	antidiarrheals
ロペラミド塩酸塩	loperamide hydrochloride《ロペミン》
タンニン酸アルブミン	albumin tannate《タンナルビン》
ラモセトロン塩酸塩	ramosetron hydrochloride《イリボー》
ポリカルボフィルカルシウム	polycarbophil calcium《コロネル》
駆虫薬, 虫下し	anthelmintic, vermifuge
利胆薬	choleretic, cholagogue
胆石溶解薬	stone dissolvent
ウルソデオキシコール酸	ursodeoxycholic acid (UDCA)《ウルソ》
ケノデオキシコール酸	chenodeoxycholic acid (CDCA)《チノ》
サラゾスルファピリジン	salazosulfapyridine (SASP)《サラゾピリン》
メサラジン	mesalazine《ペンタサ》
インフリキシマブ	infliximab (IFX)《レミケード》
インターフェロン	interferon (IFN)《スミフェロン, フエロン》
ペグインターフェロン	peginterferon (PEG-IFN)《ペガシス》
ラミブジン	lamivudine《ゼフィックス》
アデホビルピボキシル	adefovir pivoxil《ヘプセラ》
エンテカビル水和物	entecavir hydrate《バラクルード》
リバビリン	ribavirin《レベトール》
分枝鎖アミノ酸	branched-chain amino acid (BCAA)
タンパク分解酵素阻害薬	protease inhibitor
胃洗浄	gastric lavage, gastric irrigation
経鼻胃管	nasogastric (NG) tube
レヴィン管	Levin tube

⟨a nasogastric tube for gastric decompression⟩

ミラー・アボット管 かん　Miller-Abbott tube
⟨a double-channel intestinal tube, one with an inflatable balloon and the other with a metallic tip, for decompression of the small intestine⟩

ゼングスターケン・ブレークモア管 かん　Sengstaken-Blakemore (SB) tube
⟨a three-lumen tube, one for gastric drainage and two for inflation of gastric and esophageal balloons, used for the tamponade of bleeding esophageal varices⟩

経管栄養 けいかんえいよう　tube feeding
強制経管栄養 きょうせいけいかんえいよう　gastrogavage, gavage
経腸栄養 けいちょうえいよう　enteral nutrition
経静脈高カロリー輸液 けいじょうみゃくこう──ゆえき　intravenous hyperalimentation (IVH)
血球除去療法 けっきゅうじょきょりょうほう　cytapheresis
白血球除去療法 はっけっきゅうじょきょりょうほう　leukocytapheresis
人工肝補助療法 じんこうかんほじょりょうほう　artificial liver support (ALS)
ストーマケア　stoma care
注射硬化療法 ちゅうしゃこうかりょうほう　injection sclerotherapy
フェノール　phenol 《パオスクレー》
硫酸アルミニウムカリウム・タンニン酸 りゅうさん──さん　aluminum potassium sulfate-tannic acid (ALTA) 《ジオン》
内視鏡下手術 ないしきょうかしゅじゅつ　endoscopic operation, endoscopic surgical procedure
内視鏡的止血 ないしきょうてきしけつ　endoscopic hemostasis
内視鏡的ポリープ切除術 ──てき──せつじょじゅつ　endoscopic polypectomy
大腸内視鏡のポリープ切除術 だいちょう──てきせつじょじゅつ　colonoscopic polypectomy
内視鏡的粘膜切除術 ──てきねんまくせつじょじゅつ　endoscopic mucosal resection (EMR)
内視鏡的粘膜下層剥離術 ──てきねんまくかそうはくりじゅつ　endoscopic submucosal dissection (ESD)
内視鏡的静脈瘤硬化療法 ──てきじょうみゃくりゅうこうかりょうほう　endoscopic injection sclerotherapy (EIS) for varices
内視鏡的静脈瘤結紮術 ──てきじょうみゃくりゅうけっさつじゅつ　endoscopic variceal ligation (EVL)
内視鏡的乳頭切開術 ──てきにゅうとうせっかいじゅつ　endoscopic papillotomy (EPT)
内視鏡的乳頭括約筋切開　endoscopic sphincterotomy (EST)

術	
内視鏡的経鼻胆道ドレナージ	endoscopic nasobiliary drainage (ENBD)
内視鏡的逆行性胆道ドレナージ	endoscopic retrograde biliary drainage (ERBD)
内視鏡的拡張器	endoscopic dilator
拡張性金属ステント	expandable metallic stent (EMS)
腹腔・静脈短絡術	peritoneovenous (PV) shunt
デンバーシャント	Denver shunt
用手補助腹腔鏡手術	hand-assisted laparoscopic surgery (HALS)
腹腔鏡下胆嚢摘出術	laparoscopic cholecystectomy (LC)
経皮的内視鏡下胃瘻造設術	percutaneous endoscopic gastrostomy (PEG)
経皮経肝胆汁ドレナージ	percutaneous transhepatic biliary drainage (PTBD)
経皮経肝胆嚢ドレナージ	percutaneous transhepatic gallbladder drainage (PTGBD)
経皮経肝食道静脈瘤塞栓術	percutaneous transhepatic obliteration (PTO) of esophageal varices
経頸静脈性肝内門脈体循環短絡	transjugular intrahepatic portosystemic shunt (TIPS)
バルーン閉塞下逆行性経静脈の塞栓術	balloon-occluded retrograde transvenous obliteration (BRTO)
経カテーテル動脈塞栓術	transcatheter arterial embolization (TAE)
経カテーテル動脈化学塞栓術	transcatheter arterial chemoembolization (TACE)
部分的脾動脈塞栓術	partial splenic embolization (PSE)
肝動脈注入療法	transhepatic arterial infusion (TAI)
肝動脈持続動注療法	continuous hepatic arterial infusion (CHAI)
経皮的エタノール注入療法	percutaneous ethanol injection therapy (PEIT)
経皮的マイクロ波凝固療	percutaneous microwave coagulation

法	therapy (PMCT)
ラジオ波焼灼療法	radiofrequency ablation (RFA)
開腹術	laparotomy
試験開腹術	exploratory laparotomy
食道切除術	esophagectomy
噴門筋切開術, ヘラー手術	cardiomyotomy, Heller operation

⟨surgical division of circular muscles of the lower esophagus for the treatment of achalasia⟩

ニッセン噴門形成術	Nissen fundoplication

⟨antireflux procedure using complete wrap of the gastric fundus around the distal esophagus⟩

胃切除術	gastrectomy
胃全摘術	total gastrectomy
胃亜全摘術	subtotal gastrectomy
ビルロートⅠ法	Billroth Ⅰ (BⅠ)

⟨distal gastrectomy with gastroduodenostomy⟩

ビルロートⅡ法	Billroth Ⅱ (BⅡ)

⟨distal gastrectomy with gastrojejunostomy⟩

幽門形成術	pyloroplasty
腹腔鏡下胃緊縛術	laparoscopic gastric banding (LGB)
胃空腸吻合術	gastrojejunostomy
ルー・ワイ吻合	Roux-en-Y anastomosis

⟨Y-shaped anastomosis of the jejunum used in esophago-, gastro-, hepatico-, or pancreaticojejunostomy⟩

選択的迷走神経切離術	selective vagotomy
虫垂切除術	appendectomy
結腸切除術	colectomy
腹腔鏡補助下結腸切除術	laparoscopic-assisted colectomy (LAC)
腹会陰式直腸切除術, マイルズ手術	abdominoperineal resection of rectum, Miles operation

⟨combined abdominal and perineal resection for rectal cancer with a permanent colostomy⟩

ハルトマン手術	Hartmann operation

⟨sigmoid resection at the peritoneal reflexion with closure of the rectal stump and descending colostomy⟩

造瘻術	ostomy

腸瘻造設術 ちょうろうぞうせつじゅつ	enterostomy
人工肛門造設術 じんこうこうもんぞうせつじゅつ	colostomy
痔核切除術 じかくせつじょじゅつ	hemorrhoidectomy
直腸脱・内痔核手術 ちょくちょう・だつないじかくしゅじゅつ	procedure for prolapse and hemorrhoids (PPH)
肝切除術 かんせつじょじゅつ	hepatectomy
胆嚢摘出術 たんのうてきしゅつじゅつ	cholecystectomy
総胆管十二指腸吻合術 そうたんかんじゅうにしちょうふんごうじゅつ	choledochoduodenostomy
総胆管空腸吻合術 そうたんかんくうちょうふんごうじゅつ	choledochojejunodenostomy
門脈下大静脈吻合術 もんみゃくかだいじょうみゃくふんごうじゅつ	portacaval shunt (PCS)
肝移植 かんいしょく	liver transplantation
膵頭十二指腸切除術 すいとうじゅうにしちょうせつじょじゅつ	pancreaticoduodenectomy (PD)
膵体尾部切除術 すいたいびぶせつじょじゅつ	distal pancreatectomy
膵空腸吻合術 すいくうちょうふんごうじゅつ	pancreaticojejunostomy
ウィップル手術 ―しゅじゅつ	Whipple operation

⟨radical pancreaticoduodenectomy with distal gastrectomy, gastrojejunostomy, choledochojejunostomy, and pancreaticojejunostomy⟩

ピュストー術式 ―じゅつしき	Puestow procedure

⟨side-to-side pancreaticojejunostomy for relief of pain in chronic pancreatitis⟩

脾摘出術 ひてきしゅつじゅつ	splenectomy
ヘルニア縫合術 ―ほうごうじゅつ	herniorrhaphy

Tidbits

Bristol stool form scale

便の形状を表現するのに soft と hard だけでは能がない．腸管機能障害を評価するために提案された Bristol stool form scale (O'Donnell LJD et al, Br Med J 1990; 300: 439-440) が参考になる．Type 1: separate hard lumps like nuts (difficult to pass), Type 2: sausage-shaped but lumpy, Type 3: like a sausage but with cracks on its surface, Type 4: like a sausage or snake, smooth and soft, Type 5: soft blobs with clear-cut edges (passed easily), Type 6: fluffy pieces with ragged edges, a mushy stool, Type 7: watery, no solid pieces, entirely liquid の7型のうち，Type 1, 2 は constipation, Type 6, 7 は diarrhea と判断する．'blob' とは，'a small round mass of liquid or sticky substance' で，ぶよぶよの塊のことである．

9. 腎・泌尿器系

● 愁訴・症状　Complaints / Symptoms ●

腎臓病 じんぞうびょう	kidney trouble
下部尿路症状 かぶにょうろしょうじょう	lower urinary tract symptoms (LUTS)
むくみ	swelling, puffiness, edema
まぶたの腫れ —は	puffy eyelids
腰痛 ようつう	low back pain
側腹部痛 そくふくぶつう	flank pain
腎仙痛 じんせんつう	renal colic
恥骨上痛 ちこつじょうつう	suprapubic pain
会陰痛 えいんつう	perineal pain
前立腺痛 ぜんりつせんつう	prostatodynia
排尿痛 はいにょうつう	pain on urination, micturition pain, urodynia
尿道痛 にょうどうつう	urethralgia
排尿 はいにょう	urination, micturition, [動]pass (void) urine, urinate, micturate
尿量 にょうりょう	volume of urine, urinary output
血尿 けつにょう	bloody urine, hematuria
混濁尿 こんだくにょう	cloudy (nebulous, turbid) urine
排尿困難 はいにょうこんなん	difficulty in urination, dysuria
尿線 にょうせん	urinary stream
尿線途絶 にょうせんとぜつ	interrupted urinary stream
尿線細少 にょうせんさいしょう	poor urinary stream
尿勢低下 にょうせいていか	decreased force of the urinary stream, weak urinary stream
尿滴下 にょうてきか	dribbling of urine, [動]dribble
排尿遅延 はいにょうちえん	hesitancy in voiding
尿を漏らす にょう—	lose urine, wet one's pants
尿失禁 にょうしっきん	urinary incontinence, [形]incontinent of urine
腹圧性排尿 ふくあつせいはいにょう	straining to void
排尿時灼熱感 はいにょうじしゃくねつかん	burning on urination, urine ardor
尿意 にょうい	urge (desire) to urinate, micturition desire
尿意を催す にょうい—	have an urge to urinate
尿意切迫 にょうせっぱく	urinary urgency, urgency of micturition
残尿感 ざんにょうかん	sensation of incomplete emptying
尿閉 にょうへい	urinary retention, ischuria
頻尿 ひんにょう	urinary frequency, pollakiuria

9. 腎・泌尿器系

夜間頻尿 やかんひんにょう	frequent urination during the night, nocturia
夜間多尿 やかんたにょう	nycturia
多尿 たにょう	polyuria
乏尿 ぼうにょう	oliguria
無尿 むにょう	anuria
夜尿症 やにょうしょう	bed-wetting, enuresis
国際前立腺症状スコア こくさいぜんりつせんしょうじょう―	international prostate symptom score (IPSS)

● 診察所見・徴候 Physical findings / Signs ●

尿毒症性口臭 にょうどくしょうせいこうしゅう	uremic fetor, uremic breath
眼瞼浮腫 がんけんふしゅ	palpebral edema, blepharedema
下腿圧痕浮腫 かたいあっこんふしゅ	pretibial pitting edema
末梢浮腫 まっしょうふしゅ	peripheral edema
全身浮腫 ぜんしんふしゅ	anasarca, generalized massive edema
胸水 きょうすい	pleural effusion
腹水 ふくすい	ascites
高血圧 こうけつあつ	hypertension
肋骨脊柱角圧痛 ろっこつせきちゅうかくあっつう	costovertebral angle (CVA) tenderness
腎触知 じんしょくち	palpable kidney
一側性腎腫瘤 いっそくせいじんしゅりゅう	unilateral renal mass
腎血管雑音 じんけっかんざつおん	renal bruit
溢流性尿失禁 いつりゅうせいにょうしっきん	overflow incontinence
奇異性尿失禁 きいせい―	paradoxical incontinence
切迫性尿失禁 せっぱくせい―	urge incontinence, urgency incontinence
緊張性尿失禁 きんちょうせい―	stress incontinence
反射性尿失禁 はんしゃせい―	reflex incontinence
受動失禁 じゅどうしっきん	passive incontinence
膀胱拡張 ぼうこうかくちょう	distended bladder
陰嚢腫脹 いんのうしゅちょう	scrotal swelling
陰嚢腫瘤 いんのうしゅりゅう	scrotal mass
前立腺腫大硬結 ぜんりつせんしゅだいこうけつ	swollen and indurated prostate
前立腺マッサージ ぜんりつせん―	prostatic massage
前立腺液 ぜんりつせんえき	prostatic secretions
尿道分泌物 にょうどうぶんぴつぶつ	urethral discharge

● 検査法 Examination ●

検尿 けんにょう	urinalysis (UA), examination of urine
中間尿 ちゅうかんにょう	midstream urine

清潔採取尿 せいけつさいしゅにょう	clean-voided urine, clean catch urine
カテーテル尿 にょう	catheterized urine
24時間尿検体 24じかんにょうけんたい	24-hour urine specimen
尿試験紙 にょうしけんし	dipstick
肉眼的血尿 にくがんてきけつにょう	gross hematuria, macroscopic hematuria
顕微鏡的血尿 けんびきょうてきけつにょう	microscopic hematuria
ヘモグロビン尿 にょう	hemoglobinuria
糖尿 とうにょう	glycosuria, glucosuria
タンパク尿 にょう	proteinuria
微量アルブミン尿 びりょうにょう	microalbuminuria
白血球尿 はっけっきゅうにょう	leukocyturia
好酸球尿 こうさんきゅうにょう	eosinophiluria
膿尿 のうにょう	pyuria
細菌尿 さいきんにょう	bacteriuria, bacilluria
円柱尿 えんちゅうにょう	cylindruria
結晶尿 けっしょうにょう	crystalluria
乳び尿 にゅうびにょう	chyluria
ビリルビン尿 にょう	bilirubinuria
ウロビリノーゲン尿 にょう	urobilinogenuria
アミノ酸尿 にょうさん	aminoaciduria
尿酸尿 にょうさんにょう	uricaciduria
ケトン尿 にょう	ketonuria
尿沈渣 にょうちんさ	urinary sediment
シュウ酸塩	oxalate
炭酸塩	carbonate
リン酸塩	phosphate
赤血球円柱 せっけっきゅうえんちゅう	red blood cell cast
白血球円柱 はっけっきゅうえんちゅう	white blood cell cast, leukocyte cast
顆粒円柱 かりゅうえんちゅう	granular cast
上皮円柱 じょうひえんちゅう	epithelial cast
硝子円柱 しょうしえんちゅう	hyaline cast
蝋様円柱 ろうようえんちゅう	waxy cast
脂肪円柱 しぼうえんちゅう	fatty cast
細菌円柱 さいきんえんちゅう	bacterial cast
シュウ酸カルシウム結石 けっせき	calcium oxalate calculus
尿酸結石 にょうさんけっせき	urate calculus
シスチン結石 けっせき	cystine calculus
ストルビット結石 けっせき	struvite calculus

⟨<*HCG von Struve; a urinary calculus composed of magnesium ammonium phosphate; associated with infection caused by urea-*

splitting bacteria such as Proteus⟩

サンゴ状結石 けつじょう	staghorn calculus
尿比重測定 にょうひじゅうそくてい	urinometry
低張尿 ていちょうにょう	hyposthenuria
尿培養 にょうばいよう	urine culture
大腸菌 だいちょうきん	*Escherichia coli*
緑膿菌 りょくのうきん	*Pseudomonas aeruginosa*
腸球菌 ちょうきゅうきん	*Enterococcus*
腐性ブドウ球菌 ふせいきゅうきん	*Staphylococcus saprophyticus*
尿細胞診 にょうさいぼうしん	urine cytology
N-アセチルグルコサミニダーゼ	N-acetylglucosaminidase (NAG)
β_2 ミクログロブリン	β_2-microglobulin
血清クレアチニン けっせい	serum creatinine (Cr)
血液尿素窒素 けつえきにょうそちっそ	blood urea nitrogen (BUN)
高窒素血症 こうちっそけっしょう	azotemia
シスタチンC	cystatin C
高カリウム血症 こうけっしょう	hyperkalemia
低ナトリウム血症 ていけっしょう	hyponatremia
代謝性アシドーシス たいしゃせい	metabolic acidosis
尿毒症性アシドーシス にょうどくしょうせい	uremic acidosis
陰イオンギャップ いん	anion gap (AG)
低タンパク血症 ていけっしょう	hypoproteinemia
酸性ホスファターゼ さんせい	acid phosphatase (ACP)
前立腺酸性ホスファターゼ ぜんりつせん	prostatic acid phosphatase (PAP)
血漿レニン活性 けっしょうかっせい	plasma renin activity (PRA)
抗好中球細胞質抗体 こうこうちゅうきゅうさいぼうしつこうたい	antineutrophil cytoplasmic antibody (ANCA)
抗好中球細胞質ミエロペルオキシダーゼ抗体 こうこうちゅうきゅうさいぼうしつこうたい	antineutrophil cytoplasmic myeloperoxidase antibody (MPO-ANCA)
前立腺特異抗原 ぜんりつせんとくいこうげん	prostate-specific antigen (PSA)
腎機能検査 じんきのうけんさ	renal function test
糸球体濾過量 しきゅうたいろかりょう	glomerular filtration rate (GFR)
推算糸球体濾過量 すいさんしきゅうたいろかりょう	estimated glomerular filtration rate (eGFR)
単一ネフロン糸球体濾過量 たんいつしきゅうたいろかりょう	single nephron glomerular filtration rate (SNGFR)
クレアチニンクリアランス	creatinine clearance (Ccr)

コッククロフト・ゴールト式 しき	Cockcroft-Gault formula

⟨*a formula for calculation of creatinine clearance; the value is reduced by 15% for women*⟩

イヌリンクリアランス	inulin clearance
イヌリード	Inulead
腎血漿流量 じんけっしょうりゅうしつりょう	renal plasma flow (RPF)
腎血流量 じんけつりゅうりょう	renal blood flow (RBF)
濾過分画 ろかぶんかく	filtration fraction (FF)
尿細管最大輸送量 にょうさいかんさいだいゆそうりょう	maximum capacity of tubular transport
フェノールスルホンフタレイン試験 けんし	phenolsulfonphthalein (PSP) test
パラアミノ馬尿酸クリアランス ばにょうさんにょ	p-aminohippurate (PAH) clearance
フィッシュバーグ濃縮試験 のうしゅくしけん	Fishberg concentration test

⟨*after overnight fluid deprivation, specific gravity of 3 urine samples, morning void and after 1 and 2 hours, is measured; <1.024 indicates impaired renal concentration*⟩

ナトリウム排泄分画 はいせつぶんかく	fractional excretion of sodium (FENa)
尿流動態検査法 にょうりゅうどうたいけんさほう	urodynamics, urodynamic study (UDS)
尿流測定 にょうりゅうそくてい	uroflowmetry
尿流計 にょうりゅうけい	uroflowmeter, uroflometer
尿流量 にょうりゅうりょう	urinary flow rate
最大尿流率 さいだいにょうりゅうりつ	maximum urinary flow rate
平均尿流率 へいきんにょうりゅうりつ	average urinary flow rate
残尿 ざんにょう	residual urine
膀胱内圧測定 ぼうこうないあつそくてい	cystometry
腹圧下尿漏出圧 ふくあつかにょうろうしゅつあつ	abdominal leak point pressure (ALPP)
経直腸的超音波検査 けいちょくちょうてきちょうおんぱけんさ	transrectal ultrasonography (TRUS)
静脈性腎盂造影法 じょうみゃくせいじんうぞうえいほう	intravenous pyelography (IVP)
点滴静注腎盂造影法 てんてきじょうちゅうじんうぞうえいほう	drip infusion pyelography (DIP)
逆行性腎盂造影法 ぎゃっこうせいじんうぞうえいほう	retrograde pyelography (RP)
逆行性尿路造影法	retrograde urography, cystoscopic urog-

	raphy
逆行性尿道造影法	retrograde urethrography
排尿時膀胱尿道造影法	voiding cystourethrography (VCUG)
腎動脈造影法	renal arteriography
腎シンチグラフィー	renal scintigraphy
ラジオアイソトープレノグラム	radioisotope renogram
膀胱鏡検査	cystoscopy
尿道鏡検査	urethroscopy
腎生検	renal biopsy
経尿道的生検	transurethral biopsy
グリソンスコア	Gleason score

⟨*a grading of localized adenocarcinoma of the prostate by evaluating glandular differentiation*⟩

● 疾患名　Diseases ●

急性糸球体腎炎	acute glomerulonephritis (AGN)
溶連菌感染後急性糸球体腎炎	poststreptococcal acute glomerulonephritis (PSAGN)
急速進行性糸球体腎炎	rapidly progressive glomerulonephritis (RPGN)
抗糸球体基底膜腎炎	anti-glomerular basement membrane (GBM) nephritis
グッドパスチャー症候群	Goodpasture syndrome

⟨*glomerulonephtiris, pulmonary hemorrhage, and circulating anti-glomerular basement membrane antibodies*⟩

慢性糸球体腎炎	chronic glomerulonephritis (CGN)
膜性増殖性糸球体腎炎	membranoproliferative glomerulonephritis (MPGN)
半月体形成性糸球体腎炎	crescentic glomerulonephritis
膜性腎症	membranous nephropathy (MN)
IgA腎症，ベルジェ病	IgA nephropathy, Berger disease

⟨*focal glomeruronephritis caused by IgA deposits in the glomerular mesangium, marked by hematuria and sometimes associated with upper respiratory infection*⟩

ループス腎炎	lupus nephritis
ネフローゼ症候群	nephrotic syndrome

微小変化型ネフローゼ症候群	minimal change nephrotic syndrome (MCNS)
微小変化群	minimal change disease (MCD), nil disease
巣状糸球体硬化症	focal glomerulosclerosis (FGS)
キンメルスチール・ウィルソン症候群	Kimmelstiel-Wilson syndrome

⟨*nephrotic syndrome and hypertension in diabetics, associated with nodular glomerulosclerosis*⟩

急性間質性腎炎	acute interstitial nephritis (AIN)
慢性間質性腎炎	chronic interstitial nephritis (CIN)
尿細管間質性腎炎	tubulointerstitial nephritis (TIN)
糖尿病性腎症	diabetic nephropathy
アルポート症候群	Alport syndrome

⟨*progressive nephritis, sensorineural hearing loss, and ocular abnormalities; hereditary*⟩

急性尿細管壊死	acute tubular necrosis (ATN)
圧挫症候群	crush syndrome
尿細管性アシドーシス	renal tubular acidosis (RTA)
肝腎症候群	hepatorenal syndrome
腎動脈血栓症	renal artery thrombosis
腎動脈狭窄	renal artery stenosis
腎静脈血栓症	renal vein thrombosis (RVT)
腎血管性高血圧	renovascular hypertension (RVH)
多発性嚢胞腎疾患	polycystic kidney disease (PKD)
常染色体優性多発嚢胞腎症	autosomal dominant polycystic kidney disease (ADPKD)
常染色体劣性多発嚢胞腎症	autosomal recessive polycystic kidney disease (ARPKD)
慢性腎臓病	chronic kidney disease (CKD)
心腎貧血症候群	cardio-renal-anemia syndrome
急性腎不全	acute renal failure (ARF)
急性腎障害	acute kidney injury (AKI)
慢性腎不全	chronic renal failure (CRF)
末期腎不全	end-stage renal disease (ESRD)
後天性嚢胞性腎疾患	acquired cystic disease of kidney

先天性嚢胞腎疾患	(ACDK)
腎硬化	nephrosclerosis
尿毒症	uremia
石灰化尿毒症性細動脈症	calcific uremic arteriolopathy (CUA), calciphylaxis
腎性骨異栄養症	renal osteodystrophy (ROD)
水腎症	hydronephrosis
萎縮腎	renal atrophy, contracted kidney
重複腎盂	duplicated renal pelvis, double renal pelvis
尿路結石症	urolithiasis, urinary lithiasis
腎結石	renal stone, kidney calculus, kidney stone
遊走腎	floating kidney
腎下垂	renal ptosis, nephroptosis
尿路感染症	urinary tract infection (UTI)
腎盂腎炎	pyelonephritis
尿管炎	ureteritis
前立腺炎	prostatitis
膀胱炎	cystitis
尿道炎	urethritis
尿道下裂	hypospadias, hypospadia
前立腺肥大症	benign prostatic hypertrophy (BPH)
前立腺結石	prostatolithiasis
膀胱下閉塞	bladder outlet obstruction (BOO)
膀胱尿管逆流	vesicoureteral reflux (VUR)
神経因性膀胱	neurogenic bladder
無抑制収縮	uninhibited contraction (UIC)
過活動膀胱	overactive bladder (OAB)
排尿筋・括約筋協調不全	detrusor-sphincter dyssynergia (DSD)
腎細胞癌, グラヴィッツ腫瘍	renal cell carcinoma (RCC), hypernephroma, Grawitz tumor
ストファー症候群	Stauffer syndrome
⟨*hepatic dysfunction without hepatic metastasis in patients with RCC*⟩	
腎血管筋脂肪腫	renal angiomyolipoma
前立腺上皮内腫瘍	prostatic intraepithelial neoplasia (PIN)
前立腺癌	prostatic cancer
膀胱腫瘍	bladder tumor (BT)
精巣腫瘍	testicular tumor

精上皮腫	seminoma
後腹膜線維症	retroperitoneal fibrosis
透析困難症候群	disdialysis syndrome
透析アミロイドーシス	dialysis amyloidosis, hemodialysis-associated amyloidosis
透析関節症	dialysis arthropathy
破壊性脊椎関節症	destructive spondyloarthropathy (DSA)
透析脳症	dialysis encephalopathy
被包性腹膜硬化症	encapsulating peritoneal sclerosis (EPS)

● 治療法　Treatment ●

低タンパク食	low protein diet, protein restricted diet
利尿薬	diuretic, diuretic agent
降圧薬	antihypertensive
抗ムスカリン薬	antimuscarinic agent
イミダフェナシン	imidafenacin《ウリトス》
タムスロシン塩酸塩	tamsulosin hydrochloride《ハルナール》
ナフトピジル	naftopidil《フリバス》
デュタステリド	dutasteride《アボルブ》
遺伝子組み換えヒトエリスロポエチン	recombinant human erythropoietin (r-HuEPO)
アンドロゲン欠損療法	androgen deprivation therapy (ADT)
LH-RH アゴニスト	luteinizing hormone-releasing hormone (LHRH) agonist
最大アンドロゲン遮断	maximum androgen blockade (MAB)
ゴセレリン酢酸塩	goserelin acetate《ゾラデックス》
ビカルタミド	bicalutamide《カソデックス》
ソラフェニブトシル酸塩	sorafenib tosilate《ネクサバール》
導尿，尿道カテーテル法	urethral catheterization
清潔間欠導尿	clean intermittent catheterization (CIC)
清潔間欠自己導尿	clean intermittent self-catheterization (CISC)
ネラトンカテーテル　〈*flexible catheter made of rubber*〉	Nélaton catheter
尿道ステント留置	urethral stent

9. 腎・泌尿器系

留置カテーテル りゅう―	indwelling catheter
フォーリーカテーテル	Foley catheter
	⟨an indwelling catheter with a retaining balloon⟩
膀胱洗浄 ぼうこうせんじょう	bladder irrigation
血液浄化法 けつえきじょうかほう	blood purification
人工透析 じんこうとうせき	artificial dialysis
人工腎 じんこうじん	artificial kidney (AK)
血液透析 けつえきとうせき	hemodialysis (HD)
透析器 とうせき	dialyzer
透析液 とうせき	dialysate
血液濾過 けつえきろか	hemofiltration (HF)
直接血液灌流 ちょくせつけつえきかんりゅう	direct hemoperfusion (DHP)
持続性静脈静脈血液濾過 じぞくせいじょうみゃくじょうみゃくけつえきろか	continuous venovenous hemofiltration (CVVH)
持続性動静脈血液濾過 じぞくせいどうじょうみゃくけつえきろか	continuous arteriovenous hemofiltration (CAVH)
血液濾過透析 けつえきろかとうせき	hemodiafiltration (HDF)
持続性血液濾過透析 じぞくせいけつえきろかとうせき	continuous hemodiafiltration (CHDF)
限外濾過 げんがいろか	ultrafiltration
体外限外濾過法 たいがいげんがいろかほう	extracorporeal ultrafiltration method (ECUM)
腹膜透析 ふくまくとうせき	peritoneal dialysis (PD)
連続携行式腹膜透析 れんぞくけいこうしきふくまくとうせき	continuous ambulatory peritoneal dialysis (CAPD)
連続サイクル式腹膜透析 れんぞく――しきふくまくとうせき	continuous cyclic peritoneal dialysis (CCPD)
間欠的腹膜透析 かんけつてきふくまくとうせき	intermittent peritoneal dialysis (IPD)
自動腹膜透析 じどうふくまくとうせき	automated peritoneal dialysis (APD)
血漿交換 けっしょうこうかん	plasmapheresis, plasma exchange (PE)
二重濾過血漿分離交換法 にじゅうろかけっしょうぶんりこうかんほう	double-filtration plasmapheresis (DFPP)
体外衝撃波砕石術 たいがいしょうげきはさいせきじゅつ	extracorporeal shock wave lithotripsy (ESWL)
経皮的腎切石術 けいひてきじんせっせきじゅつ	percutaneous nephrolithotomy (PNL)
経皮腎尿管切石術 けいひじんにょうかんせっせきじゅつ	percutaneous nephroureteral lithotomy
経皮腎瘻造設術 けいひじんろうぞうせつじゅつ	percutaneous nephrostomy (PNS)
経皮経管的腎動脈形成術 けいひけいかんてきじんどうみゃくけいせいじゅつ	percutaneous transluminal renal angioplasty (PTRA)
経尿道的砕石術 けいにょうどうてきさいせきじゅつ	transurethral lithotripsy (TUL)

経尿道的尿管砕石術	transurethral ureterolithotripsy
恥骨上切石術	suprapubic lithotomy
経尿道的針焼灼療法	transurethral needle ablation (TUNA)
経尿道的前立腺蒸散術	transurethral vaporization of the prostate (TUVP)
経尿道的極超短波温熱療法	transurethral microwave thermotherapy (TUMT)
高密度焦点式超音波療法	high-intensity focused ultrasound (HIFU)
経尿道的レーザー前立腺切除術	transurethral laser-induced prostatectomy (TULIP)
直視下レーザー前立腺切除術	visual laser ablation of the prostate (VLAP)
ホルミウムレーザー前立腺核出術	holmium laser enucleation of the prostate (HoLEP)
ホルミウムレーザー前立腺蒸散術	holmium laser ablation of the prostate (HoLAP)
腎摘除術	nephrectomy
腎固定術	nephropexy
尿管切除術	ureterectomy
膀胱摘除術	cystectomy
経尿道的切除術	transurethral resection (TUR)
経尿道的前立腺切除術	transurethral resection of the prostate (TURP), transurethral prostatectomy
経尿道的膀胱腫瘍切除術	transurethral resection of bladder tumor (TURBT)
尿道形成術	urethroplasty
切除鏡	resectoscope
マーシャル・マーケティ・クランツ手術	Marshall-Marchetti-Krantz operation ⟨*an operation for urinary stress incontinence*⟩
後腹膜リンパ節郭清	retroperitoneal lymph node dissection (RPLND)
腎移植	kidney transplantation, renal transplantation
死体腎	cadaveric kidney
生体臓器提供者	living donor
生体血縁臓器提供者	living related donor

9. 腎・泌尿器系　*227*

Tidbits

NOTES

略語も APSGN, HHNKC, PDGFR などと長くなると覚えにくいが, NANDA, APACHE のように発音できると理解しやすく, 最近では NOTES (natural orifice transluminal endoscopic surgery) という例がある. GRACE (Global Registry of Acute Coronary Events) は文字通り洗練されているが, ACCOMPLISH (Avoiding Cardiovascular Events through Combination Therapy in Patients Living with Systolic Hypertension) は少々無理がある. 達成感はある. SICCA (Sjögren's International Collaborative Clinical Alliance) は秀逸.

10. 生殖器系

●愁訴・症状 Complaints / Symptoms●

性欲 せいよく	sexual desire, libido
性交 せいこう	sexual intercourse, coitus, coition
インポテンス，性交不能症 せいこうふのうしょう	impotence, 〔形〕impotent
勃起 ぼっき	erection, 〔動〕erect, become (stand) erect
持続勃起 じぞくぼっき	priapism
射精 しゃせい	ejaculation
早漏 そうろう	premature ejaculation
逆行性射精 ぎゃっこうせいしゃせい	retrograde ejaculation
遺精 いせい	pollution
夢精 むせい	nocturnal pollution (emission), wet dream
自慰 じい	masturbation, onanism
よこね	bubo, 〔形〕bubonic
精巣痛 せいそうつう	orchialgia, orchiodynia, testicular pain, pain in a testis
会陰痛 えいんつう	perineal pain
骨盤痛 こつばんつう	pelvic pain
月経 げっけい	menstruation, menses, periods, menstrual periods
初経 しょけい，初潮 しょちょう	menarche, onset of menses
最終月経 さいしゅうげっけい	last menstrual period (LMP)
月経不順 げっけいふじゅん	irregular menstruation
月経前症候群 げっけいぜんしょうこうぐん	premenstrual syndrome (PMS)
月経困難 げっけいこんなん	dysmenorrhea, painful menstruation
無月経 むげっけい	amenorrhea, missed periods
過多月経 かたげっけい	menorrhagia, hypermenorrhea, excessive menstrual bleeding, excessive flow
過少月経 かしょうげっけい	hypomenorrhea, scanty menstruation
希発月経 きはつげっけい	oligomenorrhea, infrequent menstruation
頻発月経 ひんぱつげっけい	polymenorrhea, abnormally frequent menstruation
月経痛 げっけいつう	menstrual pains, menorrhalgia
月経中間疼痛 げっけいちゅうかんとうつう	intermenstrual pain, middle pain, mittelschmerz
排卵痛 はいらんつう	ovulatory pain
腟分泌物 ちつぶんぴつぶつ，白色帯下	vaginal discharge, leukorrhea, whites,

白帯下 (はくたいげ)	white flow
外陰掻痒症 (がいいんそうようしょう)	vulvar pruritus
腟出血 (ちつしゅっけつ)	vaginal bleeding, vaginal spotting
子宮出血 (しきゅうしゅっけつ)	metrorrhagia, uterine bleeding
接触出血（性交時）(せっしょくしゅっけつ（せいこうじ）)	contact bleeding
性交疼痛 (せいこうとうつう)	dyspareunia, painful sexual intercourse
腟痙 (ちつけい)	vaginismus, painful spasm of the vagina
不感症 (ふかんしょう)	frigidity, 〔形〕frigid
性快感消失 (せいかいかんしょうしつ)	anhedonia
強姦 (ごうかん)	rape
閉経後出血 (へいけいごしゅっけつ)	postmenopausal bleeding
月経間出血 (げっけいかんしゅっけつ)	intermenstrual bleeding, intermenstrual spotting
更年期 (こうねんき)	climacteric, change of life, 〔形〕climacteric
閉経(期) (へいけい(き))	menopause
更年期障害 (こうねんきしょうがい)	menopausal disorder
火照り (ほてり)	hot flashes
中年の危機 (ちゅうねんのきき)	midlife crisis
空巣症候群 (からのすしょうこうぐん)	empty-nest syndrome
妊娠 (にんしん)	pregnancy, conception, 〔動〕conceive, be (become, get) pregnant, be expecting
妊婦 (にんぷ)	pregnant woman, expectant mother
初妊婦 (しょにんぷ)	primigravida
経妊婦 (けいにんぷ)	multigravida
妊娠 1（2, 3, 4）回 (にんしん——かい)	gravida I (II, III, IV), primigravida (secundigravida, tertigravida, quadrigravida)
妊娠～ヵ月である (にんしん——かげつ)	be in the ~ month of pregnancy
つわり，悪阻 (おそ)	morning sickness, nausea and vomiting of pregnancy
不妊 (ふにん)	sterility, barrenness, infertility, inability to conceive, 〔形〕sterile, barren
多胎妊娠 (たたいにんしん)	multiple pregnancy
双子 (ふたご)	twins
三つ子 (みつご)	triplets
流産 (りゅうざん)	abortion, miscarriage, 〔動〕have a miscarriage
人工流産 (じんこうりゅうざん)，妊娠中	induced abortion, artificial abortion, in-

230　IV章　診療録用語

絶 にんしんちゅうぜつ	terruption of pregnancy
避妊 ひにん	contraception, birth control
避妊する ひにん	prevent conception, practice birth control
経口避妊薬 けいこうひにんやく	pills, oral contraceptives (OC)
コンドーム	condom
陣痛 じんつう	labor, labor pains
陣痛抑制 じんつうよくせい	tocolysis
産婦 さんぷ	woman in labor, parturient woman
初産婦 しょさんぷ	primipara
経産婦 けいさんぷ	multipara
出産1 (2, 3, 4) 回 しゅっさん	para I (II, III, IV), primipara (secundipara, tertipara, quadripara)
出産 しゅっさん, 分娩 ぶんべん	childbirth, delivery, 〔動〕give birth to, be delivered of
出産予定日 しゅっさんよていび	expected date of confinement (EDC), due date
分娩予定日 ぶんべんよていび	expected date of delivery (EDD), estimated delivery date
ネーゲレ法則 ほうそく	Nägele rule

〈*prediction of the delivery date; add 7 days to the first day of the last menstrual period, subtract 3 months, and add 1 year*〉

異常分娩 いじょうぶんべん	dystocia, abnormal labor, difficult labor
安産（難産）する あんざん（なんざん）	have an easy (difficult) delivery
ラマーズ法 ほう	Lamaze method

〈*a psychoprophylactic method for childbirth involving breathing exercises and relaxation techniques*〉

早産 そうざん	premature birth, preterm delivery
早産児 そうざんじ	premature infant, preterm infant, preterm
満期自然分娩 まんきしぜんぶんべん	full-term spontaneous delivery
鉗子分娩 かんしぶんべん	forceps delivery
逆子出産 さかごしゅっさん, 骨盤位分娩 こつばんいぶんべん	breech delivery
出生前の しゅっせいぜんの	prenatal
周産期の しゅうさんきの	perinatal
産褥 さんじょく	childbed, confinement, puerperium, puerperal period
産褥熱 さんじょくねつ	puerperal fever
産休 さんきゅう	maternity leave, 〔動〕take maternity leave

10. 生殖器系　231

| 同性愛 どうせいあい | homosexuality, 〔形〕homosexual, gay, (女性) lesbian |
| 乳房自己検診 にゅうぼうじこけんしん | breast self-examination (BSE) |

● 診察所見・徴候　Physical findings / Signs ●

基礎体温 きそたいおん	basal body temperature (BBT)
宦官症 かんがんしょう	eunuchism
類宦官 るいかんがん	eunuchoid
包茎 ほうけい	phimosis, tightening of the foreskin (prepuce) of the penis
恥垢 ちこう	smegma
球海綿体反射 きゅうかいめんたいはんしゃ	bulbocavernosus reflex (BCR)
下疳 げかん	chancre
橙皮様皮膚 とうひようひふ	peau d'orange
内診 ないしん	pelvic examination
双手内診 そうしゅないしん	bimanual pelvic examination
直腸腟診 ちょくちょうちつしん	rectovaginal examination
骨盤底 こつばんてい	pelvic floor
ダグラス窩 か	Douglas cul-de-sac, excavatio rectouterina, rectouterine pouch
腟鏡診 ちつきょうしん	speculum examination
腟円蓋 ちつえんがい	fornix of vagina, vaginal vault, fornix vaginae
ナボット囊胞 のうほう	nabothian cyst

⟨<Martin Naboth; translucent nodules on the uterine cervix caused by occlusion of the mucous glands⟩

子宮付属器圧痛 しきゅうふぞくきあっつう	tenderness on palpation of the uterine adnexa
陰部潰瘍 いんぶかいよう	genital ulcer
妊娠線 にんしんせん	striae gravidarum
チャドウィック徴候	Chadwick sign

⟨dark bluish congested appearance of vaginal and cervical mucosa, associated with pregnancy⟩

| ヘガール徴候 ちょうこう | Hegar sign |

⟨softening of the lower segment of the uterus in the first trimester of pregnancy⟩

仰臥位低血圧症候群 ぎょうがいていけつあつしょうこうぐん	supine hypotensive syndrome (SHS)
胎児胎盤系 たいじたいばんけい	fetoplacental unit (FPU)
胎芽 たいが	embryo, 〔形〕embryonic, embryonal
胎児 たいじ	fetus, 〔形〕fetal
胎囊 たいのう	gestational sac (GS)

232　Ⅳ章　診療録用語

子宮内発育遅延 (しきゅうないはついくちえん)	intrauterine growth retardation (IUGR)
頭殿長 (とうでんちょう)	crown-rump length (CRL)
大横径 (だいおうけい)	biparietal diameter (BPD)
頭囲 (とうい)	head circumference (HC)
腹囲 (ふくい)	abdominal circumference (AC)
大腿骨長 (だいたいこつちょう)	femur length (FL)
児頭骨盤不均衡 (じとうこつばんふきんこう)	cephalopelvic disproportion (CPD)
胎動 (たいどう)	fetal movement, quickening
胎児心音 (たいじしんおん)	fetal heart tone
胎児心拍数 (たいじしんぱくすう)	fetal heart rate (FHR)
胎児切迫仮死 (たいじせっぱくかし)	fetal distress
胎児機能不全 (たいじきのうふぜん)	nonreassuring fetal status (NRFS)
子宮内胎児死亡 (しきゅうないたいじしぼう)	intrauterine fetal death (IUFD)
双胎間輸血症候群 (そうたいかんゆけつしょうこうぐん)	twin-twin transfusion syndrome (TTTS)
胎盤 (たいばん)	placenta, 〔形〕placental
臍帯 (さいたい)	umbilical cord
羊膜 (ようまく)	amnion, 〔形〕amniotic, amnionic
絨毛膜 (じゅうもうまく)	chorion, 〔形〕chorionic
破水 (はすい)	rupture of the amniotic sac (the bag of waters), membrane rupture
胎位 (たいい)	fetal presentation
頭位 (とうい)	cephalic presentation, head presentation
骨盤位 (こつばんい)	pelvic presentation, breech presentation
横位 (おうい)	transverse presentation
顔位 (がんい)	face presentation
額位 (がくい)	brow presentation
産道 (さんどう)	birth canal, obstetric canal, parturient canal
骨産道 (こつさんどう)	bony birth canal
骨盤上口 (こつばんじょうこう)	pelvic inlet, apertura pelvis superior
骨盤下口 (こつばんかこう)	pelvic outlet, apertura pelvis inferior
腟口 (ちつこう)	introitus
経産 (けいさん)	parity, 〔形〕parous
催乳反射 (さいにゅうはんしゃ)	let-down reflex, milk ejection reflex
レオポルド操作 (そうさ)	Leopold maneuvers

　〈*four maneuvers to determine fetal position and presentation*〉

フィッツヒュー・カーティス症候群 (しょうこうぐん)	Fitz-Hugh and Curtis syndrome

　〈*perihepatitis in women as a complication of gonococcal or chlamydial infection*〉

10. 生殖器系

メーグス症候群 こうこん　　Meigs syndrome
　〈ovarian fibromyoma with ascites and hydrothorax〉
クーパーネイル徴候　　Coopernail sign
　〈ecchymoses on the perineum, scrotum, or labia in pelvic fractures〉
ヘルクスハイマー反応　　Herxheimer reaction
んのう
　〈a febrile reaction after antibiotic treatment of syphilis probably due to release of treponemal antigens〉
クルーケンベルク腫瘍　　Krukenberg tumor
ゅよう
　〈carcinoma of the ovary, usually metastatic from the stomach, which contains signet-ring cells with mucus〉

● 胎位　Fetal presentation ●

頭位 とうい　　　　　　　　cephalic presentation
　左前方後頭位 ひだりぜんぽうこうとうい　　left occipitoanterior (LOA)
　（第1頭位第1分類）
　左後方後頭位 ひだりこうほうこうとうい　　left occipitoposterior (LOP)
　（第1頭位第2分類）
　右前方後頭位 みぎぜんぽうこうとうい　　right occipitoanterior (ROA)
　（第2頭位第1分類）
　右後方後頭位 みぎこうほうこうとうい　　right occipitoposterior (ROP)
　（第2頭位第2分類）
骨盤位 こつばんい　　　　　　pelvic presentation
　左前方仙骨位 ひだりぜんぽうせんこつい　　left sacroanterior (LSA)
　（第1骨盤位第1分類）
　左後方仙骨位 ひだりこうほうせんこつい　　left sacroposterior (LSP)
　（第1骨盤位第2分類）
　右前方仙骨位 みぎぜんぽうせんこつい　　right sacroanterior (RSA)
　（第2骨盤位第1分類）
　右後方仙骨位 みぎこうほうせんこつい　　right sacroposterior (RSP)
　（第2骨盤位第2分類）
横位 おうい　　　　　　　　transverse presentation
　左前方肩甲位 ひだりぜんぽうけんこうい　　left scapuloanterior (LScA)
　（第1横位第1分類）
　左後方肩甲位 ひだりこうほうけんこうい　　left scapuloposterior (LScP)
　（第1横位第2分類）
　右前方肩甲位 みぎぜんぽうけんこうい　　right scapuloanterior (RScA)
　（第2横位第1分類）
　右後方肩甲位 みぎこうほうけんこうい　　right scapuloposterior (RScP)
　（第2横位第2分類）

●検査法 Examination●

耐熱性アルカリホスファターゼ	heat-stable alkaline phosphatase (HSAP)
ホスファチジルグリセロール	phosphatidylglycerol (PG)
ヒト絨毛性ゴナドトロピン	human chorionic gonadotropin (HCG)
ヒト胎盤性乳腺刺激ホルモン	human placental lactogen (hPL)
性腺刺激ホルモン	gonadotropic hormone (GTH)
性腺刺激ホルモン放出ホルモン	gonadotropin-releasing hormone (GnRH)
ヒト閉経期ゴナドトロピン	human menopausal gonadotropin (hMG)
黄体形成ホルモン	luteinizing hormone (LH)
卵胞刺激ホルモン	follicle-stimulating hormone (FSH)
プロラクチン	prolactin (PRL)
プロラクチン放出因子	prolactin-releasing factor (PRF)
黄体形成ホルモン放出ホルモン試験	luteinizing hormone-releasing hormone (LHRH) test
エストロゲン	estrogen
エストロン	estrone (E1)
エストラジオール	estradiol (E2)
エストリオール	estriol (E3)
エステトロール	estetrol (E4)
プロゲステロン	progesterone
プレグナンジオール	pregnanediol
テストステロン	testosterone
ジヒドロテストステロン	dihydrotestosterone (DHT)
性ホルモン結合グロブリン	sex hormone-binding globulin (SHBG)
妊娠関連血漿タンパクA	pregnancy-associated plasma protein A (PAPP-A)
エストロゲン受容体	estrogen receptor (ER)
ヒト上皮増殖因子受容体2型, HER2タンパク	human epidermal growth factor receptor type 2 (HER2)
消退出血	withdrawal bleeding
骨盤計測	pelvimetry

10. 生殖器系

妊娠反応 にんしんはんのう	pregnancy test
頸管粘液 けいかんねんえき	cervical mucus (CM)
絨毛生検 じゅうもうせいけん	chorionic villi sampling (CVS)
羊水指数 ようすいしすう	amniotic fluid index (AFI)
胎児心拍陣痛図 たいじしんぱくじんつうず	cardiotocography (CTG)
ノンストレステスト	non-stress test (NST)
収縮ストレステスト しゅうしゅく―	contraction stress test (CST)
胎児機能評価 たいじきのうひょうか	biophysical profile score (BPS)
オキシトシン負荷試験 ―ふかしけん	oxytocin challenge test (OCT)
胎児振動音刺激試験 たいじしんどうおんしげきしけん	vibro-acoustic stimulation test (VAST)
陣痛計 じんつうけい	tocodynamometer, tokodynamometer (TKD)
パパニコロー・スミア試験 ―しけん	Papanicolaou smear, Pap test, Pap smear ⟨an exfoliative cytological staining procedure for detection of cancer of the uterine cervix⟩
性交後試験 せいこうごしけん	postcoital test (PCT)
ヒューナー試験 ―しけん	Huhner test ⟨postcoital test of cervical mucus to evaluate the number and activity of spermatozoa⟩
生殖子 せいしょくし, 配偶子 はいぐうし	gamete, 〔形〕gametic
精子 せいし	spermatozoon, sperm, 〔複〕spermatozoa
卵子 らんし	ovum, 〔複〕ova
精液検査 せいえきけんさ	sperm function test
精子膨化試験 せいしぼうかしけん	hypo-osmotic swelling test (HOS)
乏精子症 ぼうせいししょう	oligospermia, oligozoospermia
無精子症 むせいししょう	azoospermia
ヤング症候群 ―しょうこうぐん	Young syndrome ⟨obstructive azoospermia associated with sinusitis and bronchitis⟩
夜間勃起 やかんぼっき	nocturnal penile tumescence (NPT)
性腺機能低下 せいせんきのうていか	hypogonadism
淋菌 りんきん	*Neisseria gonorrhoeae*, gonococcus
梅毒トレポネーマ ばいどく―	*Treponema pallidum*
トラコーマクラミジア	*Chlamydia trachomatis*
ガードネレラ・バジナリス	*Gardnerella vaginalis*
カンジダ・アルビカンス	*Candida albicans*
腟トリコモナス ちつ―	*Trichomonas vaginalis*
ヒトパピローマウイルス	*Human papillomavirus* (HPV)
クラミジア封入体 ―ふうにゅうたい	chlamydial inclusion bodies

236　IV章　診療録用語

梅毒血清検査	serologic test for syphilis (STS)
性病研究所梅毒血清反応	Venereal Disease Research Laboratory (VRDL) test
血漿レアギン迅速試験	rapid plasma reagin (RPR) test
梅毒トレポネーマ蛍光抗体吸収試験	fluorescent treponemal antibody absorption (FTA-ABS) test
梅毒トレポネーマ運動制御試験	Treponema pallidum immobilization (TPI) test
梅毒トレポネーマ赤血球凝集試験	Treponema pallidum hemagglutination (TPHA) test
暗視野顕微鏡検査	dark-field microscopy
出生前検査	prenatal screening
羊水穿刺	amniocentesis
経腟超音波検査	endovaginal ultrasonography
腟鏡検査	vaginoscopy
コルポスコピー	colposcopy
羊水鏡検査	amnioscopy
クルドスコピー	culdoscopy
子宮鏡検査	hysteroscopy
卵管鏡検査	salpingoscopy
子宮内膜生検	endometrial biopsy
ダグラス窩穿刺術	culdocentesis
卵管通気性(疎通性)検査	test for tubal patency
子宮卵管造影法	hysterosalpingography (HSG)
骨盤動脈造影法	pelvic arteriography (PAG)
乳房X線撮影法	mammography
センチネルリンパ節生検	sentinel lymph node biopsy

● 疾患名　Diseases ●

精巣炎	orchitis, inflammation of a testis
精巣上体炎	epididymitis
精嚢炎	seminal vesiculitis
精索炎	funiculitis, inflammation of the spermatic cord
潜伏精巣	cryptorchidism, cryptorchism, unde-

	scended testis
陰嚢水瘤 (いんのうすいりゅう)	hydrocele testis
フルニエ壊疽 (えそ)	Fournier gangrene
	⟨*idiopathic gangrene of the scrotum; necrotizing fasciitis of the scrotum, penis, and perineum, caused by gram-positive bacteria, enteric bacilli, or anaerobes*⟩
包茎 (ほうけい)	phimosis
勃起不全 (ぼっきふぜん)	erectile dysfunction (ED)
加齢男性性腺機能低下 (かれいだんせいせいせんきのうていか)	late-onset hypogonadism (LOH)
亀頭炎 (きとうえん)	balanitis, inflammation of the glans penis
ペイロニー病 (びょう)	Peyronie disease
	⟨*localized fibrotic thickening of the corpus cavernosum of the penis, causing penile angulation and pain on erection*⟩
尖圭コンジローマ (せんけいー)	condyloma acuminatum
性病 (せいびょう)	venereal disease (VD)
性感染症 (せいかんせんしょう)	sexually transmitted disease (STD)
淋病 (りんびょう)	gonorrhea
梅毒 (ばいどく)	syphilis
ハッチンソン三徴 (ちょうさん)	Hutchinson triad
	⟨*Hutchinson teeth, interstitial keratitis, and labyrinthine disease causing deafness, seen in congenital syphilis*⟩
軟性下疳 (なんせいげかん)	chancroid, soft chancre
鼠径リンパ肉芽腫 (そけいーにくげしゅ)	lymphogranuloma venereum
鼠径肉芽腫 (そけいにくげしゅ)	granuloma inguinale
エイズ	acquired immunodeficiency syndrome (AIDS)
性器ヘルペス (せいき)	genital herpes, genital herpes simplex
クラミジア尿道炎 (どうえん)	chlamydial urethritis
月経前神経不安障害 (げっけいぜんしんけいふあんしょうがい)	premenstrual dysphoric disorder (PMDD)
妊娠悪阻 (にんしんおそ)	hyperemesis gravidarum
子宮外妊娠 (しきゅうがいにんしん)	ectopic pregnancy, extrauterine pregnancy
卵管妊娠 (らんかんにんしん)	tubal pregnancy, fallopian pregnancy, salpingocyesis
腹腔妊娠 (ふくくうにんしん)	abdominal pregnancy, intraperitoneal pregnancy, abdominocyesis
子宮胎盤機能不全 (しきゅうたいばんきのうふぜん)	uteroplacental insufficiency (UPI)
胎盤機能不全症候群	placental dysfunction syndrome (PDS)

IV章 診療録用語

妊娠中毒	toxemia of pregnancy
子癇前症	preeclampsia
子癇	eclampsia
妊娠高血圧	gestational hypertension
妊娠高血圧症候群	pregnancy-induced hypertension (PIH)
HELLP症候群	HELLP syndrome (*h*emolysis, *e*levated *l*iver enzymes, *l*ow *p*latelet count)
習慣流産	habitual abortion
切迫流産	threatened abortion
稽留流産	missed abortion
石児	lithopedion
早期破水	premature rupture of membranes (PROM)
絨毛膜羊膜炎	chorioamnionitis (CAM)
前置胎盤	placenta previa
胎盤早期剝離	placental abruption, abruptio placentae
胞状奇胎	hydatidiform mole, hydatid mole
腟炎	vaginitis, colpitis
外陰炎	vulvitis
細菌性腟症	bacterial vaginosis
バルトリン腺炎	bartholinitis

⟨<*Casper Thomèson Bartholin, Jr.; inflammation of Bartholin glands*⟩

子宮頸管炎	cervicitis
子宮内膜炎	endometritis
卵管炎	salpingitis
卵管留水症	hydrosalpinx
卵管留膿症	pyosalpinx
卵巣炎	oophoritis
骨盤内炎症性疾患	pelvic inflammatory disease (PID)
骨盤腹膜炎	pelvic peritonitis
卵巣囊胞	ovarian cyst
黄体囊胞	corpus luteum cyst
多嚢胞性卵巣症候群, シュタイン・レーベンタール症候群	polycystic ovary syndrome (PCOS), Stein-Leventhal syndrome

⟨*polycystic ovaries with amenorrhea, infertility, obesity, and variable hirsutism*⟩

10. 生殖器系

黄体化未破裂卵胞症候群	luteinized unruptured follicle syndrome (LUFS)
卵巣過剰刺激症候群	ovarian hyperstimulation syndrome (OHSS)
機能性子宮出血	functional uterine bleeding (FUB)
機能不全性不正子宮出血	dysfunctional uterine bleeding (DUB)
破綻出血	breakthrough bleeding
早期卵巣不全	premature ovarian failure (POF)
子宮頸部びらん	cervical erosion
子宮頸管裂傷	cervical laceration
子宮頸管ポリープ	cervical polyp
子宮筋腫	uterine myoma, leiomyoma of the uterus
線維筋腫	fibromyoma, fibroid
子宮内膜症	endometriosis
卵巣子宮内膜症	ovarian endometriosis
子宮留血症	hematometra
子宮腔癒着	intrauterine adhesion
アッシャーマン症候群	Asherman syndrome

⟨*intrauterine fibrous adhesions caused by uterine curettage*⟩

子宮後傾	retroversion of the uterus, retroverted uterus
子宮脱	uterine prolapse
膀胱瘤	cystocele
直腸瘤	rectocele
子宮癌	uterine cancer
子宮体癌	uterine corpus carcinoma
子宮内膜癌	endometrial carcinoma
子宮頸癌	uterine cervix cancer, cervical carcinoma
子宮頸部上皮内腫瘍	cervical intraepithelial neoplasia (CIN)
扁平上皮内病変	squamous intraepithelial lesion (SIL)
付属器腫瘍	adnexal tumor
ブレンナー腫瘍	Brenner tumor

⟨*ovarian fibroepithelial tumor with slight malignant potential*⟩

卵巣癌	ovarian cancer
嚢胞腺癌	cystadenocarcinoma
絨毛癌	choriocarcinoma

胎盤部トロホブラスト腫瘍	placental site trophoblastic tumor (PSTT)
半陰陽	hermaphroditism, hermaphrodism
仮性半陰陽	pseudohermaphroditism
性同一性障害	gender identity disorder
女性化症候群	feminizing syndrome
男性化	masculinization, virilism
副腎性器症候群	adrenogenital syndrome (AGS)
アンドロゲン不応症候群	androgen-insensitivity syndrome
カルマン症候群	Kallmann syndrome

⟨hypogonadism with anosmia; decreased secretion of GnRH, usually autosomal recessive and some X-linked⟩

ターナー症候群　　Turner syndrome

⟨gonadal dysgenesis associated with absence of second sex chromosome; marked by dwarfism, undifferentiated gonads, webbed neck, cubitus valgus, and cardiac defects⟩

ヌーナン症候群　　Noonan syndrome

⟨the phenotype of Turner syndrome characterized by short stature, hypogonadism, webbed neck, pulmonary stenosis, and ptosis; autosomal dominant inheritance⟩

クラインフェルター症候群　　Klinefelter syndrome

⟨XXY syndrome with male phenotype; characterized by seminiferous tubule dysgenesis, eunuchoid habitus, gynecomastia, and elevated urinary gonadotropin⟩

ライフェンスタイン症候群　　Reifenstein syndrome

⟨male pseudohermaphroditism due to incomplete androgen resistance with hypospadias, gynecomastia, infertility, and cryptorchism⟩

乳腺炎	mastitis
乳腺症	mastopathy
線維腺腫	fibroadenoma
乳癌	breast cancer
乳房パジェット病	Paget disease of breast

⟨intraductal carcinoma of the breast infiltrating the nipple and areola⟩

非浸潤性乳管癌	ductal carcinoma in situ (DCIS)
非浸潤性小葉癌	lobular carcinoma in situ (LCIS)

● 治療法 Treatment ●

子宮筋弛緩薬	uterine muscle relaxant
子宮筋刺激薬	uterine muscle stimulant
オキシトシン	oxytocin《アトニン-O》
プロスタグランジン	prostaglandin《プロスタルモン》
陣痛抑制薬	tocolytic agent
誘導分娩	induced delivery
タンポン	tampon
受胎調節	contraception, birth control
避妊薬	contraceptive, contraceptive agent
経口避妊薬	oral contraceptive pill (OCP)
低用量ピル	low-dose oral contraceptive, minipill
避妊器具	contraceptive device
子宮内器具	intrauterine device (IUD)
子宮内避妊器具	intrauterine contraceptive device (IUCD)
ペッサリー	pessary, diaphragm
緊急避妊薬	emergency contraceptive, postcoital contraceptive
排卵誘発法	ovulation induction
ホルモン補充療法	hormone replacement therapy (HRT)
エストロゲン代償療法	estrogen replacement therapy
エストラジオール	estradiol《ジュリナ》《エストラダーム》
プロゲステロン	progesterone《プロゲホルモン》
メドロキシプロゲステロン酢酸エステル	medroxyprogesterone acetate《ヒスロン》
性腺刺激ホルモン放出ホルモン作動薬	gonadotropin-releasing hormone agonist
クロミフェンクエン酸塩	clomiphene citrate《クロミッド》
カウフマン療法	Kaufmann therapy ⟨*periodic administration of estrogen and progestin to treat amenorrhea*⟩
ブロモクリプチンメシル酸塩	bromocriptine mesylate《パーロデル》
ダナゾール	danazol《ボンゾール》
トラスツズマブ	trastuzumab《ハーセプチン》
選択的エストロゲン受容体修飾薬	selective estrogen receptor modulator (SERM)
タモキシフェンクエン酸	tamoxifen citrate (TAM)《ノルバデックス》

242　IV章　診療録用語

シルデナフィルクエン酸塩	sildenafil citrate《バイアグラ》
精液銀行（せいえきぎんこう）	semen bank, sperm bank
ヒトパピローマウイルスワクチン，子宮頸癌ワクチン（しきゅうけいがん──）	human papillomavirus vaccine《サーバリックス》
環状切除（かんじょうせつじょ），割礼（かつれい）	circumcision, 〔動〕circumcise
精巣固定術（せいそうこていじゅつ）	orchiopexy, orchidopexy
精巣摘除術（せいそうてきじょじゅつ）	orchiectomy, orchidectomy
精管切除術（せいかんせつじょじゅつ）	vasectomy
治療的流産（ちりょうてきりゅうざん）	therapeutic abortion
頸管拡張術および搔爬術（けいかんかくちょうじゅつ──そうはじゅつ）	dilatation and curettage (D&C)
生殖補助医療（せいしょくほじょいりょう）	assisted reproductive technology (ART)
排卵誘発法（はいらんゆうはつほう）	ovulation induction
人工授精（じんこうじゅせい）	artificial insemination
配偶者間人工授精（はいぐうしゃかんじんこうじゅせい）	artificial insemination by husband (AIH), homologous insemination
非配偶者間人工授精（ひはいぐうしゃかんじんこうじゅせい）	artificial insemination by donor (AID), heterologous insemination
体外受精（たいがいじゅせい）	in vitro fertilization (IVF)
体外受精胚移植（たいがいじゅせいはいいしょく）	in vitro fertilization and embryo transfer (IVF-ET)
配偶子卵管内移植（はいぐうしらんかんないいしょく）	gamete intrafallopian transfer (GIFT)
受精卵卵管内移植（じゅせいらんらんかんないいしょく）	zygote intrafallopian transfer (ZIFT)
卵細胞質内精子注入法（らんさいぼうしつないせいしちゅうにゅうほう）	intracytoplasmic sperm injection (ICSI)
囲卵腔内精子注入法（いらんくうないせいしちゅうにゅうほう）	subzonal insemination (SUZI)
子宮鏡下卵管内精子注入法（しきゅうきょうからかんないせいしちゅうにゅうほう）	hysteroscopic insemination into tube (HIT)
精巣上体精子回収法（せいそうじょうたいせいしかいしゅうほう）	microsurgical epididymal sperm aspiration (MESA)
精巣内精子回収法（せいそうないせいしかいしゅうほう）	testicular sperm extraction (TESE)
卵管結紮術（らんかんけっさつじゅつ）	tubal ligation
子宮鏡下選択的卵管通水法（しきゅうきょうかせんたくてきらんかんつうすいほう）	hysteroscopic selective hydrotubation

10. 生殖器系

会陰切開	episiotomy
帝王切開	cesarean section (CS)
帝王切開後経腟分娩	vaginal birth after cesarean section (VBAC)
腹式子宮全摘術	total abdominal hysterectomy (TAH)
腟式子宮全摘術	total vaginal hysterectomy (TVH)
広汎性子宮全摘術	radical hysterectomy
腹腔鏡補助下腟式子宮摘出術	laparoscopically assisted vaginal hysterectomy (LAVH)
子宮卵管切除術	hysterosalpingectomy
卵管卵巣摘出術	salpingo-oophorectomy
子宮筋腫摘出術	uterine myomectomy, fibroidectomy
子宮固定術	hysteropexy
テンションフリー腟メッシュ	tension-free vaginal mesh (TVM)
乳房切除術	mastectomy, mammectomy, excision of the breast
根治的乳房切除術, ハルステッド手術	radical mastectomy, Halsted operation ⟨*excision of the entire breast, as well as the pectoral muscles, axillary lymph nodes, subcutaneous fat, and skin*⟩
乳房温存手術	breast-conserving surgery
腫瘍切除術	lumpectomy
乳房再建術	breast reconstruction
乳房形成術	mammaplasty
腋窩リンパ節郭清	axillary lymph node dissection

11. 内分泌・代謝系

● 愁訴・症状　Complaints / Symptoms ●

成長，発育	growth, development
成長障害	growth disorder
発育遅延	delayed growth, growth retardation
成熟	maturity, maturation, 〔形〕mature
未成熟の	immature
早熟の	precocious
性的早熟	sexual precocity
思春期，青年期	puberty, adolescence
老年，老衰	senility, 〔形〕senile
男性化	virilism, vilirization, masculinization, 〔形〕virile, masculine
女性化	feminism, feminization, 〔形〕feminine
頭痛	headache
肥満	obesity, 〔形〕obese
栄養不良	malnutrition, undernourishment, 〔形〕undernourished
るいそう	emaciation, 〔形〕emaciated
糖尿	glycosuria
口渇	thirst, 〔形〕thirsty
のどが渇く	feel (be) thirsty
多飲	polydipsia
多食	polyphagia
多尿	polyuria
血糖上昇指数	glycemic index (GI)
発汗	perspiration
動悸	palpitation
眼の突出	bulging of the eyes
嗄声	hoarseness
声変わり	the change of voice
声変わりする	one's voice changes (breaks, cracks)
暑がりの	sensitive to the heat, unable to stand the heat, intolerant of the heat
寒がりの	sensitive to the cold
薄着する	be lightly dressed
厚着する	be heavily dressed (clothed), wear many clothes
痛風発作	gouty attack

●診察所見・徴候　Physical findings / Signs●

肥満指数 (ひまんしすう)	body mass index (BMI)
除脂肪体重 (じょしぼうたいじゅう)	lean body mass (LBM)
低身長 (ていしんちょう)	short stature
高身長 (こうしんちょう)	tall stature
巨人症 (きょじんしょう)	gigantism
低身長症 (ていしんちょうしょう)	dwarfism
脂肪過多 (しぼうかた)	adiposity, adiposis
皮下脂肪 (ひかしぼう)	subcutaneous fat, panniculus adiposus
上腕三頭筋皮下脂肪厚 (じょうわんさんとうきんひかしぼうこう)	triceps skinfold (TSF) thickness
脂肪織炎 (しぼうしきえん)	panniculitis
内臓脂肪 (ないぞうしぼう)	visceral fat
中心性肥満 (ちゅうしんせいひまん)	central obesity
体幹肥満 (たいかんひまん)	truncal obesity
有痛脂肪症 (ゆうつうしぼうしょう), ダーカム病 (びょう)	adiposis dolorosa, Dercum disease

〈*tender or painful subcutaneous masses of fat, usually seen in older obese women*〉

多毛 (たもう)	hypertrichosis, polytrichia, hairiness, 〔形〕hairy, shaggy
男性型多毛症 (だんせいがたたもうしょう)	hirsutism, 〔形〕hirsute
脱毛 (だつもう)	loss of hair, depilation, epilation
脱毛症 (だつもうしょう)	baldness, alopecia
腋毛欠如 (えきもうけつじょ)	lack of axillary hair
成人陰毛 (せいじんいんもう)	adult pubic hair
色素沈着 (しきそちんちゃく)	pigmentation
痤瘡 (ざそう)	acne
黄色腫 (おうしょくしゅ)	xanthoma
眼瞼黄色腫 (がんけんおうしょくしゅ)	xanthelasma
線状皮膚萎縮 (せんじょうひふいしゅく)	linear atrophy, striae distensae, atrophoderma striatum
多汗症 (たかんしょう)	hyperhidrosis
二次性徴 (にじせいちょう)	secondary sex characteristics
満月顔貌 (まんげつがんぼう)	moon face, moon-shaped face
老人環 (ろうじんかん)	arcus senilis
顎前突症 (がくぜんとつしょう)	prognathism, protrusion of the jaws
不正咬合 (ふせいこうごう)	malocclusion
巨大舌 (きょだいぜつ)	macroglossia
肢端腫大 (したんしゅだい)	acral enlargement
頻脈 (ひんみゃく)	tachycardia
振戦 (しんせん)	tremor

眼球突出 （がんきゅうとっしゅつ）　　prominent eyes, exophthalmos
甲状腺腫大 （こうじょうせんしゅだい）　　goiter
甲状腺結節 （こうじょうせんけっせつ）　　thyroid nodules
メルセブルグ三徴候 （—さんちょうこう）　　Merseburg triad
〈*exophthalmos, goiter, tachycardia in Graves disease*〉
メビウス徴候 （—ちょうこう）　　Moebius sign
〈*inability to keep the eyeballs converged in Graves disease*〉
グレーフェ徴候 （—ちょうこう）　　Graefe sign
〈*lid lag associated with Graves disease*〉
シュテルワーグ徴候　　Stellwag sign
〈*infrequent and partial blinking due to retraction of eyelids, seen in Graves disease*〉
ジョフロイ徴候 （—ちょうこう）　　Joffroy sign
〈*failure to wrinkle the forehead when gaze is quickly moved upward; seen in Graves disease*〉
バレー徴候 （—ちょうこう）　　Ballet sign
〈*external ophthalmoplegia in Graves disease and hysteria*〉
女性化乳房 （じょせいかにゅうぼう）　　gynecomastia
乳汁漏出 （にゅうじゅうろうしゅつ）　　galactorrhea
野牛の肩瘤 （やぎゅうのけんりゅう）　　buffalo hump
指圧痕のない浮腫 （しあつこんのないふしゅ）　　nonpitting edema
痛風結節 （つうふうけっせつ）　　tophus
クスマウル呼吸 （—こきゅう）　　Kussmaul respiration
〈*deep and rapid respiration seen in DKA or coma*〉
テタニー　　tetany
クボステック徴候 （—ちょうこう）　　Chvostek sign
〈*spasm of the facial muscles elicited by tapping the facial nerve in tetany*〉
トルソー徴候 （—ちょうこう）　　Trousseau sign
〈*carpopedal spasm elicited when the upper arm is compressed by a tourniquet in tetany*〉
ウィップル三徴 （—さんちょう）　　Whipple triad
〈*hypoglycemia in insulinoma; the attack during the fast, FBS of 40 mg/dL or less, immediate recovery by glucose*〉

● 検査法　Examination ●

基礎代謝率 （きそたいしゃりつ）　　basal metabolic rate (BMR)
空腹時血糖 （くうふくじけっとう）　　fasting blood sugar (FBS)
低血糖 （ていけっとう）　　hypoglycemia
高血糖 （こうけっとう）　　hyperglycemia
暁現象 （あかつきげんしょう）　　dawn phenomenon, early-morning hyperglycemia

11. 内分泌・代謝系

ソモジー現象 げんしょう	Somogyi phenomenon
	⟨rebound hyperglycemia after an episode of hypoglycemia⟩
ブドウ糖負荷試験 とうのかしけん	glucose tolerance test (GTT)
経口ブドウ糖負荷試験 けいこうーとうふかしけん	oral glucose tolerance test (OGTT)
耐糖能異常 たいとうのういじょう	impaired glucose tolerance (IGT)
空腹時血糖異常 くうふくじけっとういじょう	impaired fasting glucose (IFG)
血糖上昇指数 けっとうじょうしょうしすう	glycemic index
ヘモグロビン A1c	hemoglobin A1c (HbA1c), glycated hemoglobin, glycosylated hemoglobin
グリコアルブミン	glycoalbumin (GA)
1,5-アンヒドログルシトール	1,5-anhydroglucitol (1,5-AG)
最終糖化産物 さいしゅうとうかさんぶつ	advanced glycation end product (AGE)
ケトン体 たい	ketone body
ケトアシドーシス	ketoacidosis
C ペプチド	C-peptide, connecting peptide
免疫反応性 C ペプチド めんえきはんのうせいーペプチド	C-peptide immunoreactivity (CPR)
免疫反応性インスリン めんえきはんのうせいー	immunoreactive insulin (IRI)
インスリン抗体 こうたい	insulin antibody
インスリン抵抗性 ていこうせい	insulin resistance
インスリン抵抗性指標 ていこうせいしひょう	homeostasis model assessment of insulin resistance (HOMA-R)
免疫反応性グルカゴン めんえきはんのうせいー	immunoreactive glucagon (IRG)
インクレチン	incretin
胃抑制ポリペプチド いよくせい	gastric inhibitory polypeptide (GIP)
グルカゴン様ペプチド よう	glucagon-like peptide (GLP)
抗グルタミン酸デカルボキシラーゼ抗体 こうーさんーこうたい	anti-glutamic acid decarboxylase antibody, anti-GAD antibody
膵島細胞抗体 すいとうさいぼうこうたい	islet cell antibody (ICA)
膵島細胞膜抗体 すいとうさいぼうまくこうたい	islet cell surface antibody (ICSA)
甲状腺機能検査 こうじょうせんきのうけんさ	thyroid function test (TFT)
サイロキシン	thyroxine, tetraiodothyronine (T4)
トリヨードサイロニン	triiodothyronine (T3)
遊離サイロキシン ゆうり	free thyroxine (FT4)
遊離サイロキシン指数	free thyroxine index (FTI)

248 Ⅳ章 診療録用語

遊離トリヨードサイロニン	free triiodothyronine (FT3)
サイログロブリン	thyroglobulin (Tg)
モノヨードチロシン	monoiodotyrosine (MIT)
ジヨードチロシン	diiodotyrosine (DIT)
サイロキシン結合グロブリン	thyroxine-binding globulin (TBG)
甲状腺刺激ホルモン	thyroid-stimulating hormone (TSH), thyrotropin
ヒトチロトロピンアルファ	thyrotropin human alfa《タイロゲン》
持続性甲状腺刺激物質	long-acting thyroid stimulator (LATS)
甲状腺刺激免疫グロブリン	thyroid stimulating immunoglobulin (TSI)
甲状腺刺激ホルモン受容体抗体	thyroid-stimulating hormone receptor antibody (TRAb)
甲状腺刺激ホルモン結合阻害免疫グロブリン	thyrotropin-binding inhibitory immunoglobulin (TBII)
抗サイログロブリン抗体	antithyroglobulin antibody (TgAb)
抗ミクロソーム抗体	antimicrosomal antibody
抗甲状腺ペルオキシダーゼ抗体	anti-thyroid peroxidase antibody (TPOAb)
トリヨードサイロニンレジン摂取率	triiodothyronine resin uptake, resin sponge uptake (RSU)
放射性ヨウ素摂取試験	radioactive iodine uptake (RAIU) test
カルシトニン	calcitonin (CT)
プロカルシトニン	procalcitonin (PCT)
副甲状腺ホルモン	parathyroid hormone (PTH), parathormone
副甲状腺ホルモン関連タンパク質	parathyroid hormone-related hormone (PTHrP)
副腎皮質刺激ホルモン, コルチコトロピン	adrenocorticotropic hormone (ACTH), corticotropin
コルチコトロピン放出ホルモン	corticotropin-releasing hormone (CRH)
コルチコトロピン様中葉	corticotropin-like intermediate lobe pep-

11. 内分泌・代謝系

ペプチド	tide (CLIP)
成長ホルモン	growth hormone (GH), somatotropin
成長ホルモン放出ホルモン	growth hormone-releasing hormone (GRH)
成長ホルモン分泌抑制ホルモン	growth hormone-inhibiting hormone (GHIH)
インスリン様成長因子, ソマトメジン	insulinlike growth factors (IGF), somatomedin
インスリン様成長因子Ⅰ, ソマトメジンC	insulinlike growth factor-I (IGF-I), somatomedin C
プロラクチン	prolactin (PRL)
プロラクチン放出ホルモン	prolactin-releasing hormone (PRH)
プロラクチン抑制ホルモン	prolactin-inhibiting hormone (PIH)
黄体形成ホルモン	luteinizing hormone (LH)
間質細胞刺激ホルモン	interstitial cell-stimulating hormone (ICSH)
黄体形成ホルモン放出ホルモン	luteinizing hormone-releasing hormone (LHRH)
卵胞刺激ホルモン	follicle-stimulating hormone (FSH)
抗利尿ホルモン	antidiuretic hormone (ADH), vasopressin
アルギニンバゾプレシン	arginine vasopressin (AVP)
オキシトシン	oxytocin
メラトニン	melatonin
コルチゾール	cortisol
11-デオキシコルチコステロン	11-deoxycorticosterone (DOC)
17-ケトステロイド	17-ketosteroid (17-KS)
17-ヒドロキシコルチコステロイド	17-hydroxycorticosteroid (17-OHCS)
アルドステロン	aldosterone
血漿アルドステロン濃度	plasma aldosterone concentration (PAC)
アルドステロン・レニン活性比	aldosterone to renin activity ratio (ARR)
コルチコトロピン放出ホルモン試験	corticotropin-releasing hormone test
デキサメタゾン抑制試験	dexamethasone suppression test (DST)

メチラポン試験	metyrapone test
水制限試験	water deprivation test
インスリン感受性試験	insulin sensitivity test
インスリン負荷試験	insulin tolerance test (ITT)
エルスワース・ハワード試験	Ellsworth-Howard test

〈measurement of urinary phosphorus and cAMP after intravenous administration of parathyroid hormone to test renal tubular response; used in the diagnosis of pseudohypoparathyroidism〉

エチレンジアミン四酢酸負荷試験	ethylenediaminetetraacetic acid (EDTA) infusion test
副腎アンドロゲン	adrenal androgen
アンギオテンシン	angiotensin
カテコールアミン	catecholamine
アドレナリン	adrenaline, epinephrine
ノルアドレナリン	noradrenaline, norepinephrine
ドーパミン	dopamine
セロトニン	serotonin
5-ヒドロキシインドール酢酸	5-hydroxyindoleacetic acid (5-HIAA)
ポルフォビリノーゲン	porphobilinogen (PBG)
ワトソン・シュウォーツ試験	Watson-Schwartz test

〈a qualitative screening test for the diagnosis of acute intermittent porphyria; based on the insolubility of porphobilinogen aldehyde in butanol and chloroform〉

脂質	lipid
総コレステロール	total cholesterol (TC)
高比重リポタンパクコレステロール	high-density-lipoprotein (HDL) cholesterol
低比重リポタンパクコレステロール	low-density-lipoprotein (LDL) cholesterol
トリグリセリド, 中性脂肪	triglyceride (TG)
リポタンパク質	lipoprotein
アポリポタンパク質	apolipoprotein (Apo)
カイロミクロン	chylomicron
リポタンパク質リパーゼ	lipoprotein lipase (LPL)
アディポネクチン	adiponectin
高尿酸血症	hyperuricemia

11. 内分泌・代謝系　251

高ナトリウム血症	hypernatremia
低ナトリウム血症	hyponatremia
高カリウム血症	hyperkalemia
低カリウム血症	hypokalemia
高カルシウム血症	hypercalcemia
腫瘍由来体液性高カルシウム血症	humoral hypercalcemia of malignancy (HMM)
低カルシウム血症	hypocalcemia
高リン酸血症	hyperphosphatemia
低リン酸血症	hypophosphatemia
高マグネシウム血症	hypermagnesemia
低マグネシウム血症	hypomagnesemia
頭蓋X線撮影	skull radiography
トルコ鞍	sella turcica
骨生検	bone biopsy

● 疾患名　Diseases ●

甲状腺機能亢進症	hyperthyroidism
甲状腺中毒症	thyrotoxicosis
バセドウ病, グレーヴス病	Basedow disease, Graves disease

⟨*hyperthyroidism caused by diffuse hyperplasia of the thyroid*⟩

| 自律性機能性甲状腺結節 | autonomously functioning thyroid nodule (AFTN) |
| プラマー病 | Plummer disease |

⟨*hyperthyroidism due to nodular toxic goiter*⟩

非中毒性甲状腺腫	nontoxic goiter
甲状腺機能低下症	hypothyroidism
粘液水腫	myxedema
クレチン病	cretinism
粘液水腫性昏睡	myxedema coma
急性甲状腺炎	acute thyroiditis
亜急性甲状腺炎	subacute thyroiditis
慢性甲状腺炎	chronic thyroiditis
無痛性甲状腺炎	painless thyroiditis, silent thyroiditis
橋本病	Hashimoto disease, Hashimoto thyroidi-

tis

⟨*autoimmune thyroiditis with lymphocytic infiltration of the gland*⟩

リーデル甲状腺腫　　　　　Riedel thyroiditis

⟨*chronic fibrous thyroiditis, fibrosis involving one lobe and compressing the trachea to cause stridor*⟩

腺腫様甲状腺腫	adenomatous goiter
濾胞腺腫	follicular adenoma
甲状腺癌	thyroid carcinoma
髄様癌	medullary carcinoma
副甲状腺機能亢進症	hyperparathyroidism
副甲状腺機能低下症	hypoparathyroidism
偽性副甲状腺機能低下症	pseudohypoparathyroidism
オールブライト遺伝性骨形成異常症	Albright hereditary osteodystrophy (AHO)

⟨*short stature, oval facies, mental retardation, brachydactyly, heterotopic calcification, and pseudohypoparathyroidism; heterogeneous inheritance*⟩

マッキューン・オールブライト症候群　　McCune-Albright syndrome

⟨*polyostotic fibrous dysplasia, irregular brown pigmentation, and endocrine dysfunction with precocious puberty, seen in females*⟩

下垂体機能亢進症	hyperpituitarism
下垂体機能低下症	hypopituitarism
汎下垂体機能低下	panhypopituitarism
シーハン症候群	Sheehan syndrome

⟨*postpartum hypopituitarism as a result of necrosis of the anterior pituitary*⟩

下垂体腺腫	pituitary adenoma
クッシング病	Cushing disease

⟨*hyperadrenocorticism secondary to excessive secretion of corticotropin; usually pituitary adenomas*⟩

成長ホルモン分泌下垂体腺腫	growth hormone-secreting pituitary adenoma
先端巨大症	acromegaly

11. 内分泌・代謝系

下垂体性巨人症 かすいたいせいきょじんしょう	pituitary gigantism
下垂体性小人症 かすいたいせいしょうじんしょう	pituitary dwarfism, hypophyseal dwarf
フレーリッヒ症候群	Fröhlich syndrome

〈*adiposogenital dystrophy; obesity, hypogonadism, and visual loss, commonly due to pituitary and hypothalamic neoplasms*〉

ローレンス・ムーン・ビードル症候群 こうぐん	Laurence-Moon-Biedle syndrome

〈*an autosomal recessive disorder characterized by obesity, retinitis pigmentosa, polydactylia, mental retardation, hypogonadism, and spastic paraplegia*〉

高ソマトトロピン分泌症 こう——ぶんぴしょう	hypersomatotropism
高プロラクチン血症 こう——けつしょう	hyperprolactinemia
キアリ・フロンメル症候群 こうぐん	Chiari-Frommel syndrome

〈*galactorrhea-amenorrhea syndrome after pregnancy unrelated to infant's nursing; hyperprolactinemic amenorrhea*〉

尿崩症 にょうほうしょう	diabetes insipidus (DI)
抗利尿ホルモン不適切分泌症候群 こうりにょう——ふてきせつぶんぴしょうこうぐん	syndrome of inappropriate secretion of antidiuretic hormone (SIADH)
副腎皮質機能亢進症 ふくじんひしつきのうこうしんしょう	hyperadrenocorticism, adrenocortical hyperfunction, hypercorticalism
クッシング症候群 こうぐん	Cushing syndrome

〈*syndrome caused by hyperadrenocorticism; characterized by moon face, trunkal obesity, striae, hypertension, diabetes, osteoporosis, amenorrhea, and hirsutism*〉

ネルソン症候群 こうぐん	Nelson syndrome

〈*development of ACTH-secreting tumors after bilateral aderenalectomy for Cushing syndrome*〉

異所性 ACTH 産生症候群 いしょせい——さんせいしょうこうぐん	ectopic ACTH syndrome
原発性アルドステロン症, コン症候群 げんぱつせい——しょう	primary aldosteronism, Conn syndrome

〈*headaches, polyuria, hypertension, hypokalemic alkalosis, hypervolemia, and decreased renin secretion; caused by excessive secretion of aldosterone from adrenocortical adenomas*〉

アルドステロン産生腺腫 ——さんせいせんしゅ	aldosterone-producing adenoma (APA)
特発性高アルドステロン症 とくはつせい——しょう	idiopathic hyperaldosteronism (IHA)

リドル症候群 こうぐん　　　Liddle syndrome
　〈*pseudoprimary aldosteronism caused by non-aldosterone mineralcorticoid excess; characterized by hypertension, hypokalemia, and metabolic alkalosis with excessive sodium reabsorption and decreased activity of renin and aldosterone; autosomal dominant*〉

低アルドステロン症　　　hypoaldosteronism

偽性低アルドステロン症　pseudohypoaldosteronism (PHA), Gordon syndrome
ゴードン症候群
　〈*pseudohypoaldosteronism type 2; normal GFR, tubular metabolic acidosis, hyperkalemia without salt wasting, and low renin and aldosterone levels; autosomal dominant*〉

バーター症候群 こうぐん　Bartter syndrome
　〈*juxtaglomerular cell hyperplasia with secondary hypokalemic alkalosis and hyperaldosteronism; usually seen in children*〉

ギテルマン症候群 こうぐん　Gitelman syndrome
　〈*a familial disorder with juxtaglomerular cell hyperplasia similar to Bartter syndrome; characterized by hypokalemia, hypomagnesemia, and hypocalciuria; usually seen in adolescents or young adults*〉

グルココルチコイド反応性アルドステロン症　glucocorticoid-remediable aldosteronism (GRA)

褐色細胞腫 かっしょくさいぼうしゅ　　pheochromocytoma
思春期早発症 ししゅんきそうはつしょう　precocious puberty
半陰陽 はんいんよう　　　　　hermaphroditism, hermaphrodism, intersexuality
性腺機能低下症 せいせんきのうていかしょう　hypogonadism
副腎機能不全 ふくじんきのうふぜん　adrenal insufficiency
副腎皮質機能低下症　hypoadrenocorticism, adrenocortical insufficiency
ふくじんひしつきのうていかしょう

アジソン病 しょう　　Addison disease
　〈*chronic adrenocortical insufficiency; characterized by weakness, weight loss, hypotension, anorexia, vomiting, and hyperpigmentation of the skin*〉

副腎クリーゼ ふくじん　　adrenal crisis
副腎性器症候群 ふくじんせいきしょうこうぐん　adrenogenital syndrome (AGS)
先天性副腎過形成　congenital adrenal hyperplasia (CAH)
せんてんせいふくじんかけいせい

アシャール・チール症候群 こうぐん　Achard-Thiers syndrome
　〈*masculinization with hirsutism, obesity and diabetes mellitus in postmenopausal women, caused by overproduction of adrenocortical*

11. 内分泌・代謝系

androgens⟩

男性型多毛症	hirsutism
副腎偶発腫	adrenal incidentaloma
シュミット症候群	Schmidt syndrome

⟨*polyglandular autoimmune syndrome type 2; hypofunction of thyroid, adrenals, gonads, and endocrine pancreas*⟩

多発性内分泌腺腫症	multiple endocrine adenomatosis (MEA)
多発性内分泌腫瘍1型,ウェルマー症候群	multiple endocrine neoplasia (MEN) type 1, Wermer syndrome

⟨*pituitary, parathyroid, and pancreatic islet cell tumors; autosomal dominant*⟩

多発性内分泌腫瘍2型	multiple endocrine neoplasia (MEN) type 2
シップル症候群	Sipple syndrome

⟨*MEN 2A; medullary thyroid carcinoma, parathyroid hyperplasia, and pheochromocytoma; autosomal dominant*⟩

インスリノーマ	insulinoma
膵島細胞腺腫	islet cell adenoma
WDHA症候群,バーナー・モリソン症候群	WDHA syndrome (*w*atery *d*iarrhea, *h*ypokalemia, *a*chlorhydria), Verner-Morrison syndrome, VIPoma
ゾリンジャー・エリソン症候群	Zollinger-Ellison syndrome (ZES)

⟨*gastric hypersecretion, intractable peptic ulcers, and gastrinoma of the pancreas or duodenum*⟩

カルチノイド症候群	carcinoid syndrome
銀親和性細胞腫	argentaffinoma
骨粗鬆症	osteoporosis
骨軟化症	osteomalacia
腫瘍性骨軟化症	oncogenic osteomalacia, tumor-induced osteomalacia
糖尿病	diabetes mellitus (DM)
1型糖尿病,インスリン依存性糖尿病	type 1 diabetes mellitus, insulin-dependent DM (IDDM)
若年型糖尿病	juvenile-onset diabetes mellitus (JODM)
劇症1型糖尿病	fulminant type 1 diabetes mellitus
2型糖尿病,インスリン非依存性糖尿病	type 2 diabetes mellitus, non-insulin-dependent DM (NIDDM)
若年性成人発症型糖尿病	maturity-onset diabetes of youth

じゃくねんせいせいじんはっしょうがた――	(MODY)
成人発症型糖尿病	adult-onset diabetes mellitus（AODM）
妊娠糖尿病 にんしんとうにょうびょう	gestational diabetes mellitus（GDM）
糖尿病網膜症 もうまくしょう	diabetic retinopathy（DR）
糖尿病性腎症 じんしょう	diabetic nephropathy
糖尿病性ニューロパチー	diabetic neuropathy
糖尿病性微小血管症 びしょうけっかんしょう	diabetic microangiopathy
糖尿病性昏睡 こんすい	diabetic coma
糖尿病性ケトアシドーシス	diabetic ketoacidosis（DKA）
高血糖性高浸透圧性昏睡 こうけっとうせいこうしんとうあつせいこんすい	hyperglycemic hyperosmolar nonketotic coma（HHNKC）
高浸透圧性非ケトン性昏睡 こうしんとうあつせいひーせいこんすい	hyperosmolar nonketotic coma（HNKC, HONK）
不安定糖尿病 ふあんていとうにょうびょう	brittle diabetes
低血糖昏睡 ていけっとうこんすい	hypoglycemic coma
脂質異常症 ししついじょうしょう	dyslipidemia
高脂血症 こうしけっしょう	hyperlipidemia
高コレステロール血症 こう――けっしょう	hypercholesterolemia
家族性複合型高脂血症 かぞくせいふくごうがたこうしけっしょう	familial combined hyperlipidemia（FCHL）
高リポタンパク血症 こう――けっしょう	hyperlipoproteinemia
高トリグリセリド血症 こう――けっしょう	hypertriglyceridemia
無ベータリポタンパク血症，バッセン・コーンツヴァイク症候群 む――けっしょう	abetalipoproteinemia（ABL），Bassen-Kornzweig syndrome

⟨*low-density β-lipoproteins absent; marked by ataxia, malabsorption, retinal pigmentary degeneration, decreased vitamin A, and acanthocytes; autosomal recessive*⟩

メタボリック症候群	metabolic syndrome
脂質蓄積症 ししつちくせきしょう	lipidosis
黄色腫症 おうしょくしゅしょう	xanthomatosis
ウォールマン病 びょう	Wolman disease

⟨*cholesterol ester storage disease caused by deficiency of the lysosomal acid lipase, with infantile onset, xanthomatosis, hepatosplenomegaly, anemia, and adrenal calcification*⟩

| タンパク質・エネルギー | protein-calorie malnutrition, protein- |

11. 内分泌・代謝系

栄養失調症	energy malnutrition
痛風	gout
糖原病	glycogen storage disease, glycogenosis
糖原病Ⅰ型, フォンギールケ病	glycogen storage disease type Ⅰ, von Gierke disease

⟨*hepatorenal glycogenosis; glucose-6-phosphatase deficiency*⟩

糖原病Ⅱ型, ポンペ病	glycogen storage disease type Ⅱ, Pompe disease

⟨*defect in acid maltase metabolism resulting in glycogen deposition in the heart, muscle, liver and nervous system; autosomal recessive*⟩

糖原病Ⅲ型, コーリー病	glycogen storage disease type Ⅲ, Cori disease

⟨*glycogen debrancher deficiency; amylo-1,6-glucosidase deficiency*⟩

糖原病Ⅳ型, アンダースン病	glycogen storage disease type Ⅳ, Andersen disease

⟨*deficiency of 1,4-α-glucan branching enzyme; early cirrhosis with liver failure*⟩

糖原病Ⅴ型, マッカードル病	glycogen storage disease type Ⅴ, McArdle disease

⟨*deficiency of muscle glycogen phosphorylase*⟩

ヘモクロマトーシス	hemochromatosis
アミロイドーシス	amyloidosis
ポルフィリン症	porphyria
急性間欠性ポルフィリン症	acute intermittent porphyria (AIP)
異型ポルフィリン症	variegate porphyria (VP)
遺伝性コプロポルフィリン症	hereditary coproporphyria (HCP)
ゴーシェ病	Gaucher disease

⟨*abnormal retention of glucocerebroside in RES; type 1, chronic nonneuronopathic adult, type 2, acute neuronopathic infantile, type 3, subacute neuronopathic juvenile*⟩

ニーマン・ピック病	Niemann-Pick disease

⟨*sphingomyelin accumulation in RES due to a lack of sphingomyelinase; five types*⟩

テイ・サックス病	Tay-Sachs disease (TSD)

⟨*accumulation of GM2 ganglioside in lysosomes due to a lack of hexosaminidase A; cherry-red macular spots*⟩

● 治療法 Treatment ●

血糖自己測定	self-monitoring of blood glucose (SMBG)

持続血糖測定	continuous glucose monitoring (CGM)
糖尿病食	diabetic diet
食品交換表	food substitution table
経口血糖降下薬	oral hypoglycemic agent, oral antihyperglycemic drug
スルホニルウレア薬	sulfonylurea (SU) compound
アセトヘキサミド	acetohexamide《ジメリン》
グリベンクラミド	glibenclamide《オイグルコン》
グリメピリド	glimepiride《アマリール》
ビグアナイド薬	biguanide
メトホルミン塩酸塩	metformin hydrochloride《グリコラン》
チアゾリジンジオン誘導体	thiazolidinedione (TZD) derivative
ピオグリタゾン塩酸塩	pioglitazone hydrochloride《アクトス》
ナテグリニド	nateglinide《ファスティック》
αグルコシダーゼ阻害薬	α-glucosidase inhibitor
アカルボース	acarbose《グルコバイ》
ミグリトール	miglitol《セイブル》
シタグリプチン	sitagliptin《ジャヌビア, グラクティブ》
エパルレスタット	epalrestat《キネダック》
速効型インスリン	rapid-acting insulin, short-acting insulin
持効型インスリン	long-acting insulin
中間型インスリン	intermediate-acting insulin
インスリングルリシン	insulin glulicine《アピドラ》
インスリングラルギン	insulin glargin《ランタス》
経口血糖降下剤と基礎インスリン注射併用	basal supported oral therapy (BOT)
持続インスリン皮下注入療法	continuous subcutaneous insulin infusion (CSII)
埋め込み型インスリンポンプ	implantable insulin pump
ジアゾキシド	diazoxide《アログリセム》
抗甲状腺薬	antithyroid agent, thyroid antagonist
プロピルチオウラシル	propylthiouracil (PTU)《チウラジール》
メチマゾール, チアマゾール	methimazole, thiamazole (MMI)《メルカゾール》
ヨウ化カリウム	potassium iodide
放射性ヨウ素	radioactive iodine (RAI)
乾燥甲状腺	desiccated thyroid gland《チラーヂン》
レボチロキシンナトリウム	levothyroxine sodium《チラーヂンS》
オクトレオチド酢酸塩	octreotide acetate《サンドスタチン》

11. 内分泌・代謝系 259

ドーパミン作動薬	dopamine agonist
ブロモクリプチン	bromocriptine《パーロデル》
デスモプレシン酢酸塩	desmopressin acetate, 1-deamino-8-D-AVP (DDAVP)《デスモプレシン》
バゾプレシン	vasopressin《ピトレシン》
スタチン系薬	statins
ヒドロキシメチルグルタリル補酵素A還元酵素阻害薬	hydroxymethylglutaryl-Coenzyme A (HMG-CoA) reductase inhibitor
プラバスタチンナトリウム	pravastatin sodium《メバロチン》
陰イオン交換樹脂	anion exchange resin
コレスチラミン	colestyramine《クエストラン》
小腸コレステロールトランスポーター阻害薬	inhibitor of intesitinal cholesterol transporter
エゼチミブ	ezetimibe《ゼチーア》
フィブラート	fibrates, fibric acid derivatives
ベザフィブラート	bezafibrate《ベザトール SR》
ニコチン酸	nicotinic acid
ニコモール	nicomol《コレキサミン》
プロブコール	probucol《シンレスタール》
イコサペント酸エチル	ethyl icosapentate《エパデール》
コルヒチン	colchicine《コルヒチン》
プロベネシド	probenecid《ベネシッド》
ベンズブロマロン	benzbromarone《ユリノーム》
ブコローム	bucolome《パラミヂン》
アロプリノール	allopurinol《ザイロリック》
甲状腺切除術	thyroidectomy
副甲状腺摘出術	parathyroidectomy
胸腺摘除術	thymectomy
下垂体切除術	hypophysectomy
副腎摘除術	adrenalectomy
膵切除術	pancreatectomy
人工膵臓	artificial pancreas
膵島移植	islet transplantation

―Tidbits―

bariatric surgery

肥満の治療のために行われる消化管手術のことで, weight loss surgery, obesity surgery とも呼ばれる. 肥満学 bariatrics という語は, barometer (気圧計, バロメーター) の bar(o)- (weight, pressure の意味の連結形) と iatrics (medical treatment) から成る. 肥満学者のことは bariatrician という.

術式としては, 胃バイパス術 gastric bypass, 垂直遮断式胃形成術 vertical banded gastroplasty (VBG), 腹腔鏡下胃緊縛術 laparoscopic gastric banding (LGB), 袖状胃切除術 sleeve gastrectomy, 胆膵バイパス術 biliopancreatic diversion などがある.

なお日本肥満学会は, Japan Society for the Study of Obesity (JASSO) と呼称するが, 米国には American Society for Metabolic and Bariatric Surgery (ASMBS) がある.

12. 血液・造血器系

● 愁訴・症状　Complaints / Symptoms ●

造血器系 ぞうけつきけい	hematopoietic system
造血臓器 ぞうけつぞうき	blood-forming organs, hematopoietic organs
血液疾患 けつえきしっかん	diseases of blood, blood dyscrasias
血性 けっせい	bloody
貧血 ひんけつ	anemia, 〔形〕anemic
蒼白 そうはく	pallor, 〔形〕pale, sallow, pasty, pallid, waxy
動悸 どうき	palpitation
息切れ いきぎれ	shortness of breath
めまい	light-headedness
筋力低下 きんりょくていか	muscle weakness
偏食 へんしょく	unbalanced diet
菜食主義 さいしょくしゅぎ	vegetarianism, veganism（極端な菜食主義）
菜食主義者 さいしょくしゅぎしゃ	vegetarian, vegan
異食 いしょく	pica
土食症 どしょくしょう	dirt-eating, geophagia
氷食症 ひょうしょくしょう	craving for ice, pagophagia
舌痛 ぜっつう	sore tongue, glossodynia, glossalgia
舌灼熱感 ぜっしゃくねっかん	burning tongue, glossopyrosis
出血 しゅっけつ	bleeding, hemorrhage, 〔形〕hemorrhagic, 〔動〕bleed
噴出性出血 ふんしゅつせいしゅっけつ	spurting bleeding, projectile bleeding
にじみ出る ―で	〔形〕oozing, oozy, 〔動〕ooze
出血傾向 しゅっけつけいこう	bleeding (hemorrhagic) tendency
出血性素因 しゅっけつせいそいん	bleeding (hemorrhagic) diathesis
歯肉出血 しにくしゅっけつ	gum bleeding
鼻血 はなぢ	nosebleed, nasal hemorrhage, epistaxis
点状出血 てんじょうしゅっけつ	petechia, petechial hemorrhage, 〔複〕petechiae
紫斑 しはん	purpura
斑状出血 はんじょうしゅっけつ	ecchymosis, blot hemorrhage, 〔複〕ecchymoses
打撲傷 だぼくしょう, 打ち身 うちみ―	bruise
青あざ あお―	black-and-blue mark
打ち身ができ易い	easy bruising, 〔名〕easy bruisability
血腫 けっしゅ	hematoma
潜血陽性便 せんけつようせいべん	occult-blood positive stool

262　IV章　診療録用語

溶血 ようけつ	hemolysis, 〔形〕hemolytic
止血 しけつ	hemostasis, 〔形〕hemostatic
血液凝固 けつえきぎょうこ	blood coagulation
凝固する ぎょう	coagulate
凝固能 ぎょうこのう	coagulating ability
凝血塊 ぎょうけつかい	blood clot, coagulum, 〔複〕coagula
献血 けんけつ	blood donation

● 診察所見・徴候　Physical findings / Signs ●

起立性低血圧 きりつせいていけつあつ	orthostatic hypotension
結膜蒼白 けつまくそうはく	conjunctival pallor
結膜溢血 けつまくいっけつ	conjunctival suffusion
手掌皮線蒼白 しゅしょうひせんそうはく	pale palmar creases
黄疸 おうだん	jaundice
顔面紅潮 がんめんこうちょう	facial plethora
歯肉肥大 しにくひだい	gum hypertrophy, gingival hypertophy
舌炎 ぜつえん	glossitis
ハンター舌炎 —ぜつえん	Hunter glossitis (cf. p.151)
舌乳頭萎縮 ぜつにゅうとういしゅく	atrophy of lingual papillae
口角びらん こうかく—	angular cheilitis, perleche
リンパ節腫 —せつしゅ	lymphadenopathy
リンパ節腫大 —せつしゅだい	enlarged lymph nodes
脾腫 ひしゅ	splenomegaly
ケール徴候 —ちょうこう	Kehr sign

⟨severe pain in the left shoulder in rupture of the spleen⟩

肝腫大 かんしゅだい	hepatomegaly
乳び腹水 にゅう—ふくすい	chylous ascites
匙状爪 さじじょうつめ	spoon nail, koilonychia
位置覚低下 いちかくていか	decreased position sense
振動覚消失 しんどうかくしょうしつ	loss of vibratory sensation
ペル・エプスタイン熱	Pel-Ebstein fever

⟨remittent fever in Hodgkin disease; several days' febrile periods alternating with afebrile periods for days or weeks⟩

ルンペル・レーデ現象 —げんしょう　　Rumpel-Leede phenomenon

⟨appearance of petechiae after application of a tourniquet, indicating capillary fragility or thrombocytopenia⟩

プラマー・ヴィンソン症候群 —こうぐん　　Plummer-Vinson syndrome

⟨dysphagia, atrophic glossitis, and perleche in iron deficiency anemia⟩

FAB分類 —ぶんるい　　French-American-British (FAB) classifi-

	cation
REAL 分類 ぶんるい	Revised European-American Lymphoma (REAL) classification
リンパ腫 WHO 分類 ぶんるい	WHO classification of lymphoid neoplasms
国際予後指標 こくさいよごしひょう	International Prognostic Index (IPI)

● 検査法　Examination ●

ベンスジョーンズタンパク質 しつ	Bence Jones proteins (BJP) ⟨*abnormal protein consisting of monoclonal immunoglobulin light chains, found in the urine in multiple myeloma and macroglobulinemia; unusual thermosolubility*⟩
血球計算器 けっきゅうけいさんき	blood cell counter
コールターカウンター	Coulter counter ⟨*an automated blood cell counter, based on the principle that cells are poor electrical conductors*⟩
全血球計算 ぜんけっきゅうけいさん	complete blood count (CBC), complete blood cell count
赤血球数 せっけっきゅうすう	red blood cell (RBC) count, erythrocyte count
ヘモグロビン，血色素 けっしきそ	hemoglobin (Hb, Hgb)
ヘマトクリット	hematocrit (Hct)
平均赤血球容積 へいきんせっけっきゅうようせき	mean corpuscular volume (MCV)
赤血球容積分布幅 せっけっきゅうようせきぶんぷはば	red cell distribution width (RDW)
平均赤血球ヘモグロビン量 へいきんせっけっきゅう―りょう	mean corpuscular hemoglobin (MCH)
平均赤血球ヘモグロビン濃度 へいきんせっけっきゅう―のうど	mean corpuscular hemoglobin concentration (MCHC)
網赤血球 もうせっけっきゅう	reticulocyte
白血球数 はっけっきゅうすう	white blood cell (WBC) count, leukocyte count
白血球分画 はっけっきゅうぶんかく	differential blood count
血小板数 けっしょうばんすう	blood platelet count, thrombocyte count
低色素血 ていしきそけつ	hypochromia, 〔形〕hypochromic
高色素血 こうしきそけつ	hyperchromia, 〔形〕hyperchromic
小球性（大球性）貧血 しょうきゅうせい（だいきゅうせい）ひんけつ	microcytic (macrocytic) anemia
赤血球大小不同	anisocytosis

異型赤血球増加	poikilocytosis
球状赤血球	spherocyte
球状赤血球症	spherocytosis
破砕赤血球	fragmented red blood cell
分裂赤血球症	schistocytosis
好塩基性斑点	basophilic stippling
標的細胞	target cell
有棘赤血球	acanthocyte, spur cell
有棘赤血球増加	acanthocytosis
金平糖状赤血球	crenocyte, echinocyte, crenated erythrocyte, burr cell
多染性	polychromasia
ハウエル・ジョリー小体	Howell-Jolly body

⟨remnants of nuclear chromatin found as inclusion bodies in erythrocytes after splenectomy or in megaloblastic or hemolytic anemia⟩

ハインツ小体	Heinz body

⟨intracellular inclusion bodies formed by denatured hemoglobin; seen in thalassemia, unstable hemoglobinopathies, and after splenectomy⟩

連銭形成	rouleau formation
網状赤血球	reticulocyte
顆粒球	granulocyte
好中球	neutrophil
多形核好中球	polymorphonuclear neutrophil (PMN)
杆状核好中球	band neutrophil, rod neutrophil, stab neutrophil
分節核好中球	segmented neutrophil
デーレ封入体	Döhle inclusion body

⟨ovoid blue-staining inclusions seen in the neutrophil cytoplasm, consisting of RNA from RER; found in sepsis, burns, aplastic anemia, and some toxic states⟩

ペルゲル・フエット核異常	Pelger-Huët nuclear anomaly

⟨defective lobulation of the nuclei of neutrophils, appearing bilobulate or dumbbell-shaped; autosomal dominant inheritance⟩

核左方(右方)移動	shift to the left (right)
好酸球	eosinophil
好塩基球	basophil
リンパ球	lymphocyte

12. 血液・造血器系

異型リンパ球 (いけい—きゅう)	atypical lymphocyte
大顆粒リンパ球 (だいかりゅう—きゅう)	large granular lymphocyte (LGL)
単球 (たんきゅう)	monocyte
形質細胞 (けいしつさいぼう)	plasma cell
赤血球増加 (せっけっきゅうぞうか)	erythrocytosis
網赤血球増加 (もうせっけっきゅうぞうか)	reticulocytosis
白血球増加 (はっけっきゅうぞうか)	leukocytosis
白血球減少 (はっけっきゅうげんしょう)	leukopenia
好中球減少 (こうちゅうきゅうげんしょう)	neutropenia
顆粒球減少 (かりゅうきゅうげんしょう)	granulocytopenia
無顆粒球症 (むかりゅうきゅうしょう)	agranulocytosis
末梢血リンパ球 (まっしょうけつ—きゅう)	peripheral blood lymphocyte (PBL)
総リンパ球数 (そう—きゅうすう)	total lymphocyte count (TLC)
リンパ球減少 (—きゅうげんしょう)	lymphopenia, lymphocytopenia
好酸球増加 (こうさんきゅうぞうか)	eosinophilia
血小板増加 (けっしょうばんぞうか)	thrombocytosis
血小板減少 (けっしょうばんげんしょう)	thrombocytopenia
汎血球減少 (はんけっきゅうげんしょう)	pancytopenia
好中球アルカリホスファターゼ (こうちゅうきゅう—)	neutrophil alkaline phosphatase (NAP)
白血球アルカリホスファターゼ (はっけっきゅう—)	leukocyte alkaline phosphatase (LAP)
細網内皮系 (さいもうないひけい)	reticuloendothelial system (RES)
マクロファージ	macrophage
食細胞 (しょくさいぼう)	phagocyte
血小板活性化因子 (けっしょうばんかっせいかいんし)	platelet-activating factor (PAF)
凝固因子 (ぎょうこいんし)	coagulation factor
出血時間 (しゅっけつじかん)	bleeding time (BT)
凝固時間 (ぎょうこじかん)	coagulation time
活性凝固時間 (かっせいぎょうこじかん)	activated coagulation time (ACT)
血小板凝集試験 (けっしょうばんぎょうしゅうしけん)	platelet aggregation test (PAT)
血餅収縮 (けっぺいしゅうしゅく)	clot retraction
プロトロンビン時間 (—じかん)	prothrombin time (PT)
トロンビン時間 (—じかん)	thrombin time
トロンボテスト	thrombotest (TT)
部分トロンボプラスチン時間 (ぶぶん—じかん)	partial thromboplastin time (PTT)
活性化部分トロンボプラスチン時間 (かっせいかぶぶん—じかん)	activated partial thromboplastin time (APTT)
ヘパプラスチンテスト	hepaplastin test (HPT)

フィブリノゲン	fibrinogen
Dダイマー	D dimer
フィブリン分解産物	fibrin degradation product (FDP)
アンチトロンビンIII	antithrombin III (AT-III)
トロンビン・アンチトロンビンIII複合体	thrombin-antithrombin III complex (TAT)
ハプトグロビン	haptoglobin (Hp)
プロテインC	protein C (PC)
活性化プロテインC	activated protein C (APC)
プロテインS	protein S (PS)
トロンボモジュリン	thrombomodulin
プラスミン	plasmin
プラスミノーゲン	plasminogen
プラスミン・αプラスミンインヒビター複合体	plasmin-αplasmin inhibitor complex (PPIC)
プラスミノーゲンアクチベーターインヒビター1	plasminogen activator inhibitor-1 (PAI-1)
ユーグロブリン溶解時間	euglobulin lysis time
フォンウィルブランド因子	von Willebrand factor (vWF)

⟨a coagulant glycoprotein produced by endothelial cells that is complexed to factor VIII in plasma; mediates platelet adhesion to damaged epithelial surfaces⟩

凝固能亢進	hypercoagulability
凝固能低下	hypocoagulability
毛細管脆弱	capillary fragility
浸透圧脆弱性試験	osmotic fragility test
赤血球沈降速度	erythrocyte sedimentation rate (ESR), blood sedimentation
骨髄抑制	bone marrow suppression
骨髄穿刺	bone marrow puncture
骨髄穿刺液	bone marrow aspirate
骨髄生検	bone marrow biopsy
赤芽球	erythroblast
骨髄球	myelocyte
骨髄芽球	myeloblast
巨核球	megakaryocyte

巨核芽球	megakaryoblast
細網細胞	reticulum cell
鉄芽球	sideroblast
環状鉄芽球	ringed sideroblast
ヒトTリンパ球向性ウイルス1型	human T-lymphotropic virus 1 (HTLV-1)
ヒトTリンパ球向性ウイルス2型	human T-lymphotropic virus 2 (HTLV-2)
末端デオキシヌクレオチド転移酵素	terminal deoxynucleotidyl transferase (TdT)
血液型	blood group, blood type
ABO血液型	ABO blood group
Rh血液型	Rh blood group
交差適合試験	cross match
血液型不適合	blood group incompatibility
クームス試験	Coombs test, antiglobulin test (AGT)

⟨*a test for nonagglutinating antibodies against red blood cells, using anti-human globulin antibody*⟩

間接抗グロブリン試験, 間接クームス試験	indirect antiglobulin test, indirect Coombs test (ICT)
直接抗グロブリン試験, 直接クームス試験	direct antiglobulin test (DAT), direct Coombs test (DCT)
一酸化炭素ヘモグロビン	carboxyhemoglobin
ポール・バンネル試験	Paul-Bunnell test

⟨*detection of heterophile antibodies in infectious mononucleosis; determines the most dilute serum capable of agglutinating sheep RBC's*⟩

エプスタイン・バーウイルス	Epstein-Barr virus (EBV)

⟨*DNA virus associated with infectious mononucleosis, Burkitt lymphoma, and nasopharyngeal carcinoma*⟩

抗EBV-VCA抗体	anti-EBV-viral capsid antigen (VCA) antibody
抗EBNA抗体	anti-EBV-nuclear antigen (EBNA) antibody
抗EBV-EA抗体	anti-EBV-early antigen (EA) antibody
細胞マーカー	cell marker
染色体分析	chromosome analysis
フィラデルフィア染色体	Philadelphia chromosome (Ph)

細胞化学 cytochemistry
ミエロペルオキシダーゼ myeloperoxidase (MPO)
血小板ペルオキシダーゼ platelet peroxidase (PPO)
免疫表現型判定 immunophenotyping
白血球関連抗原 leukocyte common antigen (LCA)
急性リンパ芽球性白血病共通抗原 common acute lymphoblastic leukemia antigen (CALLA)
抗ヒトリンパ球向性ウイルス1型抗体 anti-human T-lymphotropic virus 1 antibody
高非抱合型ビリルビン血症 unconjugated hyperbilirubinemia
エリスロポエチン erythropoietin (EPO)
血清鉄 serum iron
フェリチン ferritin
トランスフェリン transferrin (Tf)
トランスフェリン受容体 transferrin receptor
総鉄結合能 total iron-binding capacity (TIBC)
不飽和鉄結合能 unsaturated iron-binding capacity (UIBC)
内因子 intrinsic factor
ビタミン B_{12} vitamin B_{12}
葉酸 folic acid
寒冷赤血球凝集素 cold hemagglutinin
ハム試験 Ham test
  ⟨*acidified serum hemolysis test to detect paroxysmal nocturnal hemoglobinuria*⟩
ドナート・ランドシュタイナー試験 Donath-Landsteiner test
  ⟨*hemolysis occurs if blood sample is cooled to 5°C and then rewarmed; for the diagnosis of paroxysmal hemoglobinuria*⟩
シリング試験 Schilling test
  ⟨*determination of urinary excretion of vitamin B_{12} using radioactively labeled cyanocobalamine; used in the diagnosis of pernicious anemia and intestinal malabsorption*⟩

12. 血液・造血器系　269

放射性クロム標識赤血球半減期	half-life for radiochromium-labeled red blood cells (^{51}Cr)
血漿鉄交代率	plasma iron turnover rate (PITR)
赤血球鉄利用率	red cell iron utilization (RCU)
造骨性病変	osteoblastic lesion
溶骨性病変	osteolytic lesion
リード・ステルンベルグ細胞	Reed-Sternberg cell

⟨*giant histiocytic cells, multinucleated, with amphophilic* cytoplasm; diagnostic of Hodgkin disease*⟩ *stainable with either acid or basic dyes

● 疾患名　Diseases ●

慢性疾患に伴う貧血	anemia of chronic disease (ACD)
鉄欠乏性貧血	iron-deficiency anemia (IDA)
悪性貧血	pernicious anemia (PA)
巨赤芽球性貧血	megaloblastic anemia
再生不良性貧血	aplastic anemia (AA)
鉄芽球性貧血	sideroblastic anemia
先天性溶血性貧血	congenital hemolytic anemia
遺伝性球状赤血球症	hereditary spherocytosis (HS)
遺伝性楕円赤血球症	hereditary elliptocytosis
遺伝性非球状赤血球性溶血性貧血	hereditary nonspherocytic hemolytic anemia (HNSHA)
ヘモグロビン症	hemoglobinopathy
地中海貧血	thalassemia
クーリー貧血	Cooley anemia

⟨*thalassemia major; homozygous β-thalassemia characterized by severe anemia, hepatosplenomegaly, cardiomegaly, and skeletal deformation*⟩

鎌状赤血球貧血	sickle cell anemia
先天性赤血球生成不全性貧血	congenital dyserythropoietic anemia (CDA)
酸性化血清陽性を伴う遺伝性赤芽球多形核症	hereditary erythroblastic multinuclearity associated with positive acidified serum (HEMPAS)

270　IV章　診療録用語

後天性溶血性貧血	acquired hemolytic anemia (AHA)
自己免疫性溶血性貧血	autoimmune hemolytic anemia (AIHA)
寒冷凝集素症	cold agglutinin disease (CAD)
発作性寒冷血色素尿症	paroxysmal cold hemoglobinuria (PCH)
発作性夜間血色素尿症	paroxysmal nocturnal hemoglobinuria (PNH)
微小血管障害性溶血性貧血	microangiopathic hemolytic anemia (MHA)
脾機能亢進症	hypersplenism
バンチ症候群	Banti syndrome 〈*congestive splenomegaly with anemia caused by portal hypertension*〉
不応性貧血	refractory anemia (RA)
芽球増加性不応性貧血	refractory anemia with excess blasts (RAEB)
赤芽球癆	pure red cell aplasia (PRCA)
後天性免疫不全症候群	acquired immunodeficiency syndrome (AIDS)
骨髄増殖性疾患	myeloproliferative disorders (MPD)
慢性骨髄増殖性疾患	chronic myeloproliferative disorders (CMPD)
骨髄異形成症候群	myelodysplastic syndrome (MDS)
白血病	leukemia, 〔形〕leukemic
急性骨髄性白血病	acute myelogenous leukemia (AML)
急性前骨髄球性白血病	acute promyelocytic leukemia (APL)
急性骨髄単球性白血病	acute myelomonocytic leukemia (AMMoL)
急性単球性白血病	acute monocytic leukemia
赤白血病	erythroleukemia
急性巨核球性白血病	acute megakaryocytic leukemia
急性リンパ性白血病	acute lymphocytic leukemia (ALL)
急性非リンパ性白血病	acute nonlymphocytic leukemia (ANLL)

12. 血液・造血器系

慢性骨髄性白血病	chronic myelocytic leukemia (CML)
慢性骨髄単球性白血病	chronic myelomonocytic leukemia (CMML)
慢性リンパ性白血病	chronic lymphocytic leukemia (CLL)
リクター症候群	Richter syndrome

⟨*transformation of CLL to diffuse large cell lymphoma*⟩

急性好塩基球性白血病	acute basophilic leukemia
急性好酸球性白血病	acute eosinophilic leukemia
慢性好中球性白血病	chronic neutrophilic leukemia (CNL)
成人T細胞白血病	adult T-cell leukemia (ATL)
成人T細胞白血病リンパ腫	adult T-cell leukemia/lymphoma (ATLL)
毛髪様細胞白血病, 白血病性細網内皮症	hairy-cell leukemia (HCL), leukemic reticuloendotheliosis (LRE)
くすぶり白血病	smoldering leukemia
肥満細胞白血病	mast cell leukemia
前白血病	preleukemia
微少残存病変	minimal residual disease (MRD)
好酸球増加症候群	hypereosinophilic syndrome (HES)
骨髄線維症	myelofibrosis
真性多血症	polycythemia vera (PV)
ガイスベック症候群	Gaisböck syndrome

⟨*stress polycythemia; mild polycythemia without splenomegaly in obese hypertensive middle-aged men*⟩

本態性血小板血症	essential thrombocythemia (ET)
伝染性単核球症	infectious mononucleosis (IM)
伴性リンパ増殖症候群, ダンカン病	X-linked lymphoproliferative syndrome (XLP), Duncan disease

⟨*an X-linked recessive immunodeficiency disease characterized by defective immune response to EBV infection resulting in fulminant infectious mononucleosis*⟩

巨大リンパ節増殖症, キャッスルマン病 giant lymph node hyperplasia, Castleman disease
⟨*solid tumor secondary to reactive proliferation of B-cell lymphocytes; two types, benign mediastinal and premalignant multicentric*⟩

悪性リンパ腫 malignant lymphoma (ML)

ホジキン病 Hodgkin disease (HD)
⟨*malignant lymphoma with progressive generalized lymphadenopathy and splenomegaly; presence of Reed-Sternberg cells is characteristic*⟩

ホジキンリンパ腫 Hodgkin lymphoma (HL)
⟨*syn. Hodgkin disease*⟩

非ホジキンリンパ腫 non-Hodgkin lymphoma (NHL)
⟨*malignant lymphomas other than Hodgkin disease, the most recent classification being the REAL; Reed-Sternberg cells are absent*⟩

びまん性大細胞B細胞リンパ腫 diffuse large B cell lymphoma (DLBCL)

濾胞性リンパ腫 follicular lymphoma (FL)

バーキットリンパ腫 Burkitt lymphoma
⟨*small noncleaved cell lymphoma caused by Epstein-Barr virus; reported in central Africa*⟩

皮膚T細胞性リンパ腫 cutaneous T-cell lymphoma (CTCL)

異常タンパク血症を伴う血管免疫芽球性リンパ節症 angioimmunoblastic lymphadenopathy with dysproteinemia (AILD)

シェディアック・東症候群 Chédiak-Higashi syndrome
⟨*a rare autosomal recessive condition with abnormal lysosomes appearing as giant cytoplasmic granules; characterized by partial albinism, photophobia, recurrent infections, and susceptibility to lymphoma*⟩

菌状息肉症 mycosis fungoides (MF)

カポジ肉腫 Kaposi sarcoma
⟨*multiple idiopathic hemorrhagic sarcoma found in HIV-infected men*⟩

血球貪食症候群 hemophagocytic syndrome (HPS)

血球貪食性リンパ組織球症 hemophagocytic lymphohistiocytosis (HLH)

良性単クローン性免疫グロブリン症 benign monoclonal gammopathy (BMG)

12. 血液・造血器系

多発性骨髄腫	multiple myeloma (MM)
ワルデンシュトレーム・マクログロブリン血症	Waldenström macroglobulinemia

⟨a malignant disease of B cells that secrete an IgM paraprotein; marked by lymphadenopathy, anemia, bleeding tendency, cryoglobulinemia, visual disturbance, and peripheral neuropathy⟩

クロウ・深瀬症候群, POEMS症候群	Crow-Fukase syndrome, POEMS syndrome

⟨plasma cell dyscrasia with progressive neuropathy; polyneuropathy, organomegaly, endocrinopathy, M-proteins, and skin changes⟩

重鎖病	heavy chain disease (HCD)
意義不明の単クローングロブリン血症	monoclonal gammopathy of uncertain significance (MGUS)
分類不能型免疫不全症	common variable immunodeficiency (CVID)
特発性血小板減少性紫斑病	idiopathic thrombocytopenic purpura (ITP)
エヴァンス症候群	Evans syndrome

⟨idiopathic thrombocytopenia with autoimmune hemolytic anemia⟩

血栓性微小血管症	thrombotic microangiopathy (TMA)
血栓性血小板減少性紫斑病	thrombotic thrombocytopenic purpura (TTP)
ヘパリン起因性血小板減少症	heparin-induced thrombocytopenia (HIT), white clot syndrome
グランツマン病	Glanzmann disease

⟨hereditary hemorrhagic thrombasthenia characterized by prolonged bleeding time, defective clot retraction, and failure of platelet aggregation⟩

巨大血小板症候群	giant platelet syndrome
ベルナール・スーリエ症候群	Bernard-Soulier syndrome

⟨giant platelet syndrome; enlarged platelets with membranes lacking glycoprotein receptor for von Willebrand factor; platelet adhesion decreased, causing epistaxis, purpura, and prolonged bleeding time⟩

フォンウィルブランド病	von Willebrand disease (vWD)

⟨a congenital hemorrhagic diathesis of autosomal dominant inheritance associated with deficiency of von Willebrand factor⟩

溶血性尿毒症症候群	hemolytic uremic syndrome (HUS)

274　Ⅳ章　診療録用語

血友病 ようけつせいにょうどくしょうしょうこうぐん／けつゆうびょう	hemophilia
クリスマス病 びょう	Christmas disease

〈＜*Christmas, a patient's name; hemophilia B, congenital deficiency of factor IX*〉

遺伝性出血性末梢血管拡張症 いでんせいしゅっけつせいまっしょうけっかんかくちょうしょう	hereditary hemorrhagic telangiectasia, Osler-Weber-Rendu disease
播種性血管内凝固 はしゅせいけっかんないぎょうこ	disseminated intravascular coagulation (DIC)
移植片対宿主病 いしょくへんたいしゅくしゅびょう	graft-versus-host disease (GVHD)
輸血副作用 ゆけつふくさよう	transfusion reaction
脾摘後重症感染症 ひてきごじゅうしょうかんせんしょう	overwhelming postsplenectomy infection (OPSI)

● 治療法　Treatment ●

造血薬 ぞうけつやく	hematinics
鉄剤 てつざい	iron preparations
ビタミン B₁₂	vitamin B₁₂
葉酸 ようさん	folic acid
ビタミン B₆	vitamin B₆
遺伝子組み換えヒトエリスロポエチン いでんしくみかえ	recombinant human erythropoietin (r-HuEPO)
エポエチンアルファ	epoetin alfa《エスポー》
エポエチンベータ	epoetin beta《エポジン》
ダルベポエチンアルファ	darbepoetin alfa《ネスプ》
フィルグラスチム	filgrastim《グラン》
ミリモスチム	mirimostim《ロイコプロール》
タンパク同化ステロイド どうか	anabolic steroid
免疫抑制薬 めんえきよくせいやく	immunosuppressant
アントラサイクリン	anthracycline
ダウノルビシン塩酸塩	daunorubicin hydrochloride (DNR)《ダウノマイシン》
ビンクリスチン硫酸塩	vincristine sulfate《オンコビン》
メシル酸イマチニブ	imatinib mesilate《グリベック》
ボルテゾミブ	bortezomib《ベルケイド》
サリドマイド	thalidomide《サレド》
サリドマイド製剤安全管理手順 せいざいあんぜんかんりてじゅん	Thalidomide Education and Risk Management System (TERMS)
デシタビン	decitabine (DAC)
デフェロキサミン	deferoxamine (DFO)《エクジェイド》

12. 血液・造血器系

高活性抗レトロウイルス療法	highly active antiretroviral therapy (HAART)
ヌクレオシド系逆転写酵素阻害薬	nucleoside reverse transcriptase inhibitor (NRTI)
アジドチミジン, ジドブジン	azidothymidine (AZT), zidovudine《レトロビル》
ジデオキシイノシン, ジダノシン	dideoxyinosine (ddI), didanosine《ヴァイデックス》
ジデオキシシチジン, ザルシタビン	dideoxycytidine (ddC), zalcitabine《ハイビッド》
テノホビルジソプロキシルフマル酸	tenofovir disoproxil fumarate (TDF)《ビリアード》
エムトリシタビン	emtricitabine (FTC)《エムトリバ》
非ヌクレオシド系逆転写酵素阻害薬	nonnucleoside reverse transcriptase inhibitor (NNRTI)
エファビレンツ	efavirenz (EFV)《ストックリン》
プロテアーゼ阻害薬	protease inhibitor
ホスアンプレナビルカルシウム	fosamprenavir calcium (FPV)《レクシヴァ》
ダルテパリンナトリウム	dalteparin sodium《フラグミン》
ダナパロイドナトリウム	danaparoid sodium《オルガラン》
アンチトロンビンⅢ	antithrombin Ⅲ《ノイアート》
セリンプロテアーゼインヒビター	serine protease inhibitor (SPI)
ナファモスタットメシル酸塩	nafamostat mesilate《フサン》
トロンボモジュリン	thrombomodulin《リコモジュリン》
輸血	blood transfusion
血液銀行	blood bank
自己輸血	autotransfusion, autologous transfusion
術前貯血式自己血輸血	predeposit autologous transfusion
全血	whole blood
保存血	preserved blood, banked blood
クエン酸塩添加血	citrated blood
ヘパリン添加血	heparinized blood
成分輸血	blood component transfusion
赤血球濃厚液	packed red blood cells, concentrated red blood cells (CRC)

IV章 診療録用語

凍結融解赤血球（とうけつゆうかいせっけっきゅう）	frozen-thawed red blood cells
洗浄赤血球（せんじょうせっけっきゅう）	washed red blood cells
新鮮凍結血漿（しんせんとうけつけっしょう）	fresh frozen plasma (FFP)
顆粒球輸血（かりゅうきゅうゆけつ）	granulocyte transfusion
ドナーリンパ球輸注（——きゅうゆちゅう）	donor lymphocyte infusion
血小板濃縮液（けっしょうばんのうしゅくえき）	platelet concentrate (PC)
血漿交換（けっしょうこうかん）	plasmapheresis, plasma exchange
血球除去療法（けっきゅうじょきょりょうほう）	cytapheresis
抗リンパ球グロブリン（こう——きゅう）	antilymphocyte globulin (ALG)
抗胸腺細胞グロブリン（こうきょうせんさいぼう）	antithymocyte globulin (ATG)《サイモグロブリン》
顆粒球マクロファージコロニー刺激因子（かりゅうきゅう——しげきいんし）	granulocyte-macrophage colony-stimulating factor (GM-CSF)
シクロスポリン	cyclosporin A (CsA)
骨髄移植（こつずいいしょく）	bone marrow transplantation (BMT)
同種骨髄移植（どうしゅこつずいいしょく）	allogenic bone marrow transplantation
自己骨髄移植（じここつずいいしょく）	autologous bone marrow transplantation (ABMT)
全身放射線照射（ぜんしんほうしゃせんしょうしゃ）	total body irradiation (TBI)
幹細胞移植（かんさいぼういしょく）	stem cell transplantation
造血幹細胞移植（ぞうけつかんさいぼういしょく）	hematopoietic stem cell transplantation (HSCT)
自己幹細胞移植（じこかんさいぼういしょく）	autologous stem cell transplantation (ASCT)
末梢血幹細胞移植（まっしょうけつかんさいぼういしょく）	peripheral blood stem cell transplantation (PBSCT)
臍帯血幹細胞移植（さいたいけつかんさいぼういしょく）	cord blood stem cell transplantation (CBSCT)
瀉血（しゃけつ）	phlebotomy, bloodletting
骨髄抑制療法（こつずいよくせいりょうほう）	myelosuppressive therapy
脾摘出術（ひてきしゅつじゅつ）	splenectomy
リンパ節摘除術（——せつてきじょじゅつ）	lymphadenectomy, lymph node excision
全リンパ節照射（ぜん——せつしょうしゃ）	total nodal irradiation (TNI)

12. 血液・造血器系　*277*

Ⅳ章

―――Tidbits―――

six-pack

2008年のアメリカ大統領選挙では，Joe the Plumber と Joe Six-Pack が話題になったが，working-class, small-town Americans, つまり普通の庶民の味方であることを示すために用いられた．six-pack はビールなどの半ダースパックのことで，「普通のアメリカ人」が愛用している．Joe（<Joseph）は，guy, fellow の意味で「普通の人」（GI Joe は米兵のこと）．他に平均的市民を指す言葉として John Q. Public がある．また six-pack はその形状からよく発達した腹筋を指す（six-pack abs; abs は abdominal muscles）．割れた腹筋を目指す腹筋運動は six-pack abs workout である．

13. 筋・骨格系

● 愁訴・症状 Complaints / Symptoms ●

筋骨格系疾患 きんこっかくけいしっかん	diseases of the musculoskeletal system
運動器官系 うんどうきかんけい	locomotor system
運動器官症候群 うんどうきかんしょうこうぐん	locomotor syndrome
関節痛 かんせつつう	arthralgia, joint pain
膝関節痛 しつかんせつつう	gonalgia, pain in the knee
関節炎 かんせつえん	arthritis
関節腫脹 かんせつしゅちょう	swelling of joints, joint swelling
関節変形 かんせつへんけい	deformity of a joint
荷重関節 かじゅうかんせつ	weight-bearing joint
脱臼 だっきゅう	dislocation, 〔動〕be dislocated, be out of joint, be put out of joint
捻挫 ねんざ	sprain, 〔動〕sprain
くるぶしをくじく	sprain (wrench, twist) one's ankle, have a sprain in one's ankle
骨折 こっせつ	fracture, 〔動〕break a bone, suffer a broken (fractured) bone
骨折評価ツール こっせつひょうかツール	Fracture Risk Assessment Tool (FRAX)
拘縮 こうしゅく	contracture
背骨 せぼね, 脊柱 せきちゅう	backbone, spine, spinal column
脊柱変形 せきちゅうへんけい	spinal deformity
猫背 ねこぜ	humpback, 〔形〕humpbacked
リウマチ	rheumatism, 〔形〕rheumatic
朝のこわばり あさのこわばり	morning stiffness
腰痛 ようつう	low backache, low back pain (LBP), lumbago
筋肉痛 きんにくつう	muscle pain (ache), myalgia, sore muscle
筋肉圧痛 きんにくあっつう	muscular tenderness, tenderness of the muscle
筋萎縮 きんいしゅく	muscular atrophy
筋肉の痩せ きんにくのやせ	muscular wasting
筋脱力 きんだつりょく	muscular weakness
握力 あくりょく	grip
筋違い すじちがい	muscle strain, 〔動〕have a strain
筋がつる すじがつる	have a cramp, be cramped, cramp
肉離れ にくばなれ	torn muscle, pull
寝違える ねちがえる	have a stiff neck
肩こり かたこり	stiffness in a shoulder, stiff shoulder
五十肩 ごじゅうかた	frozen shoulder, scapulohumeral periar-

13. 筋・骨格系

	thritis
こむらがえり	cramp in the calf, leg cramp, 〔話〕charley horse
下肢むずむず症候群 かし——しょうこうぐん	restless legs syndrome (RLS)
ジャンパー膝 ひざ	jumper's knee
膝蓋大腿機能障害 しつがいだいたいきのうしょうがい	patellofemoral dysfunction (PFD)
テニス肘 ひじ	tennis elbow
むち打ち症 しょう	whiplash, whiplash injury, sprain of the cervical spine
むち打ち症になる	get (suffer from) whiplash injury
ぎっくり腰 こし	strained back
ぎっくり腰になる	have a strained back, put (throw) one's back out
突き指 つきゆび	sprained finger
添え木 そえぎ, 副子 ふくし	splint
ギプス	cast, plaster cast, plaster of Paris
ギプスをはめている	wear a cast, be in plaster
杖 つえ	cane, walking stick
松葉杖 まつばづえ	crutch
松葉杖で歩く まつばづえであるく	walk on crutches
義肢 ぎし	artificial limb, prosthesis
義手 ぎしゅ	artificial arm (hand), prosthetic arm
義足 ぎそく	artificial leg, prosthetic foot

● 診察所見・徴候　Physical findings / Signs ●

屈曲 くっきょく	flexion
伸展 しんてん	extension
過伸展 かしんてん	hyperextension
外転 がいてん	abduction
内転 ないてん	adduction
回内 かいない	pronation
回外 かいがい	supination
内旋 ないせん	internal rotation
外旋 がいせん	external rotation
疼痛回避歩行 とうつうかいひほこう	antalgic gait
股関節痛歩行 こかんせつつうほこう	coxalgic gait
骨盤傾斜 こつばんけいしゃ	pelvic obliquity
屈曲変形 くっきょくへんけい	flexion deformity
O脚 ——きゃく, 内反膝 ないはんしつ	bowlegs, genu varum
大腿脛骨角 だいたいけいこつかく	femorotibial angle (FTA)

骨幹端・骨幹角	metaphyseal-diaphyseal angle (MDA)
X脚, 外反膝	knock-knees, genu valgum
扁平足	flatfoot, pes planus
凹足	hollow foot, talipes cavus
尖足	drop foot, talipes equinus
内反足	clubfoot, talipes equinovarus (TEV)
踵足	talipes calcaneus
外反母趾	hallux valgus
ハンマー状足趾	hammer toe
膝蓋跳動	floating patella, ballottement of the patella
関節水症	hydrarthrosis
関節血症	hemarthrosis
引き出し徴候	drawer sign
関節ねずみ	joint mouse, joint loose body
パンヌス	pannus (inflammatory synovial tissue that covers the cartilages of rheumatoid joints)
関節可動性	joint mobility
関節可動域	range of motion (ROM)
対称性関節腫脹	symmetric joint swelling

シャルコー関節　Charcot joint
〈*neuropathic arthropathy; commonly seen in tabes dorsalis or diabetic neuropathy*〉

ベイカー嚢胞　Baker cyst
〈*synovial cyst of the popliteal space; seen in middle-aged women with osteoarthritis or rheumatoid arthritis*〉

踵骨隆起関節角, ベーラー角　Böhler angle
〈*measurement of talocalcaneal joint on lateral radiographic view; the angle reduced in crush fractures of calcaneum*〉

内反肘	cubitus varus
外反肘	cubitus valgus
三角線維軟骨複合体	triangular fibrocartilage complex (TFCC)

ヘバーデン結節　Heberden nodes
〈*osteophytic overgrowth at the distal interphalangeal joints associated with osteoarthritis*〉

ブシャール結節　Bouchard nodes
〈*marginal osteophytes at the proximal interphalangeal joints in degenerative joint disease*〉

皮下結節	subcutaneous nodules

リウマトイド結節	rheumatoid nodule
ボタン穴変形	boutonnière deformity, buttonhole deformity
陥入爪	ingrown toenail, ingrowing toenail, ingrown nail
ラセーグ徴候	Lasègue sign

⟨with the hip flexed and the knee extended, dorsiflexion of the foot causing pain in the back or leg indicates nerve root irritation⟩

下肢伸展挙上テスト	straight leg raising test (SLR)
交叉下肢伸展挙上試験	well leg raising test (WLRT)
ゲンズレン徴候	Gaenslen sign

⟨positive for sacroiliac cause of backache if pain occurs on hyperextension of the hip with the pelvis fixed by flexion of the opposite hip⟩

トーマス試験	Thomas test

⟨flexion contracture of the hip is indicated, if bringing the knee of the uninvolved side to the chest results in bending of the opposite leg,⟩

徒手筋力テスト	manual muscle test (MMT)
脊柱側彎	scoliosis
脊柱前彎	lordosis
脊柱後彎	kyphosis
突背	gibbosity, gibbus
瘢痕拘縮	cicatricial contracture
伸展拘縮	extension contracture
屈曲拘縮	flexion contracture
虚血性拘縮	ischemic contracture
筋拘縮	muscular contracture
デュピュイトラン拘縮	Dupuytren contracture

⟨flexion contracture of a finger caused by fibrosis of the palmar fascia⟩

フォルクマン拘縮	Volkmann contracture

⟨ischemic contracture of the forearm flexor muscles⟩

スワン・ネック変形	swan-neck deformity
関節拘縮	arthrogryposis
裂離	avulsion
完全骨折	complete fracture
不全骨折	incomplete fracture
開放骨折, 複雑骨折	open fracture, compound fracture

282　IV章　診療録用語

皮下骨折（ひかこっせつ），閉鎖骨折（へいさこっせつ）	closed fracture
亀裂骨折（きれつこっせつ）	fissure fracture
粉砕骨折（ふんさいこっせつ）	comminuted fracture
剥離骨折（はくりこっせつ）	avulsion fracture
圧迫骨折（あっぱくこっせつ）	compression fracture
陥没骨折（かんぼつこっせつ）	depressed fracture
嵌入骨折（かんにゅうこっせつ）	impacted fracture
疲労骨折（ひろうこっせつ）	stress fracture, fatigue fracture
脆弱性骨折（ぜいじゃくせいこっせつ）	insufficiency fracture
病的骨折（びょうてきこっせつ）	pathologic fracture, secondary fracture
若木骨折（わかぎこっせつ）	greenstick fracture
コレス骨折（―こっせつ）	Colles fracture

⟨fracture of the lower end of the radius with dorsal displacement of the distal fragment⟩

スミス骨折（―こっせつ）　　　Smith fracture

⟨reverse Colles fracture; fracture of the lower end of the radius with volar displacement of the distal fragment⟩

ポット骨折（―こっせつ）　　　Pott fracture

⟨spiral fracture of the distal fibula and of the malleolus of the tibia⟩

モンテジア骨折（―こっせつ）　Monteggia fracture

⟨fracture of the ulna with dislocation of the head of radius⟩

大腿骨頚部骨折（だいたいこつけいぶこっせつ）	femoral neck fracture
偽関節（ぎかんせつ）	false joint, pseudoarthrosis, pseudarthrosis
骨再造形（こつさいぞうけい）	bone remodeling
ルドロフ徴候（―ちょうこう）	Ludloff sign

⟨swelling and ecchymosis in the femoral triangle and inability to raise the thigh in a sitting position; seen in avulsion of the greater trochanter⟩

絞扼性ニューロパチー（こうやくせい―）　entrapment neuropathy

ファレン試験（―けん）　　　Phalen test

⟨a test for carpal tunnel syndrome; press the back of both hands with the wrists in acute flexion; positive if numbness and tingling occur⟩

アドソン試験（―けん）　　　Adson test

⟨a test for thoracic outlet syndrome; positive if radial pulse is obliterated when the head is turned toward the affected side during inhalation⟩

切断四肢重症度スコア（せつだんししじゅうしょうど―）　mangled extremity severity score (MESS)

●検査法 Examination●

クレアチンキナーゼ	creatine kinase (CK)
アルドラーゼ	aldolase
乳酸デヒドロゲナーゼ	lactate dehydrogenase (LDH)
ミオグロビン	myoglobin
リウマトイド因子	rheumatoid factor (RF)
抗核抗体	antinuclear antibody (ANA)
関節リウマチ赤血球凝集試験	rheumatoid arthritis hemagglutination test (RAHA)
抗ガラクトース欠損 IgG 抗体	anti-agalactosyl IgG antibody
マトリックスメタロプロテイナーゼ3	matrix metalloproteinase-3 (MMP-3)
抗環状シトルリン化ペプチド抗体	anti-cyclic citrullinated peptide (CCP) antibody
抗 Jo-1 抗体	anti-Jo-1 antibody
抗 Ku 抗体	anti-Ku antibody
抗ストレプトリジン O	antistreptolysin O (ASO)
骨型アルカリホスファターゼ	bone-specific alkaline phosphatase
オステオカルシン	osteocalcin
ヒドロキシプロリン	hydroxyproline (Hyp)
筋力計	dynamometer
握力計	grip dynamometer, squeeze dynamometer
角度計	goniometer, arthrometer
筋電図	electromyogram (EMG)
表面電極	surface electrode
針電極	needle electrode
単一筋線維筋電図	single fiber electromyogram (SFEMG)
神経筋単位	neuromuscular unit (NMU)
誘発筋電図	evoked electromyogram
神経伝導速度	nerve conduction velocity
骨密度検査	bone densitometry
若年成人平均値	young adult mean (YAM)
二重エネルギーX線吸収法	dual-energy x-ray absorptiometry (DEXA)
定量的 CT	quantitative computed tomography (QCT)

骨減少	osteopenia
関節穿刺	arthrocentesis
滑液分析	synovial fluid analysis
偏光顕微鏡検査	polarizing microscopy
尿酸結晶	urate crystal
痛風結晶	monosodium urate monohydrate (MSUM)
ピロリン酸カルシウム	calcium pyrophosphate dihydrate (CPPD)
塩基性リン酸カルシウム	basic calcium phosphate (BCP)
単純写真	plain films
骨棘	osteophyte
靱帯骨棘形成	syndesmophyte
腰椎化	lumbarization
仙椎化	sacralization
シュモール結節	Schmorl nodule

⟨a defect in the vertebral endplate due to prolapse of the nucleus pulposus⟩

楔状椎	wedging vertebra
関節裂隙狭細	joint space narrowing
ヒル・サックス病変	Hill-Sachs lesion

⟨an indentation of the humeral head after anterior dislocation of the shoulder; caused by impaction of the humeral head on the anterior edge of the glenoid fossa⟩

腐骨	sequestrum
腐骨形成	sequestration
関節造影法	arthrography
脊髄造影法	myelography
椎間板造影法	diskography
骨シンチグラフィー	bone scintigraphy
関節鏡検査	arthroscopy
筋生検	muscle biopsy
骨生検	bone biopsy

● 疾患名　Diseases ●

肩関節周囲炎	scapulohumeral periarthritis
肩腱板損傷	rotator cuff injury
インピンジメント症候群	impingement syndrome
胸郭出口症候群	thoracic outlet syndrome (TOS)

13. 筋・骨格系

頚腕症候群 けいわんしょうこうぐん	cervicobrachial syndrome, brachial plexopathy
肘部管症候群 ちゅうぶかんしょうこうぐん	cubital tunnel syndrome
手根管症候群 しゅこんかんしょうこうぐん	carpal tunnel syndrome (CTS)
むち打ち損傷関連障害 うーそんしょうかんれんしょうがい	whiplash-associated disorders (WAD)
バレー・リエウ症候群	Barré-Liéou syndrome

⟨*posterior cervical sympathetic syndrome; arthritis of the 3rd and 4th cervical disks with the 5th to 8th CN irritation resulting in headache, eye pain, tinnitus, vertigo, and vasomotor disturbance of the face*⟩

反復運動過多損傷 はんぷくうんどうかたそんしょう	repetitive strain (stress) injury (RSI)
絞扼性ニューロパチー こうやくせい──	entrapment neuropathy
モートン病 ─びょう	Morton disease

⟨*Morton metatarsalgia; neuralgia of the foot caused by compression of the interdigital nerve by the metatarsophalangeal joint*⟩

筋炎 きんえん	myositis
多発性筋炎 たはつせいきんえん	polymyositis (PM)
骨化性筋炎 こつかせいきんえん	myositis ossificans
封入体筋炎 ふうにゅうたいきんえん	inclusion body myositis (IBM)
横紋筋融解症 おうもんきんゆうかいしょう	rhabdomyolysis
好酸球性筋膜炎, シュルマン症候群 こうさんきゅうせいきんまくえん, ──しょうこうぐん	eosinophilic fasciitis, Shulman syndrome

⟨*inflammation and thickening of the skin and fascia after physical exertion, associated with eosinophilia and hypergammaglobulinemia*⟩

腱鞘炎 けんしょうえん	tenosynovitis, tendovaginitis
滑液包炎 かつえきほうえん	bursitis
キーンベック病 ─びょう	Kienböck disease

⟨*lunatomalacia; avascular necrosis of the lunate bone in the wrist*⟩

ばね指 ─ゆび	snapping finger, trigger finger
ドケルバン病 ─びょう	de Quervain disease

⟨*painful tenosynovitis of thumb extensors*⟩

槌指 つちゆび	mallet finger
ガングリオン	ganglion
アキレス腱断裂 ─けんだんれつ	Achilles tendon rupture
斜頚 しゃけい	torticollis, wryneck
骨関節炎 こつかんせつえん	osteoarthritis (OA)
変形性関節症 へんけいせいかんせつしょう	osteoarthrosis deformans, degenerative arthritis (DA)
変形性股関節症 へんけいせいこかんせつしょう	coxarthrosis, hip osteoarthritis

変形性膝関節症	gonarthrosis, knee osteoarthritis
骨パジェット病 〈*osteitis deformans*〉	Paget disease of bone
関節リウマチ	rheumatoid arthritis (RA)
フェルティー症候群 〈*rheumatoid arthritis with splenomegaly and leukopenia*〉	Felty syndrome
スティル病 〈*juvenile rheumatoid arthritis characterized by high fever and systemic signs before the onset of arthritis*〉	Still disease
リウマチ性多発筋痛症	polymyalgia rheumatica (PMR)
線維筋痛症	fibromyalgia (FM)
好酸球増多・筋痛症候群	eosinophilia-myalgia syndrome (EMS)
痛風性関節炎	gouty arthritis
足部痛風	podagra
偽痛風	pseudogout
結晶性関節炎	crystal-induced arthritis
感染性関節炎	infectious arthritis
化膿性関節炎	suppurative arthritis, pyogenic arthritis, septic arthritis
淋菌性関節炎	gonococcal arthritis, gonorrheal arthritis
乾癬性関節炎	psoriatic arthritis
血友病関節炎	hemophilic arthritis
反応性関節炎	reactive arthritis
ライター症候群 〈*urethritis, conjunctivitis, mucocutaneous lesions, and aseptic arthritis; seen in young men with increased levels of HLA-B27*〉	Reiter syndrome
膝関節炎	gonitis
仙腸骨炎	sacroiliitis
膝内障	internal derangement of the knee joint (IDK)
離断性骨軟骨炎	osteochondritis dissecans (OCD)
色素性絨毛結節性滑膜炎	pigmented villonodular synovitis (PVS)
特発性大腿骨頭壊死症	idiopathic osteonecrosis of the femoral head
骨軟骨症	osteochondrosis, epiphysial ischemic necrosis
レッグ・カルベ・ペルテ	Legg-Calvé-Perthes disease (LCP)

ス病 ―びょう
⟨aseptic osteonecrosis of the proximal femoral capital epiphysis in children; osteochondritis deformans juvenilis⟩

オスグッド・シュラッタ ―病 ―びょう Osgood-Schlatter disease
⟨osteochondrosis of the tuberosity of the tibia⟩

ブラウント病 ―びょう Blount disease
⟨aseptic necrosis of the medial tibial condyle; can cause bowlegs⟩

ショイエルマン病 ―びょう Scheuermann disease
⟨juvenile kyphosis; osteochondrosis of vertebral epiphysis⟩

大腿骨頭すべり症 だいたいこっとう―しょう slipped capital femoral epiphysis (SCFE)

先天性股関節脱臼 せんてんせいこかんせつだっきゅう congenital dislocation of the hip (CDH), luxatio coxae congenita (LCC)

環軸関節脱臼 かんじくかんせつだっきゅう atlantoaxial dislocation (AAD)

環軸関節亜脱臼 かんじくかんせつあだっきゅう atlantoaxial sublaxation (AAS)

強直性脊椎炎 きょうちょくせいせきついえん, マリー・シュトリュンペル病 ―びょう ankylosing spondylitis (AS), Marie-Strümpell disease

結核性脊椎炎 けっかくせいせきついえん, ポット病 ―びょう tuberculous spondylitis, Pott disease

化膿性脊椎炎 かのうせいせきついえん pyogenic spondylitis

強直性脊椎骨増殖症 きょうちょくせいせきついこつぞうしょくしょう, フォレスティエ病 ―びょう ankylosing spinal hyperostosis (ASH), Forestier disease
⟨hypertrophy of the anterolateral vertebral column, resulting in ankylosis; seen in the elderly⟩

散在性特発性骨増殖症 さんざいせいとくはつせいこつぞうしょくしょう diffuse idiopathic skeletal hyperostosis (DISH)

頚椎症性脊髄症 けいついしょうせいせきずいしょう cervical spondylotic myelopathy (CSM)

頚椎症性神経根症 けいついしょうせいしんけいこんしょう cervical spondylotic radiculopathy (CSR)

後縦靭帯骨化症 こうじゅうじんたいこっかしょう ossification of posterior longitudinal ligament (OPLL)

前縦靭帯骨化症 ぜんじゅうじんたいこっかしょう ossification of anterior longitudinal ligament (OALL)

黄色靭帯骨化症 おうしょくじんたいこっかしょう ossification of yellow ligament (OYL), ossification of ligamentum flavum (OLF)

椎間板ヘルニア ついかんばん― herniated intervertebral disk, herniated nucleus pulposus (HNP)

脊柱管狭窄症	spinal canal stenosis
腰部脊柱管狭窄症	lumbar spinal canal stenosis (LSCS)
脊椎すべり症	spondylolisthesis
脊椎分離症	spondylolysis
脊椎分離すべり症	spondylolytic spondylolisthesis
変形性脊椎症	spondylosis deformans
脊髄損傷	spinal cord injury (SCI)
骨粗鬆症	osteoporosis
骨軟化症	osteomalacia (OM)
骨形成不全症	osteogenesis imperfecta (OI)
馬尾腫瘍	cauda equina tumor
巨細胞腫	giant cell tumor (GCT)
動脈瘤性骨嚢胞	aneurysmal bone cyst (ABC)
横紋筋肉腫	rhabdomyosarcoma
骨肉腫	osteosarcoma
ユーイング肉腫	Ewing sarcoma

⟨*a highly malignant tumor of bones of the extremities, usually occurring in children or adolescents*⟩

| 内軟骨腫症 | enchondromatosis |
| オリエ病 | Ollier disease |

⟨*unilateral enchondromatosis; hamartomatous proliferation of cartilage in the metaphyses of bones of the hands and feet; chondrosarcoma may develop*⟩

| 軟骨肉腫 | chondrosarcoma |

● 治療法　Treatment ●

アセチルサリチル酸	acetylsalicylic acid (ASA)
非ステロイド系抗炎症薬	nonsteroidal antiinflammatory drug (NSAID)
金製剤	gold salts
病態修飾性抗リウマチ薬	disease-modifying antirheumatic drug (DMARD)
サラゾスルファピリジン	salazosulfapyridine (SASP)《アザルフィジン EN》
ブシラミン	bucillamine《リマチル》
メトトレキセート	methotrexate (MTX)《リウマトレックス》
タクロリムス水和物	tacrolimus hydrate《プログラフ》
レフルノミド	leflunomide《アラバ》
エタネルセプト	etanercept《エンブレル》

インフリキシマブ	infliximab (IFX)《レミケード》
トシリズマブ	tocilizumab《アクテムラ》
アダリムマブ	adalimumab《ヒュミラ》
筋弛緩薬	muscle relaxant
ヒアルロン酸ナトリウム	hyaluronate sodium《アルツ》
ビスホスフォネート	bisphosphonate (BP)
アレンドロン酸ナトリウム水和物	alendronate sodium hydrate《フォサマック》
ミノドロン酸水和物	minodronic acid hydrate《ボノテオ》
選択的エストロゲン受容体修飾薬	selective estrogen receptor modulator (SERM)
ラロキシフェン塩酸塩	raloxifene hydrochloride《エビスタ》
ビタミンD	vitamin D《アルファロール》
カルシトニン	calcitonin《エルシトニン》
安静, 氷冷, 圧迫, 挙上	rest, ice, compression, elevation (RICE)
マッサージ	massage
脊柱指圧療法	chiropractic
圧迫包帯	compress
温パック	hot pack
氷パック	ice pack
冷罨法	cold compress
パラフィン浴	paraffin bath
水治療法	hydrotherapy
灌注法	douche
徒手整復	manipulation, manipulative reduction
非観血的整復	closed reduction
テーピング法	taping
吊り包帯, 三角巾	sling
ギプス固定法	casting
体幹ギプス	body cast
吊り下げギプス包帯	hanging arm cast
下敷きギプス包帯	padded cast
無褥ギプス包帯	unpadded cast
長下肢ギプス包帯	long leg cast
短下肢ギプス包帯	short leg cast
装具	orthosis
機能装具	functional orthosis, functional brace

13. 筋・骨格系　289

IV章

短下肢装具 たんかしそうぐ	ankle-foot orthosis (AFO), short leg brace (SLB)
長下肢装具 ちょうかしそうぐ	knee-ankle-foot orthosis (KAFO), long leg brace (LLB)
膝蓋腱支持 しつがいけんしじ	patellar tendon bearing (PTB)
頚椎装具 けいついそうぐ	cervical orthosis, neck brace
胸骨・後頭骨・下顎骨固定用装具 きょうこつ・こうとうこつ・かがくこつこていようそうぐ	sternal-occipital-mandibular immobilizer (SOMI)
腰仙椎装具 ようせんついそうぐ	lumbosacral orthosis (LSO)
手関節指装具 しゅかんせつしそうぐ	wrist-hand orthosis (WHO)
ショックパンツ	military antichock trousers (MAST), pneumatic antichock garment (PASG)
双面副子 そうめんふくし	coaptation splint
動的副子 どうてきふくし	dynamic splint
手関節背屈副子 しゅかんせつはいくつふくし	wrist cock-up splint
顎間固定法 がくかんこていほう	intermaxillary fixation (IMF)
歩行器 ほこうき	walker
運動療法 うんどうりょうほう	therapeutic exercise, corrective exercise
受動運動 じゅどううんどう	passive exercise
持続的他動運動 じぞくてきたどううんどう	continuous passive motion (CPM)
自発的運動練習 じはつてきうんどうれんしゅう	active exercise
関節可動域訓練 かんせつかどういきくんれん	range of motion exercise
等尺性運動 とうしゃくせいうんどう	isometric exercise, static exercise
等張性運動 とうちょうせいうんどう	isotonic exercise
等速性運動 とうそくせいうんどう	isokinetic exercise
伸縮反復筋力増強法 しんしゅくはんぷくきんりょくぞうきょうほう	plyometrics
漸増抵抗運動 ぜんぞうていこううんどう	progressive resistance (resistive) exercise (PRE)
固有受容体神経筋促進法 こゆうじゅようたいしんけいきんそくしんほう	proprioceptive neuromuscular facilitation (PNF)
水中運動 すいちゅううんどう	underwater exercise
ハバードタンク	Hubbard tank

⟨*a large tank filled with warm water used for underwater exercise*⟩

腰痛体操 ようつうたいそう	low back exercise
コドマン体操 —たいそう	Codman exercise

⟨*stooping exercise to increase range of motion in frozen shoulder; with knees extended the body bent forward, and the affected arm passively swung like a pendulum*⟩

| 牽引療法 けんいんりょうほう | traction therapy |

13. 筋・骨格系

頭蓋牽引 とうがいけんいん	skull traction
頸椎牽引 けいついけんいん	cervical traction
頭蓋輪骨盤牽引 とうがいりんこつばんけんいん	halo-pelvic traction
腰椎牽引 ようついけんいん	lumbar traction
骨直達牽引 こつちょくたつけんいん	skeletal traction
皮膚介達牽引 ひふかいたつけんいん	skin traction
懸垂牽引 けんすいけんいん	suspended traction
持続牽引 じぞくけんいん	continuous traction
機能的電気刺激 きのうてきでんきしげき	functional electrical stimulation (FES)
経皮的髄核摘出術 けいひてきずいかくてきしゅつじゅつ	percutaneous nucleotomy (PN)
観血的整復 かんけつてきせいふく	open reduction
観血的整復内固定術 かんけつてきせいふくないこていじゅつ	open reduction and internal fixation (ORIF)
骨切り術 こつきりじゅつ	osteotomy
骨接合術 こつせつごうじゅつ	osteosynthesis
骨延長術 こつえんちょうじゅつ	bone elongation
髄内釘固定法 ずいないていこていほう	intramedullary nailing
開窓術 かいそうじゅつ	fenestration
椎弓切除術 ついきゅうせつじょじゅつ	laminectomy
部分的椎弓切除術 ぶぶんてきついきゅうせつじょじゅつ	laminotomy
椎弓形成術 ついきゅうけいせいじゅつ	laminoplasty
椎間板切除術 ついかんばんせつじょじゅつ	diskectomy
脊椎固定術 せきついこていじゅつ	spinal fusion, spondylodesis
前方椎体間固定術 ぜんぽうついたいかんこていじゅつ	anterior interbody fusion (AIF)
後方進入腰椎椎体間固定術 こうほうしんにゅうようついついたいかんこていじゅつ	posterior lumbar interbody fusion (PLIF)
滑膜切除術 かつまくせつじょじゅつ	synovectomy
腱鞘滑膜切除術 けんしょうかつまくせつじょじゅつ	tenosynovectomy
関節半月板切除術 かんせつはんげつばんせつじょじゅつ	meniscectomy
関節固定術 かんせつこていじゅつ	arthrodesis
関節形成術 かんせつけいせいじゅつ	arthroplasty
関節置換術 かんせつちかんじゅつ	replacement arthroplasty, joint replacement
股関節全置換術 こかんせつぜんちかんじゅつ	total hip arthroplasty (THA), total hip replacement (THR)
膝関節全置換術 しつかんせつぜんちかんじゅつ	total knee arthroplasty (TKA), total knee replacement (TKR)

IV章 診療録用語

肘関節全置換術 <small>ちゅうかんせつぜんちかんじゅつ</small>	total elbow arthroplasty, total elbow replacement
中間物挿入関節形成術 <small>ちゅうかんぶつそうにゅうかんせつけいせいじゅつ</small>	interposition arthroplasty
ガードルストーン手術	Girdlestone operation

⟨removal of the femoral head and neck for severe hip infections⟩

人工関節 <small>じんこうかんせつ</small>	artificial joint
臼蓋形成術 <small>きゅうがいけいせいじゅつ</small>	shelf operation
高位脛骨骨切り術 <small>こういけいこつこつきり——じゅつ</small>	high tibial osteotomy (HTO)
切断術 <small>せつだん</small>	amputation
上腕切断術 <small>じょうわんせつだんじゅつ</small>	above-elbow (A-E) amputation, trans-humeral amputation
大腿切断術 <small>だいたいせつだんじゅつ</small>	above-knee (A-K) amputation, transfemoral amputation
前腕切断術 <small>ぜんわんせつだんじゅつ</small>	below-elbow (B-E) amputation, transradial amputation
下腿切断術 <small>かたいせつだんじゅつ</small>	below-knee (B-K) amputation, transtibial amputation
サイム切断術 <small>——せつだんじゅつ</small>	Syme amputation

⟨ankle disarticulation with removal of both malleoli⟩

骨移植 <small>こついしょく</small>	bone grafting, bone transplantation

---

─ Tidbits ─

regimen

「レジメン」とは,"a strictly regulated schedule of diet, exercise, medication, or lifestyle designed to improve the health of a patient"であり,食事,運動,生活様式などの規制による摂生,養生法を意味し,投薬計画も含まれる.ラテン語の regere (=rule) に由来し「統治,管理」の意味がある.紛らわしい綴りに regime (政体,政権) と regiment (連隊) があり,regime というと西洋史で学んだアンシャンレジーム l'Ancient Régime (フランス革命前の政体) が思い出される.養生法の意味では regimen が正しいが,しばしば regime も用いられている.

14. 精神・神経系

●愁訴・症状 Complaints / Symptoms●

神経系 しんけいけい	nervous system
精神 せいしん	mind, psyche, 〔形〕psychic
意識 いしき	consciousness, awareness
意識のある（ない） いしき—	conscious (unconscious)
意識混濁 いしきこんだく	clouding of consciousness
意識不明 いしきふめい	loss of consciousness, unconsciousness
意識を失う いしき—, 失神する しっしん	lose consciousness, become unconscious, faint, swoon
失神 しっしん, 気絶 きぜつ	fainting, syncope, 〔形〕syncopal, syncopic
意識が明瞭である いしき—めいりょう—	have a clear consciousness
意識がもうろうとしている いしき—	have an indistinct (a dim) consciousness
意識を回復する いしき—かいふく—	recover (regain) consciousness
めまい	dizziness, vertigo, light-headedness, 〔形〕dizzy, vertiginous
めまいがする	feel dizzy, have a dizzy spell, feel the room spin, have a swimming head
立ちくらみする た—	feel dizzy on standing up
幻覚 げんかく	hallucination
幻聴 げんちょう	auditory hallucination
幻覚を感じる げんかく—かん—	hallucinate, have hallucinations
既視感 きしかん	déjà vue
妄想 もうそう	delusion
妄想を抱く もうそう—いだ—	fall into a delusion, nurse delusions, be under a delusion (that ~)
被害（誇大）妄想にとりつかれる ひがい（こだい）もうそう—	be obsessed by delusions of persecution (grandeur)
痙攣 けいれん	convulsion, cramp, spasm, 〔形〕convulsive, spasmodic
痙攣を起こす（全身） けいれん—お—（ぜんしん）	have a convulsive fit, go into convulsions
痙攣を起こす（脚） けいれん—お—（あし）	get a cramp in the leg (calf)
書痙 しょけい	writer's cramp
てんかん	epilepsy, 〔形〕epileptic
てんかん発作 —ほっさ	an epileptic seizure (attack), a seizure

前兆（ぜんちょう）	aura
てんかん患者（かんじゃ）	an epileptic
麻痺（まひ）	paralysis,〔動〕be paralyzed
しびれ感（かん）	numbness,〔動〕be numbed
小児麻痺（しょうにまひ）	infantile paralysis
顔面神経麻痺（がんめんしんけいまひ）	facial paralysis
半身不随（はんしんふずい）	hemiplegia
半身不随になる（はんしんふずい――）	be paralyzed on one side, become hemiplegic
脳卒中（のうそっちゅう）	apoplexy, stroke
一過性脳卒中（いっかせいのうそっちゅう）	transient ischemic attack, ministroke
ふるえ	tremor, trembling,〔動〕tremble, shake
不随意運動（ふずいいうんどう）	involuntary motion, involuntary movement
歩行困難（ほこうこんなん）	gait disturbance, difficulty in walking
歩行が困難である（ほこう――こんなん――）	have difficulty in walking, find it hard to walk
跛行する（はこう――）	limp, walk with a limp, hobble (along)
歩幅が広い（狭い）（ほはば――ひろ――（せま――））	walk with long (short) steps
よろめく	stagger, reel, falter
よたよた歩く（――あ――）	walk with unsteady (waddling) steps
千鳥足で歩く（ちどりあし――ある――）	walk zigzag, walk with an unsteady gait (with faltering steps), reel along
つまずく	stumble
石につまずいて転ぶ（いし――ころ――）	stumble over a stone
すり足で歩く（――あし――――）	shuffle (along), slide one's feet (along)
言語障害（げんごしょうがい）	disturbance of speech
発語困難（はつごこんなん）	difficulty in speech
舌がもつれる（した）	speak thickly, have a thick voice, be inarticulate
どもる	stammer, stutter
神経痛（しんけいつう）	neuralgia
神経因性疼痛（しんけいいんせいとうつう）	neuropathic pain
視床痛（ししょうつう）	thalamic pain
異痛（いつう）	allodynia
麻痺性疼痛（まひせいとうつう）	anesthesia dolorosa
筋萎縮（きんいしゅく）	atrophy of muscle
右利き（みぎき）	right-handedness,〔形〕right-handed
左利き（ひだりき）	left-handedness,〔形〕left-handed
知覚消失（ちかくしょうしつ）	loss of sensation, numbness, anesthesia

14. 精神・神経系

感覚を失う（かんかくを―）, しびれる	become numb (senseless, insensible), be benumbed, go to sleep, lose sensibility
じんじんする	tingle, 〔名〕tingle, tingling, a tingling sensation
かじかむ	be numbed with cold
足がしびれる（あし―）	one's legs are asleep (go to sleep)
記憶（きおく）	memory, remembrance
記憶力減退（きおくりょくげんたい）	memory loss
記憶する（きおく―）	remember, memorize
記憶が良い（きおく―）	have a good (strong) memory
記憶が悪い（きおく―）, 忘れっぽい（わす―）	have a poor (bad) memory, be forgetful
物忘れ（ものわす―）	forgetfulness, 〔動〕forget
健忘（けんぼう）	amnesia
もうろくした	senile, in one's dotage
認知症（にんちしょう）, 痴呆（ちほう）	dementia
老年痴呆（ろうねんちほう）	senile dementia
認知症の行動・心理症状（にんちしょう―こうどう・しんりしょうじょう）	behavioral and psychological symptoms of dementia (BPSD)
性格（せいかく）	character, personality
気分（きぶん）	mood, feeling
気質（きしつ）, 気性（きしょう）	temperament, temper
神経質（しんけいしつ）	nervousness
神経質の（しんけいしつ―）, 神経過敏の（しんけいかびん―）, 怒りっぽい（おこ―）	nervous, sensitive, touchy
神経衰弱（しんけいすいじゃく）	nervous breakdown (exhaustion)
意気消沈した（いきしょうちん―）	depressed, in low spirits
憂うつな（ゆう―）	gloomy, melancholic, depressive
うつ状態（―じょうたい）	a state of depression
緊張した（きんちょう―）	tense
気分（きぶん）	mood, feeling
不安（ふあん）	anxiety, 〔形〕anxious, apprehensive, uneasy
情動不安（じょうどうふあん）	restlessness, 〔形〕restless
情緒不安定（じょうちょふあんてい）	emotional lability, emotional instability
機嫌の良い（きげん―）	in good mood, cheerful, euphoric
気分の変わり易い（きぶん―か―やす―）	unstable, labile, capricious
興奮し易い（こうふん―やす―）	excitable, easily excited, irritable
無関心の（むかんしん―）	indifferent, nonchalant, unconcerned

Ⅳ章 診療録用語

恐怖症 きょうふしょう	phobia, [形]phobic
自閉症 じへいしょう	autism, [形]autistic
アルコール依存 ぜん	alcohol dependence
アルコール依存症 いぞんしょう	alcoholism
性欲過剰 せいよくかじょう	hypersexuality, [形]hypersexual
内向性の人 ないこうせいひと	introvert
外向性の人 がいこうせいひと	extrovert
社交的な しゃこう	sociable, [名]sociability
劣等感 れっとうかん	inferiority complex, a feeling of inferiority
ヒステリー	hysteria, [形]hysterical
自殺念慮 じさつねんりょ	suicidal thought, suicidal ideation
自殺企図 じさつきと	suicide attempt
自殺行為 じさつこうい	suicidal behavior
自殺未遂 じさつみすい	attempted suicide

● 恐怖症　Phobias ●

悪魔恐怖症 あくまきょうふしょう	demonophobia, satanophobia
異性恐怖症 いせい	genophobia
犬恐怖症 いぬ	cynophobia
汚物恐怖症 おぶつ	mysophobia
癌恐怖症 がん	cancerophobia, cancerphobia
恐糞症 きょうふんしょう	coprophobia
魚類恐怖症 ぎょるい	ichthyophobia
くも恐怖症	arachnephobia, arachnophobia
暗闇恐怖症 くらやみ	nyctophobia
群集恐怖症 ぐんしゅう	demophobia, ochlophobia
結婚恐怖症 けっこん	gamophobia
嫌気症 けんきしょう	aerophobia
高所恐怖症 こうしょ	acrophobia
孤独恐怖症 こどく	monophobia
昆虫恐怖症 こんちゅう	entomophobia
細菌恐怖症 さいきん	bacteriophobia
自己恐怖症 じこ	autophobia
死体恐怖症 したい	necrophobia
失敗恐怖症 しっぱい	hamartophobia
疾病恐怖症 しっぺい	nosophobia, pathophobia
食物恐怖症 しょくもつ	cibophobia, phagophobia
女性恐怖症 じょせい	gynephobia, gynophobia
赤面恐怖症 せきめん	erythrophobia
他人恐怖症 たにん	xenophobia
男性恐怖症 だんせい	androphobia

動物恐怖症 どうぶつ	zoophobia
猫恐怖症 ねこ	ailurophobia, galeophobia
乗物恐怖症 のりもの	amaxophobia
針恐怖症 はり	belonephobia
火恐怖症 ひ	pyrophobia
微小物恐怖症 びしょうぶつ	microphobia
広場恐怖症 ひろば	agoraphobia
閉所恐怖症 へいしょ	claustrophobia
蛇恐怖症 へび	ophidiophobia
夜間恐怖症 やかん	noctiphobia
雷鳴恐怖症 らいめい	brontophobia
裸体恐怖症 らたい	gymnophobia, nudophobia

● 診察所見・徴候　Physical findings / Signs ●

意識レベル いしき	level of consciousness
昏睡 こんすい	coma, 〔形〕comatose
昏迷 こんめい	stupor, 〔形〕stuporous
傾眠 けいみん	somnolence, sleepiness, drowsiness, 〔形〕somnolent, sleepy, drowsy
嗜眠 しみん	lethargy, 〔形〕lethargic
錯乱 さくらん	confusion, distraction, 〔形〕confused, distracted, distraught
発作後錯乱 ほっさごさくらん	postictal confusion
せん妄 もう	delirium, 〔形〕delirious
焦点性てんかん しょうてんせい	focal epilepsy
全般てんかん ぜんぱん	generalized epilepsy
大発作てんかん だいほっさ	grand mal epilepsy
ジャクソン型てんかん がた	jacksonian epilepsy

⟨<John Hughlings Jackson; focal motor seizures with unilateral clonic movements, usually without loss of consciousness; secondary to motor area lesion⟩

小発作てんかん しょうほっさ	petit mal epilepsy
欠神てんかん けっしん	absence epilepsy
複雑部分発作 ふくざつぶぶんほっさ	complex partial seizure (CPS)
トッド麻痺 まひ	Todd paralysis

⟨postepileptic paralysis; temporary paralysis of the limb involved in jacksonian epilepsy⟩

植物状態 しょくぶつじょうたい	vegetative state
脳死 のうし	brain death
日本式昏睡尺度 にほんしきこんすいしゃくど	Japan Coma Scale (JCS)
グラスゴー昏睡尺度 こんすいしゃくど	Glasgow Coma Scale (GCS)

298　Ⅳ章　診療録用語

NIH 脳卒中尺度	NIH Stroke Scale (NIHSS)
脳卒中障害評価法	Stroke Impairment Assessment Set (SIAS)
除脳硬直	decerebrate rigidity
ケルニヒ徴候	Kernig sign

⟨straightening knee with the thigh flexed causes pain in the lower back and posterior thigh; suggestive of meningeal irritation⟩

ブルジンスキー徴候	Brudzinsky sign

⟨neck flexion causes involuntary hip flexion, seen in meningitis⟩

クッシング三主徴	Cushing triad

⟨bradycardia, hypertension, and irregular respiration seen in increased intracranial pressure⟩

レルミット徴候	Lhermitte sign

⟨sudden transient electric-like shocks spreading down the body with neck flexion; seen in multiple sclerosis and cervical cord compression⟩

シャルコー三主徴	Charcot triad

⟨nystagmus, intention tremor, and staccato speech; associated with multiple sclerosis⟩

正座不能	akathisia, acathisia
鶏歩	steppage gait, drop-foot gait
運動失調性歩行	ataxic gait
痙性歩行	spastic gait
片麻痺歩行	hemiplegic gait
跛行	limp, limping
つぎ足歩行	tandem gait
はさみ脚歩行	scissors gait
ひきずり歩行	shuffling gait
動揺歩行	swaying gait, cerebellar gait
加速歩行	festinating gait, festination
猿手	ape hand
鷲手	clawhand, main en griffe
助産師手位	obstetrician's hand
下垂手	wristdrop, drop hand
項部固縮	nuchal rigidity
眼球沈下運動	ocular bobbing
人形の目徴候	doll's eye sign
カフェオレ斑点	café-au-lait spot
麻痺	paralysis, palsy, 〔形〕paralytic
不全麻痺	paresis, 〔形〕paretic
痙性麻痺	spastic paralysis
弛緩性麻痺	flaccid paralysis

14. 精神・神経系

単麻痺 たんまひ	monoplegia
片麻痺 へんまひ	hemiplegia, 〔形〕hemiplegic
同側片麻痺 どうそくへんまひ	ipsilateral hemiplegia
対側片麻痺 たいそくへんまひ	contralateral hemiplegia
交代性片麻痺 こうたいせいへんまひ	alternating hemiplegia
ミラール・ギュブレ症候群 こうこうぐん	Millard-Gubler syndrome

⟨alternating hemiplegia; contralateral hemiplegia, ipsilateral facial palsy, and ipsilateral abducens palsy⟩

フォヴィーユ症候群　　Foville syndrome

⟨similar to the Millard-Gubler syndrome; there is paralysis of conjugate eye movement in addition⟩

ウェーバー症候群 こうこうぐん　Weber syndrome

⟨ipsilateral oculomotor nerve paresis with contralateral hemiplegia due to midbrain tegmentum lesion; syn. alternating oculomotor hemiplegia⟩

ベネディクト症候群　　Benedikt syndrome

⟨ipsilateral oculomotor paralysis and contralateral hemiparesis with hyperkinesia and tremor; the nucleus ruber and corticospinal tract involved⟩

両麻痺 りょうまひ	diplegia
対麻痺 ついまひ	paraplegia, 〔形〕paraplegic
四肢麻痺 ししまひ	quadriplegia
ベル麻痺 まひ	Bell palsy

⟨unilateral facial paralysis due to lesion of the facial nerve⟩

ハント症候群 こうこうぐん　Hunt syndrome

⟨Ramsay Hunt syndrome; facial paralysis, otalgia, and vesicles of the external ear resulting from herpes zoster infection of the facial nerve and geniculate ganglion⟩

ブラウン-セカール症候群 こうこうぐん　Brown-Séquard syndrome

⟨unilateral spinal cord lesions, resulting in ipsilateral paralysis and vibration loss, and contralateral loss of pain and temperature sensation⟩

ガワース徴候 ちょうこう　Gowers sign

⟨a sign of pseudohypertrophic muscular dystrophy with pelvic girdle weakness; to rise from supine position, the patient first rolls onto side, kneels, and then pushes up with hands against shins, knees, and thighs⟩

運動緩慢 うんどうかんまん	bradykinesia
運動失調 うんどうしっちょう	ataxia, 〔形〕ataxic, atactic
錐体外路症候群 すいたいがいろしょうこうぐん	extrapyramidal syndrome (EPS)
舞踏病 ぶとうびょう	chorea, 〔形〕choreic
アテトーシス	athetosis

300　IV章　診療録用語

舞踏アテトーシス ぶとう	choreoathetosis
舞踏病性歩行不能 ぶとうびょうせいほこうふのう	choreic abasia
バリズム	ballism, ballismus
片側バリズム へんそく	hemiballism
チック	tic
ミオクローヌス	myoclonus
失行 しっこう	apraxia, 〔形〕apractic, apraxic
反響言語 はんきょうげんご	echolalia
同語反復 どうごはんぷく	palilalia
汚言 おげん	coprolalia
ロンベルグ試験 ——しけん	Romberg test

　〈swaying of the body when standing with feet together and eyes closed indicates bathyanesthesia; for differentiating peripheral ataxia from cerebellar ataxia〉

協調運動障害 きょうちょううんどうしょうがい	incoordination
指鼻試験 ゆびはなしけん	finger-nose test, finger-to-nose test
踵膝試験 しゅうしつしけん	heel-knee test, heel-to-knee test
反復拮抗運動不能 はんぷくきっこううんどうふのう	adiadochokinesis
ホームズ現象 ——げんしょう	Holmes phenomenon

　〈rebound phenomenon; loss of coordination between antagonistic muscles in cerebellar disease; on sudden removal of passive resistance the arm jerks back〉

反射 はんしゃ	reflex
腱反射 けんはんしゃ	tendon reflex
深部腱反射 しんぶけんはんしゃ	deep tendon reflex (DTR)
二頭筋反射 にとうきんはんしゃ	biceps reflex
三頭筋反射 さんとうきんはんしゃ	triceps reflex
腕橈骨筋反射 わんとうこつきんはんしゃ	brachioradialis reflex
膝蓋腱反射 しつがいけんはんしゃ	patellar tendon reflex (PTR), patellar reflex, knee jerk (KJ), quadriceps reflex
アキレス腱反射 ——けんはんしゃ	Achilles tendon reflex (ATR), Achilles reflex, ankle jerk (AJ), triceps surae reflex
イエンドラシック操作 ——そうさ	Jendrassik maneuver

　〈a method of emphasizing the patellar reflex〉

クローヌス，間代 かんたい	clonus
ウェストファール徴候	Westphal sign

　〈loss of knee jerk in tabes dorsalis〉

膝クローヌス しつ	patellar clonus, knee clonus
足クローヌス あし	ankle clonus, foot clonus
表在反射 ひょうざいはんしゃ	superficial reflex
角膜反射 かくまくはんしゃ	corneal reflex
咽頭反射 いんとうはんしゃ	pharyngeal reflex
腹壁反射 ふくへきはんしゃ	abdominal reflex
精巣挙筋反射 せいそうきょきんはんしゃ	cremasteric reflex
足底反射 そくていはんしゃ	plantar reflex
病的反射 びょうてきはんしゃ	pathologic reflex
バビンスキー反射 はんしゃ	Babinski reflex

⟨dorsiflexion of the great toe with fanning of the other toes to plantar stimulation, indicative of pyramidal tract lesions⟩

チャドック反射 はんしゃ Chaddock reflex

⟨extension of the great toe to stimulation below the external malleolus, indicative of pyramidal tract lesions⟩

ゴードン反射 はんしゃ Gordon reflex

⟨paradoxical flexor reflex; dorsiflexion of the great toe by pressure to the calf; seen in pyamidal tract disease⟩

オッペンハイム反射 はんしゃ Oppenheim reflex

⟨dorsiflexion of the great toe by downward stroking of the medial aspect of the shin, seen in pyramidal tract disease⟩

口とがらせ反射 くちはんしゃ	snout reflex
ホフマン徴候 ちょうこう	Hoffmann sign

⟨flexion of the terminal phalanx of the thumb on flicking the nail of the index or middle finger, indicating pyramidal tract involvement⟩

バリント症候群 しょうこうぐん Balint syndrome

⟨optic ataxia and disturbed visual attention due to bilateral parietooccipital lesions⟩

パリノー症候群 しょうこうぐん Parinaud syndrome

⟨dorsal midbrain syndrome; paralysis of conjugate upward gaze due to midbrain lesions such as pineal tumors⟩

皮膚知覚帯 ひふちかくたい	dermatome
知覚減退 ちかくげんたい	hypesthesia
知覚消失 ちかくしょうしつ	anesthesia
知覚過敏 ちかくかびん	hyperesthesia
知覚異常 ちかくいじょう	paresthesia
共感覚 きょうかんかく	synesthesia
痛覚鈍麻 つうかくどんま	hypalgesia, hypalgia, hypoalgesia
痛覚消失 つうかくしょうしつ	analgesia
痛覚過敏 つうかくかびん	hyperalgesia, hyperalgia
温度覚 おんどかく	temperature sense, temperature sensation, thermesthesia
温度覚消失 おんどかくしょうしつ	thermanesthesia

深部感覚 しんぶかんかく	deep sensation, bathyesthesia
固有感覚 こゆうかんかく	proprioception, proprioceptive sensation
深部感覚消失 しんぶかんかくしょうしつ	bathyanesthesia
位置覚 いちかく	position sense
関節覚 かんせつかく	joint sense, arthresthesia
運動覚 うんどうかく	motion sense, movement sense
振動覚 しんどうかく	vibration sense, pallesthesia
立体覚 りったいかく	stereognosis, stereognostic perception
立体覚認知障害 りったいかくにんちしょうがい	astereognosis
内臓知覚 ないぞうちかく	visceral sense, visceral sensation
複合性局所疼痛症候群 ふくごうせいきょくしょとうつうしょうこうぐん	complex regional pain syndrome
レム睡眠時行動障害 ――すいみんじこうどうしょうがい	REM sleep behavior disorder (RBD)
発語緩慢 はつごかんまん	bradylalia
断続言語 だんぞくげんご	staccato speech
失語症 しつごしょう	aphasia
運動性失語症 うんどうせいしつごしょう, ブローカ失語症 ――しつごしょう	motor aphasia, Broca aphasia

⟨*expressive aphasia; impaired speech and writing due to a lesion in the motor speech center*⟩

| 受容性失語症 じゅようせいしつごしょう, ウェルニッケ失語症 ――しつごしょう | receptive aphasia, Wernicke aphasia |

⟨*sensory aphasia; rapid, voluble, and incomprehensible speech; impaired naming, writing, and reading comprehension; due to a lesion in auditory and visual word centers*⟩

失声症 しっせいしょう	aphonia
構音障害 こうおんしょうがい	dysarthria
読字困難 どくじこんなん	dyslexia
計算障害 けいさんしょうがい	dyscalculia
失算 しっさん	acalculia
失書 しっしょ	agraphia
失認 しつにん	agnosia
作話 さくわ	confabulation
学習障害 がくしゅうしょうがい	learning disability (LD)
ゲルストマン症候群	Gerstmann syndrome

⟨*finger agnosia, agraphia, acalculia, and right-left disorientation; caused by a lesion in the angular gyrus of the dominant hemisphere*⟩

| 一過性全健忘 いっかせいぜんけんぼう | transient global amnesia (TGA) |
| コルサコフ症候群 ――しょうこうぐん | Korsakoff syndrome |

⟨*confusion, memory loss, especially for recent events, and confabula-*

tion; classically associated with chronic alcoholism with nutritional deficiencies⟩

多発ニューロパチー たはつ	polyneuropathy
離脱症候群 りだつしょうこうぐん	substance withdrawal syndrome
ティネル徴候 ちょうこう	Tinel sign

⟨*distal tingling on percussion at the site of a divided nerve, indicating early regeneration of the nerve*⟩

フロマン徴候 ちょうこう	Froment sign

⟨*grip is achieved by flexion of the thumb when a piece of paper is held between the thumb and index finger, indicating ulnar nerve palsy*⟩

精神遅滞 せいしんちたい	mental retardation (MR)
精神障害の診断と統計の手引き せいしんしょうがい――しんだん――とうけい――てびき	Diagnostic and Statistical Manual of Mental Disorders (DSM)

● 検査法　Examination ●

抗アセチルコリン受容体抗体 こう――じゅようたいこうたい	anti-acetylcholine receptor antibody
コーネル医学指数 いがくしすう	Cornell Medical Index (CMI)
知能検査 ちのうけんさ	intelligence test
知能指数 ちのうしすう	intelligence quotient
簡易認知機能検査 かんいにんちきのうけんさ	Mini-Mental State Examination (MMSE)
臨床的認知症尺度 りんしょうてきにんちしょうしゃくど	clinical dementia rating (CDR)
ウェクスラー成人用知能検査 ――せいじんようちのうけんさ	Wechsler Adult Intelligence Scale (WAIS)

⟨*measurement of general intelligence in adults*⟩

前頭葉機能検査 ぜんとうようきのうけんさ	frontal assessment battery (FAB)
アルツハイマー病評価スケール ――びょうひょうか	Alzheimer disease assessment scale (ADAS)
ミネソタ多面的性格検査 ――ためんてきせいかくけんさ	Minnesota Multiphasic Personality Inventory (MMPI)
顕在性不安尺度 けんざいせいふあんしゃくど	manifest anxiety scale (MAS)
ハミルトンうつ病評価尺度 ――びょうひょうかしゃくど	Hamilton depression rating scale (HDRS)

⟨*questioning depression-related symptoms to score the severity of depression*⟩

矢田部・ギルフォード性格検査 やたべ・――せいかくけんさ	Yatabe-Guilford (YG) Personality Inventory

⟨*a psychological test designed to evaluate personality traits; 120 questions covering 12 aspects*⟩

ロールシャッハテスト	Rorschach test

⟨a projective psychological test; the subject is asked to relate what is seen in each of 10 inkblot pictures⟩

感情障害ならびに統合失調症面接基準 (かんじょうしょうがい——とうごうしっちょうしょうめんせつきじゅん)	Schedule for Affective Disorders and Schizophrenia (SADS)
標準失語症検査 (ひょうじゅんしつごしょうけんさ)	standard language test of aphasia (SLTA)
文章完成法検査 (ぶんしょうかんせいほうけんさ)	sentence completion test (SCT)
脳血流量 (のうけつりゅうりょう)	cerebral blood flow (CBF)
脳灌流圧 (のうかんりゅうあつ)	cerebral perfusion pressure (CPP)
脳血管抵抗 (のうけっかんていこう)	cerebral vascular resistance (CVR)
脳酸素代謝率 (のうさんそたいしゃりつ)	cerebral metabolic rate of oxygen (CMRO$_2$)
脳波記録法 (のうはきろくほう)	electroencephalography
脳波 (のうは)	electroencephalogram (EEG)
深部脳波 (しんぶのうは)	depth electroencephalogram (DEEG)
皮質脳波 (ひしつのうは)	electrocorticogram (ECC)
光刺激 (ひかりしげき)	photic stimulation
体性感覚誘発電位 (たいせいかんかくゆうはつでんい)	somatosensory evoked potential (SEP)
神経伝導速度 (しんけいでんどうそくど)	nerve conduction velocity (NCV)
神経活動電位 (しんけいかつどうでんい)	nerve action potential (NAP)
筋活動電位 (きんかつどうでんい)	muscle action potential (MAP)
感覚神経活動電位 (かんかくしんけいかつどうでんい)	sensory nerve action potential (SNAP)
複合筋活動電位 (ふくごうきんかつどうでんい)	compound muscle action potential (CMAP)
神経興奮性検査 (しんけいこうふんせいけんさ)	nerve excitability test (NET)
皮膚電気反射 (ひふでんきはんしゃ)	galvanic skin reflex (GSR)
脳磁図法 (のうじずほう)	magnetoencephalography (MEG)
睡眠ポリグラフ計 (すいみん——けい)	polysomnography
睡眠潜時反復検査 (すいみんせんじはんぷくけんさ)	multiple sleep latency test (MSLT)
レム睡眠 (——すいみん)	rapid eye movement (REM) sleep
ノンレム睡眠 (——すいみん)	non-rapid eye movement (NREM) sleep, slow wave sleep (SWS)
頭蓋内圧 (とうがいないあつ)	intracranial pressure (ICP)
頭蓋内圧亢進 (とうがいないあつこうしん)	intracranial hypertension (ICH)
脳脊髄液 (のうせきずいえき)	cerebrospinal fluid (CSF)
髄液圧 (ずいえきあつ)	cerebrospinal fluid pressure
圧力計 (あつりょくけい)	manometer

14. 精神・神経系

髄液細胞増加	pleocytosis
髄液タンパク	cerebrospinal fluid protein
ミエリン塩基性タンパク	myelin basic protein (MBP)
クエッケンシュテット試験	Queckenstedt test

⟨*compression of the jugular vein in healthy persons causes a rapid rise in the CSF pressure, and a rapid fall to normal on release of the pressure; when there is a block in the vertebral canal, the pressure is not affected.*⟩

キサントクロミー	xanthochromia, 〔形〕xanthochromic
塩化エドロホニウム（テンシロン）試験	edrophonium chloride (Tensilon) test
単一探触子ドプラ超音波診断法	duplex Doppler ultrasonography
経頭蓋ドプラ超音波診断法	transcranial Doppler ultrasonography (TCD)
内膜肥厚	intimal thickening
内中膜複合体厚	intima-media thickness (IMT)
脳室周囲低吸収域	periventricular lucency (PVL)
気脳造影法	pneumoencephalography (PEG)
脳室造影法	ventriculography
気脳室造影法	pneumoventriculography
脳血管造影法	cerebral angiography
頚動脈造影法	carotid angiography (CAG)
椎骨動脈造影法	vertebral angiography (VAG)
脳室鏡検査法	ventriculoscopy
レヴィ小体	Lewy body

⟨*intracytoplasmic inclusion in pigmented neurons; seen in locus ceruleus and substantia nigra in Parkinson disease*⟩

グリア線維性酸性タンパク質	glial fibrillary acidic protein (GFAP)
ネグリ小体	Negri bodies

⟨*spherical inclusion bodies found in nerve cells containing the virus of rabies; pathognomonic for rabies*⟩

アミロイドβタンパク質	amyloid β-protein (Aβ)
アミロイド前駆体タンパク質	amyloid precursor protein (APP)

● 疾患名 Diseases ●

水頭症	hydrocephalus
正常圧水頭症	normal-pressure hydrocephalus (NPH)
脳浮腫	brain edema, cerebral edema
高地脳浮腫	high-altitude cerebral edema (HACE)
脳脊髄液減少症	cerebrospinal fluid hypovolemia
脳性麻痺	cerebral palsy
痙性両麻痺, リトル病	spastic diplegia, Little disease

⟨*a form of cerebral palsy due to defective development of the pyramidal tracts; bilateral spasticity, more severe in the lower extremities*⟩

アーノルド・キアリ奇形	Arnold-Chiari malformation

⟨*malformed rhombenchephalon with caudad displacement into the spinal canal; 4 types*⟩

良性頭蓋内圧亢進症	benign intracranial hypertension (BIH)
一過性脳虚血発作	transient ischemic attack (TIA)
脳血管障害	cerebral vascular accident (CVA)
脳梗塞	cerebral infarction (CI)
ラクナ梗塞	lacunar infarction
椎骨脳底動脈循環不全	vertebrobasilar insufficiency (VBI)
ワーレンベルグ症候群	Wallenberg syndrome

⟨*lateral medullary syndrome due to vertebral artery thrombosis near the posterior inferior cerebellar artery; marked by ipsilateral loss of facial pain and temperature sensations, ipsilateral ataxia, dysphagia, nystagmus and Horner syndrome, and contralateral loss of body pain and temperature sensations*⟩

回復性虚血性神経脱落候	reversible ischemic neurological deficit (RIND)
遅発性虚血性神経脱落候	delayed ischemic neurological deficit (DIND)
脳出血	cerebral hemorrhage
脳内出血	intracerebral hemorrhage (ICH)
脳振盪	cerebral concussion
脳振盪後症候群	postconcussion syndrome, postconcussional syndrome
脳損傷	brain injury
外傷性脳損傷	traumatic brain injury (TBI)

脳外傷	
脳動脈瘤, いちご状動脈瘤	cerebral aneurysm, berry aneurysm
頭蓋内動脈瘤	intracranial aneurysm
脳室内出血	intraventricular hemorrhage (IVH)
硬膜外出血	epidural hemorrhage
硬膜外血腫	epidural hematoma
硬膜下血腫	subdural hematoma (SDH)
くも膜下出血	subarachnoid hemorrhage (SAH)
頭蓋内血腫	intracranial hematoma (ICH)
脳アミロイド血管症	cerebral amyloid angiopathy (CAA)
びまん性軸索損傷	diffuse axonal injury
内頸動脈海綿静脈洞瘻	carotid cavernous fistula (CCF)
もやもや病	moyamoya disease, spontaneous occlusion of the circle of Willis
硬膜炎	pachymeningitis
トロサ・ハント症候群	Tolosa-Hunt syndrome

⟨*cavernous sinus syndrome due to idiopathic granuloma; retroorbital pain and ophthalmoplegia caused by palsy of central nerves III, IV, V-I, and VI*⟩

髄膜炎	meningitis
脳炎	encephalitis
単純ヘルペス脳炎	herpes simplex encephalitis (HSE)
亜急性硬化性全脳炎	subacute sclerosing panencephalitis (SSPE)
急性散在性脳脊髄炎	acute disseminated encephalomyelitis (ADEM)
進行性多巣性白質脳症	progressive multifocal leukoencephalopathy (PML)
ウシ海綿状脳症	bovine spongiform encephalopathy (BSE)
亜急性壊死性脳脊髄症, リー病	subacute necrotizing encephalomyelopathy (SNE), Leigh disease

⟨*similar pathological changes to Wernicke encephalopathy; infantile and adult forms; ataxia, seizures, spasticity, ophthalmoplegia, and dementia; autosomal recessive*⟩

異染性白質ジストロフィー	metachromatic leukodystrophy (MLD)
脳膿瘍	brain abscess

IV章 診療録用語

神経梅毒 しんけいばいどく	neurosyphilis
脊髄癆 せきずいろう	tabes dorsalis
アルツハイマー病 びょう	Alzheimer disease (AD)

⟨progressive dementia marked by diffuse atrophy of the cerebral cortex with neurofibrillary tangles and senile plaques⟩

ピック病 びょう	Pick disease

⟨progressive circumscribed cerebral atrophy manifested as dementia; loss of neurons confined to the frontal and temporal lobes⟩

パーキンソン病 びょう	Parkinson disease (PD)

⟨an extrapyramidal disease in late life resulting from a reduction in dopamine caused by degeneration of the basal ganglia⟩

ペリー症候群 しょうこうぐん	Perry syndrome

⟨hereditary mental depression and parkinsonism with taurine deficiency, autosomal dominant⟩

線条体黒質変性症 せんじょうたいこくしつへんせいしょう	striatonigral degeneration
進行性核上性麻痺 しんこうせいかくじょうせいまひ, スティール・リチャードソン・オルゼウスキー症候群	progressive supranuclear palsy (PSP), Steele-Richardson-Olszewski syndrome

⟨parkinsonism plus supranuclear ophthalmoplegia and pseudobulbar palsy due to degeneration of the upper brainstem⟩

進行性球麻痺 しんこうせいきゅうまひ	progressive bulbar palsy (PBP)
偽性球麻痺 ぎせいきゅうまひ	pseudobulbar palsy
筋萎縮性側索硬化症 きんいしゅくせいそくさくこうかしょう	amyotrophic lateral sclerosis (ALS)
原発性側索硬化症 げんぱつせいそくさくこうかしょう	primary lateral sclerosis (PLS)
亜急性連合性脊髄変性症 あきゅうせいれんごうせいせきずいへんせいしょう	subacute combined degeneration of spinal cord
振戦せん妄 しんせんもう	delirium tremens (DT)
多発性硬化症 たはつせいこうかしょう	multiple sclerosis (MS)
視神経脊髄炎 ししんけいせきずいえん, デビック病 びょう	optic neuromyelitis, Devic disease

⟨bilateral demyelination of the optic nerve and spinal cord⟩

先天性筋ジストロフィー せんてんせいきん	congenital muscular dystrophy (CMD)
進行性筋ジストロフィー しんこうせいきん	progressive muscular dystrophy (PMD)
偽性肥大性筋ジストロフィー ぎせいひだいせいきん	pseudohypertrophic muscular dystrophy
デュシェンヌ型筋ジストロフィー きんがた	Duchenne muscular dystrophy

⟨*progressive muscular weakness in the pelvic and shoulder girdles, pseudohypertrophy of the calf, and a peculiar swaying gait; X-linked recessive*⟩

ベッカー型筋ジストロフィー	Becker muscular dystrophy

⟨*similar to Duchenne type, but with milder symptoms and later onset; X-linked recessive*⟩

進行性脊髄性筋萎縮症	progressive spinal muscular atrophy (PSMA)
球脊髄性筋萎縮症	spinobulbar muscular atrophy (SBMA)
スモン, 亜急性脊髄視神経障害	subacute myelo-optico-neuropathy (SMON)
水俣病	Minamata disease

⟨*methyl mercury poisoning causing peripheral paresthesias, tremors, ataxia, dysarthria, and visual and hearing loss*⟩

HTLV-1 関連脊髄障害	HTLV-1-associated myelopathy (HAM)
傍腫瘍性神経症候群	paraneoplastic neurological syndrome (PNS)
傍腫瘍性小脳変性症	paraneoplastic cerebellar degeneration (PCD)
傍腫瘍性多発ニューロパチー	paraneoplastic polyneuropathy
多巣性運動ニューロパチー	multifocal motor neuropathy (MMN)
急性炎症性脱髄性多発ニューロパチー	acute inflammatory demyelinating polyneuropathy (AIDP)
慢性炎症性脱髄性多発ニューロパチー	chronic inflammatory demyelinating polyneuropathy (CIDP)
遺伝性運動感覚ニューロパチー	hereditary motor and sensory neuropathy (HMSN)
遺伝性感覚自律性ニューロパチー	hereditary sensory and autonomic neuropathy (HSAN)
家族性アミロイド多発ニューロパチー	familial amyloid polyneuropathy (FAP)
橋中心髄鞘崩壊症	central pontine myelinolysis (CPM)
脊髄小脳変性症	spinocerebellar degeneration (SCD)

晩発性小脳皮質萎縮症 late cortical cerebellar atrophy (LCCA)

オリーブ橋小脳萎縮症 olivopontocerebellar atrophy (OPCA)

多系統萎縮症 multiple system atrophy (MSA)

重症筋無力症 myasthenia gravis (MG)

ハンチントン病，ハンチントン舞踏病 Huntington disease (HD), Huntington chorea

〈an autosomal dominant neurodegenerative disorder, characterized by chronic progressive chorea and dementia〉

シデナム舞踏病 Sydenham chorea

〈postinfectious chorea in children or pregnant women, linked with rheumatic fever; involuntary movements of distal limbs and emotional lability〉

有棘赤血球を伴う舞踏病 chorea with acanthocytes

ジルドラトゥレット症候群 Gilles de la Tourette syndrome

〈chronic relapsing motor and voice tics in children associated with obsessive-compulsive behavior, distractibility, coprolalia, echolalia, and palilalia〉

ギラン・バレー症候群 Guillain-Barré syndrome (GBS)

〈acute idiopathic polyneuritis characterized by rapidly progressive ascending motor neuron paralysis; often preceded by a respiratory or enteric infection〉

フィッシャー症候群 Fisher syndrome

〈Miller Fisher syndrome; a variant of Guillain-Barré syndrome marked by ophthalmoplegia, ataxia, and areflexia secondary to infection〉

シャイ・ドレーガー症候群 Shy-Drager syndrome

〈autonomic nervous system failure marked by orthostatic hypotension, impotence, bowel and bladder dysfunction, and anhidrosis, followed by parkinsonian syndrome〉

シャルコー・マリー・トゥース病 Charcot-Marie-Tooth disease (CMT)

〈hereditary motor and sensory neuropathy, characterized by progressive muscle weakness and atrophy in distal extremities; peroneal muscular atrophy〉

フリードライヒ運動失調症 Friedreich ataxia

〈hereditary ataxia marked by ataxia, speech impairment, cardiomyopathy, absent reflexes, scoliosis, talipes cavus, and sclerosis of the

14. 精神・神経系

posterior and lateral columns of the spinal cord⟩

レフスム病 ―びょう　　Refsum disease
⟨*an autosomal recessive disorder due to a disturbance in phytanic acid metabolism; manifested by retinitis pigmentosa, polyneuropathy, cerebellar ataxia, deafness, and ichthyosis*⟩

メージ症候群 ―しょうこうぐん　　Meige syndrome
⟨*focal dystonia of facial muscles with blepharospasm, lip retraction, and tongue protrusion, usually seen in older women*⟩

クロイツフェルト・ヤコブ病 ―びょう　　Creutzfeldt-Jakob disease (CJD)
⟨*subacute spongiform encephalopathy caused by a prion protein in sporadic, familial, and infectious forms; characterized by ataxia, progressive dementia, myoclonus, and diagnostic EEG changes*⟩

ゲルストマン・ストロイスラー・シャインカー病 ―びょう　　Gerstmann-Sträussler-Scheinker disease (GSS)
⟨*a chronic cerebellar form of spongiform encephalopathy marked by cerebellar ataxia; autosomal dominant*⟩

ウェルニッケ脳症 ―のうしょう　　Wernicke encephalopathy
⟨*confusion, ataxia, ophthalmoplegia, and nystagmus, caused by thiamine deficiency due to chronic alcohol abuse*⟩

ミトコンドリア脳筋症 ―のうきんしょう　　mitochondrial encephalomyopathy

メラス症候群 ―しょうこうぐん　　MELAS syndrome (*m*itochondrial *m*yopathy, *e*ncephalopathy, *l*actic *a*cidosis, and *s*troke-like episodes)

赤ぼろ線維を伴うミオクローヌスてんかん
あか―せんい―ともな―　　myoclonus epilepsy with ragged red fibers (MERRF)

周期性四肢麻痺 しゅうきせいししまひ　　periodic paralysis

腕神経叢障害 わんしんけいそうしょうがい　　brachial plexus neuropathy (BPN)

反射性交感神経性ジストロフィー はんしゃせいこうかんしんけいせい―　　reflex sympathetic dystrophy (RSD)

脳血管性認知症 のうけっかんせいにんちしょう　　vascular dementia, multi-infarct dementia

ビンスワンガー病 ―びょう　　Binswanger disease
⟨*progressive subcortical arteriosclerotic encephalopathy; dementia due to subcortical demyelination and lacunar infarcts caused by arteriosclerotic arteries in the white matter*⟩

アルツハイマー型認知症 ―がたにんちしょう　　dementia of the Alzheimer type (DAT)

前頭側頭型認知症 ぜんとうそくとうがたにんちしょう　　frontotemporal dementia (FTD)

IV章 診療録用語

レヴィ小体型認知症	dementia with Lewy bodies (DLB)
統合失調症	schizophrenia
躁うつ病	manic-depressive psychosis
双極性障害	bipolar disorder
大うつ病性障害	major depressive disorder, major depression
単極性うつ病	unipolar depression
脳卒中後うつ状態	post-stroke depression (PSD)
気分変調性障害	dysthymic disorder
気分障害	mood disorder
強迫神経症	obsessive-compulsive neurosis
不安障害	anxiety disorder
全般性不安障害	generalized anxiety disorder (GAD)
適応障害	adjustment disorder
パニック障害	panic disorder
解離性障害	dissociative disorder
転換性障害	conversion disorder
物質依存	substance dependence
心身症	psychosomatic disease (PSD), psychophysiological disorder
身体表現性障害	somatoform disorder
心的外傷後ストレス障害	posttraumatic stress disorder (PTSD)
摂食障害	eating disorder
神経性食欲不振症	anorexia nervosa (AN)
神経性大食症	bulimia nervosa
クライネ・レヴィン症候群	Kleine-Levin syndrome

⟨*periodic hypersomnia and bulimia, common in young men*⟩

クリューバー・ビューシー症候群	Klüver-Bucy syndrome

⟨*hyperphagia, hypersexuality, and compulsive licking, caused by bilateral temporal lobe lesion*⟩

ナルコレプシー	narcolepsy
過眠症	hypersomnia
概日リズム睡眠障害	circadian rhythm sleep disorder

14. 精神・神経系

人格障害 じんかくしょうがい	personality disorder
境界性人格障害 きょうかいせい―	borderline personality disorder (BPD)
演技性人格障害 えんぎせい―	histrionic personality disorder (HPD)
反社会的人格障害 はんしゃかいてき―	antisocial personality disorder (ASPD)
自己愛性人格障害 じこあいせい―	narcissistic personality disorder (NPD)
注意欠陥多動障害 ちゅういけっかんたどうしょうがい	attention-deficit hyperactivity disorder (ADHD)
反抗挑戦性障害 はんこうちょうせんせいしょうがい	oppositional defiant disorder (ODD)
広汎性発達障害 こうはんせいはったつしょうがい	pervasive developmental disorder (PDD)
自閉性障害 じへいせいしょうがい	autistic disorder
アスペルガー症候群	Asperger syndrome

⟨a pervasive developmental disorder resembling autistic disorder, characterized by severe impairment in social skills and by restricted behaviors and interests⟩

| レット症候群 ―しょうこうぐん | Rett syndrome |

⟨a PDD in girls characterized by autistic attitude, ataxia, loss of purposeful hand skills, seizures, and mental retardation⟩

| ミュンヒハウゼン症候群 | Munchausen syndrome |

⟨<Münchhausen; a factitious disorder with physical symptoms characterized by self-infliction of harm to induce illness requiring hospital treatment⟩

脳腫瘍 のうしゅよう	cerebral tumor, brain tumor (BT)
髄膜腫 ずいまくしゅ	meningioma
神経鞘腫 しんけいしょうしゅ, シュワン細胞腫 ―さいぼうしゅ	neurinoma, schwannoma

⟨<Theodor Schwann; a benign neoplasm originating from Schwann cells of the myelin sheath of neurons⟩

下垂体腺腫 かすいたいせんしゅ	hypophyseal adenoma
空虚トルコ鞍症候群 くうきょ―あんしょうこうぐん	empty sella syndrome
頭蓋咽頭腫 とうがいいんとうしゅ	craniopharyngioma
星状細胞腫 せいじょうさいぼうしゅ	astrocytoma
神経膠腫 しんけいこうしゅ	glioma
膠芽腫 こうがしゅ	glioblastoma
神経線維腫症 しんけいせんいしゅしょう, フォンレックリングハウゼン病 ―びょう	neurofibromatosis, von Recklinghausen disease

⟨neurofibromatosis type 1; multiple neurofibromas and hyperpigmented skin patches, café-au-lait spots; autosomal dominant⟩

| フォンヒッペル・リンダウ病 ―びょう | von Hippel-Lindau disease (VHL) |

⟨hereditary phakomatosis characterized by retinal hemangiomas and cerebellar hemangioblastomas; sometimes with tumors or cysts of kidneys, pancreas, or adrenal gland; autosomal dominant⟩

悪性症候群, 神経遮断薬による悪性症候群	malignant syndrome, neuroleptic malignant syndrome (NMS)

● 治療法 Treatment ●

抗精神病薬	antipsychotic agent
精神安定薬	tranquilizer, ataractic
神経遮断薬	neuroleptic
鎮静薬	sedative
抗痙攣薬	anticonvulsant, anticonvulsive
抗不安薬	antianxiety agent
催眠薬	hypnotic
バルビツレート	barbiturate
ベンゾジアゼピン	benzodiazepine
ジアゼパム	diazepam《セルシン》
トリアゾラム	triazolam《ハルシオン》
クアゼパム	quazepam《ドラール》
抗うつ薬	antidepressant, antidepressive drug
三環系抗うつ薬	tricyclic antidepressant (TCA)
イミプラミン塩酸塩	imipramine hydrochloride《トフラニール》
選択的セロトニン再取り込み阻害薬	selective serotonin reuptake inhibitor (SSRI)
パロキセチン塩酸塩水和物	paroxetine hydrochloride hydrate《パキシル》
セロトニン・ノルアドレナリン再取り込み阻害薬	serotonin-noradrenaline reuptake inhibitor (SNRI)
ミルナシプラン塩酸塩	milnacipran hydrochloride《トレドミン》
ノルアドレナリン作動性・特異的セロトニン作動性抗うつ薬	noradrenergic and specific serotonergic antidepressant (NaSSA)
ミルタザピン	mirtazapine《レメロン, リフレックス》
精神刺激薬	psychostimulant
メチルフェニデート塩酸塩	methylphenidate hydrochloride《リタリン》《コンサータ》
抗ウイルス薬	antiviral agent
抗血小板薬	platelet inhibitor

14. 精神・神経系

チクロピジン塩酸塩	ticlopidine hydrochloride《パナルジン》
クロピドグレル硫酸塩	clopidogrel sulfate《プラビックス》
シロスタゾール	cilostazol《プレタール》
組織プラスミノーゲン活性化因子	tissue plasminogen activator (t-PA)
遺伝子組み換え組織プラスミノーゲン活性化因子	recombinant tissue plasminogen activator (rt-PA)
アルテプラーゼ	alteplase《グルトパ》
フリーラディカルスカベンジャー	free radical scavenger
エダラボン	edaravone《ラジカット》
A型ボツリヌス毒素	Botulinum A toxin《ボトックス》
レボドーパ製剤	levodopa, L-dopa《ドパストン》
ドーパミン作動薬	dopamine (DA) agonist
ブロモクリプチンメシル酸塩	bromocriptine mesilate《パーロデル》
ペルゴリドメシル酸塩	pergolide mesilate《ペルマックス》
カベルゴリン	cabergoline《カバサール》
ロピニロール塩酸塩	ropinirole hydrochloride《レキップ》
COMT阻害薬	COMT inhibitor
エンタカポン	entacapone《コムタン》
モノアミンオキシダーゼ阻害薬	monoamine oxidase inhibitor (MAOI)
セレギリン塩酸塩	selegiline hydrochloride《エフピー》
抗コリン作動薬	anticholinergic agent
ビペリデン	biperiden《アキネトン》
アマンタジン塩酸塩	amantadine hydrochloride《シンメトレル》
ドロキシドーパ	droxidopa《ドプス》
ゾニサミド	zonisamide (ZNS)《トレリーフ》
リルゾール	riluzole《リルテック》
マンニトール	mannitol
ドネペジル塩酸塩	donepezil hydrochloride《アリセプト》
アフェレシス	apheresis
髄腔内バクロフェン投与	intrathecal baclofen (ITB)《ギャバロン》
抗てんかん薬	antiepileptic drug (AED)
フェニトイン	phenytoin (PHT)《アレビアチン》
カルバマゼピン	carbamazepine (CBZ)《テグレトール》
フェノバルビタール	phenobarbital (PB)《フェノバール》

316 Ⅳ章 診療録用語

プリミドン	primidone (PRM)《プリミドン》
バルプロ酸	valproic acid (VPA)《デパケン》
エトスクシミド	ethosuximide (ESM)《エピレオプチマル》
クロナゼパム	clonazepam (CZP)《ランドセン》
ゾニサミド	zonisamide (ZNS)《エクセグラン》
ガバペンチン	gabapentin《ガバペン》
トピラマート	topiramate《トピナ》
ラモトリギン	lamotrigine《ラミクタール》
ダントロレンナトリウム水和物	dantrolene sodium hydrate《ダントリウム》
セロトニン・ドーパミン拮抗薬	serotonin-dopamine antagonist (SDA)
リスペリドン	risperidone《リスパダール》
クロザピン	clozapine《クロザリル》
アリピプラゾール	aripiprazole《エビリファイ》
多元受容体標的化抗精神薬	multiacting receptor targeted antipsychotic (MARTA)
カウンセリング	counseling
社会生活技能訓練	social skills training (SST)
精神分析	psychoanalysis
交流分析	transactional analysis (TA)
自律訓練法	autogenic training (AT)
認知行動療法	cognitive behavioral therapy (CBT)
言語療法	speech therapy
断酒会	Alcoholics Anonymous (AA)
電気痙攣療法	electroconvulsive therapy (ECT)
電気ショック療法	electric shock therapy, electroshock therapy (EST)
深部脳刺激法	deep brain stimulation (DBS)
迷走神経刺激法	vagal nerve stimulation (VNS)
機能的神経筋刺激法	functional neuromuscular stimulation (FNS)
硬膜外血液パッチ法	epidural blood patch (EBP)
頸動脈内膜切除術	carotid endarterectomy (CEA)
頸動脈ステント留置術	carotid artery stenting (CAS)
浅側頭動脈・中大脳動脈吻合術	superficial temporal artery-middle cerebral artery (STA-MCA) anastomosis

14. 精神・神経系　*317*

頭蓋内外バイパス	extracranial-intracranial (EC-IC) bypass
経皮経管血管形成術	percutaneous transluminal angioplasty (PTA)
定位手術的照射	stereotactic radiosurgery (SRS)
ガンマナイフ	Gamma Knife
開頭クリッピング	surgical clipping
コイル塞栓術	coil embolization
脳硬膜動脈血管癒合術	encephaloduroarteriosynangiosis (EDAS)
脳室ドレナージ	ventricular drainage
脳室穿刺	ventricular puncture, ventriculopuncture
脳室腹腔シャント	ventriculoperitoneal (VP) shunt
脳室腹腔短絡形成術	ventriculoperitoneostomy
脳室心房短絡	ventriculoatrial shunt
穿頭孔	burr hole
開頭	craniotomy
経蝶形骨洞手術	transsphenoidal surgery (TSS)
胸腺摘除術	thymectomy

Tidbits

mnemonic

「ニマニック」と発音し，記憶を助ける工夫のこと．医学論文に必要なことは CAPERS であると Edith Schwager は述べた (*c*larity, *a*ccuracy, *p*reciseness, *e*conomy, *r*eflectiveness, *s*implicity)．一語としての意味と共に記憶に残る名言である．臨床医学でも ABC (*a*irway, *b*reathing, *c*irculation) をはじめ種々の mnemonic aids が工夫されている．Parkinson disease の症状は TRAP (*t*remor, *r*igidity, *a*kinesia, *p*ostural instability), multiple sclerosis の診断は INSULAR (*i*ntention tremor, *n*ystagmus, *s*canning speech, *u*rinary difficulties, *l*oss of *a*bdominal *r*eflexes), Apgar score は APGAR (*a*ppearance, *p*ulse, *g*rimace, *a*ctivity, *r*espirations) など．

15. 皮膚

●愁訴・症状　Complaints / Symptoms●

皮膚 ひふ	skin, cutis, dermis, integument, 〔形〕cutaneous, dermal, integumentary
発疹 ほっしん	eruption, rash, exanthema, exanthem
(発疹が) 出る	break out, appear
青あざ あお	bruise
赤あざ あか	birthmark
あかぎれ	chaps, cracks
あせも	prickly heat, heat rashes
いぼ	warts
いんきんたむし	ringworm, jockstrap itch
うおのめ	corn, clavus
打ち身 うみ	bruise
おでき	boil, furuncle
おむつかぶれ	diaper rash
かさぶた	scab, crust, slough
かすり傷 きず	graze
切り傷 きず	cut, gash
しもやけ	chilblain, frostbite
しらくも	favus, scald head, honeycomb ringworm
シラミ	louse
蕁麻疹 じんま	hives, urticaria
そばかす	freckles
たこ	callus
ただれ	sore, erosion, festering
床ずれ とこ, 褥瘡 じょくそう	bedsore, pressure sores, decubitus
とびひ	impetigo
なまず	tinea versicolor
にきび	pimple, acne
日焼け ひや	sunburn
日焼け止め指数 ひやしすう	sun protection factor (SPF)
ふけ	dandruff, scurf
ほくろ	mole
みみず腫れ ば	welt, wheal, wale
水ぶくれ みず	blister
水虫 みずむし	athlete's foot, ringworm of the feet
虫刺され むしさ	insect bite
やけど	burn
鳥肌が立つ とりはだた	get gooseflesh, get goosebumps

15. 皮膚 319

痒み かゆ, 掻痒感 そうようかん	itching, pruritus, 〔形〕itchy, itching, pruritic
掻く か	scratch
かぶれる	be poisoned [with lacquer]
膿む う	fester, form pus, suppurate
滲出する しんしゅつ, じくじくする	exude, ooze, weep
股擦れがする またず	have a thigh sore, have chafing in the groin
脱毛 だつもう	loss of hair, falling-out of hair
毛が抜ける けぬ	lose one's hair, hair falls (comes out, drops out)
毛のない け	hairless, bald
毛の薄い うす	thinly-haired
毛深い けぶか, 多毛の たもう	hairy, thickly haired, shaggy, hirsute
白髪 しらが	gray hair
禿頭 とくとう	baldness, bald-headedness, bald head

● 診察所見・徴候　Physical findings / Signs ●

ガラス圧診法 あっしんほう	diascopy
皮膚描記症 ひふびょうきしょう	dermography, dermographism, dermatographism
潮紅 ちょうこう	flushing
母斑 ぼはん	nevus, birthmark
紅斑 こうはん	erythema
蝶形紅斑 ちょうけいこうはん	butterfly rash
ヘリオトロープ疹 しん	heliotrope eruption
紫斑 しはん	purpura
白斑 はくはん	vitiligo, leukoderma
肝斑 かんぱん	chloasma
色素斑 しきそはん	pigmented spot
色素沈着 しきそちんちゃく	pigmentation
黒皮症 こくひしょう	melanosis, melanism
メラニン減少症 げんしょうしょう	hypomelanosis, 〔形〕hypomelanotic
雀卵斑 じゃくらんはん	ephelis, 〔複〕ephelides, freckles
黒子 ほくろ	lentigo, 〔複〕lentigines
さめ皮様皮膚 かわようひふ	shagreen skin
紅皮症 こうひしょう	erythroderma, erythrodermia
湿疹 しっしん	eczema
痒疹 ようしん	prurigo
丘疹 きゅうしん	papule
種粒腫 ひりゅうしゅ	milium, 〔複〕milia

膨疹（ぼうしん）	wheal
蕁麻疹（じんま しん）	urticaria
蕁麻疹誘発（じんましん ゆうはつ）	urtication
ダリエー徴候（ちょうこう）	Darier sign

⟨urtication and itching on rubbing lesions of urticaria pigmentosa⟩

クインケ浮腫（ふしゅ）	Quincke edema

⟨angioedema, angioneurotic edema⟩

光線過敏症（こうせんかびんしょう）	photosensitivity
汗疹（かんしん）	miliaria
水疱（すいほう）	bulla, bleb
小水疱（しょうすいほう）	vesicle, blister
膿疱（のうほう）	pustule
面皰（めんぽう）	comedo
びらん	erosion
潰瘍（かいよう）	ulcer
擦過傷（さっかしょう）	abrasion
表皮剥脱（ひょうひはくだつ）	excoriation
裂傷（れっしょう）	laceration
熱傷（ねっしょう）	burn
第1度熱傷（だい1どねっしょう）	first-degree burn, epidermal burn
第2度熱傷（だい2どねっしょう）	second-degree burn, partial-thickness burn
第3度熱傷（だい3どねっしょう）	third-degree burn, full-thickness burn
第4度熱傷（だい4どねっしょう）	fourth-degree burn
9の法則（9のほうそく）	rule of nines
凍傷（とうしょう）	congelation, frostbite
凍瘡（とうそう）	pernio, chilblain
痂皮（かひ）	crust, scab
膿痂疹（のうかしん）	impetigo
落屑（らくせつ）	desquamation
鱗屑（りんせつ）	scale
粃糠疹（ひこうしん）	pityriasis
苔癬化（たいせんか）	lichenification
ウィッカム線条（せんじょう）	Wickham striae

⟨whitish lines on the surface of the papules in lichen planus⟩

表皮肥厚（ひょうひひこう）	acanthosis
間擦疹（かんさつしん）	intertrigo
魚鱗癬（ぎょりんせん）	ichthyosis
疣贅（ゆうぜい）	verruca, wart
胼胝（べんち）	callus, tyloma
角化（かっか）	keratinization
角化症（かっかしょう）	keratosis

角皮症 かくひしょう	keratodermia
多毛症 たもうしょう	hypertrichosis, polytrichosis
白毛 はくもう	poliosis
いれずみ	tattoo
わきが腋臭 えきしゅう	hircismus
臭汗症 しゅうかんしょう	osmidrosis
無汗症 むかんしょう	anhidrosis, adiaphoresis
多汗症 たかんしょう	hyperhidrosis
乾皮症 かんぴしょう	xerosis, xeroderma
匙状爪 さじじょうづめ	spoon nail, koilonychia
爪下血腫 そうかけっしゅ	subungual hematoma
爪剥離症 そうはくりしょう	onycholysis
爪甲白斑 そうこうはくはん	leukonychia
爪裂症 そうれつしょう	onychorrhexis
ボー線 せん	Beau lines

⟨transverse grooves in the nail plate associated with growth arrest during acute severe illness; tend to appear about one month after the event⟩

ミーズ線 せん	Mees lines

⟨transverse while lines on the fingernails after exposure to arsenic and heavy metals⟩

レイノー現象 げんしょう	Raynaud phenomenon

⟨blanching, paresthesia, and pain of the fingers and toes induced by cold; caused by intermittent spasm of small arteries⟩

ケブナー現象 げんしょう	Koebner phenomenon

⟨isomorphic* response to trauma in uninvolved areas of patients with psoriasis and lichen planus⟩ *similar in form

ニコルスキー徴候 ちょうこう	Nikolsky sign

⟨ready separation of the epidermis by rubbing in pemphigus vulgaris⟩

アウスピッツ徴候 ちょうこう	Auspitz sign

⟨pinpoint bleeding after removal of a scale; typical of psoriasis⟩

ゴットロン徴候 ちょうこう	Gottron sign

⟨violet, flat papules over the extensor surfaces of interphalangeal joints; pathognomonic of dermatomyositis⟩

レーザー・トレラー徴候	Leser-Trélat sign

⟨marked increase in the number of seborrheic keratoses; a sign of gastrointestinal and other malignancies⟩

● 検査法　Examination ●

抗核抗体 こうかくこうたい	antinuclear antibody (ANA)
LE 細胞 さいぼう	LE cell
抗 DNA 抗体 こうたい	anti-DNA antibody

抗Sm抗体	anti-Sm antibody
抗二本鎖DNA抗体	anti-double stranded DNA antibody
抗ENA抗体	anti-extractable nuclear antigen (ENA) antibody
抗リン脂質抗体	anti-phospholipid antibody
抗カルジオリピン抗体	anti-cardiolipin antibody (ACL)
ループス抗凝固因子	lupus anticoagulant (LA)
抗トポイソメラーゼⅠ抗体	antitopoisomerase I antibody
抗セントロメア抗体	anticentromere antibody (ACA)
循環免疫複合体	circulating immune complex (CIC)
連鎖球菌発熱外毒素	streptococcal pyrogenic exotoxin (SPE)
毒素性ショック症候群毒素	toxic shock syndrome toxin (TSST-1)
単純ヘルペスウイルス	herpes simplex virus (HSV)
抗単純ヘルペスウイルス抗体	anti-herpes simplex virus antibody
水痘帯状疱疹ウイルス	varicella-zoster virus (VZV)
抗水痘帯状疱疹ウイルス抗体	anti-varicella-zoster virus antibody
ワイル・フェリックス反応	Weil-Felix reaction

⟨*a test for typhus and other rickettsial diseases; the patient's serum tested for the presence of antibodies against Proteus vulgaris,* OX19, OXK, OX2, *based on agglutination*⟩

ダーモスコピー	dermoscopy, epiluminescence microscopy
経表皮水分喪失	transepidermal water loss (TEWL)
サーモグラフィー	thermography
ウッド灯	Wood lamp

⟨*a nickel-oxide filtered UV light source; used to demonstrate fluorescence caused by Microsporum canis, tinea capitis, or Corynebacterium minutissimum, erythrasma*⟩

即時型過敏反応	immediate hypersensitivity reaction

15. 皮膚

遅延型過敏反応 (ちえんがたかびんはんのう)	delayed-type hypersensitivity reaction (DTH)
遅延型皮膚過敏症 (ちえんがたひふかびんしょう)	delayed cutaneous hypersensitivity (DCH)
アルサス反応 (——はんのう)	Arthus reaction

⟨edema, hemorrhage, and necrosis at the injection site of antigen in a previously sensitized animal; caused by deposition of antigen-antibody complexes⟩

免疫グロブリン E	immunoglobulin E (IgE)
ヒト TARC 定量	thymus and activation-regulated chemokine (TARC)
単刺試験 (たんししけん)	prick test
プリック・プリック試験 (——しけん)	prick-to-prick test
掻破試験 (そうはしけん)	scratch test
皮内テスト (ひない)	intradermal test
スポロトリキン試験 (——しけん)	sporotrichin test
ディック試験 (——しけん)	Dick test

⟨an intradermal test of susceptibility to erythrogenic toxin of Group A streptococci responsible for the rash of scarlet fever⟩

フライ試験 (——しけん)	Frei test

⟨a skin test for diagnosis of lymphogranuloma venereum using suspension of inactivated chlamydiae⟩

クベイム試験 (——しけん)	Kveim test

⟨an intradermal test for sarcoidosis using antigen from sarcoid spleen and performing biopsy within 6 weeks⟩

パッチテスト	patch test
密封貼布試験 (みっぷうちょうふしけん)	closed patch test
開放貼布試験 (かいほうちょうふしけん)	open patch test
ジニトロクロロベンゼン試験 (——しけん)	dinitrochlorobenzene (DNCB) test
多項目抗原同時検査 (たこうもくこうげんどうじけんさ)	multiple antigen simultaneous test (MAST)
放射性アレルゲン吸着試験 (ほうしゃせい——きゅうちゃくしけん)	radioallergosorbent test (RAST)
放射性免疫吸着試験 (ほうしゃせいめんえききゅうちゃくしけん)	radioimmunosorbent test (RIST)
リンパ球刺激試験 (——きゅうしげきしけん)	lymphocyte stimulation test (LST)
薬剤誘発リンパ球刺激試験 (やくざいゆうはつ——きゅうしげきしけん)	drug-induced lymphocyte stimulation test (DLST)
光線過敏試験 (こうせんかびんしけん)	photosensitivity test
光線貼布試験 (こうせんちょうふしけん)	photopatch test

最小紅斑量 さいしょうこうはんりょう　minimal erythema dose (MED)
受動皮膚アナフィラキシー じゅどうひふ　passive cutaneous anaphylaxis (PCA)
皮膚電位図 ひふでんいず　electrodermogram (EDG)
皮膚生検 ひふせいけん　skin biopsy
ツァンク試験 けんし　Tzanck test
〈sampling of cells from the floor of vesicular or bullous lesions; multinucleated giant cells indicate varicella, herpes simplex, herpes zoster, or pemphigus〉

● 疾患名　Diseases ●

皮膚炎 ひふえん　dermatitis
接触皮膚炎 せっしょくひふえん　contact dermatitis (CD)
アトピー性皮膚炎 せいひふえん, ベスニエ痒疹 ようしん　atopic dermatitis (AD), Besnier prurigo
接触蕁麻疹 せっしょくじんましん　contact urticaria
ラテックスアレルギー　latex allergy
脂漏性皮膚炎 しろうせいひふえん　seborrheic dermatitis
放射線皮膚炎 ほうしゃせんひふえん　radiodermatitis, radiation dermatitis
薬疹 やくしん　drug eruption, dermatitis medicamentosa
脂漏性角化症 しろうせいかくかしょう　seborrheic keratosis
日光角化症 にっこうかくかしょう　actinic keratosis, solar keratosis
毛包性角化症 もうほうせいかくかしょう, ダリエー病 びょう　follicular keratosis, Darier disease
〈an autosomal dominant disorder of keratinization characterized by keratotic papules on seborrheic areas of the body〉
進行性指掌角皮症 しんこうせいししょうかくひしょう　keratodermia tylodes palmaris progressiva (KTPP)
色素性蕁麻疹 しきそせいじんましん　urticaria pigmentosa
遺伝性血管神経性浮腫 いでんせいけっかんしんけいせいふしゅ, 遺伝性血管浮腫 いでんせいけっかんふしゅ　hereditary angioneurotic edema (HANE), hereditary angioedema (HAE)
単純ヘルペス たんじゅん　herpes simplex
帯状疱疹 たいじょうほうしん　herpes zoster
デューリング病 びょう　Duhring disease
〈dermatitis herpetiformis; a symmetrical pruritic eruption of vesicles and papules in groups; associated with celiac disease〉
汗疱 かんぽう　pompholyx
伝染性膿痂疹 でんせんせいのうかしん　impetigo contagiosa
褥瘡 じょくそう　decubitus
尋常性痤瘡 じんじょうせいざそう　acne vulgaris

15. 皮膚

脂漏症 しろうしょう	seborrhea
ばら色粃糠疹 いろこうしん	pityriasis rosea
色素性乾皮症 しきそせいかんぴしょう	xeroderma pigmentosum (XP)
尋常性魚鱗癬 じんじょうせいぎょりんせん	ichthyosis vulgaris
ネザートン症候群 しょうこうぐん	Netherton syndrome

⟨congenital ichthyosis associated with atopy, bamboo-like hairs, aminoaciduria, and mental retardation; probably autosomal recessive⟩

扁平苔癬 へんぺいたいせん	lichen planus
慢性単純性苔癬 まんせいたんじゅんせいたいせん, ヴィダール苔癬 たいせん	lichen simplex chronicus, lichen Vidal
硬化性萎縮性苔癬 こうかせいいしゅくせいたいせん	lichen sclerosus et atrophicus (LSA)
硬結性紅斑 こうけつせいこうはん, バザン病 びょう	erythema induratum, Bazin disease

⟨recurrent hard subcutaneous nodules on the calves in young and middle-aged women; may form necrotic ulcers⟩

レオパード症候群 しょうこうぐん	LEOPARD syndrome (multiple lentigines syndrome; *l*entigines, *E*CG abnormalities, *o*cular hypertension, *p*ulmonary stenosis, *a*bnormal genitalia, *r*etardation of growth, and *d*eafness; autosomal dominant)
麻疹 ましん	measles
風疹 ふうしん	rubella
水痘 すいとう	varicella
白癬 はくせん	tinea, trichophytia, ringworm
頭部白癬 とうぶはくせん	tinea capitis
体幹白癬 たいかんはくせん	tinea corporis
股部白癬 こぶはくせん	tinea cruris
足部白癬 そくぶはくせん	tinea pedis
手掌白癬 しゅしょうはくせん	tinea manus, tinea manuum
爪白癬 そうはくせん	tinea unguinum
癜風 でんぷう	tinea versicolor, pityriasis versicolor
疥癬 かいせん	scabies
紅色陰癬 こうしょくいんせん	erythrasma
シラミ症 しょう	pediculosis
爪周囲炎 そうしゅういえん	paronychia
毛嚢炎 もうのうえん	folliculitis
毛瘡 もうそう	sycosis
蜂巣炎 ほうそうえん	cellulitis

丹毒 たんどく	erysipelas
ひょう疽 そ	felon, whitlow
円形脱毛症 えんけいだつもうしょう	alopecia areata
裂毛症 れつもうしょう	trichothiodystrophy (TTD)
毛巣嚢胞 もうそうのうほう	pilonidal cyst
血管腫 けっかんしゅ	hemangioma
カサバッハ・メリット症候群 こうぐん	Kasabach-Merritt syndrome

⟨thrombocytopenic purpura, DIC, and bleeding associated with extensive hemangiomas; platelets are trapped in the tumor⟩

尋常性白斑 じんじょうせいはくはん	vitiligo vulgaris
白皮症 はくひしょう	albinism
太田母斑 おおたぼはん	nevus of Ota

⟨oculodermal melanosis; unilateral blue pigmentation of the conjunctiva and skin around the eye⟩

眼皮膚型白皮症 がんひふがたはくひしょう	oculocutaneous albinism (OCA)
母斑症 ぼはんしょう	phakomatosis, phacomatosis
結節性硬化症 けっせつせいこうかしょう, ブルヌヴィーユ病 びょう, プリングル病 びょう	tuberous sclerosis, Bourneville disease, Pringle disease, epiloia

⟨phakomatosis with neurologic and skin manifestations such as seizures, mental retardation, facial angiofibromas, hypomelanotic macules, shagreen patches, and periungual fibromas; autosomal dominant⟩

結節性紅斑 けっせつせいこうはん	erythema nodosum
多形紅斑 たけいこうはん	erythema multiforme
多形滲出性紅斑 たけいしんしゅつせいこうはん	erythema multiforme exudativum, erythema exudativum multiforme (EEM)
スチーブンス・ジョンソン症候群 こうぐん	Stevens-Johnson syndrome

⟨erythema multiforme exudativum involving large areas of the skin and oral, genital, and colonic mucous membranes in reaction to drugs and toxins⟩

粘膜皮膚眼症候群 ねんまくひふがんしょうこうぐん	mucocutaneous ocular syndrome (MCOS)
中毒性表皮壊死症候群 ちゅうどくせいひょうひえししょうこうぐん, ライエル症候群	toxic epidermal necrolysis (TEN), Lyell syndrome

⟨nonstaphylococcal scalded skin syndrome; full-thickness epidermal necrosis as a severe reaction to drugs, infections, or chemicals⟩

毒素性ショック症候群 どくそせいしょうこうぐん	toxic shock syndrome (TSS)
毒素性ショック様症候群	toxic shock-like syndrome (TSLS)

| 薬剤性過敏症症候群 | drug-induced hypersensitivity syndrome (DIHS) |
| スウィート病 | Sweet disease |

〈*acute febrile neutrophilic dermatosis; sudden onset of painful erythema on the neck, trunk, and limbs with fever*〉

尋常性乾癬	psoriasis vulgaris
掌蹠膿疱症	palmoplantar pustulosis, pustulosis palmaris et plantaris (PPP)
異型線維黄色腫	atypical fibroxanthoma (AFX)
皮膚筋炎	dermatomyositis (DM)
表皮水疱症	epidermolysis bullosa (EB)
尋常性天疱瘡	pemphigus vulgaris
水疱性類天疱瘡	bullous pemphigoid (BP)
進行性色素性皮膚症, シャンバーグ病	Schamberg disease

〈*progressive pigmentary dermatosis; characterized by pigmented purpura of the legs in young men*〉

播種性表在性光線性汗孔角化症	disseminated superficial actinic porokeratosis (DSAP)
黒色表皮腫	acanthosis nigricans (AN)
基底細胞癌	basal cell carcinoma (BCC)
ゴーリン症候群	Gorlin syndrome

〈*nevoid basal cell carcinoma syndrome; BCCs, pitted depression of the hands and feet, and bone anomalies with hypoplastic maxilla and frontal bossing; autosomal dominant*〉

| ボーエン病 | Bowen disease |

〈*intraepidermal squamous cell carcinoma*〉

悪性黒色腫	malignant melanoma (MM)
菌状息肉症	mycosis fungoides (MF), cutaneous T-cell lymphoma
セザリー症候群	Sézary syndrome

〈*cutaneous T-cell lymphoma with exfoliative erythroderma and intense pruritus*〉

皮膚良性リンパ節症	lymphadenosis benigna cutis (LABC), cutaneous lymphoid hyperplasia
全身性エリテマトーデス	systemic lupus erythematosus (SLE)
円板状エリテマトーデス	discoid lupus erythematosus (DLE)
皮膚エリテマトーデス	cutaneous lupus erythematosus (CLE)

顔面播種状粟粒性狼瘡 (ひふ / がんめんはしゅじょうぞくりゅうせいろうそう) — lupus miliaris disseminatus faciei (LMDF)

CREST症候群 (こうぐん) — *c*alcinosis cutis, *R*aynaud phenomenon, *e*sophageal dysfunction, *s*clerodactyly, *t*elangiectasia (CREST) syndrome

混合性結合組織病 (こんごうせいけつごうそしきびょう) — mixed connective tissue disease (MCTD)

進行性全身性強皮症 (しんこうせいぜんしんせいきょうひしょう) — progressive systemic sclerosis (PSS)

強皮症腎クリーゼ (きょうひしょうじん——) — scleroderma renal crisis (SRC)

弾力線維性仮性黄色腫 (だんりょくせんいせいかせいおうしょくしゅ) — pseudoxanthoma elasticum (PXE)

ハンセン病 (——びょう) — Hansen disease
〈*leprosy; a chronic granulomatous infection caused by Mycobacterium leprae*〉

晩発性皮膚ポルフィリン症 (ばんぱつせいひふ——しょう) — porphyria cutanea tarda (PCT)

● 治療法 Treatment ●

軟膏 (なんこう) — ointment
乳剤性軟膏 (にゅうざいせいなんこう) — emulsion ointment
親水軟膏 (しんすいなんこう) — hydrophilic ointment (HO)
吸水軟膏 (きゅうすいなんこう) — absorption ointment (AO)
油脂性軟膏 (ゆしせいなんこう) — oleaginous ointment
ワセリン — vaseline
亜鉛華軟膏 (あえんかなんこう) — zinc oxide ointment
泥膏 (でいこう) — paste
ローション剤 — lotion
塗布剤 (とふざい) — liniment
噴霧剤 (ふんむざい) — spray
皮膚軟化剤 (ひふなんかざい) — emollient
湿潤剤 (しつじゅんざい) — moisturizer, moistening agent
硬膏 (こうこう) — plaster
絆創膏 (ばんそうこう) — adhesive bandage
タクロリムス水和物 (——すいわぶつ) — tacrolimus hydrate《プロトピック》
化学的除去 (かがくてきじょきょ) — chemical peeling
密封包帯法 (みっぷうほうたいほう) — occlusive dressing technique (ODT)
水痘帯状疱疹免疫グロブリン (すいとうたいじょうほうしんめんえき——) — varicella-zoster immune globulin (VZIG), zoster immune globulin (ZIG)

15. 皮膚

ケトコナゾール	ketoconazole (KCZ)《ニゾラール》
ミコナゾール	miconazole (MCZ)《フロリード F》
イトラコナゾール	itraconazole (ITCZ)《イトリゾール》
テルビナフィン塩酸塩	terbinafine hydrochloride《ラミシール》
グリセオフルビン	griseofulvin (GRF)《ポンシル FP》
アシクロビル	acyclovir (ACV)《ゾビラックス》
バラシクロビル塩酸塩	valacyclovir hydrochloride (VACV)《バルトレックス》
ビダラビン	vidarabine, adenine arabinoside (Ara-A)《アラセナ-A》
ファムシクロビル	famcicrovir (FCV)《ファムビル》
トラフェルミン	trafermin《フィブラスト》
アダパレン	adapalene《ディフェリン》
スクアラン酸ジブチルエステル	squaric acid dibutylester (SADBE)
ソラレン長波長紫外線療法 ちょうはちょうしがいせんりょうほう	psoralen-ultraviolet A (PUVA) therapy
中波長紫外線 ちゅうはちょうしがいせん	ultraviolet B (UVB)
軟 X 線 なん—	soft x-ray
冷凍療法 れいとうりょうほう	cryotherapy, frigotherapy
凍結手術 とうけつしゅじゅつ	cryosurgery
液体窒素 えきたいちっそ	liquid nitrogen
レーザー凝固 —ぎょうこ	laser coagulation
爪切除術 そうせつじょじゅつ	onychectomy, nail excision
植皮術 しょくひじゅつ	skin grafting
皮膚移植片 ひふいしょくへん	skin graft

Tidbits

uncountable noun

名詞の可算,不可算は日本人には悩みの種である.不可算名詞は複数形をとらず不定冠詞や another, many, these などをつけないが,医学論文でよく用いる不可算名詞には, advice, assistance, behavior, character, dependence, encouragement, equipment, evidence, health, help, information, knowledge, literature, progress, proof, research などがある. "many informations" は誤りで, "much information", あるいは "many items of information" としなければならない. ただし例外的に, "He has a good knowledge of Greek.", "You've been a great help." のように具体的な意味の場合に単数扱いの用法がある.複数になることはない.

16. 小児科

●愁訴・症状　Complaints / Symptoms●

発育 はついく	development, growth, 〔形〕developmental
成長曲線 せいちょうきょくせん	growth curve
新生児 しんせいじ	newborn, neonate
乳児 にゅうじ	baby, infant
幼児 ようじ	small child
学童 がくどう	schoolchild
思春期 ししゅんき	puberty
育児 いくじ	child care, child rearing
子供を育てる こども―そだ―	raise (bring up) a child
揺りかご ゆ―	cradle
ベビーベッド	crib
かごベッド	bassinet
話しかけると笑う はな―わら―	smile when spoken to
頭を持ち上げようとする あたま―も―	try to raise head
首がすわる くび	hold head steady
寝返りを打つ ねがえ―	roll over
支えなしに座る ささ―すわ―	sit unsupported
這い這いする は―	crawl
摑まり立ちする つか―た―	stand holding on
一瞬立っていられる いっしゅんた―	stand unsupported for a second or two
一人歩きをする ひとりあ―	walk unaided
よちよち歩く ―あ―	toddle
歯が生える は―	teethe
指しゃぶり ゆび	thumb-sucking
おむつかぶれ	diaper rash
はしか, 麻疹 ましん	measles, rubeola
三日ばしか みっか―, 風疹 ふうしん	German measles, three-day measles, rubella
水ぼうそう みず―, 水痘 すいとう	chickenpox, varicella
おたふくかぜ, 流行性耳下腺炎 りゅうこうせいじかせんえん	mumps, epidemic parotitis
猩紅熱 しょうこうねつ	scarlet fever, scarlatina
百日咳 ひゃくにちぜき	whooping cough, pertussis
レプリーゼ	reprise
あせも	heat rash, prickly heat
みずいぼ	molluscum contagiosum

とびひ	impetigo
しもやけ	chilblain
おねしょ	bed-wetting, enuresis
大便失禁	fecal incontinence, encopresis
ひきつけ	a fit of convulsions
夜驚症	night terrors, pavor nocturnus
小児麻痺	infantile paralysis, polio

● 診察所見・徴候　Physical findings / Signs ●

アプガースコア	Apgar score

⟨*evaluation of the condition of a newborn infant, at 1 minute after birth, based on heart rate, respiratory effort, muscle tone, reflex irritability, and skin color*⟩

未熟児	premature infant
低出生体重児	low birth weight (LBW) infant
極低出生体重児	very low birth weight (VLBW) infant
超低出生体重児	extremely low birth weight (ELBW) infant
在胎期間軽小児	small-for-gestational-age (SGA) infant, small-for-dates (SFD) infant
在胎期間相当体重児	appropriate-for-gestational-age (AGA) infant, appropriate-for-dates (AFD) infant
在胎期間過大児	large-for-gestational-age (LGA) infant, large-for-dates (LFD) infant
無頭体	acephalus
無脳体	anencephalus
低身長	short stature
発育不全	failure to thrive (FTT)
カウプ指数	Kaup index

⟨*body mass index in infants; weight (g) × 10 / body length (cm) squared; normal range 15-18*⟩

ローレル指数	Röhrer index

⟨*measure of nutritional status in schoolchildren; weight (g) × 100 / height (cm) cubed; normal range 110-160*⟩

発達指数	developmental quotient (DQ)
蒙古斑	mongolian spot, mongolian blue spot
乳幼児突発性危急事態	apparent life-threatening event (ALTE)
熱性痙攣	febrile convulsions, febrile seizure
痙攣重積	status convulsivus, convulsive status

	epilepticus
点頭てんかん	infantile spasm, West syndrome
レノックス・ガストー症候群	Lennox-Gastaut syndrome

⟨*petit mal variant characterized by tonic, atonic, or clonic seizures, mental retardation, and slow spike waves*⟩

産瘤	caput succedaneum
大頭症	macrocephalus, macrocephaly
小頭症	microcephalus, microcephaly
水頭症	hydrocephalus, hydrocephaly
尖頭症	acrocephaly
船状頭蓋症	scaphocephalus, scaphocephaly
大泉門	anterior fontanelle (fontanel), fonticulus major
小泉門	posterior fontanelle (fontanel), fonticulus minor
大泉門閉鎖	closure of the anterior fontanelle
オプソクロヌス, 眼間代	opsoclonus
副耳	accessory ear
小耳症	microtia
上皮真珠	epithelial pearls
エプシュタイン真珠	Epstein pearls

⟨*small, whitish milia found in the midline of the hard plate of the newborn, which disappear within a few weeks*⟩

舌小帯短縮	short lingual frenulum
先天性エプーリス	congenital epulis
リガ・フェーデ病	Riga-Fede disease

⟨*sublingual ulceration in teething infants; caused by erupted lower central incisors*⟩

ベドナーアフタ	Bednar aphtha

⟨*symmetric excoriation of hard plate, probably due to sucking*⟩

口唇裂	cleft lip
口蓋裂	cleft palate, uranoschisis, palatoschisis
小顎症	micrognathia, micromandible
ピエール・ロバン症候群	Pierre Robin syndrome

⟨*cleft palate, micrognathia, glossoptosis, and frequent upper airway obstruction; autosomal recessive*⟩

斜頸	torticollis, wryneck
翼状頸	webbed neck, pterygium colli
ルーカス徴候	Lucas sign

⟨*abdominal distention in early rickets*⟩

多指症	polydactyly

16. 小児科

合指症 ごうしょう	syndactyly
体幹屈曲 たいかんくつきょく	trunk incurvation
緊張性頚反射 きんちょうせいけいはんしゃ	tonic neck reflex (TNR)
非対称性緊張性頚反射 ひたいしょうせいきんちょうせいけいはんしゃ	asymmetrical tonic neck reflex (ATNR)
モロー反射 はんしゃ	Moro reflex, Moro embrace reflex

⟨startle reflex, parachute reflex; brisk abduction of arms with extension and opening of palms and abduction and flexion of legs in response to a sudden stimulus⟩

プレー反射 はんしゃ　　Perez reflex

⟨extension of the whole body elicited by holding an infant in prone position and running a finger down the spine⟩

マキューイン徴候 ちょうこう　　Macewen sign

⟨percussion of the parietal bone produces cracked-pot sound before closure of skull sutures in normal infants; after infancy the sign indicates separation of sutures by increased intracranial pressure⟩

オルトラニ徴候 ちょうこう　　Ortolani sign

⟨a palpable click on flexing and abducting newborn's legs; positive for congenital dislocation of the hip⟩

トレンデレンブルク試験　　Trendelenburg test

⟨for detection of gluteus medius weakness in CDH or femoral neck fracture; the pelvis sags on the sound side during single leg standing on the affected side⟩

● 検査法　Examination ●

イクテロメータ	icterometer
ガスリー試験 けん	Guthrie test

⟨bacterial inhibition assay to detect serum phenylalanine⟩

チロシン尿 にょう	tyrosinuria
ミロン試験 けん	Millon test

⟨a test for proteins; tyrosine reacts with the solution of mercury and nitric acid to give a red color⟩

フェニルケトン尿 にょう	phenylketonuria (PKU)
メープルシロップ尿 にょう	maple syrup urine
分枝鎖ケト酸尿 ぶんしさけとさんにょう	branched-chain ketoaciduria
ジニトロフェニルヒドラジン試験 けん	dinitrophenylhydrazine test
ホモシスチン尿 にょう	homocystinuria
ニトロプルシド試験 けん	nitroprusside test
ガラクトース血症 けっしょう	galactosemia
尿中バニリルマンデル酸 にょうちゅう—さん	urinary vanillylmandelic acid (VMA)
尿中ホモバニル酸 にょうちゅう—さん	urinary homovanillic acid (HVA)

β溶血性連鎖球菌	β-hemolytic streptococcus
呼吸器合胞体ウイルス	respiratory syncytial virus (RSV)
抗麻疹ウイルス抗体	anti-measles virus antibody
抗風疹ウイルス抗体	anti-rubella virus antibody
抗ムンプス抗体	anti-mumps virus antibody
ヒトパルボウイルス B19	human parvovirus B19
ベロ毒素産生性大腸菌	verotoxin-producing *Escherichia coli* (VTEC)
ディック試験	Dick test

⟨*intradermal injection of group A streptococcal purified erythrogenic toxin to test susceptibility to scarlet fever*⟩

選択視法	preferential looking (PL)
行動観察聴力検査	behavioral observation audiometry
誘発耳音響放射	evoked otoacoustic emission (EOAE)
尖塔徴候	steeple sign
デンバー式発達スクリーニング検査	Denver Developmental Screening Test (DDST)
日本版デンバー式発達スクリーニング検査	Japanese edition of Denver Developmental Screening Test (JDDST)
ビネー式知能検査	Binet intelligence test

⟨*a method of testing mental capacity and mental age of children*⟩

ウェクスラー児童用知能検査	Wechsler Intelligence Scale for Children (WISC)

⟨*measurement of general intelligence in children 5 to 15 years of age*⟩

● 疾患名 Diseases ●

新生児仮死	neonatal asphyxia, asphyxia neonatorum
低酸素性虚血性脳症	hypoxic-ischemic encephalopathy (HIE)
新生児呼吸窮迫症候群	neonatal respiratory distress syndrome (RDS)
硝子膜症	hyaline membrane disease (HMD)
新生児一過性多呼吸	transient tachypnea of the newborn (TTN)

新生児黄疸	neonatal jaundice
新生児高ビリルビン血症	neonatal hyperbilirubinemia
核黄疸	kernicterus, bilirubin encephalopathy
クリグラー・ナジャール症候群	Crigler-Najjar syndrome

⟨congenital nonhemolytic jaundice due to absent glucuronosyltransferase; unconjugated bilirubinemia with kernicterus; autosomal recessive inheritance⟩

エルブ・デュシェンヌ麻痺	Erb-Duchenne paralysis

⟨upper brachial plexus paralysis due to birth injury⟩

クルンプケ麻痺	Klumpke paralysis

⟨lower brachial plexus paralysis caused by birth injury, seen in breech delivery⟩

新生児溶血性疾患	hemolytic disease of the newborn (HDN)
胎児赤芽球症	erythroblastosis fetalis (EBF)
ダイアモンド・ブラックファン貧血	Diamond-Blackfan anemia

⟨congenital hypoplastic anemia characterized by deficient erythroid precursors with normal other elements⟩

新生児同種免疫血小板減少症	neonatal alloimmune thrombocytopenia (NAIT)
先天性赤芽球性ポルフィリン症, ギュンター病	congenital erythopoietic porphyria (CEP), Günther disease

⟨increased porphyrin formation by erythroid cells in the bone marrow caused by deficiency of uroporphyrinogen-III synthase; hemolytic anemia, skin photosensitivity, and hypertrichosis; autosomal recessive⟩

赤血球産生性プロトポルフィリン症	erythropoietic protoporphyria (EPP)
ブルトン病	Bruton disease

⟨X-linked agammaglobulinemia characterized by lack of B cells with the onset of 6 months of age and recurrent pyogenic infections⟩

特発性新生児肝炎	idiopathic neonatal hepatitis
胎便吸引症候群	meconium aspiration syndrome (MAS)
非免疫性胎児水腫	nonimmune hydrops fetalis (NIHF)

新生児遷延性肺高血圧症	persistent pulmonary hypertension of the newborn (PPHN)
胎児循環遺残	persistent fetal circulation (PFC)
新生児壊死性腸炎	neonatal necrotizing enterocolitis (NEC)
新生児膿漏眼	neonatal blennorrhea
気管支肺異形成症	bronchopulmonary dysplasia (BPD)
未熟児慢性呼吸不全	chronic pulmonary insufficiency of prematurity (CPIP)
メープルシロップ尿症,楓糖尿症	maple syrup urine disease (MSUD)
クレチン病	cretinism, congenital hypothyroidism
先天性副腎過形成	congenital adrenal hyperplasia (CAH)

ディジョージ症候群　　DiGeorge syndrome
〈*congenital parathyroid and thymic hypoplasia, often with cardiac and facial anomalies*〉

ウォルフラム症候群　　Wolfram syndrome
〈*an autosomal recessive disorder, consisting of diabetes insipidus, diabetes mellitus, optic atrophy, and deafness, hence DIDMOAD*〉

軟骨異栄養症　　chondrodystrophy

ファンコーニ貧血　　Fanconi anemia
〈*congenital aplastic anemia; characterized by bone marrow hypoplasia and multiple anomalies; autosomal recessive*〉

ダウン症候群　　Down syndrome
〈*trisomy 21 associated with mental retardation, flattened skull, short nose, epicanthal folds, brachydactyly, duodenal atresia, and cardiac defects*〉

一過性異常骨髄造血　　transient abnormal myelopoiesis (TAM)

エドワーズ症候群　　Edwards syndrome
〈*trisomy 18 syndrome with low birth weight, scaphocephaly, micrognathia, congenital heart disease, spina bifida, and mental retardation*〉

ブルーム症候群　　Bloom syndrome
〈*dwarfism, photosensitivity, and butterfly telangiectatic erythema on the face; increased risk of leukemia; autosomal recessive*〉

ネコ鳴き症候群　　cat-cry syndrome, cri du chat syndrome

ファブリ病　　Fabry disease
〈*α-galactosidase A deficiency; marked by angiokeratomas, corneal*

opacities, hypohidrosis, paresthesia, vascular involvement, and retarded growth; X-linked recessive inheritance〉

クラッベ病 ［ーび］　Krabbe disease
〈*globoid cell leukodystrophy; a lysosomal storage disease marked by accumulation of galactocerebroside in the brain due to a lack of galactosylceramidase; blindness, seizures, and early death; autosomal recessive*〉

エーラス・ダンロー症候群 ［ーこうしょう］　Ehlers-Danlos syndrome
〈*a group of inherited connective tissue disorders marked by hyperextensible skin and joints, easy bruising, and posttraumatic pseudotumors; six types are distinguished*〉

マルファン症候群 ［ーこうしょう］　Marfan syndrome
〈*a congenital connective tissue disorder characterized by long limbs, arachnodactyly, joint laxity, lens subluxation, and aortic aneurysm; autosomal dominant*〉

ムコ多糖症 ［ーうしょう］　mucopolysaccharidosis (MPS)

ハーラー症候群 ［ーこうしょう］　Hurler syndrome
〈*mucopolysaccharidosis I caused by L-iduronidase deficiency; gargoylism, dwarfism, kyphosis, corneal clouding, hirsutism, hepatosplenomegaly, and mental retardation; autosomal recessive*〉

ハンター症候群 ［ーこうしょう］　Hunter syndrome
〈*mucopolysaccharidosis II caused by iduronate sulfatase deficiency; similar to Hurler syndrome but less severe and absent corneal clouding; X-linked recessive*〉

ワールデンブルグ症候群　Waardenburg syndrome
〈*hereditary deafness and pigmentary defects due to failure of melanocyte to migrate from neural crest; white forelock, leukoderma, heterochromia iridis, displacement of medial canthi, and broad nasal root; four types based on genetic and clinical features*〉

テイ症候群 ［ーこうぐん］　Tay syndrome
〈*IBIDS syndrome; ichthyosis, brittle hair, infertility, developmental delay, and short stature; autosomal recessive*〉

レッシュ・ナイハン症候群 ［ーこうしょう］　Lesch-Nyhan syndrome
〈*complete HGPRT deficiency disease; an X-linked disorder of purine metabolism due to deficient hypoxanthine-guanine phosphoribosyl transferase, characterized by mental retardation, self-mutilation, choreoathetosis, hyperuricemia, and uricaciduria; fatal in childhood*〉

くる病 ［ーび］　rickets
ビタミンD依存性くる病 ［ーいぞんせいーびょう］　vitamin D-dependent rickets (VDDR)
デトーニ・ファンコーニ　de Toni-Fanconi syndrome

症候群	⟨*renal rickets with dwarfism; the most common cause is cystinosis*⟩
胎児性アルコール症候群	fetal alcohol syndrome (FAS)
口・顔・指症候群	oral-facial-digital (OFD) syndrome
トーチ症候群	TORCH (*t*oxoplasmosis, *o*ther agents, *r*ubella, *c*ytomegalovirus, *h*erpes simplex) syndrome
プラダー・ウィリ症候群	Prader-Willi syndrome (PWS)
	⟨*short stature, obesity, mental retardation, hypogonadism, and muscular hypotonia; caused by a break in chromosome 15*⟩
唇顎口蓋裂	cheilognathopalatoschisis
先天性心疾患 (cf. 循環器系)	congenital heart disease (CHD)
左心低形成症候群	hypoplastic left heart syndrome (HLHS)
先天性風疹症候群	congenital rubella syndrome (CRS)
先天性食道閉鎖	congenital esophageal atresia
気管食道瘻	tracheoesophageal fistula (TEF)
肥厚性幽門狭窄	hypertrophic pyloric stenosis
鎖肛	anal atresia, imperforate anus
腸重積	intussusception
軸捻	volvulus
ラッド症候群	Ladd syndrome
	⟨*congenital duodenal obstruction due to peritoneal bands, Ladd bands, and cecal volvulus*⟩
ヒルシュシュプルング病	Hirschsprung disease
	⟨*congenital megacolon; colonic obstruction due to absence of ganglion cells in the rectosigmoid and rectum*⟩
先天性胆道閉鎖症	congenital biliary atresia (CBA)
先天性横隔膜ヘルニア	congenital diaphragmatic hernia (CDH)
ボックダレックヘルニア	Bochdalek hernia
	⟨*most common type of CDH due to a posterolateral diaphragmatic defect that results from failure of fusion of the pleuroperitoneal canal*⟩
モルガニーヘルニア	Morgagni hernia
	⟨*a CDH with extrusion of the abdominal contents, usually through the right retrosternal Morgagni foramen; often asymptomatic*⟩
鼠径ヘルニア	inguinal hernia

| 臍帯ヘルニア | umbilical hernia, exomphalos |
| ベックウィズ・ウィーデマン症候群, EMG症候群 | Beckwith-Wiedeman syndrome, EMG syndrome |

⟨*exomphalos-macroglossia-gigantism syndrome; autosomal dominant*⟩

腹壁破裂	gastroschisis
間欠性水腎症	intermittent hydronephrosis
幼児型多発性囊胞腎	infantile polycystic kidney
乳児突然死症候群	sudden infant death syndrome (SIDS), crib death
小児型呼吸促迫症候群	infant respiratory distress syndrome (IRDS)
ウィスコット・アルドリッチ症候群	Wiskott-Aldrich syndrome (WAS)

⟨*an immunodeficiency in male children characterized by eczema, thrombocytopenia, and susceptibility to infections; X-linked recessive*⟩

乳児湿疹	infantile eczema
水疱性口峡炎, ヘルパンギーナ	herpangina
突発性発疹	exanthema subitum, roseola infantum, sixth disease
伝染性紅斑, 第5病	erythema infectiosum, infectious erythema, fifth disease
ジアノッティ・クロスティ症候群	Gianotti-Crosti syndrome

⟨*infantile acrodermatitis; a self-limited viral disease characterized by papules on the face, buttocks and limbs, most commonly by hepatitis B virus*⟩

単純型先天表皮水疱症	epidermolysis bullosa simplex (EBS)
手足口病	hand-foot-and-mouth disease (HFMD)
ライ症候群	Reye syndrome

⟨*acute encephalopathy as a sequel of influenza or varicella infection; characterized by recurrent vomiting, disturbed consciousness, elevated ammonia and transaminase levels, and fatty liver; related to aspirin therapy*⟩

| 出血性ショック・脳症候群 | hemorrhagic shock and encephalopathy syndrome (HSE) |
| 急性小脳性失調症 | acute cerebellar ataxia |

クループ症候群 こうぐん	croup syndrome
急性喉頭気管気管支炎 きゅうせいこうとうきかんきかんしえん	acute laryngotracheobronchitis
急性喉頭蓋炎 きゅうせいこうとうがいえん	acute epiglottitis
痙性クループ けいせい	spasmodic croup
リウマチ熱 ねつ	rheumatic fever
連鎖球菌感染後急性糸球体腎炎 れんさきゅうきんかんせんごきゅうせいしきゅうたいじんえん	acute poststreptococcal glomerulonephritis (APSGN)
ヘノッホ・シェーンライン紫斑病 しはんびょう	Henoch-Schönlein purpura (HSP) ⟨allergic or anaphylactoid purpura; nonthrombocytopenic purpura associated with arthritis, abdominal pain, melena, and glomerulonephritis⟩
ウォーターハウス・フリーデリクセン症候群	Waterhouse-Friderichsen syndrome ⟨acute fulminating meningococcal septicemia with bilateral adrenal hemorrhages⟩
シャーガス病 びょう	Chagas disease ⟨South American trypanosomiasis characterized by erythematous nodule, fever, and lymphadenopathy; cardiomyopathy, achalasia, and megacolon in chronic form⟩
川崎病 かわさきびょう，皮膚粘膜リンパ節症候群 ひふねんまくせつしょうこうぐん	Kawasaki disease, mucocutaneous lymph node syndrome (MCLS) (MLNS) ⟨systemic vasculitis in children, characterized by fever, erythema of the skin and oral cavity, conjunctivitis, lymphadenopathy, and desquamation of the fingers; may develop coronary artery aneurysm⟩
乳児性骨皮質過形成，キャフィー病 にゅうじせいこつひしつかけいせい，——びょう	infantile cortical hyperostosis, Caffey disease ⟨hypertrophy of cortical bone with soft tissue swellings and fever, affecting the mandible, clavicle, and long bones⟩
若年性関節リウマチ じゃくねんせいかんせつ——	juvenile rheumatoid arthritis (JRA)
肘内障 ちゅうないしょう	internal derangement of the elbow joint
先天性股関節脱臼 せんてんせいこかんせつだっきゅう	congenital dislocation of the hip (CDH)
発育性股関節形成異常 はついくせいこかんせつけいせいいじょう	developmental dysplasia of the hip (DDH)
先天性内反足 せんてんせいないはんそく	congenital clubfoot, talipes equinovarus

16. 小児科

先天性多発性関節拘縮症	arthrogryposis multiplex congenita (AMC)
尖頭合指症	acrocephalosyndactyly
尖頭多合指症	acrocephalopolysyndactyly (ACPS)
アペール症候群	Apert syndrome

⟨acrocephalosyndactyly type 1; acrocephaly, syndactyly of 2nd-5th fingers and toes, cleft palate, and mental retardation; autosomal dominant⟩

カーペンター症候群	Carpenter syndrome

⟨acrocephalopolysyndactyly type 2; acrocephaly, polydactyly, syndactyly, obesity, hypogonadism, and mental retardation; autosomal recessive⟩

クリッペル・フェール症候群	Klippel-Feil syndrome

⟨congenital anomaly with a short neck due to fusion of cervical vertebrae; autosomal dominant, sporadic⟩

進行性骨化性線維異形成症	fibrodysplasia ossificans progressiva (FOP)
進行性骨幹異形成症, カムラチ・エンゲルマン症候群	progressive diaphyseal dysplasia, Camurati-Engelmann syndrome

⟨symmetrical fusiform enlargement of long bones due to thickening of diaphysis associated with bone pain and waddling gait⟩

遺伝性進行性関節眼症, スティックラー症候群	hereditary progressive arthro-ophthalmopathy, Stickler syndrome

⟨hypoplastic mandible, cleft palate, and skeletal dysplasia with myopia, retinal detachment, and deafness; autosomal dominant⟩

下顎顔面異形成症, トリーチャーコリンズ症候群	mandibulofacial dysostosis, Treacher Collins syndrome

⟨micrognathia, hypoplastic zygomatic arches, coloboma palpebrae, and antimongoloid slanting of the palpebral fissures⟩

起立性調節障害	orthostatic dysregulation (OD)
中心・側頭部棘波をもつ良性小児てんかん	benign epilepsy of childhood with centrotemporal spikes (BECCT)
脊髄性筋萎縮症	spinal muscular atrophy (SMA)
ウェルドニッヒ・ホフマン病	Werdnig-Hoffmann disease

⟨spinal muscular atrophy type I caused by neuron destruction;

クーゲルベルク・ウェランダー病 　Kugelberg-Welander disease
〈spinal muscular atrophy type III caused by degeneration of motor neurons in the anterior horns; onset in childhood〉

カーンズ・セイヤー症候群 　Kearns-Sayer syndrome (KSS)
〈progressive external ophthalmoplegia, retinitis pigmentosa, and cardiac conduction defect; due to mutations in mitochondrial DNA〉

脳動静脈奇形	cerebral arteriovenous malformation
二分脊椎	spina bifida
髄膜瘤	meningocele
脊髄空洞症	syringomyelia
脳室周囲白質軟化症	periventricular leukomalacia (PVL)
脳性麻痺	cerebral palsy (CP)
小児交代性片麻痺	alternating hemiplegia in infants

ランゲルハンス細胞組織球症 　Langerhans cell histiocytosis (LCH)
〈formerly histiocytosis X; a set of disorders characterized by proliferation of Langerhans cells; lytic bone lesions with involvement of the bone marrow, endocrine organs, and lungs〉

ハンド・シュラー・クリスチャン病 　Hand-Schüller-Christian disease
〈multifocal Langerhans cell histiocytosis; cholesterol accumulation and xanthomatosis; classic triad consists of bone defects, exophthalmos, and diabetes insipidus〉

レットレル・ジーベ病 　Letterer-Siwe disease
〈acute disseminated Langerhans cell histiocytosis; onset in infancy of hemorrhagic rash, anemia, lymphadenopathy, and hepatosplenomegaly; autosomal recessive〉

脳腫瘍	brain tumor
神経芽腫	neuroblastoma
網膜芽細胞腫	retinoblastoma
原始神経外胚葉性腫瘍	primitive neuroectodermal tumor (PNET)
ウィルムス腫瘍	Wilms tumor

〈nephroblastoma; embryonal adenomyosarcoma〉

スタージ・ウェーバー症候群 　Sturge-Weber syndrome
〈encephalotrigeminal angiomatosis with seizures, hemiparesis, men-

tal retardation, and meningeal calcifications⟩

微細脳機能障害	minimal brain dysfunction (MBD)
知的障害	mental retardation
発達性言語障害	developmental language disorder
注意欠陥障害	attention deficit disorder (ADD)
注意欠陥多動障害	attention-deficit hyperactivity disorder (ADHD)
自閉性障害	autistic disorder
カナー症候群	Kanner syndrome, infantile autism
小児虐待	child abuse
児童性的虐待	child molestation
代理人によるミュンヒハウゼン症候群	Munchausen syndrome by proxy (MSBP)

⟨*<Münchhausen; a factitious disorder characterized by deliberate infliction of harm on another person, usually a child, to induce illness and hospitalization for gaining attention*⟩

思春期早発症	precocious puberty
登校拒否	school refusal

● 治療法　Treatment ●

新生児集中治療	neonatal intensive care
新生児集中治療室	neonatal intensive care unit (NICU)
小児集中治療室	pediatric intensive care unit (PICU)
保育器	incubator
光線療法	phototherapy, actinotherapy
交換輸血	exchange transfusion
体外式膜型人工肺	extracorporeal membrane oxygenation (ECMO)
肺サーファクタント	pulmonary surfactant
母乳栄養	breast-feeding, 〔形〕breast-fed
人工栄養	bottle-feeding, 〔形〕bottle-fed
調合乳	formula
授乳	nursing
初乳	colostrum
哺乳瓶	nursing bottle
離乳	weaning, ablactation
離乳食	weaning food
予防接種	immunization, inoculation, vaccination
三種混合ワクチン	triple vaccine, diphtheria-tetanus-

IV章 診療録用語

	pertussis (DTP) vaccine
ポリオワクチン	poliovirus vaccine
BCGワクチン	BCG vaccine
麻疹・風疹混合ワクチン ましん・ふうし こんごう	measles-rubella vaccine
日本脳炎ワクチン にほんのう えん	Japanese B encephalitis vaccine
水痘ワクチン すいとう	varicella vaccine
流行性耳下腺炎ワクチン りゅうこうせいじ かせんえん	mumps vaccine
インフルエンザワクチン	influenza vaccine
インフルエンザ菌b型ワクチン きん がた	*Haemophilus influenzae* type b (Hib) vaccine
7価肺炎球菌結合型ワクチン かはいえんきゅう きんけつごうがた	heptavalent pneumococcal conjugate vaccine《プレベナー》
パリビズマブ	palivizumab《シナジス》
ヒト免疫グロブリン めん えき	human normal immunoglobulin
成長ホルモン せいちょ	somatotropin

Tidbits

gargoylism

「ガーゴイリズム」は，ハーラー症候群の原因がムコ多糖の蓄積と判明するまで患児の特異な顔貌が gargoyle に類似することから名付けられた呼称である．gargoyle とは，ゴシック建築の教会の屋根に作られた雨水の落とし口のグロテスクな彫像で，ノートルダム寺院のもの（gargouilles de Notre-Dame）が有名．gargoyle はフランス語の gargouille（spout, gullet のこと）に由来し語源はラテン語の garugulio である．語根の gar が swallow を意味し，「うがい」の gargle（〔仏〕gargariser）もラテン語の gargarizo に由来する．

V章

診療英会話

1. 問診の英会話

●インタビューを始める　Interview●

スミスさん，お早うございます．木村です．
　Good morning, Mr. Smith. I am Dr. Kimura.

はじめまして，ジョーンズさん．山田です．
　Hello, Mr. Jones. I'm Dr. Yamada. Nice to meet you.

今日はどういうことでしょうか？
　How can I help you today? / What can I do for you today?

今日はどんなことで受診されましたか？
　What made you come in today?
　Tell me, what made you come in?
　So, what brought you to the hospital today?

どうされましたか？
　What is the trouble? / What is your problem?
　What is wrong with you? / What seems to be the problem?

具合はいかがですか？
　How do you feel? / How are you feeling?
　How are you doing? / How are you getting along?

最近の調子はいかがですか？
　How have you been recently?

大体どんな具合でしたか？
　How have you been feeling in general?

どのような症状ですか？
　What symptoms do you have?

症状を言ってみてください．
　Tell me what symptoms you have.

病気のことを話してください．
　Tell me about your illness.

何があったのですか？
　What has happened? / Tell me what happened.

何か気になりますか？
　What is worrying you?

何か心配なことがありますか？
　Is there anything that is making you worry?

一番困る症状は何ですか？
What symptom bothers you the most?

何が一番心配ですか？
What are you most worried about?

全部お話しください．
Tell me all about it.

他に何かありましたか？
Did anything else happen?

それからどうなりましたか？
What happened next?

他に何か仰りたいことがありますか？
Is there anything else you want to mention?
Is there anything else you would like to tell me about?

● 患者の訴え　Patient's complaints ●

詳しい健診をしてください．
I think I need a complete check-up.

コレステロールを調べてください．
I want my cholesterol checked.

何週間もそこら中が痛いです
I have been aching all over for weeks.

元気がなくて疲れやすいで
I have no energy and get tired easily.

くたくたです．
I'm so tired. / I'm exhausted. / I'm worn out. / I'm dog-tired.

この2ヵ月で8キロ痩せました．
I have lost 8 kilos in the past two months.

熱があります．
I have a fever. / I'm running a fever. / I'm feverish.

寒気がします．
I have the chills.

今朝起きたら頭がずきずきしていました．
This morning I woke up with a throbbing headache.

のどが痛くて何も飲み込めません．
I have a sore throat, and cannot swallow a thing.

ひどいかぜのようです．
I seem to have a bad cold.

しつこいかぜに悩まされています．
I can't seem to shake off my nagging cold.

鼻づまりです．
I have a stuffy nose. / My nose is stuffed up.

鼻水が出ます．
I have a runny nose. / My nose is running.

耳が聞こえにくいです．
I can't hear well. / I have a hard time hearing.
I'm hard of hearing. / My hearing is poor.

耳鳴りがします．
My ears are ringing. / There is a ringing in my ears.
I have a noise in my ears.

のどに何か引っかかっている感じです．
I feel like something is stuck in my throat.

この頃胸が痛みます．
I have been having chest pains these days.

胸に重しがある感じです．
I feel like I have a heavy weight on my chest.

急いで階段を昇っているときに急に胸の圧迫感が起こりました．
All of a sudden I felt pressure in my chest when I was running up the stairs.

動悸がします．
I have palpitations. / My heart palpitates.

急ぎ足で息が切れます．
I get short of breath when I walk fast.

2ヵ月前から足首のところがむくんでいます．
My ankles have been swollen for two months.

胃がむかむかします．
I feel sick to my stomach. / I've got a queasy stomach.
I feel like I'm going to throw up.

胃がしくしく痛みます．
I have a gnawing pain in the stomach.

去年から胃の調子が悪く，今週は胸焼けがひどいです．
I've had an upset stomach since last year, and heartburn which is worse this week.

おなかが張ります．
I feel bloated. / I feel gassy.

長い間便秘に悩まされています．
I've been troubled with constipation for a long time.

夜中に4回以上排尿のために起こされます．
I have to wake up more than four times at night to urinate.

おしっこが我慢できません．
I have trouble holding my water.

めまいがします．
I feel dizzy. / I feel giddy. / My head is spinning.

急に立ち上がるとめまいがします．
I become dizzy when I stand up suddenly.

ぼやけて見えます．
Things are blurry. / My vision has become blurry.

目がしょぼしょぼします．
I have bleary eyes.

このところいつも塞ぎ込んでいて，寝付きも悪いです．
These days I feel depressed all the time and can't fall asleep easily.

コーヒーを飲むとき手が震えます．
My hand shakes when I drink my coffee.

石につまずいて前のめりに倒れました．
I stumbled over a stone and fell forward.

背中が痛みます．
I have a pain in my back. / My back hurts.

右腕の骨を折りました．
I broke my right arm.

夜中にこむらがえりが起こります．
I get cramps in my calf during the night.
I get a charley horse in my leg during the night.

長距離歩くと脚がつります．
I get leg cramps when I walk a long way.

左足首をくじいたに違いありません．
I must have sprained my left ankle.

腕が変にぴくぴく動くようになりました．
I began to notice strange jerky movements in my arms.

真夜中に右足の親指の激痛で目が覚めました．
I was awakened by severe pain in my right big toe in the middle of the night.

顔に発疹ができました．
A rash has broken out on my face.

左足の黒子が濃くなり少し大きくなりました．
The mole on my left foot appears to have become darker and a bit larger.

● 症状について尋ねる　Symptoms ●

どんな，どこ，いつ，どのように，何故？
What? Where? When? How? Why?

症状はどんな具合ですか？
What does the symptom feel like?

この症状がありますか？
Do you have this symptom?

症状についてもう少し話してください．
Tell me more about your ～.

詳しく説明してくださいますか？
Can you describe the ～ further?

その他に症状はありますか？
Do you have any other symptoms?

どのようにしてけがをしたのですか？
How did you injure yourself?

どんな時に起こりますか？
When do you have the ～?

いつ気がつきましたか？
When did you notice the ～?

いつ始まりましたか？
When did the ～ begin? / When did it start?
Since when?

1. 問診の英会話

最初にあったのはいつでしたか？
　When was the first time you had the ~?

最初気付いたとき何をしていましたか？
　What were you doing when you first noticed the ~?

どのくらい前からですか？
　How long have you had this symptom? ／ For how long?

どのくらい続きますか？
　How long does the ~ last?

いつ頃から悩んでますか？
　How long has the ~ been bothering you?

いつから具合が悪いですか？
　How long have you been ill?

きっかけは何だったようですか？
　What seems to trigger the ~?

起こる頻度はどのくらいですか？
　How often do you get the ~?
　How often does this symptom come on?

1ヵ月に何回ありますか？
　How many times a month do you get the ~?

1週間に何回ありますか？
　How often do you get the ~ in a week?

1年間に何回起こりましたか？
　How many times a year has the ~ happened?

何日間続きましたか？
　How many days did the ~ last?

どういうふうに辛いですか？
　In what way is the ~ bothering you?

どのように体にこたえますか？
　How does the ~ affect you?

どれくらい辛いですか？
　How severe is the ~?

和らげるために何かしますか？
　What do you do to relieve the ~?

仕事に影響がありますか？
　Does the ~ affect your work?

そのため仕事を休むことになりましたか？
　Have you lost time from work because of the ~?

薬を飲んでますか？
　Are you taking medicines for your ~?

原因について何か思い当たることがありますか？
　Do you have any ideas about what might be causing the ~?

● 全身状態　General ●

健康状態はいかがですか？
　How is your general health?

健康ですか？
　Are you in good health?

健康状態に何か変わりがありましたか？
　Has there been any change in your health?

疲れ易いですか？
　Do you tire easily?

疲労に悩まされてましたか？
　Have you been troubled by fatigue?

最近体重の増減はありましたか？
　Has your weight changed recently?

体重の変動に気が付きましたか？
　Have you noticed any change in your weight?

体重が増えていますか？
　Have you been gaining weight?

先月から体重が増えましたか？
　Have you put on any weight in the last month?

体重が減りましたか？
　Have you lost any weight?

どのくらい体重が減りましたか？
　How much weight have you lost?

昨年体重はいくらありましたか？
　How much did you weigh last year?

何キロ減りましたか？
　How many kilograms did you lose?

よく眠れますか？
　Do you sleep well?

眠りにくいことがありますか？
　Are you having any difficulty sleeping?
　Do you have trouble sleeping?

夜の睡眠時間はどのくらいですか？
　How many hours do you sleep at night?

昼間眠いことがありますか？
　Do you feel sleepy during the day?

寝付きが悪いですか？
　Do you have any problems falling asleep?

いびきをかきますか？
　Do you snore?

睡眠薬を飲みますか？
　Do you take any sleeping pills?

発熱していますか？
　Are you running a fever?

熱や寒気がありますか？
　Do you have a fever or chills?

どれくらいの熱でしたか？
　How high was your fever?

寝汗をかきますか？
　Do you have night sweats?

●疼痛　Pain●

痛むところがありますか？
　Do you have pain?

どこが痛みますか？
　Where is the pain? / Where does it hurt?
　Where is it sore?

痛みの場所はどこですか？
　Where is the pain located?

どこが一番痛みますか？
  Where do you feel the pain most?

正確に言うとどこに痛みがありましたか？
  Exactly where did you feel the pain?

痛む場所を示してください．
  Show me where it hurts. / Point to where you feel the pain.

どんな痛みですか？
  What kind of pain is it? / What is the pain like?

どんな痛みか説明できますか？
  Can you describe the pain?

言ってみるとずきずきする痛みですか？
  Would you describe it as a throbbing pain?

このような痛みは以前にもありましたか？
  Have you ever had a pain like this before?

似たような痛みの経験がありますか？
  Have you had a similar pain before?

痛みの程度はどれくらいでしたか？
  How severe was the pain? / How intense was the pain?

痛みはどのくらい続きますか？
  How long does the pain last?

今まで痛みはどのくらい続いていますか？
  How long have you had the pain?

痛みが治まる迄どのくらいかかりましたか？
  How long did it take for the pain to go away?

痛みの起こる頻度はどれくらいでしたか？
  How often did the pain occur?

痛みは突然きたのですか？
  Did the pain come on suddenly?

絶え間ない痛みですか，間隔がありますか？
  Is the pain constant, or does it come at intervals?

絶えず痛いですか，それとも来たりひいたりしますか？
  Is it a constant pain or does it come and go?

痛みが起きる原因が分かりますか？
  Do you know what causes the pain to start?

1. 問診の英会話

どうして痛みが起きますか？
  What brings the pain on?

痛みの場所は同じですか？
  Does the pain stay in one place?

痛みはどこかへ移動しますか？
  Does the pain go anywhere else?

痛みは他所へ広がりますか？
  Does the pain spread anywhere?

痛みが脚に下りていきますか？
  Does the pain travel down your legs?

どうすると痛みがとれますか？
  What makes the pain go away?

何かで痛みがきつくなりますか？
  Does anything make the pain worse?

痛みで睡眠が妨げられますか？
  Does the pain interfere with sleep?
  Does the pain disrupt your sleep?

頭痛で夜目が覚めますか？
  Do your headaches wake you up at night?

苦痛が減るように感じる体位がありますか？
  Does any position help you to feel more comfortable?

座ると痛みが楽になりますか？
  Does sitting up help the pain?

横になると痛みが楽になりますか？
  Does lying down ease the pain?

発作中はどうなさいますか？
  What do you do during the attack?

● 眼 Eyes ●

眼の具合が悪かったことがありますか？
  Have you had any trouble with your eyes?

視力はいかがですか？
  How is your vision?

眼がかすみますか？
  Does your vision blur? / Do you have blurred vision?

遠方が見えにくいですか？
　Do you have trouble seeing in the distance?

二重に見えますか？
　Do you see double? / Do you suffer from double vision?

眼に痛みがありますか？
　Do you have pain in your eyes?

眼の奥に痛みがありますか？
　Do you have pain behind your eyes?

黒点が見えますか？
　Do you see spots in front of your eyes?

眼の前を何か飛んでいるように見えることがありますか？
　Have you noticed things seeming to float before your eyes?

まぶたがぴくぴくしますか？
　Does your eyelids flicker?

眼鏡を掛けていますか？
　Do you wear glasses?

コンタクトレンズをしていますか？
　Are you wearing contact lenses?

目薬を差していますか？
　Are you using any eye drops?

●耳鼻咽喉　Ear, nose and throat●

耳が痛みますか？
　Do your ears hurt? / Do you have pain in your ears?

聴力はいかがですか？
　How is your hearing?

難聴がありますか？
　Do you have any difficulty hearing?

右側の耳だれはいつからですか？
　How long have you had this discharge from your right ear?

耳鳴りがありますか？
　Do you get ringing in your ears?
　Do you hear buzzing or ringing noises?

耳鳴りの時にめまいがしますか？
　Do you feel dizzy when the ringing happens?

職場で騒音に曝されることが多いですか？
　Are you often exposed to loud noises at work?

体のバランスがとれないことがありますか？
　Do you have a loss of balance?
　Do you often lose your balance?

鼻づまりがありましたか？
　Have you ever had a stuffy nose?

鼻血に悩まされたことがありますか？
　Have you been troubled with nosebleeds?

しょっちゅうくしゃみが出ますか？
　Do you have frequent sneezing?

匂いは分かりますか？
　How is your sense of smell?

嗅覚に変わりはありませんか？
　Have you noticed any change in your sense of smell?

咽頭痛や飲み込むときの痛みがありますか？
　Do you have sore throat and pain when swallowing?

首にぐりぐりがありますか？
　Do you have any swollen glands in your neck?

声が嗄れてきましたか？
　Has your voice become hoarse?

● 呼吸器・循環器系　Respiratory and circulatory systems ●

胸痛がありますか？
　Do you have a pain in your chest?

胸痛の経験がありますか？
　Have you had a pain in your chest?

胸部の圧迫を覚えたことがありますか？
　Have you had any pressure in your chest?

胸痛が始まった時に何をしていましたか？
　What were you doing when the chest pain started?

胸痛は腕や首の方に行きますか？
　Does the chest pain go into your arm or neck?

休めば胸痛は治まりますか？
　Does the chest pain settle down when you rest?

舌下錠で胸痛は治まりましたか？
　Did the sublingual tablets help to relieve the chest pain?

動悸がありますか？
　Do you have palpitations?

心臓の鼓動が速いのを感じますか？
　Do you feel your heart beating fast?

心臓の鼓動が不規則なことがありましたか？
　Have you noticed your heart beating irregularly?

心拍が早くなったり遅くなったりしましたか？
　Have you noticed your heartbeat speed up or slow down?

動悸は急に止まりましたか？
　Did the palpitations stop suddenly?

咳が出ますか？
　Do you have a cough?

咳をして何か吐き出すことがありますか？
　Do you cough anything up?
　Are you bringing up something when you cough?

咳は日中と夜とではどちらがきついですか？
　Is the cough worse during the day or at night?

血痰を出したことがありますか？
　Have you ever coughed up blood?

痰に血が付いてますか？
　Is there any blood in phlegm?

痰の中の血液に気付いたことがありますか？
　Have you noticed any blood in your sputum?

息が切れることがありますか？
　Do you have any shortness of breath?

息切れしたことがありますか？
　Have you had any trouble breathing?
　Do you ever get short of breath?

どんな時に息が切れますか？
　When do you feel short of breath?

休んでいるときに息が切れますか？
　Do you feel out of breath at rest?

階段を上がるときに息切れしますか？
Do you get short of breath when you climb stairs?

夜中に息苦しくて目が覚めることがありますか？
Do you sometimes wake up at night because you are short of breath?

ぜいぜい息をしていますか？
Have you been wheezing?

血圧が高かったことがありますか？
Have you ever had high blood pressure?

家での血圧はどれくらいですか？
What are your blood pressure readings at home?

足が腫れますか？
Do your feet swell?

足首のむくみを認めましたか？
Have you noted any swelling of your ankles?

夕方に脚がむくみますか？
Do your legs swell in the evening?

胸の写真を撮ったことがありますか？
Have you ever had a chest X-ray?

● 消化器系　Gastrointestinal system ●

最近食欲はいかがですか？
How is your appetite lately?

食欲はどんな具合ですか？
What is your appetite like?

食欲は良いですか？
Do you have a good appetite?

食欲が変わりましたか？
Has your appetite changed?

最近食が細くなりましたか？
Have you been eating less recently?

食べ物を呑み込むときに具合が悪いですか？
Do you have any trouble swallowing food?

流動物と固形物で呑み込み難いのは？
Do you have more difficulty swallowing liquids or solids?

胃痛がありますか？
　Do you have pain in your stomach?

腹痛がありますか？
　Do you have any abdominal pain?

どんな食物で痛みが強くなりますか？
　What foods aggravate your pain?

食べると痛みは軽くなりますか？
　Does the pain diminish when you eat?

油物やフライは口に合いませんか？
　Do fatty or fried foods disagree with you?

吐き気や嘔吐がありましたか？
　Have you had any nausea or vomiting?

吐き気を催しましたか？
　Did you feel nauseated?

吐き気がよくありますか？
　Do you have frequent nausea?

吐いた量はどのくらいでしたか？
　How much did you vomit?

吐物の色はどうでしたか？
　What color was the vomit?

便通の不調がありますか？
　Do you have any trouble with your bowel movements?

最近便通に変化がありましたか？
　Has your bowel habit changed recently?

1日に何回便通がありますか？
　How many bowel movements do you have per day?
　How many times do you go to the bathroom in a day?

便秘ですか？
　Are you constipated?

頻繁に下剤を使いますか？
　Do you use laxatives frequently?

便の色はどうですか？
　What color is your stool?

便の色や匂いが変なことがありましたか？
　Have your stools had an unusual color or odor?

便に血を認めたことがありますか？
　Have you noticed any blood in your stools?

黒色便のことがありましたか？
　Have you ever had black stools?

排便時いきまなければなりませんか？
　Do you have to strain to move your bowels?

白目が黄色に見えましたか？
　Did the whites of your eyes look yellow?

● 泌尿器系　Urinary system ●

尿が出にくいことがありますか？
　Do you have any difficulty urinating?

排尿時に痛みがありますか？
　Do you have pain when you pass urine?

排尿時にひりひりしますか？
　Does it burn when you urinate?

いきまないと尿がでませんか？
　Do you need to strain to urinate?

最初尿が出にくいことがありますか？
　Do you notice any difficulty when you start to urinate?
　Do you have trouble starting your flow?
　Is there a delay before you start to urinate?

排尿の勢いに何か変化がありましたか？
　Have you noticed any change in the force of the stream of urine?

排尿後に2時間以上我慢できますか？
　Can you hold urine more than two hours after you finished urinating?

夜中に排尿に起きますか？
　Do you get up at night to urinate?

夜中に排尿に起きなければなりませんか？
　Do you have to get up in the night to urinate?

夜中に何回排尿しますか？
> How often do you urinate at night?

尿の色が変わりましたか？
> Has the urine color changed?
> Have you noticed any change in the color of your urine?

尿に血液が混じったことがありますか？
> Have you ever had blood in your urine?
> Have you seen blood in the urine?

腎臓結石に罹ったことがありますか？
> Have you ever had a kidney stone?

腰の辺りの片方に痛みがありますか？
> Do you have pain in one side of the small of your back?

● 生殖器系　Reproductive system ●

生理はいかがですか？
> How are your periods?

生理は規則正しいですか？
> Are your periods regular?
> Do you have your periods regularly?

最終月経はいつでしたか？
> When was your last period?
> When did your last period begin?

初潮は何歳のときでしたか？
> How old were you when your periods started?
> At what age did you have your first menstrual period?
> At what age did you start having your period?

閉経はいつでしたか？
> When did your periods stop?
> At what age did you stop menstruating?

生理痛がありますか？
> Do you have any difficulties with your periods?
> Do you have any pain or cramps with periods?

月経の前に痛みますか？
> Do you get pain before your periods?

生理の間に出血がありましたか？
> Have you noticed any spotting between periods?

おりものがありますか？
　Do you have any vaginal discharge?

妊娠したことがありますか？
　Have you ever been pregnant?

性生活に変わりはありませんか？
　Have you noticed any change in your sex life?

性生活に何か問題がありますか？
　Do you have any sexual problems?
　Do you have any problems in your sex life?

性交時に痛いことがありますか？
　Do you have pain during intercourse?

避妊法はどうされましたか？
　What birth control methods have you used?

何か避妊薬を用いたことがありますか？
　Have you used any form of contraceptive?

ピルを使ってますか？
　Are you taking the pill?

妊娠時に高血圧がありましたか？
　Did you have high blood pressure during any pregnancy?

妊娠時に何か合併症がありましたか？
　Did you have any complications during any pregnancy?

勃起障害がありますか？
　Do you have any trouble having an erection?

勃起やその維持に問題ありと思っていますか？
　Do you feel that you are having problems with getting or maintaining an erection?

●内分泌系　Endocrine system●

暑さと寒さと，どちらがいいですか？
　Which weather do you prefer, cold or warm?
　Do you prefer hot or cold weather?

同じ部屋で他の人は快適なのにあなたは寒く感じることがありますか？
　Do you often feel cold when other people in the room are comfortable?

いつも汗かきですか？
　Do you always sweat?

発汗が増してきましたか？
　Have you noticed increased sweating?

手がふるえますか？
　Do your hands tremble (shake)?

いつから手がふるえてますか？
　How long have your hands been shaky?

最近のどが渇きますか？
　Have you been thirsty?

異常にのどが渇きますか？
　Do you feel thirsty more than usual?

毛が抜けたりしていますか？
　Have you been losing hair?

● 骨・関節・筋肉系　Musculoskeletal system ●

節々が痛みますか？
　Do you have any painful joints?

関節のこわばりがありますか？
　Do you have any stiffness in your joints?

関節が腫れることがありますか？
　Do you have any swelling in your joints?

腕や脚は大丈夫ですか？
　Do you have any problems with your arms or legs?

筋肉痛はありますか？
　Do you have any pain in your muscles?

脚の筋肉が痛んだり引きつったりしますか？
　Do you have pains or cramps in your legs?

こむらがえりで困ることがありますか？
　Are you troubled by leg cramps?

腰の具合はいかがですか？
　Do you have any back trouble?

肩が凝ることがありますか？
　Do you have any stiffness in your shoulders?

背中のどこが具合悪いですか？
　Which part of your back is affected?

背痛は何か重いものを持ち上げてからですか？
　Did the backache start after lifting something heavy?

寒いと指が痛く白くなりますか？
　Do your fingers become painful and white in the cold?

歩くのは大丈夫ですか？
　Do you have any trouble walking?

● 精神・神経系　Nervous system ●

頭痛がありますか？
　Do you get headaches? / Do you suffer from headaches?

気絶したことがありますか？
　Have you ever fainted?

失神発作の経験がありますか？
　Have you had fainting episodes?

一時意識不明になったことがありますか？
　Have you had any blackouts?

どのくらいの間意識を失ってましたか？
　For how long were you unconscious?

周囲のことは分かっていましたか？
　Were you aware of your surroundings?

ひきつけを起こしたことがありますか？
　Have you ever had a convulsion?

最近めまいがすることがありますか？
　Have you been having dizzy spells recently?

腕や脚が動きにくいことがありますか？
　Do you have any trouble moving your arms or legs?

脚に脱力やしびれがありますか？
　Have you noticed any weakness or numbness in your legs?

足がしびれてちくちくしますか？
　Do you feel pins and needles in your feet?

指がじんじんしますか？
　Do you have tingling in your fingers?

力が入らなくなりましたか？
  Have you lost any strength?

いらいらしますか？
  Do you feel nervous (irritable, restless)?

何か感情問題を経験しましたか？
  Have you ever had any emotional problems?

気分はいかがですか？
  How are your spirits? / How is your mood?

悲しくなったり憂鬱になることがありますか？
  Do you feel sad or depressed?

仕事や家庭に何か心配事がありますか？
  Are you anxious about anything at work or at home?

物覚えが悪くなりましたか？
  Have you had any memory problems?

記憶障害に気づいたことがありますか？
  Have you noted any difficulty with your memory?

忘れっぽくなりましたか？
  Have you become forgetful?

今日は何日か分かりますか？
  Do you know what day it is today? / What is today's date?

集中できないですか？
  Do you have any difficulty concentrating?

●皮膚 Skin●

発疹がありますか？
  Do you have a skin rash?
  Have you noted any rashes on your skin?

何か皮膚に問題がありますか？
  Do you have any skin problems?

このただれはいつからありますか？
  How long have you had this sore?

治りにくい傷がありますか？
  Do you have a sore that will not heal?

痒いですか？
  Do you feel itchy? / Do you itch?

皮膚に痒みがありますか？
　Any itching of the skin?

痒いところに発疹がありますか？
　Is the itching accompanied by a rash?

ほくろの様子に変わりはありませんか？
　Have you noticed any change in the look of the mole?

訳の分からない打ち身に気づいたことがありますか？
　Have you noticed bruises that appear without apparent reason?

髪の毛に変わりはありませんか？
　Have you noticed any change in your hair?

髪の毛が減ってますか？
　Are you losing your hair?

髪が薄くなってますか？
　Is your hair thinning?

頭の一部がはげることがありましたか？
　Have any bald patches appeared on your scalp?

● 患者像　Patient profile ●

仕事は何ですか？
　What do you do? / What is your occupation?
　What is your profession? / What type of work do you do?

勤め先はどちらですか？
　What company do you work for?

今どちらにお勤めですか？
　Where are you currently employed?

何をして生計を立てていますか？
　What do you do for a living?

仕事の具合はどうですか？
　How are you getting along with your job?

教育はどこで受けましたか？
　Where were you educated?

家族と一緒に住んでいますか？
　Do you live with your family?

どなたと一緒に住んでいますか？
　Who do you live with?

何か家庭内に問題がありますか？
　Do you have any family problems?
　Are you having any problems at home?

何か経済的な問題がありますか
　Do you have any financial problems?

結婚していますか？
　Are you married?

結婚してどれくらいですか？
　How long have you been married?

結婚はうまくいっていますか？
　Are you happily married?

離婚の理由は何でしたか？
　Why did you get a divorce?

この2年間に外国に行ったことがありますか？
　Have you been abroad in the last 2 years?

何かダイエットしていますか？
　Are you on a special diet?／Have you followed any diet?

一日に何本タバコを吸いますか？
　How many cigarettes do you smoke a day?

いつ禁煙しましたか？
　When did you quit smoking?

お酒を飲みますか？　量はどれくらい？
　Do you drink alcohol? How much?

アルコールは何を飲みますか？
　What do you drink?
　What type of alcoholic drinks do you consume?

1週間にどれくらい飲みますか？
　How much do you drink per week?

普段飲むときは，どれくらい飲みますか？
　How much do you usually drink on a typical drinking day?

普段の量よりも過ごすことがありますか？
　Do you ever drink more than your usual amount?

酒量を減らさなければと思ったことがありますか？
Have you ever felt the need to cut down on drinking?

寝起きに酒を飲むことがありますか？
Have you ever taken a morning drink as an eye-opener?

何か服薬していますか？
Are you taking any medications?

常用薬はありますか？
Do you take any medicine regularly?

何かアレルギーがありますか？
Do you have any allergies?

何かにアレルギー（過敏症）がありますか？
Are you allergic to anything?
Are you sensitive to anything?

薬や食べ物に当たったことがありますか？
Have you ever had any reaction to a medicine or food?

薬や注射で具合悪くなったことがありますか？
Have you ever had bad reactions to a medicine or a shot?

服用できない薬がありますか？
Are there any medications you cannot take?

化学薬品を扱う仕事をしたことがありますか？
Have you ever worked with chemicals?

普段，一日をどんな風に過ごしていますか？
Tell me how you spend your average day.

あなたらしい一日とはどのようですか？
What's a typical day like for you?

余暇には何をしますか？
What do you do in your spare time?
What do you do in your free time?

普段，運動していますか？
Do you exercise regularly?

健康のために何かしていますか？
What do you do to stay in good health?

楽しみは何ですか？
What do you do for fun?

趣味は何ですか？
> What are your hobbies?

●既往歴　Past history●

以前，大病や手術の経験はありますか？
> Have you had any serious illness or operations in the past?

大事故や怪我の経験はありますか？
> Have you had any serious accidents or injuries before?

今までに何か患ったことがありますか？
> Have you suffered from any previous illness?

心臓の具合が悪かったことがありますか？
> Have you had any troubles with your heart?

糖尿病とか肝臓病に罹ったことがありますか？
> Have you ever had diabetes or any sort of liver disease?

盲腸は取ってますか？
> Have you had your appendix taken out?

入院したことがありますか？
> Have you been hospitalized before?
> Have you ever been admitted to a hospital for anything?

入院の理由は何でしたか？
> What were you hospitalized for?

入院期間はどれくらいでしたか？
> How long were you in the hospital?

臥床期間はどれくらいでしたか？
> How long were you in bed?

休業期間はどれくらいでしたか？
> How long were you away from work?

病気で仕事を休んだことがありますか？
> Have you had time off work because of illness?

就職の時検診を受けたことがありますか？
> Have you had a medical examination for employment?

保険の検診を受けたことがありますか？
> Have you had a medical examination for insurance purposes?

何か言われましたか？
> What was the result?

● 家族歴　Family history ●

ご両親は存命ですか？　健康ですか？
Are your parents alive? Are they in good health?

お母様が亡くなられた時おいくつでしたか？
How old was your mother when she died?

亡くなられた原因は何ですか？
What was the cause of death? / What did she die of?

兄弟は何人ですか？　元気ですか？
How many brothers do you have? How are they?

きょうだいで肝炎だった人はいますか？
Have any of your siblings ever had hepatitis?

お子さんの健康はどうですか？
How is your children's health?

家族で癌の人はいますか？
Is there anyone in your family with cancer?

家族の中に誰か糖尿病の人はいますか？
Has anyone suffered from diabetes in your family?

家族に同じ問題を抱えている人がいますか？
Does anyone in your family have the same problem?

血縁内に高血圧の人がいますか？
Do you have blood relatives who have had high blood pressure?

Tidbits

tautology

類語反復 tautology とは，文字通り同じ意味の言葉を重複することで，pleonasm（冗語法）と相通ずる．causal factor, consensus of opinion, end result, future plans, true facts などがその例であり，必要以上に言葉を重ねることによる修辞学的効果はあるが科学論文では避けたほうがよい．更に red in color, small in size, round in shape, fewer in number, grouped together なども一語で十分である．もっとも "past history" も tautological だから好ましくないと言われると困る．

2. 診察の英会話

●診察前　Before examination●

これから〜の診察をします．
> I would like to examine your 〜 now.
> I need to examine your 〜 now.

着物を脱いでください．
> Take your clothes off. / Get undressed.
> Take off your shirt. / Remove your clothes.

パンツ以外は全部脱いでください．
> Take off all your clothes except your shorts.
> Take off everything but your underpants.

上半身脱いでください．
> Take off your clothes from the waist up.
> Remove the clothing above your waist.

病院のガウンを着てください．
> Put on this hospital gown.

靴を脱いで体重計に乗ってください．
> Take off your shoes and step on the scale.

●バイタルサイン　Vital signs●

熱を計ります．
> Let me take your temperature.

体温計を舌の下に入れてください．
> Put the thermometer under your tongue.

血圧を計ります．
> I am going to take your blood pressure.

右腕の袖をまくりあげてください．
> Roll up your right sleeve.

血圧の圧迫帯を膨らませると手が少し気持ち悪くなるかもしれません．
> You may feel some discomfort in your hand when the blood pressure cuff is inflated.

脈をみましょう．
> Let me check your pulse.

脈をみるので手を出してください．
> Give me your hand so that I may take your pulse.

●頭部 Head●

真っ直ぐ前を見てください.
Look straight ahead.

左の方を見てください.
Look to your left.

天井を見てください.
Look up at the ceiling.

右手で右の目を覆ってください.
Cover your right eye with your right hand.

頭を動かさないで，私の指を目で追ってください.
Keep your head still and follow my finger with your eyes.

私の指が動いているのが見えたら教えてください.
Tell me when you can see my fingers moving.

指を見つめてください.
Focus on my finger.

目をしっかり閉じてください.
Close your eyes tight. / Keep your eyes shut.

ちょっと目をつぶってください.
Close your eyes for a minute.

眉をあげてください.
Raise your eyebrows.

額に皺を寄せてください.
Wrinkle your forehead.

口を大きく開けてください. のどを調べます.
Open your mouth wide. I need to check your throat.

舌を出してください.
Stick out your tongue. / Put your tongue out.
Poke your tongue out.

舌を左右に動かしてください.
Move your tongue from side to side.

歯を食いしばってください.
Clench your teeth.

頬を膨らませてください.
Puff out your cheeks. / Blow your cheeks out.

時計の音が聞こえますか？
Can you hear the watch ticking?

振動が分かりますか？
Do you feel vibrations?

顔を右に向けてください．
Turn your head to the right.

首を動かすと痛いですか？
Is it painful to move your neck?

水を一口含んで，言ったら飲み込んでください．
Hold a mouthful of water and swallow when I say so.

●胸部　Chest●

心臓（肺）の音を聴きます．
I'm going to listen to your heart (lung).

シャツを上げてください．
Pull up your shirt.

背筋を伸ばして座ってください．
Sit up straight.

楽にして静かに座ってください．
Relax and sit quietly.

向きを変えて背中を見せてください．
Turn around and show me your back.

頭の上に手を挙げてください．
Raise your arms overhead.

口で息をしてください．
Breathe through your mouth.

深呼吸をしてください．
Breathe deeply in and out. / Breathe as deeply as you can.

息を大きく吸って止めてください．
Take a deep breath in and hold it.

息を吐き出したところで止めてください．
Hold your breath when you breathe out.

息をゆっくり口から吸ったり吐いたりしてください．
Breathe in and out slowly through your mouth.

息をすっかり吐き出してください．
  Blow it all way out. / Let it out.

咳払いしてください．
  Cough. / Clear your throat.

アー (99) と言ってください．
  Say "Ah". / Can you say "ninety-nine" for me?

● 腹部　Abdomen ●

では腹部を診ましょう．
  Now let me examine your abdomen.

仰向けになって楽にしてください．
  Lie on your back and relax.

脚を伸ばして仰向けに寝てください．
  Lie down with your legs stretched out.

じっとして横になり脇に腕をおろしてください．
  Lie still and place your arms by your sides.

膝を曲げてください．
  Bend your knees. / Draw up your knees.
  Draw up your legs.

おなかのこの辺りを押します．深呼吸してください．
  I'm going to push your belly here. Take a deep breath.

脚をまっすぐ伸ばしてください．
  Put your legs out straight.

右下に横になってください．
  Lie on your right side.

左側を下に横になってください．
  Turn over on your left side.

向きを変えて，体を丸めてください．
  Turn over and curl yourself into a ball.

うつ伏せになってください．
  Lie down on your stomach. / Roll over onto your stomach.

右手を頭の上に挙げてください．
  Put your right hand on your head.

排便の時のようにいきんでください.
　Bear down as if your want to move your bowels.
　Strain down as if you move your bowels.

ここを押さえると痛みますか？
　Does it hurt when I press here?

手を離したときに痛みを感じますか？
　Do you feel any pain when I let go?

直腸を診察します.
　I am going to examine your rectum.

直腸指診です. 指先を肛門の中に入れます.
　Now a rectal examination; I'm going to insert my fingertip into your anus.

排便したい気分になるかもしれません.
　You may feel like you want to move your bowels.

● 四肢　Extremities ●

握りこぶしを作ってください.
　Make a fist.

私の手を握ってください.
　Grip my hand. ／ Squeeze my hand.

眼を閉じたまま肘を曲げずに手を突き出してください.
　Keep your eyes closed and hold out your hands with your arms straight.

両手の指を広げてください. 紙を1枚載せます.
　Spread out your fingers of both hands. I'm going to put a sheet of paper on them.

思い切り私の手を押してください.
　Push against my hands as hard as you can.

前にかがんで, 膝は真っ直ぐのまま足の指に触ってみてください.
　Lean forward and try to touch your toes with both knees straight.

脚を挙げたときに腰や脚に痛みを感じますか？
　Do you feel any pain in your hips or legs when I raise your legs?

2. 診察の英会話   377

眼を閉じて,ピンで刺したのを鋭く感じるか鈍く感じるか言ってください.

Close your eyes and tell me whether the pinprick feels sharp or dull.

腕を伸ばしてから右手の人差し指でゆっくり自分の鼻先を触ってみてください.

Hold your arms out and try to touch the tip of your nose with the index finger of your right hand slowly.

足を組んでください.反射を調べます.

Cross your legs. I'll test your reflexes.

足の指を動かしてください.

Wiggle your toes.

親指を上向きか下向きか,どちらに動かしていますか?

Which direction am I moving your big toe, up or down?

鼠径部と足首の脈をみます.

I'm going to check the pulses in your groins and ankles.

●診察後　After examination●

これで終わりです.

That's all. / The examination is over now.

もう着ていいです.

You can get dressed now. / You can get your clothes on now. Put your clothes back on.

ご苦労さま.

Thank you for your time.

注:例文は命令形で示してあるが,もちろん実際には「命令」ではなく「依頼」であり,前か後に "please" をつけるか,"Would you ~ ?", "Could you ~ ?", "Would you mind ~ ing?" などの丁寧文を使う.

3. 患者説明の英会話

●病状・診断の説明　About diagnosis●

何も心配要りません．ひとりでによくなります．
　There's nothing to worry about. It will clear up on its own.

この類の症状は二三日でおのずと治るはずです．
　This type of symptom should resolve itself in a few days.

診断は流行性耳下腺炎，つまりおたふくかぜです．
　The diagnosis is epidemic parotitis, that is mumps.

肝臓がちょっと悪いようです．
　You seem to have a little problem with your liver.

心臓の音をよく聴いてみましたが，何も悪いところはありませんでした．
　I have listened to your heart carefully, and cannot find anything wrong with it.

咳は服用されている血圧の薬のせいのようです．
　The cough seems to be caused by the medicine you are taking for your blood pressure.

関節血症というものです．右膝の関節内に血が溜まっていて脹れています．
　You have what we call "hemarthrosis"; you have blood in your right knee joint, which is making it swell.

一過性の卒中だったようです．脳の動脈が短時間ふさがった状態です．
　You may have suffered a mini-stroke. It is a condition when an artery in your brain was blocked for a short time.

左側の腎臓結石ではないかと思います．
　I suspect that you have a stone in your left kidney.

あなたの病気は多分憩室炎というものではないかと思います．
　I feel that you are probably suffering from a condition called diverticulitis.

右の踵の骨に亀裂骨折があるようです．
　It seems that you have a fissured fracture of the right heel bone.

マイコプラズマ肺炎に罹っているようです．
　It looks like you have mycoplasma pneumonia.

3. 患者説明の英会話　379

胃酸が食道へ逆流しているようです．
> It sounds like acid from your stomach is flowing back up into your esophagus.

心内膜炎の可能性があります．
> It's possible that you might have endocarditis.

胆石が胆管に詰まって胆汁の流れを妨げています．
> Gallstones are trapped in your bile duct, and the flow of bile is blocked.

あなたの失神発作は血圧が低くて起こったのです．
> Your fainting spells were brought about by low blood pressure.

この病気は一旦治ったら二度と罹りません．
> Once you recover from the illness, it won't recur.

命にかかわることはありませんし，治療は容易です．
> This is not life-threatening and is easily treated.

傷は治りますから安心してください．
> I reassure you that there's a cure for this wound.

癌がご心配のことと思いますが，前立腺癌の徴候はありません．
> I know you are concerned about cancer, but there is no sign of prostate cancer.

長期的にみてどうなるかはまだ何とも言えません．
> It's too early to say what will happen in the long term.

再燃と軽快を繰り返す一生の病気です．
> This is a lifelong disease that repeats exacerbations and remissions.

病気が広がっているので，できるのは症状を軽くすることだけです．
> Since the disease is so widespread, all we can do is relieve the symptoms.

●検査の説明　About tests●

検尿をしましょう．
> We need to do a urine test.

便潜血の検査があります．
> You need to have a stool examination for occult blood.

腫瘍マーカーを調べるので採血をします．
I'm going to draw some blood to examine it for tumor markers.

甲状腺機能を確かめるため血液を数本採ります．
I'll take several blood samples to check your thyroid function.

念のため胸の写真を撮ってください．
I'd like you to have a chest X-ray just to make sure.

胃の内視鏡検査を受けてください．
I want you to have a gastroscopy.

おなかにしこりがあるのでエコー検査を受けてください．
Because we have found a lump in your abdomen, I think you should have an ultrasound.

ホルター心電計という心臓の鼓動を24時間記録する携帯用器具をつけてみてはいかがでしょう．
How about wearing a Holter monitor, a portable device that records your heartbeats for 24 hours?

血液検査の結果が異常ですので検査を追加する必要があります．
The results of your blood tests are abnormal, and so I feel additional tests are needed.

もう少し検査が必要です．CT スキャンの手配をします．
We need to do more tests. I'll make arrangements for a CT scan.

貧血そのものは鉄剤で治療できますが，大本の原因を突き止めなければなりません．
The anemia itself can be treated with iron tablets, but we have to identify its underlying cause.

尿の検査では糖やタンパクはおりていません．
The urine test does not show any sugar or protein.

血液検査は全部正常でした．
All of your blood tests showed normal results.

血液検査で血糖値が異常に低いことが分かりました．
Your blood test showed abnormally low blood glucose levels.

血液検査で数種類の膵酵素が高値でした．
Your blood test showed high levels of several pancreatic enzymes.

この血液検査の費用はかさみますが，健康保険がききます．
The blood test costs a lot of money, but is covered by your health insurance.

胸の写真では昔の結核の影のほかは異常ありませんでした．
Your chest X-ray was normal except for old tuberculous shadows.

脊骨のX線検査で5番目の腰椎が前方にずれています．
X-rays of the spine showed forward displacement of the fifth lumbar vertebra.

右肩のMRIをお勧めします．
I recommend you have an MRI scan done on your right shoulder.

レントゲンで腕に骨折はありませんでした．
X-rays showed no fractures in your arm.

CTスキャンで脳腫瘍の徴候はありませんでした．
There was no evidence of a brain tumor on the CT scans.

心電図で心筋梗塞の所見はありませんでした．
Your EKG did not show any sign of coronary.

残念ながら悪性腫瘍です．
Unfortunately, it is a malignant growth.

前立腺生検標本の一つから癌細胞が出たようです．
I'm afraid one of the biopsy specimens from your prostate showed cancer cells.

わきの下のこぶの生検の結果は悪性でした．
I'm afraid that the biopsy of the lump in your armpit showed you have a malignancy.

● 治療方針の説明　About treatment ●

重症ではありませんが，二三日休んでください．
This is not a serious illness, but you will need to rest for a few days.

めまいがひどいので，数日間は安静臥床が必要でしょう．
Since you have severe dizziness, you will have to rest quietly in bed for several days.

胸腔穿刺が必要です．ということは胸腔の中に針を刺して中の液を抜きます．
  You will need thoracentesis; it means passing a needle into the chest cavity and removing the fluid inside.

肝臓の中に膿瘍，すなわち膿の溜まった袋があります．管を入れて排液しなければなりません．
  You have abscesses, or pus-filled pockets, in your liver. They must be drained through the introduction of tubes.

残念ですが胆嚢を取らざるをえません．
  I'm afraid we have no choice but to take your gallbladder out.

腫瘍が増大して尿の通りが悪くなれば手術が必要になります．
  Surgery may be necessary if the mass increases in size and prevents the passage of urine.

手術は最後の手段ですが，今すぐ入院していただきましょう．
  You need to be admitted immediately, although surgery would be a last resort.

観察と追加の検査のため入院していただかねばなりません．
  I think we should admit you to the hospital for observation and more tests.

入院は要りませんし，ほとんど普段と同じ生活ができます．
  You don't require hospitalization, and can lead a close to normal life.

入院しなければならないような病状ではありません．
  This is not a condition you need to be hospitalized for.

息子さんは入院してもらわなければなりません．
  We feel your son needs to be admitted to the hospital.

感染の徴候が全部なくなってしまうまで入院していなければなりません．
  You will have to remain in the hospital until all signs of the infection have cleared up.

手術になれば最低1週間の入院が必要です．
  The operation will require at least a week's stay in the hospital.

手術中に輸血が必要です．
  It is necessary for you to receive a blood transfusion during the operation.

気が進まないのは分かりますが，必要な治療は進めなければなりません．
I understand you don't feel like doing that, but we have to proceed with any necessary treatment.

自分の母親だとしたら手術を受けるように勧めます．
If you were my mother, I would recommend that you have a surgery.

普通術後の回復は早くて全快します．
Recovery after the operation is normally quick and complete.

処置がすんだら大事をとって一晩入院していただきますが，1週間以内に仕事に戻れます．
After the procedure you will spend a night in the hospital just to be safe, and return to work in less than a week.

奥さんは今月末までには退院できるでしょう．
Your wife will be able to leave the hospital by the end of this month.

放射線療法に化学療法を併用すれば症状の軽減と延命の可能性があります．
Chemotherapy combined with radiation therapy may reduce the symptoms and prolong your life.

痛み止めを処方します．それで治まるはずです．
I'm going to prescribe a pain reliever. That should take care of your pain.

高血圧と動悸の薬を処方します．
I will give you prescriptions for high blood pressure and palpitations.

食事や減量でコレステロールの数値が下がらなければコレステロール降下薬を処方します．
I'll prescribe a cholesterol-lowering drug if diet and weight-reduction fail to lower your cholesterol levels.

この薬は，傷を早く治すのに必要な安静と冷湿布の代わりになるわけではありません．
The medicine is not a substitute for the rest and cold compresses needed for rapid healing of the wound.

血液の凝固傾向を減らして危険な凝血塊ができないようにするため抗凝固療法を始めます．
> We need to start anticoagulant therapy to reduce the blood's tendency to clot so that formation of dangerous blood clots is prevented.

ひと晩ぐっすり眠ってください．
> I recommend you have a good night's sleep.

もっと運動するようにお勧めします．
> I would like to advise you to get more exercise.

ボクシングやフットボールのような肉体的接触競技は避けなければなりません．
> You must avoid physical contact sports such as boxing and football.

食事を変えて飲酒を止めて減量しなければいけません．
> You need to lose weight by changing your diet and giving up alcoholic beverages.

脂っこい食べ物を避けて，もっと緑黄色野菜を摂るのが賢明です．
> It is advisable to avoid greasy food and eat more green and yellow vegetables.

青物を沢山食べて，塩分の多い食物を控えてください．
> Make sure to eat plenty of green vegetables and stop eating salty foods.

学校から帰ったら手を洗ってうがいをするのを忘れないで．
> Remember to wash your hands and gargle when you get home from school.

妙薬はありません．減量食，規則的な運動，温熱療法など自分でできることをしてください．
> There are no magic cures. Please try self-help measures like a weight reducing diet, regular exercise, and heat treatments.

しばらくすれば，新しい食事の決まりにきっと慣れると思います．
> After a while, I'm sure you'll get used to the new dietary formula.

家の中をきれいにして，ほこり，花粉，羽毛，家ダニ，ゴキブリなどアレルゲンの可能性があるものを除去しなければなりません．
> You should keep the house clean and remove potential allergens, such as dust, pollens, feathers, mites, and cockroaches.

整形外科医ならおそらく脊椎の手術を勧めると思います．
An orthopedic surgeon will probably recommend that you have an operation on your spine.

これ以上の検査は必要ありません．
There is no need for further tests.

今後は2年ごとに大腸内視鏡検診を必ず受けてください．
From now on, be sure to have a colonoscopic checkup every two years.

6ヵ月後くらいに肝臓を再検します．
We'd like to check your liver again in about six months.

検尿を再検するので3週間後に再受診してください．
Come back to the clinic in three weeks for a repeat urinalysis.

心臓専門医の山田先生に紹介状を書きます．
I'll write a letter referring you to a cardiologist, Dr. Yamada.

来月の予約をしておきます．
I'll make an appointment for you next month.

1週間後の再診予約をしておきましょう．
I'll give you an appointment to return in a week.

前田先生の予約は明日9時半です．お大事に．
Your appointment with Dr. Maeda is at 9:30 tomorrow. Take care, Mr. Ito.

● 服薬指導　About medication ●

あなたの処方薬を調合します．
We will fill the prescription for you.

先生の処方箋がないと調剤できません．
We cannot dispense the medicine without a doctor's prescription.

先生が処方された薬はこれです．
This is the medicine your doctor prescribed for you.

どんな薬か説明します．
I'll tell you what kind of medicine this is.

錠剤が2種類ありますが，白いのが関節痛の薬です．
There are two kinds of tablets; the white one is for your joint pain.

この薬は鼻水に効きます．
This medicine is good for a runny nose.

この薬は高いコレステロール値を下げるのに用います．
This medicine is used to bring down high cholesterol levels.

この処方は利尿剤です．体から余分の水分を取り除きます．
This prescription is for a diuretic, a water pill; it works to remove extra fluid from the body.

この薬は酸分泌を抑えて胃痛を和らげる働きがあります．
This medicine is supposed to suppress acid secretion and relieve a stomachache.

この薬は尿酸が腎臓から排泄されるのを増やします．
This medicine increases the excretion of uric acid through the kidneys.

血管を拡張して狭心症の予防と治療に使う薬です．
This is a drug that dilates blood vessels and is used to prevent and treat angina.

血液をさらさらにする薬で，心臓の中で血液が停滞して血栓ができるのを防ぎます．
This is a blood thinner that prevents the formation of blood clots due to stagnation in the heart.

これは合成ステロイドホルモンで卵巣の働きを抑えて，子宮内面の粘膜の増殖を遅らせます．
This is a synthetic steroid hormone that suppresses the activity of the ovaries and slows the growth of the mucous membrane lining the uterus.

眼圧を下げて痛みを軽くする薬です．
The drugs will help lower the pressure within the eye and relieve pain.

この錠剤は効き目が早いです．
This tablet takes effect quickly.

薬が効き始めるには2週間かかるでしょう．
It may take two weeks for this medicine to start working.

これは痛み止めです．残念ですが胃が悪くなることがあります．
This is a painkiller. Unfortunately, it may cause an upset stomach.

3. 患者説明の英会話

この薬の副作用には，むかつき，便秘，めまい，排尿困難などがあります．
Side effects of this medicine include nausea, constipation, dizziness, and difficulty urinating.

この薬を飲むと眠気を催します．
This medicine will make you sleepy.

副作用の予測はできませんが，空咳が出る人がいます．
Side effects cannot be anticipated, but some people experience a dry cough.

この薬で一番よくある副作用は下痢です．
The most frequent side effect of this medicine is diarrhea.

この薬をグレープフルーツジュースと一緒に飲むと作用が増強されますが，副作用の可能性も増えます．
Taking this medicine with grapefruit juice can increase its effect, but the likelihood of an adverse reaction increases as well.

この錠剤は習慣性になるので，できるだけ少量をできるだけ短期間用いるべきです．
These pills should be taken in as low doses as possible and for as short a time as possible, because they are habit-forming.

これ以上睡眠薬を続けると依存症になりかねません．
If you continue to use this sleep aid much longer, you may become dependent on it.

毎朝，食前に1錠飲んでください．
Take one tablet every morning before breakfast.

夜，寝る前に2錠服用してください．
Take two tablets at night, before going to bed.

1日に4回，毎食後と就寝前に2錠服用してください．
Take two tablets four times a day, after each meal and at bedtime.

この錠剤は毎日同じ時間に服用するようにしてください．
Try to take this tablet at the same time each day.

カプセル1個を1日3回，8時間毎に飲んでください．
Take one capsule three times daily, every eight hours.

1日3回，2錠ずつ，2週間飲んでください．
Take two tablets three times a day for two weeks.

今すぐ2錠服用して，今夜7時に1錠，その後は毎朝1錠服用してください．

Take two tablets now, then one tablet at 7 pm tonight and one tablet every morning thereafter.

錠剤は，コップ1杯の水（白湯1杯，食べ物か牛乳）と一緒に服用してください．

Take the pill with a glass of water (a cup of warm water, food or milk).

この薬を服用しているときは，毎日水気を沢山飲んでください．

While taking this medicine, you should drink plenty of liquids every day.

頭痛には，必要に応じてアスピリンを2錠服用してください．

Take two tablets of aspirin as needed for your headache.

必要なときだけ服用してください．

Take it only when you need it.

錠剤は飲み込まないで下さい．舌の下に入れてすっかり溶けるまでそのままにしてください．

Don't swallow the tablet. Keep it under your tongue until it is completely dissolved.

この薬はつぶしたり噛んだりしてはいけません．苦い味がしていやなにおいがありますから．

You should not crush or chew this drug because it has a bitter taste and an unpleasant odor.

定量吸入器を正しく使うには練習が要ります．

You need to practice using the metered-dose inhaler properly.

吸入器の頭を押しながら息を深く吸ってできるだけ長く息を止めてください．

While pressing the top of the inhaler, breathe in deeply and hold your breath as long as you can.

咽頭痛にはこの薬液でうがいしてください．

Gargle with this medicated solution to help your sore throat.

患部に軟膏を1日2回塗ってください．

Apply the ointment to the affected area twice a day.

温湿布を右膝に1日2回貼ってください．

Apply the hot compress to your right knee twice a day.

クリームは足の裏と足指の間に軽く擦り込んでください．
Rub the cream gently into the sole and between the toes of your foot.

一度に1滴，点眼してください．
Put it in your eyes one drop at a time.

坐薬は尖った方を先に肛門の中に指で入れてください．
Push the suppository, pointed end first, into the anus with your finger.

指示通りに服薬してください．
Take the medicine as directed.

服薬を忘れないように．
Don't forget to take your medicine.

飲み忘れに気付いたらすぐに服用してください．
Take the forgotten dose as soon as you remember.

飲み忘れたら1回とばしていつもの服用法に戻ってください．
Skip the missed dose and go back to your regular schedule.

倍量を服用しないでください．
Do not take a double dose of this medication.

抜けた薬はできるだけ早く飲んでください．でも倍量で埋め合わせようとしてはいけません．
Take the missed dose as soon as possible but never try to make it up by doubling the dose.

気分が良くなったと思っても，1日3回の薬を丸1週間は飲み続けてください．
Keep taking the medicine three times a day for a full week, even if you think you are feeling better.

この薬を飲んでいる間はアルコールはいけません．
Avoid alcohol while taking this medicine.

発疹が出たら薬を止めてください．
Stop taking the medicine if you break out in a rash

最初の二三日でふらつくようでしたら，電話してください．
If you feel light-headed during the first few days, please give me a call.

この薬を飲んだら車の運転や重機の操作をしてはいけません．
After taking this medicine you should not drive or operate heavy machinery.

ニトログリセリン貼布剤を使用しているのでこの薬は服用できません．
Because you have been using nitroglycerin patches, you should not take this medicine.

冷暗所で保存してください．
Store it in a cool, dark place.

冷蔵庫に入れなくてもいいです．室温で保管してください．
You don't have to keep it in the fridge. Store it at room temperature.

熱，日光，湿気を避けてください．
Keep it away from heat, sunlight and moisture.

子供の手が届かないところに置いてください．
Keep it out of children's reach.

Tidbits

data

data は単数か複数か？ data は datum の複数であるから，本来複数扱いが正しいが，単数扱いも多くなっている．facts と同義ならば複数，information と同義ならば単数と区別する意見もあるが，複数扱い (The data were collected by～; The clinical data were compared with～) か，単数扱い (All the data shows that～, This data agrees well with～) か，many (few) data か much (little) data か，non-native にとっては迷うところである．AMA Manual of Style (2007) では，agenda 同様単数扱いの日が近いとしながらも，今のところ「いかなる場合も複数形の使用が望ましい」としている．因みに agenda は agendum の複数であるが，現在では単数扱いが標準化していて複数形として agendas が用いられる．そのほか criteria も単数扱いのことがあるが口語的であり，bacteria, criteria, phenomena などは複数である（単数は bacterium, criterion, phenomenon）．

VI章

症例プレゼンテーション

1. 基本短文例

●症例検討　Case study●

症例提示	case presentation
口頭症例提示	oral case presentation
症例検討会	case conference
症例報告	case report

●患者紹介　Introduction / Opening statement●

- This is the first KUH admission for this 58-year-old man who was brought to our emergency department by ambulance last night, after being found unconscious in his apartment.
- This 40-year-old woman was admitted to this hospital because of a persistent fever, night sweats, and weight loss.
- This is a 35-year-old man who presented with a four-day history of pain in the right upper quadrant of the abdomen, accompanied by a low-grade fever and sore throat.
- This is the second admission to this hospital for this 44-year-old man whose problems are: No. 1 exertional dyspnea, No. 2 hacking cough, and No. 3 diabetes mellitus.
- Ms. Sato is a 62-year-old woman who came to our OPD complaining of pain in her eyes of 5 days' duration.
- Mr. Ito has been seen by us for his cirrhosis since July 1998.
- Mr. Harris is an active 70-year-old man who has been followed here regularly for his prostate and yearly checkups.
- The patient is an 84-year-old man with hypertension who presented with a one-month history of lower abdominal pain and bloody stools.
- This 55-year-old man presented to our hospital with a 3-week history of progressive swelling of the right knee, accompanied by limping.
- This 38-year-old woman came to the breast clinic after she found a lump in her right breast during self-examination.
- The patient, a 67-year-old woman, who had been well except for a 10-year history of hypertension treated with nisoldipine, developed right shoulder pain.
- This is a 56-year-old woman who complains of urinary burning and frequency beginning a week ago.
- Before admission the patient was evaluated in the GI service because of abdominal pain and weight loss.
- The patient, an unidentified man who appeared to be about 60 years of age, was brought to the ER of this hospital after a

sudden loss of consciousness.
- This 74-year-old woman came to the emergency department because of severe pain in her right wrist resulting from a fall down the stairs.
- This 55-year-old man was brought to the ED of this hospital by ambulance after a cardiac arrest while sleeping.
- The patient presented to the emergency department after the acute onset of severe substernal pain which woke him up from sleep in the early morning.
- This 67-year-old man presented with an asymptomatic swelling in the left supraclavicular fossa two years after gastrectomy for a pyloric cancer.
- This patient was first admitted to the neurology service of this hospital because of postictal memory loss and speech disturbance.
- This 31-year-old woman with systemic lupus erythematosus was readmitted to our department with a 3-week history of facial puffiness and dependent edema.
- This patient presented to the OPD describing a five-day history of sore throat, wheeze, productive cough, and shortness of breath.
- This 68-year-old man came to our hospital last week complaining of blurred vision and a unilateral throbbing headache.
- This patient presented to the emergency room with complaints of fever, headache, and photophobia that had lasted for 3 days.
- Last month the patient was studied at another hospital for weight loss of 15 kg over the previous 6 months.
- This boy was referred by his family physician to the hematology clinic because of a low-grade fever and cervical lymphadenopathy.
- This 5-year-old girl was brought in by her parents with complaint of a one-month history of intermittent vomiting.
- This patient was referred by his dentist to the oral surgery clinic of this hospital because of right mandibular swelling.
- This 80-year-old woman was referred for excisional biopsy of two pigmented moles on her left leg.
- This patient was referred to the oncology clinic for management of metastatic lung cancer.
- This 25-year-old man was referred to us for investigation of daily episodes of fainting that started 2 months PTA.
- This patient was transferred to the ICU from the Y Hospital

394 Ⅵ章 症例プレゼンテーション

with profound jaundice and diminished consciousness.
- The patient was transferred to our floor for further evaluation of generalized rash and deteriorating renal function.
- This time the patient was admitted for consideration of and preparation for liver transplantation.
- The history was obtained from the patient and his wife, and is reliable.
- The historical data were obtained from the patient's mother, and are of questionable reliability.
- The patient does not speak English well, and is a poor historian.

● 患者像　Patient profile ●
- The patient is a homemaker with four healthy children.
- He has been married for 10 years, with two children; all three family members are well.
- She is a retired nurse and has been divorced for 5 years.
- She has been a widow for 15 years.
- He is married and has two grown children who are married and live away from his home.
- He worked as a car mechanic, but has been unable to work for the past month because of his present illness.
- He works for a securities company as section manager.
- He is a retired high school teacher who gives private math lessons at home.
- The patient does not use tobacco, alcohol, or illicit drugs.
- She smokes cigarettes occasionally and denies use of alcohol or illicit drugs.
- He denies having had a problem with drinking.
- He has smoked cigarettes (a pack a day) for 30 years.
- He is a heavy smoker (3 packs of cigarettes per day) and drinks several beers on the weekend.
- The patient admitted to smoking two packs of cigarettes per day.
- She drinks alcoholic beverages only socially and smoked cigarettes in the remote past.
- He has no known contact with sick persons or recent exposures to animals.
- The patient has no allergies.
- She is allergic to nuts and shrimp.
- He is allergic to penicillin.
- The patient has no known sensitivity to food or medications.

- She has been under a lot of stress because of her child's illness and her husband's lay-off.
- The patient has no particular home problems.
- The patient usually wakes up about 7:30, eats breakfast at 8:00, works from 9 a.m. to 5 p.m. and eats dinner at home around 7:00.

●現病歴　Present illness●

- The patient was well until 2 days before admission, when acute, severe pain developed in his right great toe.
- The patient had been well until two months before admission, when she had an episode of generalized tonic-clonic seizure.
- He had been well until two months ago, when he began to have fatigue and insomnia.
- This patient was doing well until 2 years ago, when she developed progressively severe fatigue.
- The patient sustained an injury to his right ankle when he tripped and tumbled down the stairs 3 days ago.
- The patient noted no specific symptoms until five days ago, when he awoke in the morning with throbbing headache and chilly sensations.
- About a week ago, she started having lower backache associated with numbness and tingling in both legs.
- The patient who underwent cholecystectomy for "gallstones" last year has been troubled with constant fatigue and loss of appetite for the past three weeks.
- One week after the trip, the patient noted the gradual onset of severe pain in the right calf.
- About two months ago, the patient noted insidious onset of weight loss (from 65 kg to 60 kg at present), anorexia, and constipation.
- The patient had been well until two weeks PTA, when a pruritic rash appeared over his upper chest, both arms, and both thighs.
- Six months before the hospitalization limb pain developed, and has become progressively worse in the past two weeks.
- One week before admission, sore throat and hemicrania developed, and daily spiking fevers continued.
- One week ago, he stepped on a nail, and the puncture site became red and tender two days ago.
- Then the patient became short of breath on exertion and could not climb the stairs without stopping.

- Red macules appeared on his trunk overnight, and by the next day involved his arms and legs, sparing the palms and soles.
- A week later, the patient developed nausea, vomiting, and epigastralgia, and his urine became dark.
- Although he stayed away from work for three days, the symptoms have persisted and worsened.
- During the past week, he has had several episodes of right upper quadrant pain lasting 10 minutes before spontaneously subsiding.
- The lower abdominal pain lasted off and on for several hours.
- After the sudden onset of pain in his left eye 5 days ago, the vision in that eye has been deteriorating.
- The patient remained asymptomatic for two months, but then the same low backache recurred.
- The pain was relieved to some extent by sitting up and leaning forward.
- He could not sleep well for two nights because of a productive cough. He used over-the-counter cough syrup, but without relief.
- Treatment with Tosuxacin for 1 week prescribed by his general practitioner for a presumed lower urinary-tract infection had little effect on his symptoms.
- Since last May the patient has had a variety of treatments including NSAIDs and intra-articular injections, none of which produced any substantial relief.
- After two courses of chemotherapy at another hospital, the metastatic tumors of the liver remained unchanged.
- System review is essentially unchanged from his last admission.
- Review of systems revealed orthostatic vertigo, occasional tinnitus, and palpitations.
- The remainder of the history is only notable for knee pain when walking, probably due to osteoarthritis.

● 既往歴　Past history ●
- There is no significant medical history.
- The patient denies a previous history of liver disease.
- The patient has no past history of serious illnesses or major operations.
- The patient has a history of hypertension, hypercholesterolemia, and osteoarthritis.

- The patient has a 15-year history of type 2 diabetes with poor control complicated by retinopathy and peripheral neuropathy.
- His past history is significant for hypertension, with good control on amlodipine treatment (5 mg per day).
- He seems to have no relevant medical history, although he has undergone minor orthopedic operations.
- Her medical history is notable mainly for pulmonary tuberculosis, for which she was treated in 2000.
- His medical history includes coronary artery disease, hypertension, and hyperlipidemia.
- A diagnosis of type 2 diabetes mellitus, which has been controlled with diet and acarbose, was made 6 months before the current admission.
- A diagnosis of pulmonary tuberculosis was made 2 months ago, when the patient presented at a nearby hospital with a productive cough and pleuritic pain.
- Ten years ago, he was diagnosed with Crohn disease endoscopically and histologically.
- At the age of 35, the patient had an acute episode of right flank pain followed by spontaneous passage of a stone.
- At the age of 26, the patient underwent an emergency operation for rupture of the liver and multiple fractures of the legs caused by a car accident.
- The patient was hospitalized only once for appendectomy in 1990.
- She underwent hysterectomy because of fibroids at the age of 35.
- Five years ago he was hospitalized for a "heart problem", but he is not sure what the diagnosis was.
- The patient has no notable medical history except for hepatitis B, from which he completely recovered.
- Her past medical history is otherwise unremarkable.
- The past medical history is otherwise noncontributory.

● 家族歴　Family history ●
- There is no family history of diabetes, hypertension, or cancer.
- She has no family history of CVA or other neurological diseases.
- Nobody in his family has heart trouble.
- No members of his family has or has had hepatitis or liver trouble.
- None of her immediate family members has similar symptoms.

- Her family history is negative for epilepsy or mental diseases.
- Hypertension appears to run in her family.
- A tendency to form kidney stones runs in his family.
- There is no familial tendency to diabetes.
- Both parents are alive and in good health.
- Her father is well and active at age 74, while he takes medicine for BPH.
- His mother died at age 82 after prolonged hospitalization with Parkinson disease.
- His mother died at 30, unknown cause, when he was 5.
- Her stepmother, age 45, and two half-siblings are all well.
- His paternal grandfather died of a "stroke", age 60.
- The maternal grandmother and an aunt had breast cancer.
- The patient has two older brothers, one of whom has chronic hepatitis C.
- Her only sister died in infancy.
- His son died of leukemia at a young age.

● 身体所見　Physical findings ●

- On examination, the patient appeared well, and his vital signs were normal.
- Physical examination revealed a well-developed, well-nourished man who was in no distress.
- On physical examination, the patient appeared cachectic and pale, but she was not in acute distress.
- Physical exam revealed a jaundiced woman with a blood pressure of 130/70 mmHg, a pulse of 80 beats/min and a temperture of 37℃.
- On admission, the patient's vital signs were normal, his height was 165 cm, and weight 50 kg.
- On admission, his blood pressure was 90/60, his heart rate 120, and his temperature 38.5℃.
- Her vital signs were normal except for a blood pressure of 180/100 mmHg.
- The patient is normotensive.
- The patient was alert and cooperative.
- The patient was confused as to date and place.
- The patient was oriented to person and place, but not to time.
- On physical examination, the patient appeared younger than his chronological age.
- The patient appeared older than his stated age of 55 by at least five years.

- On examination, he was emaciated, febrile, and had general lymphadenopathy and hepatosplenomegaly.
- Physical examination revealed exudative pharyngitis, enlarged lymph nodes in the cervical region, and mild tenderness in the right upper quadrant of the abdomen.
- The pupils were equal, round, and reactive to light.
- There was no jugular venous distention or carotid bruits.
- The chest was clear to auscultation, and the heart sounds were normal, without murmurs.
- The heart revealed a regular rate and rhythm, without murmurs or rubs.
- A firm, smooth, mobile mass, 2 cm in diameter, was palpable in the upper outer quadrant of the left breast.
- The abdomen was soft and not distended, with normal bowel sounds.
- Her abdomen was moderately distended and showed shifting dullness.
- The abdomen was tender throughout without guarding or rebound tenderness.
- There was exquisite tenderness at McBurney point.
- There was a firm mass, about 4 cm in diameter, in the left lower quadrant.
- The liver was palpable 5 cm below the right costal margin.
- His liver was enlarged, measuring 15 cm in span, and was normal in consistency.
- The only abnormality noted during his abdominal examination was mild tenderness in the epigastrium, without any palpable mass.
- The pertinent findings were confined to the abdomen.
- Her extremities are free of pitting edema, cyanosis, and clubbing.
- There was no peripheral edema.
- There was 3+edema extending to the thighs.
- Specifically there were no splinter hemorrhages or Roth spots.
- The general physical examination revealed no abnormalities.
- A cursory physical examination at the ER showed no abnormalities.
- The rest of the physical examination was normal.
- The remainder of the physical examination, which included rectal and pelvic examination, showed no abnormalities.

●検査所見　Laboratory and imaging findings●

- The results of routine laboratory tests revealed no abnormalities.
- Results of laboratory tests are shown in tables in the handout.
- The white-cell count, platelet count, levels of liver enzymes, and the prothrombin time were within normal ranges.
- Laboratory tests revealed elevated hematocrit and leukocytosis with a shift to the left.
- The white-cell count was 18,800, with 84 percent neutrophils and 5 percent band forms.
- Results of liver function tests were within normal limits.
- The serum levels of electrolytes were normal, as were the results of renal-function tests.
- Blood tests showed severe hyponatremia (100 mmol/L), hypokalemia (2.9 mmol/L), and hypochloremia (64 mmol/L).
- The serum amylase level was three times the upper limit of the normal range.
- Serologic tests for hepatitis A, B and C were negative.
- Cultures of multiple specimens of blood and urine were negative for pathogens.
- His oxygen saturation on pulse oximetry was only 55 percent.
- The results of a complete blood count, ECG, and chest radiography were normal.
- The initial electrocardiogram showed sinus tachycardia and prolongation of the QRS interval.
- The ECG printout is available here for your review.
- Chest X-rays revealed an enlarged cardiac silhouette and bilateral pleural effusions.
- An upright chest film showed free air under the diaphragm and dilated loops of bowel under the left hemidiaphragm.
- Flat and upright abdominal films showed moderate dilatation of the small bowel.
- Radiographs of the spine, pelvis, and long bones showed diffuse osteopenia without lytic lesions or fractures.
- Abdominal ultrasonography showed mild right hydronephrosis and fluid in the right side of the pelvic cavity.
- CT scanning of the brain showed a small enhancing mass within the left temporal lobe.
- A contrast-enhanced CT study of the abdomen showed multiple tortuous vessels in the right lobe of the liver.
- MRI of the brain showed small lacunar infarcts in the right side of the thalamus.

- Coronary CT angiography showed mild proximal stenosis of the right coronary artery.
- Upper gastrointestinal endoscopy showed several nonbleeding superficial ulcers in the antrum.
- Total colonoscopy performed after admission showed no abnormalities except for a small polyp in the descending colon.

● 診断　Diagnosis ●
- My impression is that he has intrahepatic cholestasis due to phenytoin.
- I believe she has a flare-up of Crohn disease which she is known to have had for the past 10 years.
- The presence of fever, night sweats, and fatigability suggests an underlying infection.
- Substernal pain radiating to the left arm with sweating and weakness suggests myocardial infarction.
- The sudden development of a pruritic rash with periorbital edema suggests either contact dermatitis or drug-induced exanthema.
- The combination of progressive dyspnea and pleuritic pain suggests either pneumothorax or pleural effusion.
- The signs, symptoms, and laboratory abnormalities suggest an inflammatory myopathy.
- The present episode of chest pain unrelieved by nitroglycerine and associated with ST segment elevation, indicates an acute myocardial infarction.
- Although his physical examination did not show hepatosplenomegaly, palmar erythema, or vascular spiders, the prolonged prothrombin time and increased serum globulin level indicate possible development of cirrhosis.
- Biliary colic with jaundice and high fever is indicative of suppurative cholangitis.
- His clinical course is diagnostic of acute otitis media.
- His symptoms are characteristic of pericardial tamponade.
- His physical findings were nonspecific for alcoholic liver disease.
- The absence of fever makes a chronic infection less likely.
- Diabetic neuropathy is unlikely from the relatively short history of diabetes.
- It seems likely that her dependent edema is related to hypothyroidism.
- Her symptoms are likely due to endometriosis involving the

urinary bladder.
- The most likely cause of his arthralgia is gout.
- The most likely diagnosis for this patient is maxillary sinusitis.
- Hyperparathyroidism is an unlikely explanation because of normal calcium levels.
- Her high blood pressure is probably related to stress and nervous tension.
- A pulmonary embolism is a good possibility in view of the pleuritic pain with hemoptysis and diminished pulmonary vascular markings.
- Fever and headache with vomiting raise the possibility of acute bacterial meningitis.
- Hemorrhagic shock and septic shock were considered as possible causes.
- Intestinal obstruction must be considered until proven otherwise.
- A metastatic cancer could explain the dysphagia, bone pain, and reduced food intake.
- A vasculitic disorder such as polyarteritis nodosa or temporal arteritis might be an alternative explanation.
- The irregular mass seen in the left lower lung is highly suspicious for cancer.
- My differential diagnosis includes acute myocardial infarction, pulmonary embolism, and pericarditis.
- This is not a typical case of carpal tunnel syndrome.
- The diagnosis of Graves disease was supported by typical physical and laboratory findings.
- The diagnosis of rheumatoid arthritis can be readily ruled out by the history and clinical features in this patient.
- Hydronephrosis should be ruled out with abdominal ultrasonography.
- All the findings met the criteria for the diagnosis of carcinoid syndrome.
- A presumptive diagnosis of aseptic meningitis was made.
- Fine needle aspiration biopsy of the thyroid mass was consistent with papillary carcinoma.
- The x-ray findings are consistent with osteomalacia.
- High-resolution CT scans of the chest showed consolidation in both lower lobes consistent with a diagnosis of bacterial pneumonia.
- The patient lacks pathognomonic features for sarcoidosis.
- The working diagnosis of fibromyalgia is not entirely convinc-

ing.

●計画 Plans●

- Diagnostic plans: Repeat CBC and electrolytes, stool culture; schedule UGI endoscopy.
  Therapeutic plans: Adequate hydration with IV drip, clear liquids p.o., withhold antibiotics.
  Educational plans: Was told about the studies planned.
- We will check clean-voided midstream urine for culture and sensitivity.
- In addition to routine lab tests, we plan to perform total colonoscopy and CT scanning of the pelvis.
- Our diagnostic workup includes 24-hour urine collection and renogram.
- MRI of the spine was recommended to the patient who continues to have back pain unexplained by plain films.
- Because of the patient's age and rapid clinical improvement, I don't think invasive diagnostic procedures are necessary at this time.
- Our present therapeutic plans are maintenance of thrombolytic therapy and the use of elastic graduated compression stockings combined with elevation of the legs.
- The initial treatment is directed at the control of arthritis.
- The best treatment option for this patient would be a combination of irradiation and chemotherapy.
- There is a high likelihood that the cancer will respond to high-dose chemotherapy.
- We need to start vigorous therapy with high-dose corticosteroids and cyclophosphamide.
- His current medications include digoxin, potassium chloride, chlortalidone, atenolol, warfarin, and glycopyramide.
- The cardiologist advised us of the use of combined therapy with an ACE inhibitor, valsartan, plus a calcium-channel blocker, azelnidipine.
- This girl is going to be treated with zanamivir, two 5-mg inhalations twice daily for 5 days.
- An exploratory laparotomy was proposed because of suspected bacterial peritonitis due to perforation of the sigmoid colon.
- A pylorus-preserving pancreaticoduodenectomy is scheduled for next Monday.
- The patient is on continuous ventilation and is to have arterial

blood gases daily until stable.
- The patient is scheduled for CABG on October 10, 2009.
- We'll need an ophthalmological consultation about possible laser photocoagulation for his diabetic retinopathy.
- A neuropsychiatric assessment is essential before the initiation of the interferon treatment.
- The patient was instructed to continue 1600-calorie reducing diet.
- The necessity of weight reduction was stressed.
- Since he is unable to carry on normal activity or to do active work, he will require considerable assistance at home.
- I have discussed with the patient what we think is wrong and what tests he needs.

2. 実 例

● 症例提示　Case presentation ●

ID No. 12-345-67, Admission date May 18, 2009

Mr. Ichiro Kato is a 57-year-old man who was admitted to the Central Wing 6 with a three-month history of epigastralgia and anorexia. He had been in his usual state of health until last February, when he noticed an insidious onset of epigastralgia which was described as dull and constant. It was not related to meals. Occasionally he felt nauseous, but there was no actual vomiting. His appetite and intake gradually decreased, and he has lost 5 kg over the past three months. He tended to be constipated, but has not noticed tarry stools. There have been no febrile episodes.

He took OTC antacids without much relief. He has been worried he might have cancer. Because of the persisting symptoms he visited a nearby clinic last week, and was told about a gallstone, 1 cm in diameter, demonstrated by ultrasound. He was referred by the physician to our hospital for further evaluation.

Patient profile: The patient worked at a subcontract factory of Nippon Motor Company, but was laid off last December, two months before the onset of his symptoms. His daily life and eating habits became erratic after he was laid off. Apparently he has had to cut down food expenses.

He quit smoking 20 years ago (he smoked two packs per day in his twenties). He admitted to drinking "some beer" nightly, but declined to specify the amount or duration.

His past history is significant for a whiplash injury which required a week's hospitalization in June 2000 when he was involved in a car accident.

His family history is notable in that his father died of gastric cancer at 55, and his wife died of breast cancer 5 years ago, at 42. His only son, age 28, is well, works for a trading company, and is now stationed in Shanghai. There was no family history of diabetes, hypertension, cardiac disease, or mental disease.

On physical examination his vital signs were within normal limits except for elevated BP (170/100). His height was 168 cm and his weight was 54 kg. He appeared older than his stated age. He was alert and cooperative, but anxious.

Chest was clear to auscultation. There was a 2/6 systolic murmur at the left sternal border.

Abdomen was scaphoid. Bowel sounds were normal. The liver edge was palpable 10 cm below the xiphoid process, and 2 cm below the right costal margin. It was firm and nontender. There was no Murphy sign. The spleen was not palpable.

Rectal exam showed no mass or hemorrhoids. The prostate was bilaterally enlarged, and was smooth without palpable nodules. The stool was yellowish and negative for occult blood.

Available lab data are those from the OPD and are not extensive. Pertinent results were slight leukocytosis (8,500 with a normal differential) and elevated levels of AST (180) and γGT (150). ALT was 50. Platelets, PT, glucose, and CRP were within normal limits. The chest X-ray showed clear lungs and no cardiomegaly.

In summary, Mr. Kato's problems are: #1 epigastralgia, #2 cholelithiasis, #3 hepatomegaly, #4 hypertension, and #5 prostatic enlargement.

Problems #1 to #3: This patient's epigastralgia is different from biliary colic, and can be due to any of various disorders of the stomach, bile duct, pancreas and liver. Although epigastralgia with a detected gallstone appears to justify the referring diagnosis of cholelithiasis, it cannot explain the whole picture. The stone is more likely to be silent without evidence of cholecystitis or impaction in the cystic duct.

I'd rather think that hepatomegaly with moderate elevation of AST (the ratio to ALT greater than 2) and γGT suggests alcoholic liver disease. While he denies alcoholic abuse, I suspect that he might be drinking much, and will check into the exact amount and duration of alcohol use. The enlarged left lobe indicates chronic liver disease, but there were no jaundice, ascites, spider angiomas, palmar erythema, or gynecomastia.

Blood samples have been sent for hepatitis serology and AFP. Upper GI endoscopy, colonoscopy, and abdominal CT scanning with contrast are scheduled.

Problem #4 hypertension: He has been unaware he has high blood pressure. He does not have cardiac risk factors such as diabetes, history of angina pectoris or palpitations. While following his BP readings, we will assess his renal function and cardiac status, and decide treatment options after hypertension workup.

Problem #5 prostatic enlargement: He has no complaints of urinary frequency or dysuria. The prostate will be checked during the repeat abdominal ultrasound. We may ask for a urology consultation after confirming PSA.

---Tidbits---

back-formation

逆成語 back-formation とは，ある語から通常の派生語を作る手順とは逆に，その起源と思われる新語をつくること (neologism) で，James Murray (1897) の造語である．例えば，beg＜beggar, donate＜donation, edit＜editor, televise＜television, typewrite＜typewriter など動詞が多い．医学用語でも，ambulate＜ambulation, diagnose＜diagnosis, dialyze＜dialysis, injure＜injury, secrete＜secretion, sedate＜sedative, vaccinate＜vaccination などが用いられているが，adhese＜adhesion, cyanose＜cyanosis, diurese＜diuresis などはまだ口語的で一般に許容されていない．

VII章

英文紹介状

1. 基本短文例

●挨拶文句　Salutation●

Dear Dr. Jones:
Dear Doctor Jones:
Dear Drs. Bowers and Kerry:
Dear Professor Kennedy:

●本文　Text●

前　文

- I am writing to introduce Mr. Shiro Yamamoto to you.
- I would appreciate it if you could take time to examine this patient.
- I would appreciate it if you would take time to talk with Mrs. Yoshiko Ueda.
- I am referring this patient to you because of her complicated cardiac status.
- I am writing to request that you would see this patient and advise me of necessary procedures.
- This is a letter of introduction for Mr. Thomas Y. Adams who wishes to seek your opinion on his condition.
- I would be grateful if you could see Ms. Lewis who would like a second opinion about the need for a gastrectomy.
- Confirming our telephone conversation of May 20, this is to introduce to you Mrs. Patricia Roberts who has been under my care for the past 10 years.

紹介状返礼

- Thank you for referring Mr. Thomas Y. Adams.
- Thank you very much for sending your patient to see me.
- Thank you for referring Mr. John Smith to me for ophthalmologic evaluation.
- Thank you for referring Ms. Mary Kelly to the Orthopedic Clinic.
- I am writing to thank you for referring Mr. Robert Olson to me.
- Thank you for asking me to see this 65-year-old man who has an unexplained mass in the abdomen.
- Thank you for your detailed letter about this patient.
- Thank you for your helpful letter about Mr. Hiroshi Kobayashi.
- Thank you for letting me know about the results of endocrinological workup.

- It was a pleasure to see your referred patient, Mr. Taro Ishida.
- Mrs. Mary E. Jones was seen on September 9, 2008.
- Today I saw your patient, Mr. Jiro Ito, whom you referred to me on August 15, 2008.
- I saw your patient in gastroenterological consultation at your request today.

患者紹介

- The patient was first seen in September 2007, and followed up with a diagnosis of duodenal ulcer.
- This 78-year-old man has advanced Parkinson disease for several years.
- This 40-year-old lady came in stating that she has had a dry cough and dyspnea on exertion for a week.
- The patient presented to the OPD complaining of increased dizziness over the preceding week.
- This 68-year-old man with a medical history notable for diabetes, sciatica, and benign prostatic hypertrophy presented with a productive cough and shortness of breath, which he reported having had for the past 5 days.
- This patient presented to our emergency department with hematemesis and melena.
- This patient was first seen for his diabetes at our clinic on October 20, 2000.
- This is a 35-year-old single man who has been admitted to our hospital seven times since April 2004.
- The patient has been paraplegic since suffering a complete transection of the spinal cord in an automobile accident 10 years ago.
- This patient has been under my care for benign prostatic hypertrophy since May 2005.
- I have been treating Mrs. Smith for endometriosis for two years.
- This patient has a known diagnosis of chronic hepatitis C and received a 24-week course of interferon treatment last year.
- The patient is known to have chronic obstructive pulmonary disease.
- The patient was initially admitted to the Neurology floor on July 12 and was started on phenytoin 200mg a day.

所見説明

- Physical examination revealed the following: ～
- There were no significant abnormalities on physical examination.
- Physical examination was unremarkable except for varicosities of the lower legs.
- Physical examination revealed no abnormalities other than the presence of pityriasis on the trunk.
- Neurological examination was normal, aside from diminished tendon reflexes in both legs.
- Physical examination revealed cervical lymphadenopathy, splenomegaly, and erythematous plaques over the trunk.
- Positive findings on physical examination were emaciation, anemia, apical systolic murmur, and an abdominal mass.
- Initial examination disclosed moon face, trunkal obesity, abdominal striae, and kyphosis.
- On physical examination he showed no features of chronic hepatic failure.
- The only pertinent physical finding was dependent edema.
- Results of laboratory studies were as follows: ～
- Results from all of the liver function tests were within normal limits.
- Follow-up laboratory studies gave normal results.
- Laboratory studies, with the exception of liver function tests, were normal.
- Biochemical tests disclosed hypercholesterolemia and hyperamylasemia.
- Plain radiographs showed the characteristic changes of osteonecrosis of the hip: subchondral collapse, flattening of the femoral head, and acetabular changes.
- The following examinations were performed: abdominal ultrasound, upper GI series, and colonoscopy.
- The electrocardiogram, a copy of which is enclosed, showed second-degree atrioventricular block.
- Laboratory data are attached.
- A copy of the record is enclosed for your files.
- Attached is a CD-ROM of his recent MRI.
- Attached are copies of x-ray findings for your records.
- I am enclosing a copy of the surgical pathology report with this letter.
- Copies of operative report and discharge summary are enclosed.

患者説明

- I explained to him that we can treat the swelling symptomatically.
- I have explained to her that her episodes of hypoglycemia were probably caused by insulinoma.
- The therapeutic plan including IV antibiotics was explained to the patient and his wife.
- I have discussed the risks and benefits of the alternative treatment with the patient.
- I have discussed the probable cause of his condition with the patient and advised him to see the dermatologist.
- I have discussed the likelihood of an operation being necessary with the patient.
- I have reassured him that he will not need postoperative chemotherapy.
- The patient was reassured that he had several liver cysts that would not in any way affect his health.
- I have told him that he needs continued close observation of his creatinine level.
- I have educated him about elevating the head of the bed during the night.
- I urged him to get a regular amount of exercise and maintain a normal weight.
- She has been instructed to perform a breast self-examination each month.
- The patient was advised to take ample fluids during the daytime.
- I have advised him to keep track of his blood pressure twice a day.
- I have advised her to wear compression stockings and elevate the foot of her bed 20 degrees.
- The patient was cautioned against overeating and overdrinking.
- The importance of strict adherence to the prescribed dosage schedule was emphasized to the patient.
- Because of his history of gallbladder attacks I suggested he might consider laparoscopic cholecystectomy if the colic recurs.

意 見

- I believe the patient has acute interstitial pneumonia.
- It is my medical opinion that needle biopsy is indicated if

significant symptoms continue.
- In my opinion, the abnormal liver function test results are not sufficient to confirm chronic active hepatitis.
- I am of the opinion that he is a poor candidate for general anesthesia because of his age and pulmonary function.
- I think that he is definitely a candidate for immediate treatment and for further evaluation.
- I think it is most likely that this child has coronary artery aneurysm as a sequela of Kawasaki disease.
- The most likely diagnosis is patellofemoral osteoarthritis.
- My assessment is that this patient has erythema multiforme minus.
- I should point out that his dependent edema persisted unrelated to postures.
- I do not think this mass accounts for all of his symptoms.
- I do not think his general condition would permit further chemotherapy.
- I cannot rule out that some of his symptoms may be secondary to chronic renal insufficiency.
- I have no convincing explanation for his spiking fever.
- I suppose the absence of diarrhea makes the diagnosis of intestinal lymphangiectasis unlikely.
- I entirely agree with you on the diagnosis.
- I agree with the present program of anticoagulant therapy.
- I would tend to agree with the diagnosis of chronic thyroiditis.
- There is no clear-cut evidence of hemochromatosis at this point.
- The patient appears to meet the diagnostic criteria for polymyalgia rheumatica.
- This patient shows clinical features compatible with Hodgkin disease.

勧 告
- Recommendations: 1. ~ 2. ~ 3. ~
- Further immunological studies are needed to confirm the diagnosis.
- A CT scan of the pelvis is recommended for evaluation of pelvic lymph nodes.
- The patient should be on a strict low-calorie diet.
- Physical therapy is recommended to minimize deformities of upper extremities.

- I recommend that she try to use the new type of eye drops.
- I would recommend conservative management in view of his age.
- I am recommending endoscopic nasobiliary drainage.
- A course of intensity-modulated radiation therapy was recommended.
- Total hip replacement is advisable in view of unremitting pain and limited range of motion.
- I believe she would benefit from antibiotic therapy.
- One alternative might be watchful waiting in view of his cardiovascular problems and type 2 diabetes mellitus.
- I would recommend the patient returning to the OPD if hematuria recurs.
- The patient was instructed to return to the clinic if he has ankle swelling.
- The patient is to be seen in Dr. Johnson's office in 5 days for suture removal.

治療内容

- Current medications: atenolol 50 mg q.d., theophyllin 200 mg b.i.d., and erythromycin 200 mg q.i.d.
- At the present time he is taking allopurinol 100 mg a day.
- Digoxin was started on June 25 and is now maintained in a dose of 0.125 mg daily.
- Discharge medications include amlodipine 5 mg/day, valsartan 40 mg/day, and indapamide 1 mg/day.
- The patient was maintained on 500 mg twice-daily Cellcept.
- Prophylactic antihistamines were given: dimenhydrinate 50 mg to be taken orally one hour before departure, and then every 4-6 hours as needed.
- Proposed regimen is a 7-day course of treatment with lansoprazole 30 mg twice daily plus amoxicillin 750 mg twice daily and clarithromycin 400 mg twice daily.
- Prednisolone was decreased to 5 mg every other day.
- In this patient low-molecular-weight heparin is preferred for home-based therapy of deep venous thrombosis.
- The mainstay of treatment is bed rest, diuretics, and ACE inhibitors.
- The patient is due to be admitted next month for his second course of combination chemotherapy.
- For his moderate ankle sprain the applied walking cast must be left in place for 3 weeks.

- Oxygen therapy should be continued with nasal prongs to maintain $SaO_2 > 90\%$.
- The patient requires assistance in bathing, getting dressed, and going to toilet.
- The patient needs to take precautions against suffering any cuts and scrapes.

末文
- Thank you for the referral.
- Thank you very much for referring this patient to me.
- Thank you very much for the opportunity of seeing this patient.
- Thank you for allowing me to see this patient.
- I appreciate your taking the time to see this patient.
- I hope that this information is of help to you.
- I hope that the enclosed information will be of some help to you.
- I hope that this can provide you with some additional information on his problem.
- Please let me know if I can do anything more to help.
- Please give me a call if I can help you in any way.
- Please call me at 123 456-7890 if you have any questions.
- I look forward to hearing from you soon.
- I look forward to hearing your opinion.
- I look forward to your comments on his problems.
- Please keep me informed of his course.
- Please keep me updated (posted) on his progress.
- I would appreciate hearing from you, if you have any comments about his progress.
- I would very much appreciate your consideration of my request.
- I will continue the care of this patient and keep you informed of his progress.
- I will be glad to see him again at any time you feel it is necessary.

● 結びの句　Complimentary close ●

Best regards,
Sincerely,
Yours truly,

● 署名　Signature ●

Ichiro Tanaka, MD

Tidbits

Ich bin ein Berliner.

「私もベルリン市民の一人だ」とは Kennedy 大統領が述べた有名な演説の一句だが，ドイツ人には "I am a jelly doughnut."（私は菓子パンだ）と聞こえたと AP 通信は伝えた．もちろんベルリン市民は，笑うどころか "I am a Berliner." の意味と理解して喝采した．ドイツ語では英語と異なり，「〜人」，「〜っ子」，職業を示すときには無冠詞となり，"Ich bin Amerikaner.", "Er ist Berliner.", "Sie ist Lehrerin." というので，JFK は冠詞を入れないで，"Ich bin auch Berliner." と言うべきところだった．
Berliner には，Berliner Pfannkuchen ジャム入りの丸い揚げ菓子（ベルリーナ）という普通名詞がある．
日本人医師の論文に冠詞の誤用は珍しくないが，一味違う冠詞誤用のお話．

2. 実 例

● 紹介状　Referral letter ●

THOMAS F. KENT, MD
111 PARK STREET
PEYTON PLACE, NH 03333
TELEPHONE (603) 555-2222

November 10, 2008

John M. Smith, MD
Department of Gastroenterology
Stepford General Hospital
214 Alexander Street
Stepford, CT

Dear Dr. Smith:

This letter is to confirm our telephone conversation on November 8 about my referral of Mr. Robert M. Brown to you.

This 45-year-old patient was found to have mild anemia during his annual check-up on October 2. He was asymptomatic, and was working as usual. On questioning, however, he admitted that he had noticed a black-colored stool once last month.

Physical examination was non-contributory excepting that normal-colored stool obtained by DRE was positive for occult blood.
Complete blood count showed hypochromic anemia with Hgb 10.8 g/dL. Liver function tests were within normal limits. Serum iron level was 50μg/dL, TIBC 185μg/dL, UIBC 92μg/d, ferritin 30ng/mL, and transferrin 180mg/dL. Abdominal ultrasonography was essentially negative, and sigmoidoscopy excluded hemorrhoids and rectal ulcers or tumors.

My impression is that the patient suffers from iron-deficiency anemia due to chronic blood loss from the gastrointestinal tract. I believe further studies are indicated including upper gastrointestinal endoscopy and total colonoscopy. I would greatly appreciate it if you could schedule these studies and elucidate this intriguing problem.

Sincerely yours,

Thomas F. Kent, MD

TFK / ah

● 紹介状返答　Referral response ●

STEPFORD GENERAL HOSPITAL
214 ALEXANDER STREET
STEPFORD, CT 06666
TELEPHONE (203) 555-4567

December 5, 2008

Thomas F. Kent, MD
111 Park Street
Peyton Place, NH

Dear Dr. Kent:

Re: Mr. Robert M. Brown
    148 Lake Avenue
    Stepford, CT

The above patient was seen on November 15, 2008. He was complaining of slight fatigue, but no significant gastrointestinal symptoms. No black stools had been noticed in the interim.

As you indicated, endoscopic examinations of the upper gastrointestinal tract and colon were performed. Upper GI endoscopy revealed no lesions, specifically no varices or peptic ulcerations. Total colonoscopy showed several polyps in the transverse and descending colon. Polypectomy was performed for a pedunculated polyp in the descending colon. Thus, no obvious bleeding source was detected in the GI tract.

During the night while he was staying after colonoscopic polypectomy, he suddenly vomited fresh blood after several episodes of retching, and became hypotensive. Emergency upper gastrointestinal endoscopy was performed. There were no bleeding lesions in the esophagus; no erosions or Mallory-Weiss tears. The stomach was filled with fresh blood, and on the right decubitus spurting bleeding from a protruded vessel below the cardia was identified. Complete hemostasis was achieved with a Bicap probe. Although he required transfusion of 1,000 ml of blood, the subsequent course was uneventful and repeat endoscopy confirmed complete healing of the bleeding lesion.

Obviously this patient bled from a Dieulafoy ulcer, but I am not certain whether his apparent chronic blood loss was caused by this gastric vascular malformation. I think that watchful follow-up is required.

Thank you very much for referring this interesting patient to me. I would appreciate your keeping me posted about his progress.

Sincerely yours,

John M. Smith, MD
Department of Gastroenterology

Enclosures: 2

JMS: mj

―― Tidbits ――

Leggett's tree

2008年のノーベル物理学賞を日本人が受賞して大きな話題となったが，2003年のノーベル物理学賞は Anthony J Leggett ら米口3氏に贈られた．授賞理由は「超伝導と超流動の理論に関する先駆的貢献」で門外漢には理解困難であるが，Leggett の論文 "Notes on the writing of scientific English for Japanese physicists"（日本物理学会誌21：790-805, 1966）は英語で科学論文を書こうとする日本人にとって必読の文献である．英国生まれで米国籍の博士は日本語も堪能で（夫人は日本人）京大滞在中に Progress of Theoretical Physics への投稿論文査読の経験から日本人英語論文に共通する誤りを指摘した．中でも日英の思考過程の違いを示した図が印象的である．"Japanese English" では論旨が脇道にそれたり後戻りして更に分かれたりするので（図 A），一つの文章と次の文章との関係が不明でパラグラフ全体を読み直してようやく理解できる．正しくは，一本の主流に沿って論旨を進め，枝分かれは少なく短くしかも理由をその都度明確にしなければならない（図 B）．要するに "In English it is essential to be precise and unambiguous."

(A)　　　　(B)

VIII章

略号，記号

1. 医薬品略号

● 抗菌薬　Antibacterial agents ●

略号	一般名	系統・用法／商品名
ABK	arbekacin	アミノ配糖体系・注射／ハベカシン
ABPC	ampicillin	ペニシリン系・注射・内服／ビクシリン，ソルシリン
ABPC/MCIPC	ampicillin/cloxacillin	ペニシリン系合剤・注射・内服／ビクシリンS
ABPC/SBT	ampicillin/sulbactam	ペニシリン系合剤・注射／ユナシンS
ACPC	ciclacillin	ペニシリン系・内服／バストシリン
AKM	bekanamycin	アミノ配糖体系・注射／カネンドマイシン
AMK	amikacin	アミノ配糖体系・注射／ビクリン，硫酸アミカシン
AMPC	amoxicillin	ペニシリン系・内服／アモリン，サワシリン，パセトシン
AMPC/CVA	amoxicillin/clavulanic acid	ペニシリン系合剤・内服／オーグメンチン，クラバモックス
AMPH	amphotericin B	抗真菌薬・注射・内服／ファンギゾン，アムビゾーム
ASPC	aspoxicillin	ペニシリン系・注射／ドイル
ASTM	astromicin	アミノ配糖体系・注射／フォーチミシン
AZM	azithromycin	マクロライド系・内服／ジスロマック
AZT	aztreonam	モノバクタム系・注射／アザクタム
BAPC	bacampicillin	ペニシリン系・内服／ペングッド
BC	bacitracin	アミノ配糖体系・外用／バラマイシン軟膏
BIPM	biapenem	カルバペネム系・注射／オメガシン
CAM	clarithromycin	マクロライド系・内服／クラリシッド，クラリス
CAZ	ceftazidime	第3世代セフェム系・注射／モダシン
CBPZ	cefbuperazone	第2世代セフェム系・注射／ケイペラゾン，トミポラン
CCL	cefaclor	第1世代セフェム系・内服／ケフラール

1. 医薬品略号

略号	一般名	系統・用法/商品名
CDTR-PI	cefditoren pivoxil	第3世代セフェム系・内服/メイアクト MS
CDX	cefadroxil	第1世代セフェム系・内服/サマセフ
CDZM	cefodizime	第3世代セフェム系・注射/ケニセフ, ノイセフ
CET	cephalothin	第1世代セフェム系・注射/コアキシン
CETB	ceftibuten	第3世代セフェム系・内服/セフテム
CEX	cephalexin	第1世代セフェム系・内服/ケフレックス, センセファリン
CEZ	cefazolin	第1世代セフェム系・注射/セファメジン α
CFDN	cefdinir	第3世代セフェム系・内服/セフゾン
CFIX	cefixime	第3世代セフェム系・内服/セフスパン
CFPM	cefepime	第4世代セフェム系・注射/マキシピーム
CFPN-PI	cefcapene pivoxil	第3世代セフェム系・内服/フロモックス
CFS	cefsulodin	第3世代セフェム系・注射/タケスリン
CFT	cefatrizine	第1世代セフェム系・内服/タイセファコール, セフラコール
CFTM-PI	cefteram pivoxil	第3世代セフェム系・内服/トミロン
CINX	cinoxacin	キノロン系・内服/タツレキシン
CL	colistin	ポリペプチド系・内服/コリマイシン S, メタコリマイシン
CLDM	clindamycin	リンコマイシン系・注射・内服・外用/ダラシン S, ダラシン, ダラシン T ゲル
CMNX	cefminox	第2世代セフェム系・注射/メイセリン
CMX	cefmenoxime	第3世代セフェム系・注射・外用/ベストコール, ベストロン点眼液・耳科用液
CMZ	cefmetazole	第2世代セフェム系・注射/セフメタゾン
CP	chloramphenicol	クロラムフェニコール系・注射・内服・外用/クロロマイセチンサクシネート, クロロマイセチン, クロラムフェニコール点眼液, クロロマイセチン耳科用液

略号	一般名	系統・用法/商品名
CPDX-PR	cefpodoxime proxetil	第3世代セフェム系・内服/バナン
CPFX	ciprofloxacin	ニューキノロン系・注射・内服/シプロキサン
CPM	cefpiramide	第3世代セフェム系・注射/サンセファール, セパトレン
CPR	cefpirome	第4世代セフェム系・注射/ケイテン, プロアクト
CPZ	cefoperazone	第3世代セフェム系・注射/セフォビッド, セフォペラジン
CRMN	carumonam	モノバクタム系・注射/アマスリン
CS	cycloserine	抗結核薬・内服/サイクロセリン
CTM	cefotiam	第2世代セフェム系・注射/パンスポリン
CTM-HE	cefotiam hexetil	第2世代セフェム系・内服/パンスポリンT
CTRX	ceftriaxone	第3世代セフェム系・注射/ロセフィン
CTX	cefotaxime	第3世代セフェム系・注射/クラフォラン, セフォタックス
CXD	cefroxadine	第1世代セフェム系・内服/オラスポア
CXM-AX	cefuroxime axetil	第2世代セフェム系・内服/オラセフ
CZOP	cefozopran	第4世代セフェム系・注射/ファーストシン
CZX	ceftizoxime	第3世代セフェム系・外用/エポセリン坐剤
DBECPCG	benzylpenicillin benzathine	ペニシリン系・内服/バイシリンG
DKB	dibekacin	アミノ配糖体系・注射・外用/パニマイシン, パニマイシン点眼液
DMCTC	demethylchlortetracycline	テトラサイクリン系・内服・外用/レダマイシン
DOXY	doxycycline	テトラサイクリン系・内服/ビブラマイシン
DRPM	doripenem	カルバペネム系・注射/フィニバックス

略号	一般名	系統・用法/商品名
EB	ethambutol	抗結核薬・内服 / エサンブトール, エブトール
EM	erythromycin	マクロライド系・注射・内服・外用/エリスロシン, エリスロマイシン, エリスロシン軟膏
ENX	enoxacin	ニューキノロン系・内服/フルマーク
ETH	ethionamide	抗結核薬・内服/ツベルミン
EVM	enviomycin	抗結核薬・注射/ツベラクチン
FA	fusidic acid	抗生物質・外用/フシジンレオ軟膏
5-FC	flucytosine	抗真菌薬・内服/アンコチル
F-FLCZ	fosfluconazole	抗真菌薬・注射/プロジフ
FLCZ	fluconazole	抗真菌薬・注射・内服/ジフルカン
FLRX	fleroxacin	ニューキノロン系・内服/メガキサシン
FMOX	flomoxef	オキサセフェム系・注射/フルマリン
FOM	fosfomycin	ホスホマイシン系・注射・内服・外用/ホスミシン, ホスミシンS, ホスミシンS点耳液
FRM	fradiomycin	アミノ配糖体系・外用 / ソフラチュール, フラジオマイシン
FRPM	faropenem	ペネム系・内服/ファロム
GFLX	gatifloxacin	ニューキノロン系・内服・外用 / ガチフロ, ガチフロ点眼液
GM	gentamicin	アミノ配糖体系・注射・外用 / ゲンタシン, ゲンタシン点眼液・軟膏
GRF	griseofulvin	抗真菌薬・内服/ポンシルFP
GRNX	garenoxacin	ニューキノロン系・内服/ジェニナック
INH	isoniazid	抗結核薬・注射・内服 / イスコチン, ヒドラ, ヒドラジット
INMS	isoniazid sodium methanesulfonate	抗結核薬・内服/ネオイスコチン
IPM/CS	imipenem /cilastatin	カルバペネム系合剤・注射/チエナム
ISP	isepamicin	アミノ配糖体系・注射 / イセパシン, エクサシン

略号	一般名	系統・用法 / 商品名
ITCZ	itraconazole	抗真菌薬・注射・内服 / イトリゾール
JM	josamycin	マクロライド系・内服 / ジョサマイシン
KCZ	ketoconazole	抗真菌薬・外用 / ニゾラール
KM	kanamycin	アミノ配糖体系・注射・内服・外用 / カナマイシン, カナマイシン軟膏
LAPC	lenampicillin	ペニシリン系・内服 / バラシリン
LCM	lincomycin	リンコマイシン系・注射・内服 / リンコシン
LFLX	lomefloxacin	ニューキノロン系・内服・外用 / バレオン, ロメバクト, ロメフロン点眼液・耳科用液
LMOX	latamoxef	オキサセフェム系・注射 / シオマリン
LVFX	levofloxacin	ニューキノロン系・内服・外用 / クラビット, クラビット点眼液
LZD	linezolid	オキサゾリジノン系・注射・内服 / ザイボックス
MCFG	micafungin	抗真菌薬・注射 / ファンガード
MCR	micronomicin	アミノ配糖体系・注射・外用 / サガミシン, サンテマイシン点眼液
MCZ	miconazole	抗真菌薬・注射・内服・外用 / フロリード, フロリードゲル・腟坐剤
MDM	midecamycin	マクロライド系・内服 / ミオカマイシン, メデマイシン
MEPM	meropenem	カルバペネム系・注射 / メロペン
MFLX	moxifloxacin	ニューキノロン系・内服・外用 / アベロックス, ベガモックス点眼液
MINO	minocycline	テトラサイクリン系・注射・内服・外用 / ミノマイシン
MUP	mupirocin	抗 MRSA 薬・外用 / バクトロバン鼻腔用軟膏
NA	nalidixic acid	キノロン系・内服 / ウイントマイロン
NDFX	nadifloxacin	キノロン系・外用 / アクアチム軟膏・クリーム・ローション
NFLX	norfloxacin	ニューキノロン系・内服・外用 / バクシダール, バクシダール点眼液

1. 医薬品略号

略号	一般名	系統・用法/商品名
NYS	nystatin	抗真菌薬・内服/ナイスタチン
OFLX	ofloxacin	ニューキノロン系・内服・外用/タリビッド, タリビッド点眼液・耳科用液
OTC	oxytetracycline	テトラサイクリン系・外用/オキシテトラコーン
PA	piromidic acid	キノロン系・内服/パナシッド
PAPM/BP*	panipenem/betamipron	カルバペネム系合剤・注射/カルベニン
PAS-Ca	calcium para-aminosalicylate	抗結核薬・内服/ニッパスカルシウム
PCG	benzylpenicillin	ペニシリン系・注射/ペニシリンGカリウム
PIPC	piperacillin	ペニシリン系・注射/ペントシリン
PL-B	polymyxin B	ポリペプチド系・内服・外用/硫酸ポリミキシン
PMPC	pivmecillinam	ペニシリン系・内服/メリシン
PMR	pimaricin	抗真菌薬・外用/ピマリシン点眼液・眼軟膏
PPA	pipemidic acid	キノロン系・内服/ドルコール
PUFX	prulifloxacin	ニューキノロン系・内服/スオード
PZA	pyrazinamide	抗結核薬・内服/ピラマイド
PZFX	pazufloxacin	ニューキノロン系・注射/パシル, パズクロス
QPR/DPR	quinupristin/dalfopristin	ストレプトグラミン系・注射/シナシッド
RBT	rifabutin	抗結核薬・内服/ミコブテイン
RFP	rifampicin	抗結核薬・内服/リファジン, リマクタン
RKM	rokitamycin	マクロライド系・内服/リカマイシン
RSM	ribostamycin	アミノ配糖体系・注射/ビスタマイシン
RXM	roxithromycin	マクロライド系・内服/ルリッド
SBT/CPZ	sulbactam/cefoperazone	セフェム系合剤・注射/スルペラゾン
SBTPC	sultamicillin	ペニシリン系・内服/ユナシン

略号	一般名	系統・用法/商品名
SISO	sisomicin	アミノ配糖体系・外用/シセプチン点眼液
SM	streptomycin	アミノ配糖体系・注射/硫酸ストレプトマイシン
SPCM	spectinomicin	アミノ配糖体系・注射/トロビシン
SPFX	sparfloxacin	ニューキノロン系・内服/スパラ
SPM	spiramycin	マクロライド系・内服/アセチルスピラマイシン
ST	sulfamethoxazole /trimethoprim	サルファ剤合剤・内服/バクタ, バクトラミン
STFX	sitafloxacin	ニューキノロン系・内服/グレースビット
TAPC	talampicillin	ペニシリン系・内服/アセオシリン
TAZ /PIPC	tazobactam /piperacillin	ペニシリン系合剤・注射/ゾシン
TBPM-PI	tebipenem pivoxil	カルバペネム系・内服/オラペネム小児用細粒
TC	tetracycline	テトラサイクリン系・内服・外用/アクロマイシン, アクロマイシン軟膏
TEIC	teicoplanin	グリコペプチド系・注射/タゴシッド
TEL	telithromycin	ケトライド系・内服/ケテック
TFLX	tosufloxacin	ニューキノロン系・内服・外用/オゼックス, トスキサシン, オゼックス点眼液
TOB	tobramycin	アミノ配糖体系・注射・外用/トブラシン, トブラシン点眼液
TP	thiamphenicol	クロラムフェニコール系・内服/アーマイ
VCM	vancomycin	グリコペプチド系・注射・内服/塩酸バンコマイシン
VRCZ	voriconazole	抗真菌薬・注射・内服/ブイフェンド

●抗癌剤　Anticancer agents●

略号	一般名	系統・用法 / 商品名
ACNU	nimustine	アルキル化剤・注射 / ニドラン
ACR	aclarubicin	抗生物質・注射 / アクラシノン
ACT-D	actinomycin D	抗生物質・注射 / コスメゲン
ADM	doxorubicin	抗生物質・注射 / アドリアシン, ドキシル
AMR	amrubicin	抗生物質・注射 / カルセド
ANA	anastrozole	ホルモン製剤・注射 / アリミデックス
Ara-C	cytarabine	代謝拮抗物質・注射 / キロサイド
ATRA	tretinoin	分化誘導活性作用・内服 / ベサノイド
BH-AC	enocitabine	代謝拮抗物質・注射 / サンラビン
BLM	bleomycin	抗生物質・注射・外用 / ブレオ
BST	ubenimex	免疫強化剤・内服 / ベスタチン
BUS	busulfan	アルキル化剤・注射 / ブスルフェクス
BUS	busulfan	アルキル化剤・内服 / マブリン
CBDCA	carboplatin	白金製剤・注射 / パラプラチン, カルボプラチン
2-CdA	cladribine	代謝拮抗物質・注射 / ロイスタチン
CDDP	cisplatin	白金製剤・注射 / ブリプラチン, ランダ, アイエーコール
CDGP	nedaplatin	白金製剤・注射 / アクプラ
CPA	cyclophosphamide	アルキル化剤・注射・内服 / エンドキサン
CPT-11	irinotecan	トポイソメラーゼ阻害薬・注射 / カンプト, トポテシン, イリノテカン
DCF	pentostatin	代謝拮抗物質・注射 / コホリン
DES	fosfestrol	ホルモン製剤・注射・内服 / ホンバン
5'-DFUR	5'-doxifluridine	代謝拮抗物質・内服 / フルツロン
DNR	daunorubicin	抗生物質・注射 / ダウノマイシン
DOC	docetaxel	アルカロイド系・注射 / タキソテール
DTIC	dacarbazine	アルキル化剤・注射 / ダカルバジン
DTX	docetaxel	アルカロイド系・注射 / タキソテール

VIII章 略号, 記号

略号	一般名	系統・用法 / 商品名
DXR	doxorubicin	抗生物質・注射 / アドリアシン, ドキシル
EP	estramustine	ホルモン製剤・内服 / エストラサイト
EPI	epirubicin	抗生物質・注射 / ファルモルビシン, エピルビシン
ETP	etoposide	トポイソメラーゼ阻害薬・注射・内服 / ベプシド, ラステット
FLU	fludarabine	代謝拮抗物質・注射・内服 / フルダラ
FT	tegafur	代謝拮抗物質・注射・内服・外用 / フトラフール
5-FU	5-fluorouracil	代謝拮抗物質・注射・内服・外用 / 5-FU
GEM	gemcitabine	代謝拮抗物質・注射 / ジェムザール
HCFU	carmofur	代謝拮抗物質・内服 / ミフロール
HU	hydroxycarbamide	代謝拮抗物質・内服 / ハイドレア
IDR	idarubicin	抗生物質・注射 / イダマイシン
IFM	ifosfamide	アルキル化剤・注射 / イホマイド
IFN-α	interferon alfa	インターフェロン・注射 / スミフェロン
IFN-α2b	interferon alfa-2b	インターフェロン・注射 / イントロン A
IFN-β	interferon beta	インターフェロン・注射 / フエロン
IFN-γ1a	interferon gamma-1a	インターフェロン・注射 / イムノマックス-γ
IFN-γn1	interferon gamma-n1	インターフェロン・注射 / オーガンマ
L-ASP	L-asparaginase	アスパラギン分解・注射 / ロイナーゼ
l-LV	levofolinate calcium	抗癌療法補助剤・注射 / アイソボリン
L-PAM	melphalan	アルキル化剤・注射・内服 / アルケラン
L-OHP	oxaliplatin	白金製剤・注射 / エルプラット
LV	calcium folinate	抗癌療法補助剤・内服 / ロイコボリン, ユーゼル
MCNU	ranimustine	アルキル化剤・注射 / サイメリン
MIT	mitoxantrone	抗生物質・注射 / ノバントロン

1. 医薬品略号

略号	一般名	系統・用法 / 商品名
MMC	mitomycin C	抗生物質・注射 / マイトマイシン
6-MP	6-mercaptopurine	代謝拮抗物質・内服 / ロイケリン
MPA	medroxyprogesterone	ホルモン製剤・内服 / ヒスロン H，プロベラ
MPT	mepitiostane	ホルモン製剤・内服 / チオデロン
MTX	methotrexate	代謝拮抗物質・注射・内服 / メソトレキセート
NGT	nogitecan	トポイソメラーゼ阻害薬・注射 / ハイカムチン
OK-432	picibanil	免疫強化剤・注射 / ピシバニール
PCZ	procarbazine	アルキル化剤・内服 / 塩酸プロカルバジン
PEP	peplomycin	抗生物質・注射 / ペプレオ
PSK	krestin	免疫強化剤・内服 / クレスチン
PTX	paclitaxel	アルカロイド系・注射 / タキソール，パクリタキセル
SPAC	cytarabine ocfosfate	代謝拮抗物質・内服 / スタラシド
SPG	sizofiran	免疫強化剤・注射 / ソニフィラン
TAM	tamoxifen	ホルモン製剤・内服 / ノルバデックス
TESPA	thiotepa	アルキル化剤・注射 / テスパミン
TGF	tegafur	代謝拮抗物質・注射・内服・外用 / フトラフール
THP	pirarubicin	抗生物質・注射 / テラルビシン，ピノルビン
TOR	toremifene	ホルモン製剤・内服 / フェアストン
TS-1	tegafur-gimeracil-oteracil	代謝拮抗物質・内服 / ティーエスワン
TXT	docetaxel	アルカロイド系・注射 / タキソテール
UFT	tegafur-uracil	代謝拮抗物質・内服 / ユーエフティ
VCR	vincristine	アルカロイド系・注射 / オンコビン
VDS	vindesine	アルカロイド系・注射 / フィルデシン
VLB	vinblastine	アルカロイド系・注射 / エクザール

略号	一般名	系統・用法/商品名
VNR	vinorelbine	アルカロイド系・注射/ナベルビン
VP-16	etoposide	トポイソメラーゼ阻害薬・注射・内服/ベプシド, ラステット

●分子標的治療薬　Molecularly targeted medicine●

一般名	英語名	適応腫瘍	商品名
イブリツモマブ・チウキセタン	ibritumomab tiuxetan	CD20(+)NHL	ゼヴァリン
イマチニブメシル酸塩	imatinib mesilate	CML, Ph(+)ALL	グリベック
エルロチニブ	erlotinib	NSCLC	タルセバ
ゲフィチニブ	gefitinib	NSCLC	イレッサ
ゲムツズマブ・オゾガマイシン	gemtuzumab ozogamicin	AML	マイロターグ
スニチニブ	sunnitinib	RCC	スーテント
セツキシマブ	cetuximab	結腸・直腸癌	アービタックス
ソラフェニブ	sorafenib	RCC, HCC	ネクサバール
ダサチニブ	dasatinib	CML	スプリセル
トラスツズマブ	trastuzumab	乳癌	ハーセプチン
ニロチニブ	nilotinib	CML	タシグナ
ベバシズマブ	bevacizumab	結腸・直腸癌	アバスチン
ボルテゾミブ	bortezomib	MM	ベルケイド
ラパチニブ	lapatinib	乳癌	タイケルブ
リツキシマブ	rituximab	CD20(+)NHL	リツキサン
以下未承認			
イキサベピロン	ixabepilone	乳癌	Ixempra
テムシロリムス	temsirolimus	RCC	Torisel
パニツムマブ	panitumumab	結腸・直腸癌	Vectibix

2. 元素記号

原子番号	元素記号	英語名	日本語名	原子量(u)
1	H	hydrogen	水素	1.00794(7)
2	He	helium	ヘリウム	4.002602(2)
3	Li	lithium	リチウム	6.941(2)
4	Be	beryllium	ベリリウム	9.012182(3)
5	B	boron	ホウ素	10.811(7)
6	C	carbon	炭素	12.0107(8)
7	N	nitrogen	窒素	14.0067(2)
8	O	oxygen	酸素	15.9994(3)
9	F	fluorine	フッ素	18.9984032(5)
10	Ne	neon	ネオン	20.1797(6)
11	Na	sodium	ナトリウム	22.98976928(2)
12	Mg	magnesium	マグネシウム	24.3050(6)
13	Al	aluminium	アルミニウム	26.9815386(8)
14	Si	silicon	ケイ素	28.0855(3)
15	P	phosphorus	リン	30.973762(2)
16	S	sulfur	硫黄	32.065(5)
17	Cl	chlorine	塩素	35.453(2)
18	Ar	argon	アルゴン	39.948(1)
19	K	potassium	カリウム	39.0983(1)
20	Ca	calcium	カルシウム	40.078(4)
21	Sc	scandium	スカンジウム	44.955912(6)
22	Ti	titanium	チタン	47.867(1)
23	V	vanadium	バナジウム	50.9415(1)
24	Cr	chromium	クロム	51.9961(6)
25	Mn	manganese	マンガン	54.938045(5)
26	Fe	iron	鉄	55.845(2)
27	Co	cobalt	コバルト	58.933195(5)
28	Ni	nickel	ニッケル	58.6934(4)
29	Cu	copper	銅	63.546(3)
30	Zn	zinc	亜鉛	65.38(2)
31	Ga	gallium	ガリウム	69.723(1)
32	Ge	germanium	ゲルマニウム	72.64(1)
33	As	arsenic	ヒ素	74.92160(2)
34	Se	selenium	セレン	78.96(3)
35	Br	bromine	臭素	79.904(1)
36	Kr	krypton	クリプトン	83.798(2)
37	Rb	rubidium	ルビジウム	85.4678(3)

原子番号	元素記号	英語名	日本語名	原子量(u)
38	Sr	strontium	ストロンチウム	87.62(1)
39	Y	yttrium	イットリウム	88.90585(2)
40	Zr	zirconium	ジルコニウム	91.224(2)
41	Nb	niobium	ニオブ	92.90638(2)
42	Mo	molybdenum	モリブデン	95.96(2)
43	Tc	technetium	テクネチウム	[99]
44	Ru	ruthenium	ルテニウム	101.07(2)
45	Rh	rhodium	ロジウム	102.90550(2)
46	Pd	palladium	パラジウム	106.42(1)
47	Ag	silver	銀	107.8682(2)
48	Cd	cadmium	カドミウム	112.411(8)
49	In	indium	インジウム	114.818(3)
50	Sn	tin	スズ	118.710(7)
51	Sb	antimony	アンチモン	121.760(1)
52	Te	tellurium	テルル	127.60(3)
53	I	iodine	ヨウ素	126.90447(3)
54	Xe	xenon	キセノン	131.293(6)
55	Cs	caesium	セシウム	132.9054519(2)
56	Ba	barium	バリウム	137.327(7)
57	La	lanthanum	ランタン	138.90547(7)
58	Ce	cerium	セリウム	140.116(1)
59	Pr	praseodymium	プラセオジム	140.90765(2)
60	Nd	neodymium	ネオジム	144.242(3)
61	Pm	promethium	プロメチウム	[145]
62	Sm	samarium	サマリウム	150.36(2)
63	Eu	europium	ユウロピウム	151.964(1)
64	Gd	gadolinium	ガドリニウム	157.25(3)
65	Tb	terbium	テルビウム	158.92535(2)
66	Dy	dysprosium	ジスプロシウム	162.500(1)
67	Ho	holmium	ホルミウム	164.93032(2)
68	Er	erbium	エルビウム	167.259(3)
69	Tm	thulium	ツリウム	168.93421(2)
70	Yb	ytterbium	イッテルビウム	173.054(5)
71	Lu	lutetium	ルテチウム	174.9668(1)
72	Hf	hafnium	ハフニウム	178.49(2)
73	Ta	tantalum	タンタル	180.94788(1)
74	W	tungsten	タングステン	183.84(1)
75	Re	rhenium	レニウム	186.207(1)
76	Os	osmium	オスミウム	190.23(3)

原子番号	元素記号	英語名	日本語名	原子量(u)
77	Ir	iridium	イリジウム	192.217(3)
78	Pt	platinum	白金	195.084(9)
79	Au	gold	金	196.966569(4)
80	Hg	mercury	水銀	200.59(2)
81	Tl	thallium	タリウム	204.3833(2)
82	Pb	lead	鉛	207.2(1)
83	Bi	bismuth	ビスマス	208.98040(1)
84	Po	polonium	ポロニウム	[210]
85	At	astatine	アスタチン	[210]
86	Rn	radon	ラドン	[222]
87	Fr	francium	フランシウム	[223]
88	Ra	radium	ラジウム	[226]
89	Ac	actinium	アクチニウム	[227]
90	Th	thorium	トリウム	232.03806(2)
91	Pa	protactinium	プロトアクチニウム	231.03588(2)
92	U	uranium	ウラン	238.02891(3)
93	Np	neptunium	ネプツニウム	[237]
94	Pu	plutonium	プルトニウム	[244]
95	Am	americium	アメリシウム	[243]
96	Cm	curium	キュリウム	[247]
97	Bk	berkelium	バークリウム	[247]
98	Cf	californium	カリホルニウム	[251]
99	Es	einsteinium	アインスタイニウム	[252]
100	Fm	fermium	フェルミウム	[257]
101	Md	mendelevium	メンデレビウム	[258]
102	No	nobelium	ノーベリウム	[259]
103	Lr	lawrencium	ローレンシウム	[262]
104	Rf	rutherfordium	ラザホージウム	[267]
105	Db	dubnium	ドブニウム	[268]
106	Sg	seaborgium	シーボーギウム	[271]
107	Bh	bohrium	ボーリウム	[272]
108	Hs	hassium	ハッシウム	[277]
109	Mt	meitnerium	マイトネリウム	[276]
110	Ds	darmstadtium	ダームスタチウム	[281]
111	Rg	roentgenium	レントゲニウム	[280]
112	Cn	copernicium	コペルニシウム	[285]
113	Uut	ununtrium	ウンウントリウム	[284]
114	Uuq	ununquadium	ウンウンクアジウム	[289]
115	Uup	ununpentium	ウンウンペンチウム	[288]
116	Uuh	ununhexium	ウンウンヘキシウム	[293]

原子番号	元素記号	英語名	日本語名	原子量(u)
117	Uus	ununseptium	ウンウンセプチウム	[292]
118	Uuo	ununoctium	ウンウンオクチウム	[294]

3. 単 位

記号	英語名	日本語名
A	ampere	アンペア
Bq	becquerel	ベクレル
C	coulomb	クーロン
℃	degree Celsius	摂氏
cal	calorie	カロリー
cc	cubic centimeter	立方センチメートル
cd	candela	カンデラ
cm	centimeter	センチメートル
Da	dalton	ダルトン
dl/dL	deciliter	デシリットル
dyn	dyne	ダイン
F	farad	ファラド
℉	degree Fahrenheit	華氏
fl oz	fluid ounce	液量オンス
ft	foot, feet	フィート
g	gram	グラム
G	gauss	ガウス
gal	gallon	ガロン
gr	grain	グレーン
Gy	gray	グレイ
H	henry	ヘンリー
Hz	hertz	ヘルツ
in	inch	インチ
J	joule	ジュール
K	kelvin	ケルヴィン
kg	kilogram	キログラム
km	kilometer	キロメートル
l/L	liter	リットル
lb	pound	ポンド
lm	lumen	ルーメン
lx	lux	ルクス
m	meter	メートル
meq	milliequivalent	ミリグラム当量
mg	milligram	ミリグラム
mi	mile	マイル
min	minute	分
mm	millimeter	ミリメートル
mol	mole	モル

記号	英語名	日本語名
N	newton	ニュートン
ng	nanogram	ナノグラム
osmol	osmole	オスモル
oz	ounce	オンス
Pa	pascal	パスカル
pg	picogram	ピコグラム
pt	pint	パイント
qt	quart	クオート
R	roentgen	レントゲン
rad	radian	ラジアン
rpm	revolutions per min	毎分回転数
s	second	秒
S	siemens	ジーメンス
Sv	sievert	シーベルト
T	tesla	テスラ
torr	torricelli	トール
u	atomic mass unit	原子質量単位
V	volt	ボルト
W	watt	ワット
Wb	weber	ウェーバー
yd	yard	ヤード
μg	microgram	マイクログラム
Ω	ohm	オーム

IX章

人体解剖図

1. 人 体

● 頭 Head ●

頭蓋 (とうがい, ずがい)	skull, cranium, 〔形〕cranial
頭蓋冠 (とうがいかん)	calvaria, 〔形〕calvarial
頭頂 (とうちょう)	top of the head, vertex
後頭部 (こうとうぶ)	back of the head, occiput
頭皮 (とうひ)	scalp
頭髪 (とうはつ)	hair (of the head)
前髪 (まえがみ)	forelock
顔 (かお)	face
額 (ひたい)	forehead
こめかみ	temple
眼 (め)	eye
眼球 (がんきゅう)	eyeball
瞼 (まぶた)	eyelid
眉毛 (まゆげ)	eyebrow, supercilium
眉間 (みけん)	the middle of the eyebrows, glabella
もみあげ	sideburns
鼻 (はな)	nose
耳 (みみ)	ear
耳たぶ (みみ—)	earlobe
頬 (ほお)	cheek
頬骨 (ほおぼね)	cheekbone
えくぼ	dimple
口 (くち)	mouth
唇 (くちびる)	lip
上唇 (うわくちびる, じょうしん)	upper lip
下唇 (したくちびる, かしん)	lower lip
歯 (は)	tooth, 〔複〕teeth
前歯 (まえば)	front tooth
奥歯 (おくば)	back tooth
歯茎 (はぐき)	gum
のど	throat
口髭 (くちひげ)	mustache, moustache
顎 (あご)	jaw
上顎 (うわあご)	upper jaw
下顎 (したあご)	lower jaw
あご先 (—さき), 頤 (おとがい)	chin, mentum
顎鬚 (あごひげ)	beard
首 (くび)	neck
のど仏 (—ぼとけ)	Adam's apple

1. 人体   443

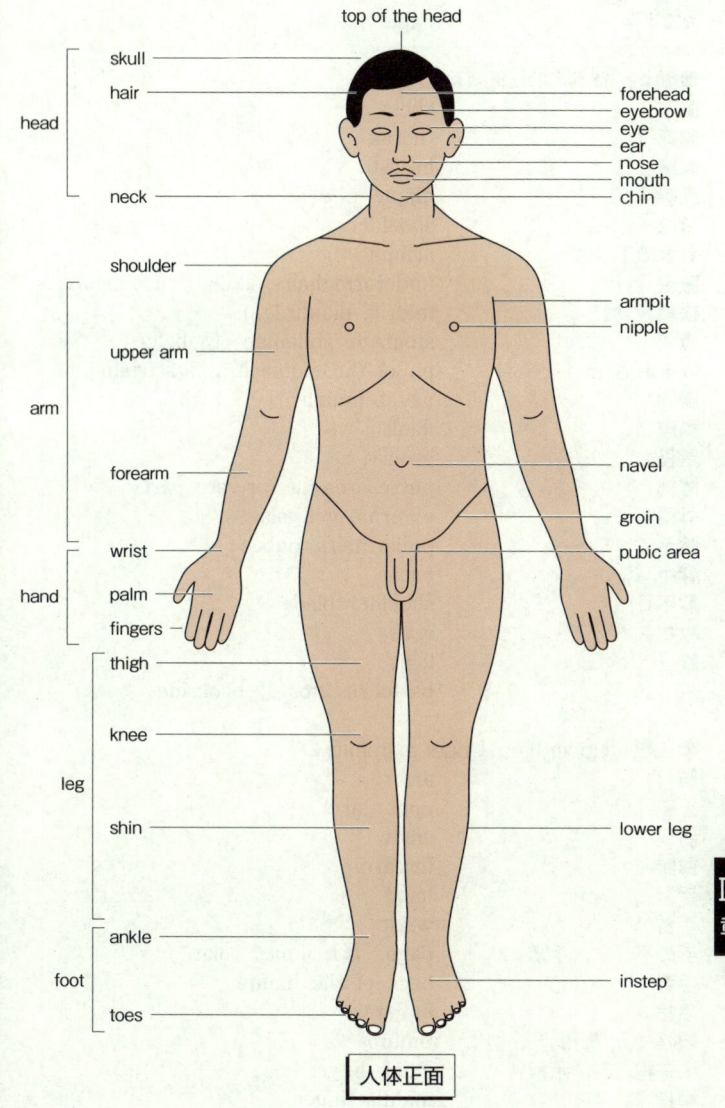

人体正面

うなじ　　　　　　　　　　　nape

● 胴体, 体幹　Trunk, Torso ●

胸 むね	chest
胸郭 きょうかく	thorax
乳房 ちぶさ, にゅうぼう	breast
乳頭 にゅうとう	nipple
肩 かた	shoulder
わきの下 した	armpit
腋毛 わきげもう	underarm hairs, axillary hairs, hirci
横隔膜 おうかくまく	midriff, diaphragm
腹 はら	stomach, abdomen, 〔話〕belly
みぞおち	pit of the stomach, epigastrium
臍 へそ	navel, umbilicus
横腹 よこばら	flank
鼠径 そけい	groin
陰部 いんぶ	pubic area, 〔話〕private parts
外陰部 がいいんぶ	external genitals
陰毛 いんもう	pubic hairs, pubes
背中 せなか	back
肩甲骨 けんこうこつ	shoulder blade
ウエスト	waist
腰 こし	loins
尻 しり	buttocks, hip, 〔話〕backside

● 上肢　Upper limb, Upper extremity ●

腕 うで	arm
上腕 じょうわん	upper arm
肘 ひじ	elbow
前腕 ぜんわん	forearm
手 て	hand
手首 てくび	wrist
手の平 てのひら, 手掌 しゅしょう	palm, 〔形〕palmar, volar
手背 しゅはい	back of the hand
手指 しゅし	fingers
親指 おやゆび, 母指 ぼし	thumb
人差指 ひとさしゆび, 示指 じし	index finger
中指 なかゆび	middle finger
薬指 くすりゆび	ring finger
小指 こゆび	little finger, pinkie
指先 ゆびさき, 指尖 しせん	fingertip
指紋 しもん	fingerprint

1. 人体　445

- back of the head
- nape
- shoulder
- shoulder blade
- elbow
- waist
- buttocks
- back of the hand
- nail
- calf
- sole
- heel

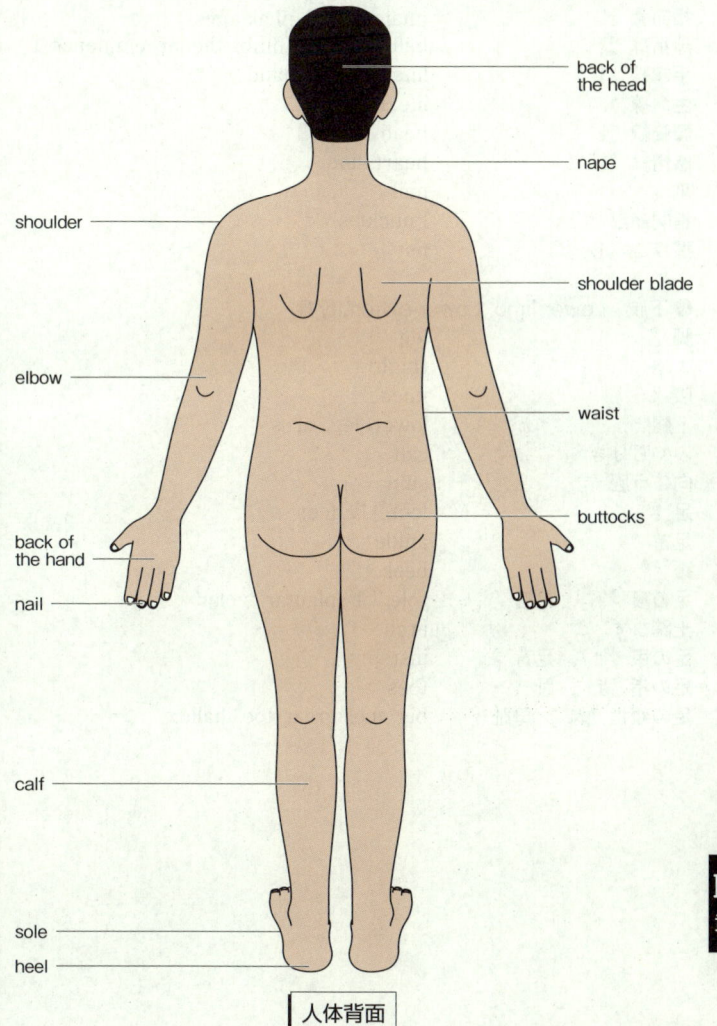

人体背面

IX章 人体解剖図

指節骨 しせつこつ	phalanx, 〔複〕phalanges
母指球 ぼしきゅう	ball of the thumb, thenar eminence
手掌線 しゅしょうせん	lines of the hand
生命線 せいめいせん	life line
頭脳線 ずのうせん	head line
感情線 かんじょうせん	heart line
爪 つめ	nail
指関節部 ゆびかんせつぶ	knuckles
握りこぶし にぎ―	fist

● 下肢 Lower limb, Lower extremity ●

脚 あし	leg
太腿 ふともも	thigh
膝 ひざ	knee
下腿 かたい	lower leg, crus
ふくらはぎ	calf
向こう脛 ―ずね	shin
足 あし	foot, 〔複〕feet
足首 あしくび	ankle
踵 かかと	heel
足の裏 あしうら―, 足底 そくてい	sole, 〔形〕plantar, volar
土踏まず つちふ―	arch
足の甲 あしこう―, 足背 そくはい	instep
足の指 あしゆび―, 趾 し	toes
足の親指 あしおやゆび―, 母趾 ぼし	big toe, great toe, hallux

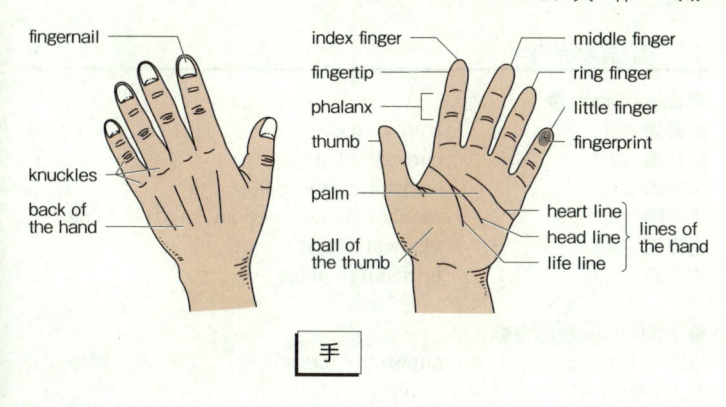

1. 人体

手

- fingernail
- knuckles
- back of the hand
- index finger
- fingertip
- phalanx
- thumb
- palm
- ball of the thumb
- middle finger
- ring finger
- little finger
- fingerprint
- heart line ⎤
- head line ⎬ lines of the hand
- life line ⎦

Tidbits

extremity

ラテン語の extremitas（先端, 末端）に由来し, extremitas sternalis claviculae 鎖骨胸骨端, extremitas superior testis 精巣上端のように細長い部分の端を意味する. 従って胴体から遠い手足 hands and feet のことになるが, extremitas superior は membrum superius と同義で upper limb, extremitas inferior は membrum inferius と同義で lower limb を指す言葉となっている. 従って上肢は upper extremity（両側であれば upper extremities）, 下肢は lower extremity (extremities), 四肢は four extremities.

口語で "an arm and a leg" は「法外な金額」のことで, "cost an arm and a leg" といえば「大変な金がかかる」ということになる (The plumber charged an arm and a leg. Good childcare costs an arm and a leg.). 2001年にガソリン価格が高騰したとき米ウィスコンシン州のあるガソリンスタンドは, 店頭に "Regular 172, Plus ARM, Premium LEG" と掲示して話題になった.

2. 表面解剖学

● 面　Planes ●

前頭面 ぜんとうめん	frontal plane
冠状面 かんじょうめん	coronal plane
矢状面 しじょうめん	sagittal plane
正中面 せいちゅうめん	median plane, median sagittal plane
垂直面 すいちょくめん	vertical plane
水平面 すいへいめん	horizontal plane

● 方向　Directions ●

上方―下方 じょうほう―かほう	superior / inferior
前方―後方 ぜんぽう―こうほう	anterior / posterior
内側―外側 ないそく―がいそく	medial / lateral
内方―外方 ないほう―がいほう	internal / external
垂直―水平 すいちょく―すいへい	vertical / horizontal
頭側―尾側 とうそく―びそく	cranial / caudal
頭側へ―尾側へ とうそくへ―びそくへ	cephalad / caudad
腹側―背側 ふくそく―はいそく	ventral / dorsal
口側―肛門側 こうそく―こうもんそく	oral / anal
中心―末梢 ちゅうしん―まっしょう	central / peripheral
近位―遠位 きんい―えんい	proximal / distal
縦―横 たて―よこ	longitudinal / transverse
橈側―尺側 とうそく―しゃくそく	radial / ulnar
脛側―腓側 けいそく―ひそく	tibial / fibular
伸展側―屈側 しんてんそく―くっそく	extensor / flexor

Tidbits

anatomical position

解剖学的肢位 anatomical position とは、人体の部位や方向を示す標準的な肢位。立位で顔を正面に向け、前腕を回外して手掌を正面に向け、足は爪先を前に向けて揃える。

2. 表面解剖学　449

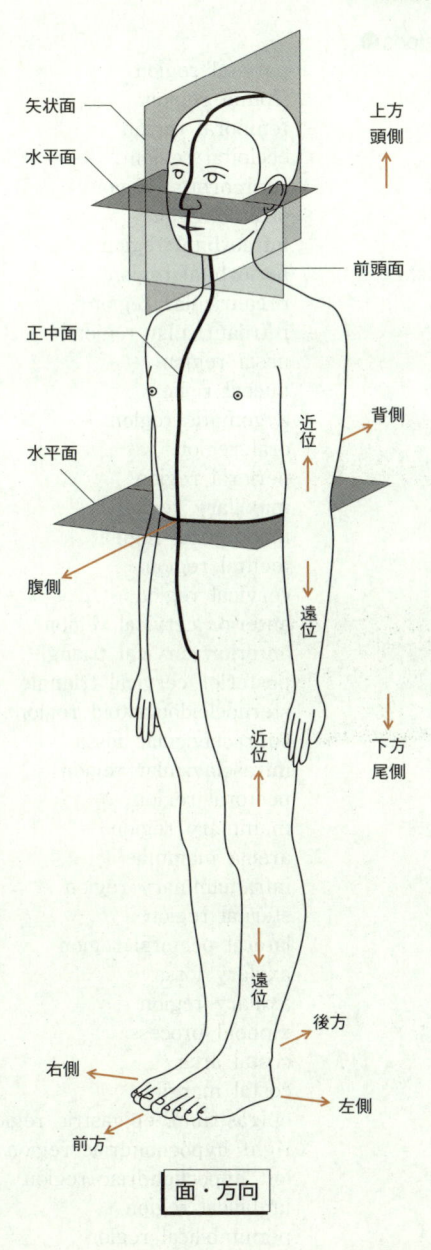

面・方向

●部位　Regions●

頭頂部 とうちょうぶ	parietal region
前頭部 ぜんとうぶ	frontal region
側頭部 そくとうぶ	temporal region
後頭部 こうとうぶ	occipital region
眼窩上部 がんかじょうぶ	supraorbital region
眼窩部 がんかぶ	orbital region
眼窩下部 がんかかぶ	infraorbital region
眼窩周囲部 がんかしゅういぶ	periorbital region
耳介前部 じかいぜんぶ	preauricular region
耳介後部 じかいこうぶ	retroauricular region
鼻部 びぶ	nasal region
頬部 きょうぶ	buccal region
頬骨部 きょうこつぶ	zygomatic region
口部 こうぶ	oral region
口周囲部 こうしゅういぶ	perioral region
上顎部 じょうがくぶ	maxillary region
下顎部 かがくぶ	mandibular region
頤部 おとがいぶ	mental region
頚部 けいぶ	cervical region
前頚部 ぜんけいぶ	anterior cervical region
前頚三角部 ぜんけいさんかくぶ	anterior cervical triangle
後頚三角部 こうけいさんかくぶ	posterior cervical triangle
胸鎖乳突筋部 きょうさにゅうとつきんぶ	sternocleidomastoid region
鎖骨上窩 さこつじょうか	supraclavicular fossa
鎖骨下部 さこつかぶ	infraclavicular region
胸部 きょうぶ	pectoral region
乳房部 にゅうぼうぶ	mammary region
乳輪 にゅうりん	areola mammae
乳房下部 にゅうぼうかぶ	inframammary region
胸骨部 きょうこつぶ	sternal region
側胸部 そくきょうぶ	lateral pectoral region
腋窩 えきか	axillary fossa
腋窩部 えきかぶ	axillary region
剣状突起 けんじょうとっき	xiphoid process
肋骨弓 ろっこつきゅう	costal arch
肋骨縁 ろっこつえん	costal margin
心窩部 しんかぶ	epigastrium, epigastric region
右下肋部 みぎかろくぶ	right hypochondriac region
左下肋部 ひだりかろくぶ	left hypochondriac region
臍部 さいぶ	umbilical region
臍周囲部 さいしゅういぶ	periumbilical region

2. 表面解剖学　451

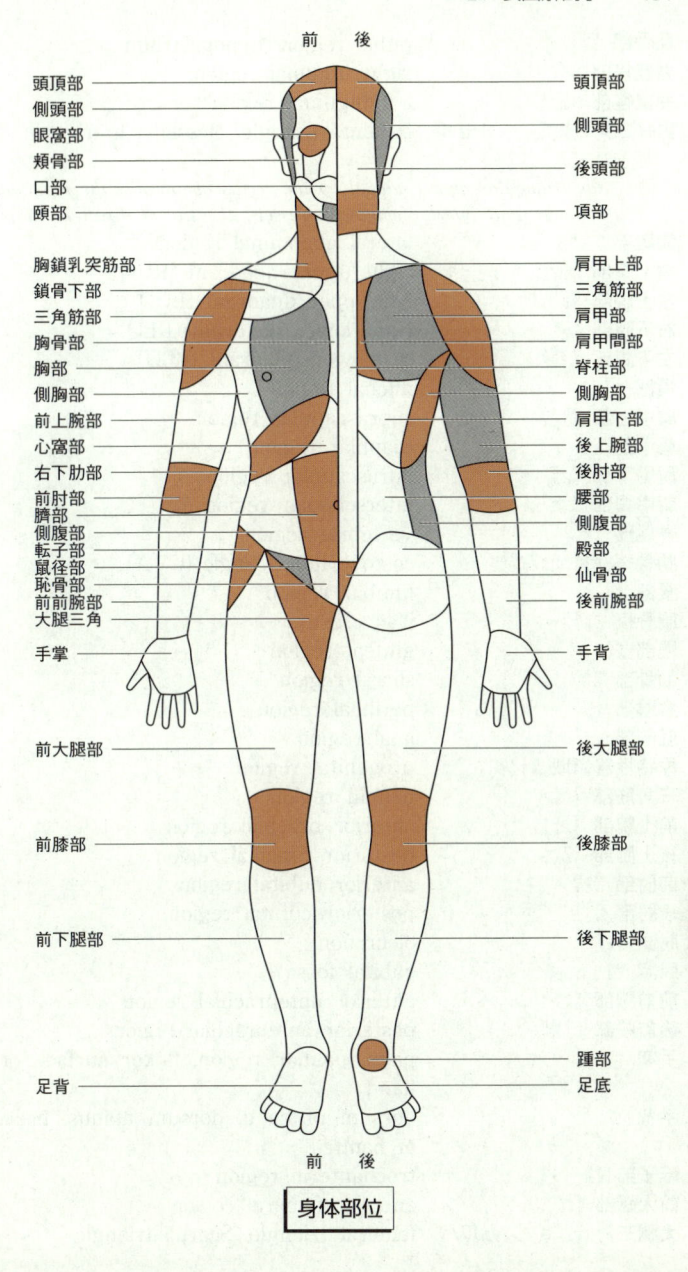

前　後

前面	後面
頭頂部	頭頂部
側頭部	側頭部
眼窩部	後頭部
頬骨部	
口部	
頤部	項部
胸鎖乳突筋部	肩甲上部
鎖骨下部	三角筋部
三角筋部	肩甲部
胸骨部	肩甲間部
胸部	脊柱部
側胸部	側胸部
前上腕部	肩甲下部
心窩部	後上腕部
右下肋部	後肘部
前肘部	腰部
臍部	側腹部
側腹部	殿部
転子部	仙骨部
鼠径部	
恥骨部	
前前腕部	後前腕部
大腿三角	
手掌	手背
前大腿部	後大腿部
前膝部	後膝部
前下腿部	後下腿部
足背	踵部
	足底

前　後

身体部位

452　IX章　人体解剖図

恥骨部 ちこつぶ	pubic region, hypogastrium
右鼠径部 みぎそけいぶ	right inguinal region
左鼠径部 ひだりそけいぶ	left inguinal region
鼠径三角 そけいさんかく, ヘッセルバッハ三角 ―さんかく	inguinal triangle, Hesselbach triangle

〈*the triangular area bounded by the rectus abdominis, the inguinal ligament, and inferior epigastric vessels; the site of direct hernia*〉

側腹部 そくふくぶ	lateral abdominal region
右上腹部 みぎじょうふくぶ	right upper quadrant (RUQ)
左上腹部 ひだりじょうふくぶ	left upper quadrant (LUQ)
右下腹部 みぎかふくぶ	right lower quadrant (RLQ)
左下腹部 ひだりかふくぶ	left lower quadrant (LLQ)
項部 こうぶ	nuchal region
肩甲上部 けんこうじょうぶ	suprascapular region
肩甲部 けんこうぶ	scapular region
肩甲下部 けんこうかぶ	infrascapular region
肩甲間部 けんこうかんぶ	interscapular region
脊柱部 せきちゅうぶ	vertebral region
肋骨脊柱角 ろっこつせきちゅうかく	costovertebral angle (CVA)
腰部 ようぶ	lumbar region
腸骨稜 ちょうこつりょう	iliac crest
殿部 でんぶ	gluteal region
仙骨部 せんこつぶ	sacral region
会陰部 えいんぶ	perineal region
肛門部 こうもんぶ	anal region
尿路性器領域 にょうろせいきりょういき	urogenital region
三角筋部 さんかくきんぶ	deltoid region
前上腕部 ぜんじょうわんぶ	anterior brachial region
後上腕部 こうじょうわんぶ	posterior brachial region
前肘部 ぜんちゅうぶ	anterior cubital region
後肘部 こうちゅうぶ	posterior cubital region
肘頭 ちゅうとう	olecranon
肘窩 ちゅうか	cubital fossa
前前腕部 ぜんぜんわんぶ	anterior antebrachial region
後前腕部 こうぜんわんぶ	posterior antebrachial region
手掌 しゅしょう	palm, palmar region, flexor surface of hand
手背 しゅはい	dorsum of hand, dorsum manus, back of hand
転子部 てんしぶ	trochanteric region
前大腿部 ぜんだいたいぶ	anterior femoral region
大腿三角 だいたいさんかく, スカルパ	femoral triangle, Scarpa triangle

2. 表面解剖学

三角 さんかく
⟨*the triangular area bounded by the inguinal ligament, the abductor longus, and the sartorius*⟩

後大腿部 こうだいたいぶ	posterior femoral region
前膝部 ぜんしつぶ	anterior knee region
後膝部 こうしつぶ	posterior knee region
膝蓋部 しつがいぶ	patellar region
膝窩 しっか	popliteal fossa
前下腿部 ぜんかたいぶ	anterior crural region
後下腿部 こうかたいぶ	posterior crural region
腓腹部 ひふくぶ	sural region
踵部 しょうぶ	calcaneal region, calx
足背 そくはい	dorsum of foot, dorsum pedis
足底 そくてい	planta, sole, undersurface of foot

IX章

454 Ⅸ章 人体解剖図

●体表面線　Surface lines●

正中線（せいちゅうせん）	midline, median line
後正中線（こうせいちゅうせん）	midspinal line
胸骨中線（きょうこつちゅうせん）	midsternal line (MSL)
胸骨線（きょうこつせん）	sternal line
傍胸骨線（ぼうきょうこつせん）	parasternal line
鎖骨中央線（さこつちゅうおうせん）	midclavicular line (MCL)
乳頭線（にゅうとうせん）	mamillary line, mammillary line
前腋窩線（ぜんえきかせん）	anterior axillary line (AAL)
腋窩中央線（えきかちゅうおうせん）	midaxillary line
後腋窩線（こうえきかせん）	posterior axillary line (PAL)
肩甲骨中央線（けんこうこつちゅうおうせん）	midscapular line
傍脊椎線（ぼうせきついせん）	paravertebral line

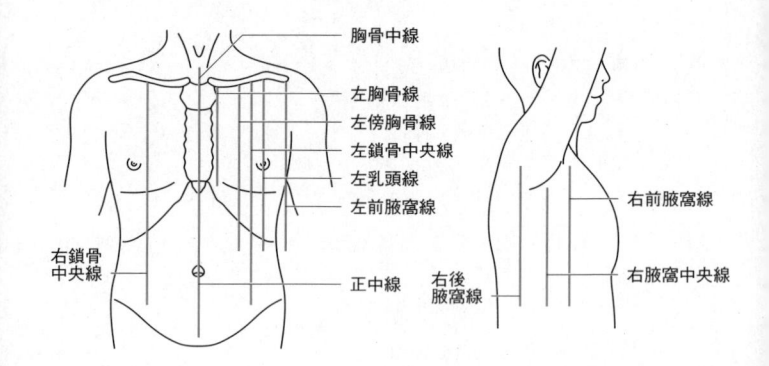

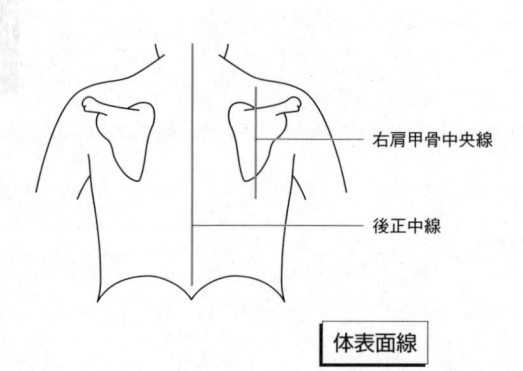

体表面線

●体腔　Body cavity●

頭蓋腔 とうがいくう	cranial cavity
脊柱管 せきちゅうかん	vertebral canal, spinal canal
胸腔 きょうくう	thoracic cavity
横隔膜 おうかくまく	diaphragm, 〔形〕diaphragmatic
腹腔 ふくくう	abdominal cavity
骨盤腔 こつばんくう	pelvic cavity

- 頭蓋骨
- 頭蓋腔
- 背柱管
- 胸腔
- 横隔膜
- 背柱
- 腹腔
- 骨盤腔

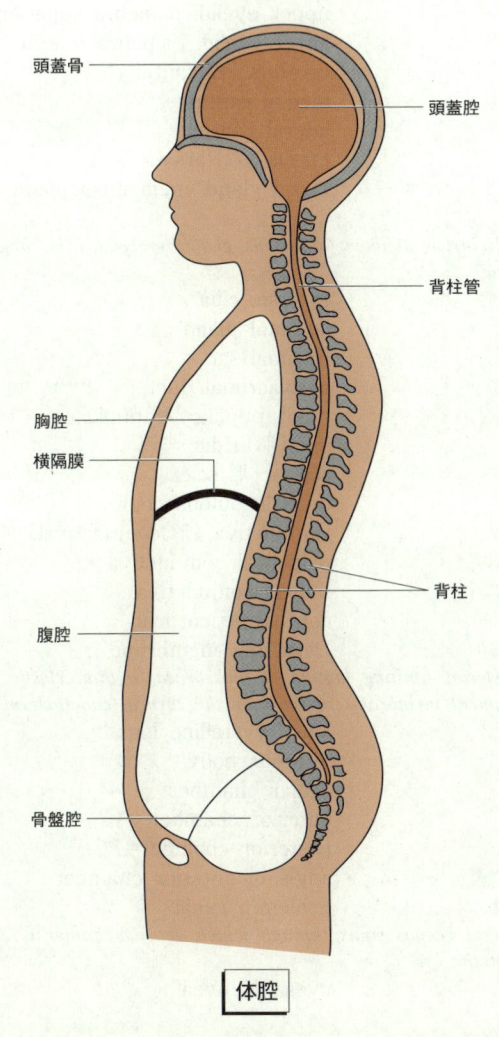

体腔

3. 感覚器

●眼 Eye●

視器 しき	visual organ
眼窩 がんか	orbit, orbita, 〔形〕orbital
眉 まゆ	eyebrow, supercilium, 〔複〕supercilia
眼瞼 がんけん	eyelid, palpebra, 〔形〕palpebral
上眼瞼 じょうがんけん	upper eyelid, palpebra superior
下眼瞼 かがんけん	lower eyelid, palpebra inferior
眼角 がんかく	canthus, 〔複〕canthi
内眼角 ないがんかく	medial canthus
外眼角 がいがんかく	lateral canthus
瞼板 けんばん	tarsus, 〔形〕tarsal
瞼板腺 けんばんせん, マイボーム腺	tarsal gland, meibomian gland

⟨<Heinrich Meibom; sebacious glands embedded in tarsal fibrous tissue⟩

睫毛 まつげ	eyelash, cilia
涙腺 るいせん	lacrimal gland
涙嚢 るいのう	lacrimal sac
鼻涙管 びるいかん	nasolacrimal duct
瞳孔 どうこう	pupil, pupilla, 〔形〕pupillary
虹彩 こうさい	iris, 〔形〕iridic
強膜 きょうまく	sclera, 〔形〕scleral
眼球 がんきゅう	eyeball, bulbus oculi
結膜 けつまく	conjunctiva, 〔形〕conjunctival
眼瞼結膜 がんけんけつまく	palpebral conjunctiva
眼球結膜 がんきゅうけつまく	bulbar conjunctiva
角膜 かくまく	cornea, 〔形〕corneal
デスメ膜 まく	Descemet membrane

⟨posterior limiting lamina of the cornea; a thin, elastic, acellular basement membrane, secreted by the corneal endothelium⟩

水晶体 すいしょうたい	lens, crystalline lens
硝子体 しょうしたい	vitreous body
眼房 がんぼう	ocular chamber
前房 ぜんぼう	anterior chamber (AC)
後房 こうぼう	posterior chamber (PC)
前房隅角 ぜんぼうぐうかく	angle of anterior chamber
シュレム管 かん	Schlemm canal

⟨scleral venous sinus through which aqueous humor is eliminated from the eye⟩

ぶどう膜 まく	uvea, 〔形〕uveal

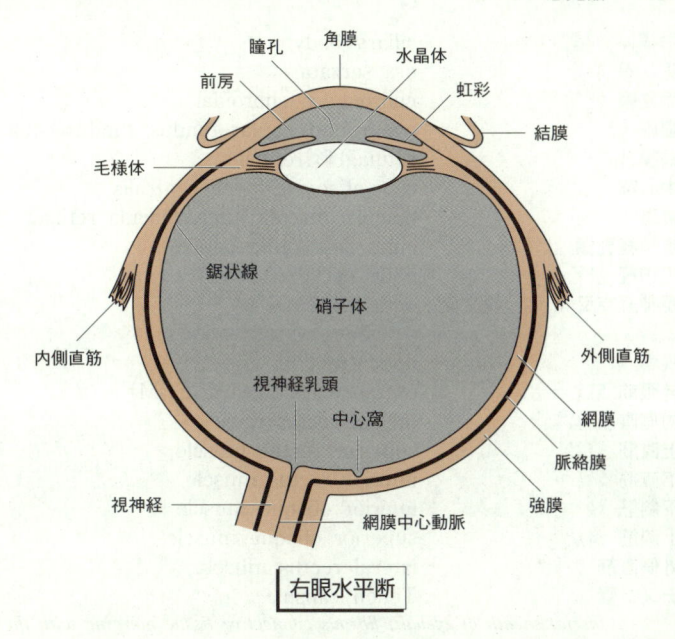

3. 感覚器　457

右眼水平断

- 瞳孔
- 角膜
- 水晶体
- 前房
- 虹彩
- 結膜
- 毛様体
- 鋸状線
- 硝子体
- 内側直筋
- 視神経乳頭
- 中心窩
- 外側直筋
- 網膜
- 脈絡膜
- 視神経
- 網膜中心動脈
- 強膜

正常眼底

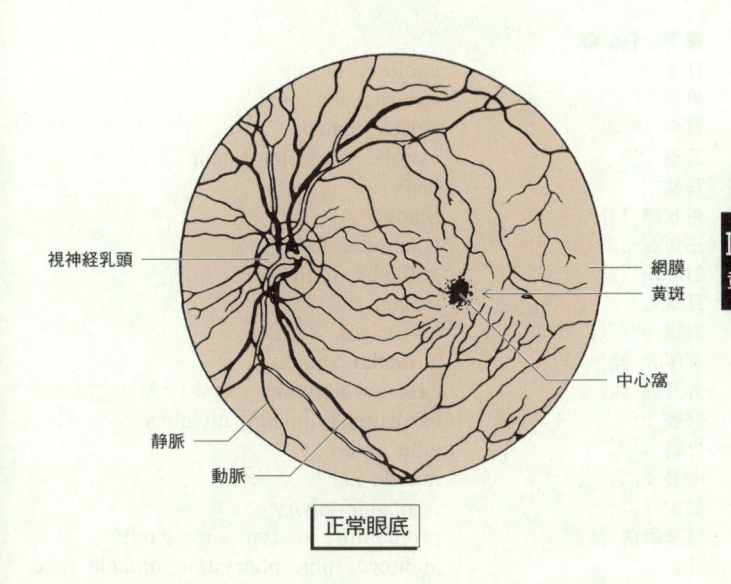

- 視神経乳頭
- 網膜
- 黄斑
- 中心窩
- 静脈
- 動脈

IX章 人体解剖図

毛様体 もうようたい	ciliary body
鋸状縁 きょじょうえん	ora serrata
脈絡膜 みゃくらくまく	choroid, 〔形〕choroidal
眼底 がんてい	eyeground, ocular fundus, fundus oculi
網膜 もうまく	retina, 〔形〕retinal
中心窩 ちゅうしんか	central fovea, fovea centralis
黄斑 おうはん	macula, macula lutea, macula retinae
視神経乳頭 ししんけいにゅうとう	optic disk, optic papilla
視神経 ししんけい	optic nerve
視神経交叉 ししんけいこうさ, 視交叉 しこうさ	optic chiasm
視索 しさく	optic tract
外眼筋 がいがんきん	extraocular muscles (EOM)
内側直筋 ないそくちょくきん	medial rectus muscle
上直筋 じょうちょくきん	superior rectus muscle
下直筋 かちょくきん	inferior rectus muscle
下斜筋 かしゃきん	inferior oblique muscle
上斜筋 じょうしゃきん	superior oblique muscle
外側直筋 がいそくちょくきん	lateral rectus muscle
テノン嚢 のう	Tenon capsule

⟨*fascial sheath of eyeball; fibrous connective tissue merging with the optic nerve sheath and the fascia of the EOMs*⟩

● 耳 Ear ●

聴器 ちょうき	auditory organ
外耳 がいじ	external ear
耳介 じかい	auricle, pinna
耳垂 じすい	earlobe, auricular lobule
耳輪 じりん	helix
舟状窩 しゅうじょうか	scapha
三角窩 さんかくか	triangular fossa
対耳輪 ついじりん	antihelix, anthelix
耳珠 じじゅ	tragus
対珠 たいじゅ	antitragus
耳甲介 じこうかい	auricular concha
外耳道 がいじどう	external auditory canal (EAC)
鼓膜 こまく	eardrum, tympanic membrane
光錐 こうすい	light reflex
中耳 ちゅうじ	middle ear
鼓室 こしつ	tympanic cavity
鼓室岬角 こしつこうかく	promontory of tympanic cavity
耳管 じかん	auditory tube, pharyngotympanic tube,

3. 感覚器

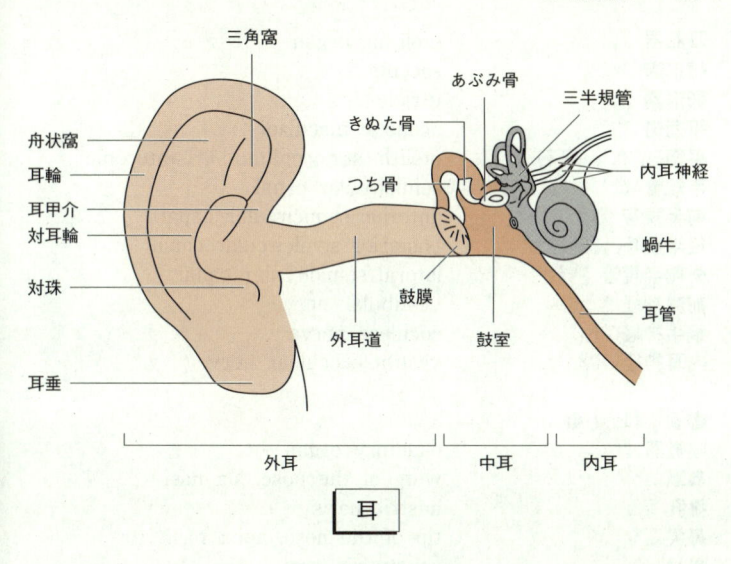

耳

外耳 / 中耳 / 内耳

ラベル: 三角窩, 舟状窩, 耳輪, 耳甲介, 対耳輪, 対珠, 耳垂, あぶみ骨, きぬた骨, つち骨, 三半規管, 内耳神経, 蝸牛, 耳管, 鼓膜, 外耳道, 鼓室

	eustachian tube 〈<*Bartolommeo Eustachio*〉
耳小骨 じしょうこつ	auditory ossicles
つち骨 こつ	malleus, hammer
きぬた骨 こつ	incus, anvil
あぶみ骨 こつ	stapes, stirrup
内耳 ないじ	internal ear
迷路 めいろ	labyrinth, 〔形〕labyrinthine
骨迷路 こつめいろ	bony labyrinth
膜迷路 まくめいろ	membranous labyrinth
蝸牛 かぎゅう	cochlea, 〔形〕cochlear
正円窓 せいえんそう	round window, fenestra cochleae
蝸牛管 かぎゅうかん	cochlear duct
コルチ器 き	organ of Corti

〈*spiral organ; specialized hearing receptors on the basilar membrane in the cochlear duct, consisting of neuroepithelial hair cells and several supporting cells; transmit sounds as nerve impulses to the brain*〉

蓋膜 がいまく	tectorial membrane
鼓室階 こしつかい	scala tympani
前庭階 ぜんていかい	scala vestibuli
前庭 ぜんてい	vestibule, 〔形〕vestibular
卵円窓 らんえんそう	oval window, fenestra vestibuli

IX章

耳石器 じせきき	otolithic organ
球形嚢 きゅうけいのう	saccule
卵形嚢 らんけいのう	utricle
平衡斑 へいこうはん	acoustic maculae
平衡砂 へいこうさ, 耳石 じせき	otolith, statoconium, 〔複〕statoconia
半規管 はんきかん	semicircular canal
前半規管 ぜんはんきかん	anterior semicircular canal
後半規管 こうはんきかん	posterior semicircular canal
外側半規管 がいそくはんきかん	lateral semicircular canal
前庭神経 ぜんていしんけい	vestibular nerve
蝸牛神経 かぎゅうしんけい	cochlear nerve
内耳神経 ないじしんけい	vestibulocochlear nerve

● 鼻 Nose ●

嗅覚器 きゅうかくき	olfactory organ
鼻翼 びよく	wing of the nose, ala nasi
鼻孔 びこう	nostril, naris
鼻尖 びせん	tip of the nose, apex nasi
鼻柱 びちゅう	columnella nasi
鼻背 びはい	dorsum of the nose
鼻根 びこん	root of the nose, radix nasi
人中 にんちゅう	philtrum
鼻腔 びくう	nasal cavity
鼻中隔 びちゅうかく	nasal septum
鼻甲介 びこうかい	turbinate, concha nasalis
上鼻甲介 じょうびこうかい	superior turbinate
中鼻甲介 ちゅうびこうかい	middle turbinate
下鼻甲介 かびこうかい	inferior turbinate
鼻道 びどう	nasal meatus
上鼻道 じょうびどう	superior nasal meatus
中鼻道 ちゅうびどう	middle nasal meatus
下鼻道 かびどう	inferior nasal meatus
鼻前庭 びぜんてい	nasal vestibule, vestibulum nasi
キーセルバッハ部位 ぶい	Kiesselbach area

⟨*an area on the anterior nasal septum above the intermaxillary bone; highly vascular and a common site of nosebleed*⟩

副鼻腔 ふくびくう	paranasal sinus
前頭洞 ぜんとう	frontal sinus
蝶形骨洞 ちょうけいこつどう	sphenoidal sinus, sphenoid sinus
上顎洞 じょうがくどう, ハイモア洞 どう	maxillary sinus, Highmore antrum
篩骨洞 しこつどう	ethmoidal sinus

3. 感覚器 461

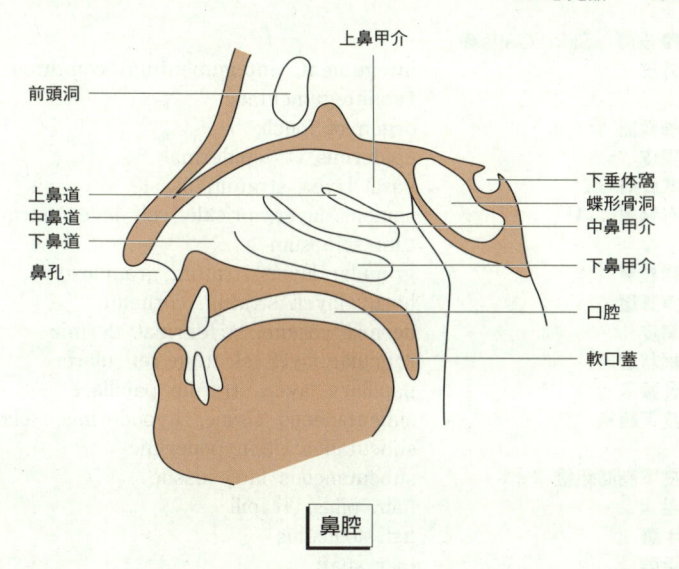

鼻腔

（図中ラベル）
- 前頭洞
- 上鼻甲介
- 上鼻道
- 中鼻道
- 下鼻道
- 鼻孔
- 下垂体窩
- 蝶形骨洞
- 中鼻甲介
- 下鼻甲介
- 口腔
- 軟口蓋

下垂体窩 かすいたいか　　hypophysial fossa, pituitary fossa

● 皮膚　Skin, Cutis ●

外皮 がいひ	integument, integumentum commune, 〔形〕integumentary
触覚器 しょっかくき	organ of touch
表皮 ひょうひ	epidermis, 〔形〕epidermal
基底層 きていそう	basal layer, stratum basale
有棘層 ゆうきょくそう	spinous layer, prickle cell layer, stratum spinosum
顆粒層 かりゅうそう	granular layer, stratum granulosum
角質層 かくしつそう	horny layer, stratum corneum
真皮 しんぴ	dermis, corium, 〔形〕dermal, dermic
網状層 もうじょうそう	reticular layer, stratum reticulare
乳頭層 にゅうとうそう	papillary layer, stratum papillare
皮下組織 ひかそしき	subcutaneous tissue, hypodermis, tela subcutanea, 〔形〕hypodermic
皮下脂肪組織 ひかしぼうそしき	subcutaneous fatty tissue
毛 け	hair, pilus, 〔複〕pili
毛嚢 もうのう	hair folliculus
毛幹 もうかん	hair shaft
毛根 もうこん	hair root
立毛筋 りつもうきん	arrector pili muscle, arrector muscles of hairs
爪 つめ	nail, unguis, 〔形〕ungual
爪根 そうこん	nail root, radix unguis
爪体 そうたい	nail body, corpus unguis
爪板 そうばん	nail plate
爪床 そうしょう	nail bed, matrix unguis
爪半月 そうはんげつ	lunula, lunule
胎生爪皮 たいせいそうひ	eponychium
汗腺 かんせん	sweat glands, sudoriferous glands
脂腺 しせん	sebaceous glands
アポクリン腺 せん	apocrine gland
エクリン腺 せん	eccrine gland
知覚性神経終末 ちかくせいしんけいしゅうまつ	sensory nerve ending
パチニ小体 しょうたい	pacinian corpuscle

〈<i>Filippo Pacini; lamellar corpuscle; encapsulated nerve endings in the deep dermis, sensitive to pressure, deep touch, and vibration</i>〉

メルケル細胞 さいぼう	Merkel cell

〈<i>tactile cells in the epidermis; tactile receptors in association with Merkel disk, sensory nerve endings</i>〉

3. 感覚器　463

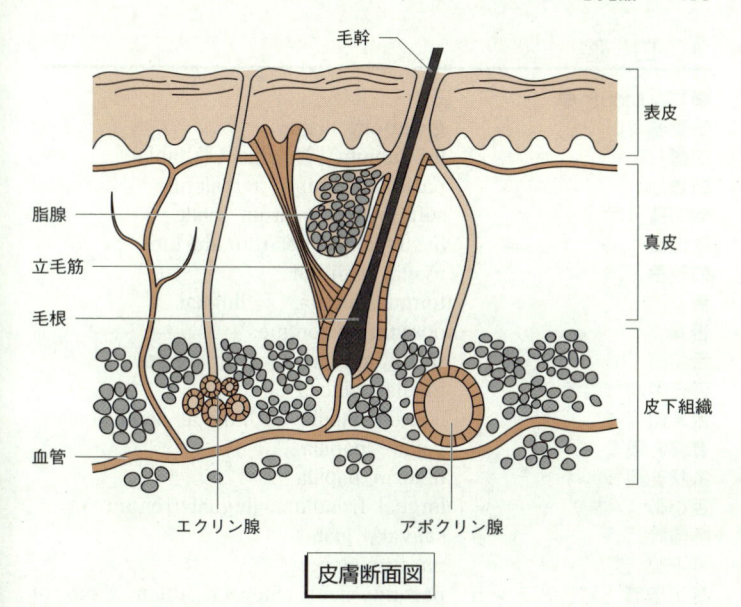

毛幹 / 表皮 / 真皮 / 皮下組織

脂腺
立毛筋
毛根
血管

エクリン腺　アポクリン腺

皮膚断面図

4. 口腔

● 口 Mouth ●

味覚器 みかくき	gustatory organ
口唇 こうしん	lip, labium, 〔複〕labia, 〔形〕labial
口蓋 こうがい	palate, palatum, 〔形〕palatine
軟口蓋 なんこうがい	soft palate, palatum molle
硬口蓋 こうこうがい	hard palate, palatum durum
口蓋垂 こうがいすい	uvula, 〔形〕uvular
舌 ぜつ	tongue, lingua, 〔形〕lingual
舌背 ぜっぱい	dorsum of tongue
舌尖 ぜっせん	tip of tongue, apex of tongue
舌正中溝 ぜっせいちゅうこう	median sulcus of tongue
舌乳頭 ぜつにゅうとう	lingual papilla, 〔複〕lingual papillae
有郭乳頭 ゆうかくにゅうとう	vallate papilla
糸状乳頭 しじょうにゅうとう	filiform papilla
舌小帯 ぜっしょうたい	lingual frenulum, lingual frenum
唾液腺 だえきせん	salivary gland
耳下腺 じかせん	parotid gland
耳下腺管 じかせんかん, ステンセン管 かん	parotid duct, Stensen duct, duct of Steno
顎下腺 がっかせん	submandibular gland, submaxillary gland
顎下腺管 がっかせんかん, ワルトン管 かん	submandibular duct, Wharton duct
舌下腺 ぜっかせん	sublingual gland

● 歯 Tooth ●

切歯 せっし	incisor, incisive tooth
犬歯 けんし	canine, canine tooth
小臼歯 しょうきゅうし	premolar tooth, bicuspid tooth
大臼歯 だいきゅうし	molar, molar tooth
智歯 ちし, 第3大臼歯 だいさんだいきゅうし	wisdom tooth, third molar tooth
歯肉 しにく	gingiva, 〔形〕gingival
歯冠 しかん	dental crown, corona dentis
歯根 しこん	dental root, radix dentis
歯根管 しこんかん	root canal
歯髄 しずい	dental pulp, pulpa dentis
象牙質 ぞうげしつ	dentin, dentinum
エナメル質 しつ	dental enamel, dentinum
セメント質 しつ	dental cement, cementum

口腔

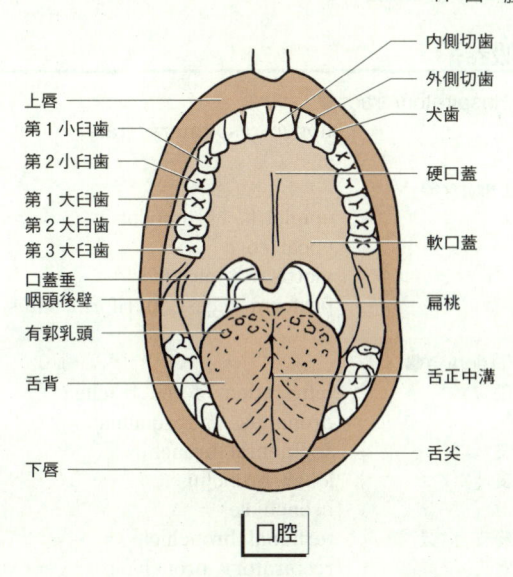

- 内側切歯
- 外側切歯
- 上唇
- 犬歯
- 第1小臼歯
- 第2小臼歯
- 硬口蓋
- 第1大臼歯
- 第2大臼歯
- 第3大臼歯
- 軟口蓋
- 口蓋垂
- 咽頭後壁
- 扁桃
- 有郭乳頭
- 舌背
- 舌正中溝
- 下唇
- 舌尖

咬頭 こうとう	dental cusp
歯根膜 しこんまく	periodontal ligament, periodontal membrane
歯槽 しそう	dental alveolus, tooth socket

● 咽頭 Pharynx ●

扁桃 へんとう	tonsil, tonsilla
扁桃窩 へんとうか	tonsillar fossa
口蓋扁桃 こうがいへんとう	palatine tonsil, faucial tonsil
舌扁桃 ぜつへんとう	lingual tonsil
咽頭扁桃 いんとうへんとう	pharyngeal tonsil
ワルダイエル輪 りん	Waldeyer tonsillar ring

⟨*circular lymphoid tissue formed by the lingual, pharyngeal, and palatine tonsils*⟩

5．呼吸器系

● 気道　Respiratory tract ●
上気道 じょうきどう　　　　　　　　　upper respiratory tract

● 喉頭　Larynx ●
喉頭蓋 こうとうがい　　　　　　　　　epiglottis, 〔形〕epiglottic
声帯 せいたい　　　　　　　　　　　vocal cord
声門 せいもん　　　　　　　　　　　glottis, 〔形〕glottic
梨状陥凹 りじょうかんおう　　　　　　piriform recess, pyriform sinus

● 気管　Trachea ●
気管分岐部 きかんぶんきぶ　　　　　　bifurcation of the trachea
気管支 きかんし　　　　　　　　　　bronchus, 〔形〕bronchial
区域気管支 くいききかんし　　　　　　segmental bronchus
肺葉気管支 はいようきかんし　　　　　lobar bronchus
細気管支 さいきかんし　　　　　　　bronchiole
終末細気管支 しゅうまつさいきかんし　terminal bronchiole
呼吸細気管支 こきゅうさいきかんし　　respiratory bronchiole
肺胞 はいほう　　　　　　　　　　　pulmonary alveolus
肺胞嚢 はいほうのう　　　　　　　　alveolar sac

● 肺　Lung ●
肺尖 はいせん　　　　　　　　　　　apex of the lung
肺門部 はいもんぶ　　　　　　　　　hilum of the lung
肺底部 はいていぶ　　　　　　　　　base of the lung
横隔膜 おうかくまく　　　　　　　　diaphragm, 〔形〕diaphragmatic
モルガニー孔 こう　　　　　　　　　Morgagni foramen, foramen of Morgagni

〈pleuroperitoneal foramen; a small defect between the sternal and costal portions of the diaphragm〉

右肺 うはい　　　　　　　　　　　　right lung
右上葉 うじょうよう　　　　　　　　right upper lobe (RUL)
右中葉 うちゅうよう　　　　　　　　right middle lobe (RML)
右下葉 うかよう　　　　　　　　　　right lower lobe (RLL)
左肺 さはい　　　　　　　　　　　　left lung
左上葉 さじょうよう　　　　　　　　left upper lobe (LUL)
左下葉 さかよう　　　　　　　　　　left lower lobe (LLL)
斜裂 しゃれつ　　　　　　　　　　　oblique fissure
水平裂 すいへいれつ　　　　　　　　horizontal fissure

5. 呼吸器系　467

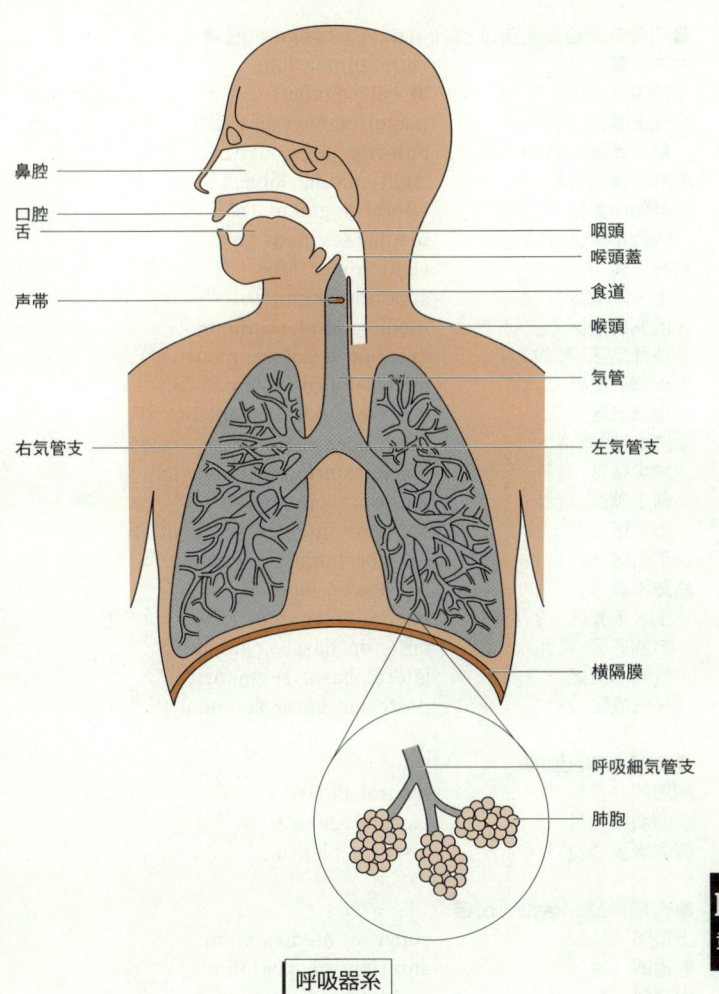

- 鼻腔
- 口腔
- 舌
- 声帯
- 右気管支
- 咽頭
- 喉頭蓋
- 食道
- 喉頭
- 気管
- 左気管支
- 横隔膜
- 呼吸細気管支
- 肺胞

呼吸器系

● 気管支肺区域　Bronchopulmonary segments ●

右肺上葉 うはいじょうよう	right upper lobe
肺尖区 はいせんく	apical segment (S^1)
後上葉区 こうじょうようく	posterior segment (S^2)
前上葉区 ぜんじょうようく	anterior segment (S^3)
右肺中葉 うはいちゅうよう	right middle lobe
外側中葉区 がいそくちゅうようく	lateral segment (S^4)
内側中葉区 ないそくちゅうようく	medial segment (S^5)
右肺下葉 うはいかよう	right lower lobe
上・下葉区 じょうかようく	superior segment (S^6)
内側肺底区 ないそくはいていく	medial basal segment (S^7)
前肺底区 ぜんはいていく	anterior basal segment (S^8)
外側肺底区 がいそくはいていく	lateral basal segment (S^9)
後肺底区 こうはいていく	posterior basal segment (S^{10})
左肺上葉 さはいじょうよう	left upper lobe
肺尖後区 はいせんこうく	apicoposterior segment (S^{1+2})
前上葉区 ぜんじょうようく	anterior segment (S^3)
上舌区 じょうぜつく	superior lingular segment (S^4)
下舌区 かぜつく	inferior lingular segment (S^5)
左肺下葉 さはいかよう	left lower lobe
上・下葉区 じょうかようく	superior segment (S^6)
前肺底区 ぜんはいていく	anterior basal segment (S^8)
外側肺底区 がいそくはいていく	lateral basal segment (S^9)
後肺底区 こうはいていく	posterior basal segment (S^{10})

● 胸膜　Pleura ●

胸膜腔 きょうまくくう	pleural cavity
壁側胸膜 へきそくきょうまく	parietal pleura
臓側胸膜 ぞうそくきょうまく	visceral pleura

● 縦隔　Mediastinum ●

上縦隔 じょうじゅうかく	superior mediastinum
前縦隔 ぜんじゅうかく	anterior mediastinum
中縦隔 ちゅうじゅうかく	middle mediastinum
後縦隔 こうじゅうかく	posterior mediastinum

5. 呼吸器系　469

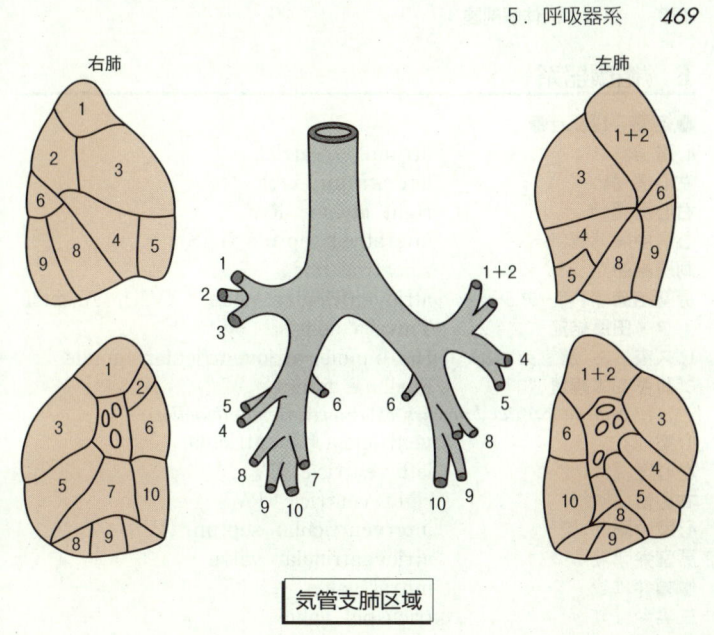

右肺　　　　　　　　　　　　　左肺

気管支肺区域

6. 循環器系

● 心臓　Heart ●

心房 しんぼう	atrium, 〔形〕atrial
左心房 さしんぼう	left atrium (LA)
右心房 うしんぼう	right atrium (RA)
心房中隔 しんぼうちゅうかく	interatrial septum (IAS)
洞房結節 どうぼうけっせつ	sinoatrial node
房室結節 ぼうしつけっせつ, アショッフ・田原結節 たわらけっせつ	atrioventricular node (AVN), Aschoff-Tawara node
ヒス束 そく, 房室束 ぼうしつそく	His bundle, atrioventricular bundle
プルキンエ線維 せんい	Purkinje fibers
〈subendocardial branches of atrioventricular bundles〉	
心室 しんしつ	ventricle, 〔形〕ventricular
左心室 さしんしつ	left ventricle (LV)
右心室 うしんしつ	right ventricle (RV)
心室中隔 しんしつちゅうかく	interventricular septum (IVS)
房室弁 ぼうしつべん	atrioventricular valve
僧帽弁 そうぼうべん	mitral valve
三尖弁 さんせんべん	tricuspid valve
腱索 けんさく	chordae tendineae
大動脈弁 だいどうみゃくべん	aortic valve
肺動脈弁 はいどうみゃくべん	pulmonary valve
心膜 しんまく	pericardium, 〔形〕pericardial
心内膜 しんないまく	endocardium, 〔形〕endocardial
心外膜 しんがいまく	epicardium, 〔形〕epicardial
心筋 しんきん	myocardium, cardiac muscle, 〔形〕myocardial
乳頭筋 にゅうとうきん	papillary muscles

6. 循環器系　471

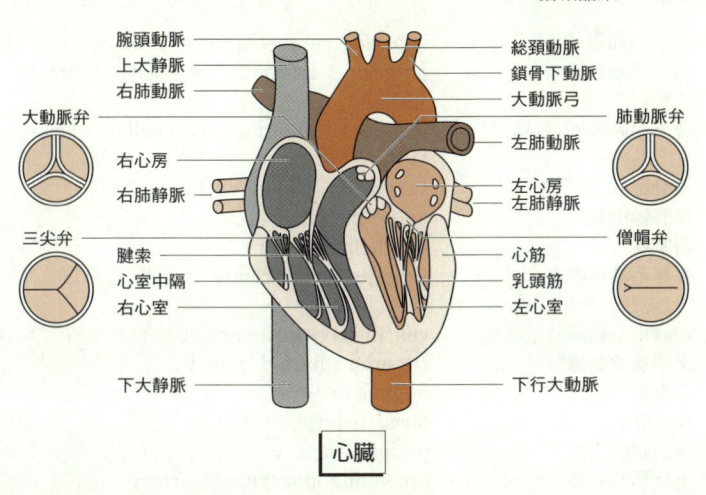

図中ラベル:
- 腕頭動脈
- 上大静脈
- 右肺動脈
- 大動脈弁
- 右心房
- 右肺静脈
- 三尖弁
- 腱索
- 心室中隔
- 右心室
- 下大静脈
- 総頚動脈
- 鎖骨下動脈
- 大動脈弓
- 肺動脈弁
- 左肺動脈
- 左心房
- 左肺静脈
- 僧帽弁
- 心筋
- 乳頭筋
- 左心室
- 下行大動脈

心臓

● 動脈　Artery (A) ●

大動脈 (だいどうみゃく)	aorta, 〔形〕aortic
上行大動脈 (じょうこうだいどうみゃく)	ascending aorta
大動脈弓 (だいどうみゃくきゅう)	aortic arch
冠動脈 (かんどうみゃく)	coronary artery
左冠動脈 (さかんどうみゃく)	left coronary artery (LCA)
左冠動脈主幹部 (さかんどうみゃくしゅかんぶ)	left main trunk (LMT)
左前下行枝 (ひだりぜんかこうし)	left anterior descending branch (LAD)
左回旋枝 (ひだりかいせんし)	left circumflex branch (LCx)
右冠動脈 (うかんどうみゃく)	right coronary artery (RCA)
肺動脈 (はいどうみゃく)	pulmonary artery (PA)
総頚動脈 (そうけいどうみゃく)	common carotid artery (CCA)
内頚動脈 (ないけいどうみゃく)	internal carotid artery (ICA)
外頚動脈 (がいけいどうみゃく)	external carotid artery (ECA)
大脳動脈輪 (だいのうどうみゃくりん)	cerebral arterial circle, circle of Willis
前大脳動脈 (ぜんだいのうどうみゃく)	anterior cerebral artery (ACA)
中大脳動脈 (ちゅうだいのうどうみゃく)	middle cerebral artery (MCA)
後大脳動脈 (こうだいのうどうみゃく)	posterior cerebral artery (PCA)
前交通動脈 (ぜんこうつうどうみゃく)	anterior communicating artery
後交通動脈 (こうこうつうどうみゃく)	posterior communicating artery
脳底動脈 (のうていどうみゃく)	basilar artery (BA)
ウィリス動脈輪 (—どうみゃくりん)	circle of Willis

⟨*cerebral arterial circle; formed by the two internal carotid, the anterior, and posterior cerebral arteries, the anterior communicating artery, and the posterior communicating arteries*⟩

IX章

IX章 人体解剖図

上小脳動脈 じょうしょうのうどうみゃく	superior cerebellar artery (SCA)
前下小脳動脈 ぜんかしょうのうどうみゃく	anterior inferior cerebellar artery (AICA)
後下小脳動脈 こうかしょうのうどうみゃく	posterior inferior cerebellar artery (PICA)
椎骨動脈 ついこつどうみゃく	vertebral artery (VA)
前脊髄動脈 ぜんせきずいどうみゃく	anterior spinal artery
眼動脈 がんどうみゃく	ophthalmic artery
長後毛様体動脈 ちょうこうもうようたいどうみゃく	long posterior ciliary artery (LPCA)
網膜中心動脈 もうまくちゅうしんどうみゃく	central retinal artery (CRA)
上甲状腺動脈 じょうこうじょうせんどうみゃく	superior thyroid artery
舌動脈 ぜつどうみゃく	lingual artery
顔面動脈 がんめんどうみゃく	facial artery
後頭動脈 こうとうどうみゃく	occipital artery
上行咽頭動脈 じょうこういんとうどうみゃく	ascending pharyngeal artery
後耳介動脈 こうじかいどうみゃく	posterior auricular artery
浅側頭動脈 せんそくとうどうみゃく	superficial temporal artery (STA)
顎動脈 がくどうみゃく	maxillary artery
腕頭動脈 わんとうどうみゃく	brachiocephalic artery
鎖骨下動脈 さこつかどうみゃく	subclavian artery
甲状頚動脈 こうじょうけいどうみゃく	thyrocervical trunk
肋頚動脈 ろくけいどうみゃく	costocervical trunk
内胸動脈 ないきょうどうみゃく	internal thoracic artery (ITA)
腋窩動脈 えきかどうみゃく	axillary artery
上腕動脈 じょうわんどうみゃく	brachial artery
橈骨動脈 とうこつどうみゃく	radial artery
尺骨動脈 しゃっこつどうみゃく	ulnar artery
浅掌動脈弓 せんしょうどうみゃくきゅう	superficial palmar arterial arch
深掌動脈弓 しんしょうどうみゃくきゅう	deep palmar arterial arch
下行大動脈 かこうだいどうみゃく	descending aorta
胸部大動脈 きょうぶだいどうみゃく	thoracic aorta
気管支動脈 きかんしどうみゃく	bronchial artery
食道動脈 しょくどうどうみゃく	esophageal artery
上横隔動脈 じょうおうかくどうみゃく	superior phrenic artery
肋間動脈 ろっかんどうみゃく	intercostal artery
腹部大動脈 ふくぶだいどうみゃく	abdominal aorta
腹腔動脈 ふくくうどうみゃく	celiac artery (CA)
総肝動脈 そうかんどうみゃく	common hepatic artery (CHA)
固有肝動脈 こゆうかんどうみゃく	proper hepatic artery
胆嚢動脈 たんのうどうみゃく	cystic artery (CA)
右肝動脈 うかんどうみゃく	right hepatic artery (RHA)

6. 循環器系　473

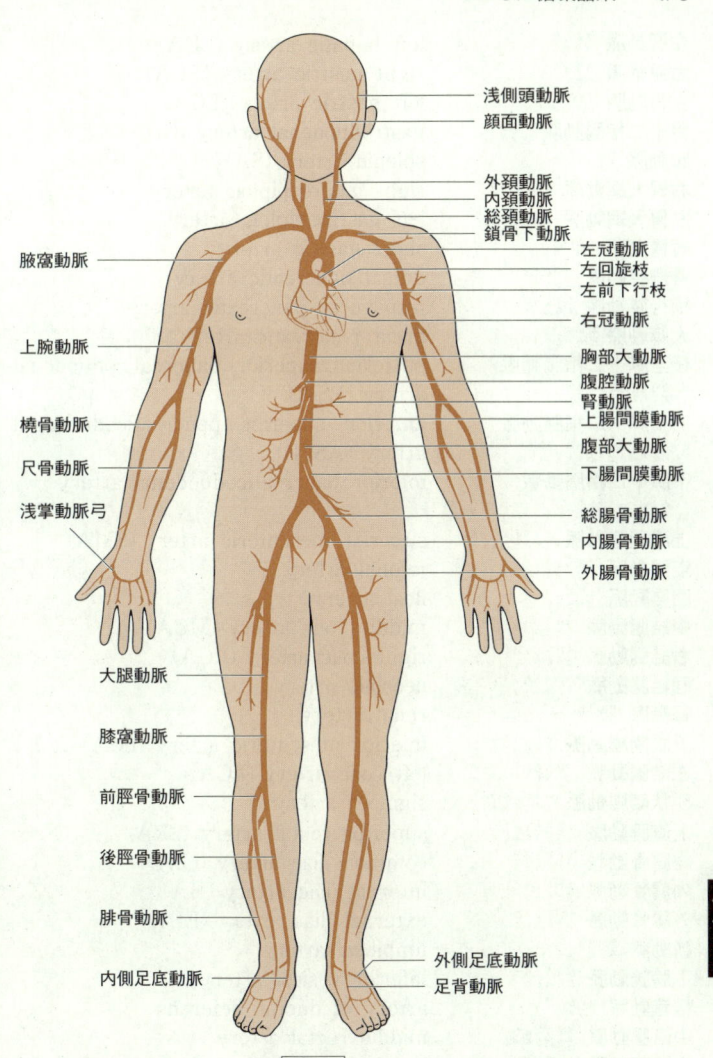

- 浅側頭動脈
- 顔面動脈
- 外頸動脈
- 内頸動脈
- 総頸動脈
- 鎖骨下動脈
- 左冠動脈
- 左回旋枝
- 左前下行枝
- 右冠動脈
- 胸部大動脈
- 腹腔動脈
- 腎動脈
- 上腸間膜動脈
- 腹部大動脈
- 下腸間膜動脈
- 総腸骨動脈
- 内腸骨動脈
- 外腸骨動脈

- 腋窩動脈
- 上腕動脈
- 橈骨動脈
- 尺骨動脈
- 浅掌動脈弓

- 大腿動脈
- 膝窩動脈
- 前脛骨動脈
- 後脛骨動脈
- 腓骨動脈
- 内側足底動脈
- 外側足底動脈
- 足背動脈

動脈

IX章

左肝動脈 さかんどうみゃく	left hepatic artery (LHA)
右胃動脈 ういどうみゃく	right gastric artery (RGA)
左胃動脈 さいどうみゃく	left gastric artery (LGA)
胃十二指腸動脈 いじゅうにしちょうどうみゃく	gastroduodenal artery (GDA)
脾動脈 ひどうみゃく	splenic artery (SA)
右胃大網動脈 ういだいもうどうみゃく	right gastroepiploic artery
左胃大網動脈 さいだいもうどうみゃく	left gastroepiploic artery
短胃動脈 たんいどうみゃく	short gastric artery
背側膵動脈 はいそくすいどうみゃく	dorsal pancreatic artery
横行膵動脈 おうこうすいどうみゃく	transverse pancreatic artery
大膵動脈 だいすいどうみゃく	great pancreatic artery
後上膵十二指腸動脈 こうじょうすいじゅうにしちょうどうみゃく	posterior superior pancreaticoduodenal artery (PSPD)
前上膵十二指腸動脈 ぜんじょうすいじゅうにしちょうどうみゃく	anterior superior pancreaticoduodenal artery (ASPD)
下膵十二指腸動脈 かすいじゅうにしちょうどうみゃく	inferior pancreaticoduodenal artery
上腸間膜動脈 じょうちょうかんまくどうみゃく	superior mesenteric artery (SMA)
空腸動脈 くうちょうどうみゃく	jejunal artery
回腸動脈 かいちょうどうみゃく	ileal artery
中結腸動脈 ちゅうけっちょうどうみゃく	middle colic artery (MCA)
右結腸動脈 うけっちょうどうみゃく	right colic artery (RCA)
回結腸動脈 かいけっちょうどうみゃく	ileocolic artery
腎動脈 じんどうみゃく	renal artery
下腸間膜動脈 かちょうかんまくどうみゃく	inferior mesenteric artery (IMA)
左結腸動脈 さけっちょうどうみゃく	left colic artery (LCA)
S状結腸動脈 エスじょうけっちょうどうみゃく	sigmoid artery
上直腸動脈 じょうちょくちょうどうみゃく	superior rectal artery (SRA)
総腸骨動脈 そうちょうこつどうみゃく	common iliac artery (CIA)
内腸骨動脈 ないちょうこつどうみゃく	internal iliac artery (IIA)
外腸骨動脈 がいちょうこつどうみゃく	external iliac artery (EIA)
臍動脈 さいどうみゃく	umbilical artery
下膀胱動脈 かぼうこうどうみゃく	inferior vesical artery
精管動脈 せいかんどうみゃく	artery of ductus deferens
中直腸動脈 ちゅうちょくちょうどうみゃく	middle rectal artery
内陰部動脈 ないいんぶどうみゃく	internal pudendal artery
閉鎖動脈 へいさどうみゃく	obturator artery
下腹壁動脈 かふくへきどうみゃく	inferior epigastric artery
深腸骨回旋動脈 しんちょうこつかいせんどうみゃく	deep circumflex iliac artery
大腿動脈 だいたいどうみゃく	femoral artery (FA)
浅大腿動脈 せんだいたいどうみゃく	superficial femoral artery (SFA)

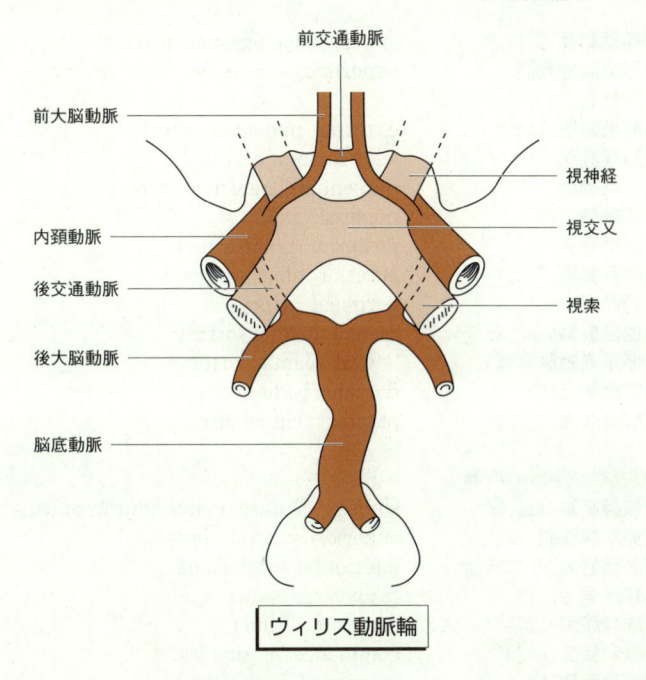

6. 循環器系　475

ウィリス動脈輪

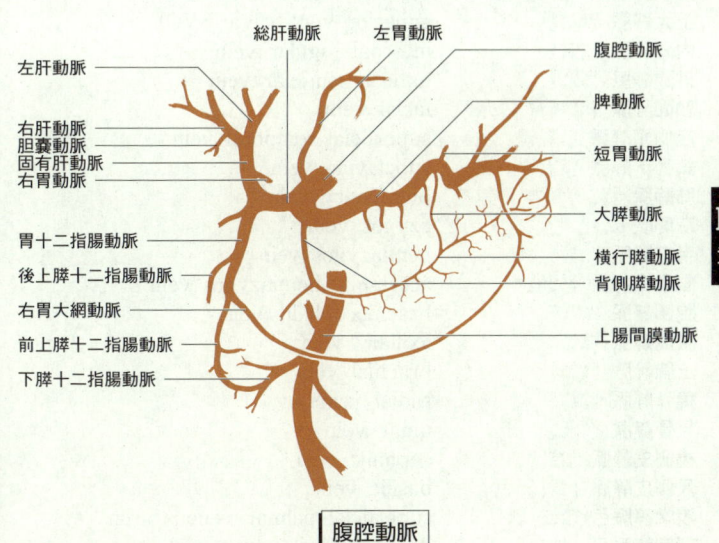

- 前交通動脈
- 前大脳動脈
- 内頸動脈
- 後交通動脈
- 後大脳動脈
- 脳底動脈
- 視神経
- 視交叉
- 視索

腹腔動脈

- 総肝動脈
- 左胃動脈
- 左肝動脈
- 右肝動脈
- 胆嚢動脈
- 固有肝動脈
- 右胃動脈
- 胃十二指腸動脈
- 後上膵十二指腸動脈
- 右胃大網動脈
- 前上膵十二指腸動脈
- 下膵十二指腸動脈
- 腹腔動脈
- 脾動脈
- 短胃動脈
- 大膵動脈
- 横行膵動脈
- 背側膵動脈
- 上腸間膜動脈

浅腹壁動脈 せんふくへきどうみゃく　　superficial epigastric artery
浅腸骨回旋動脈 せんちょうこつかいせんどうみゃく　　superficial circumflex iliac artery
外陰部動脈 がいいんぶどうみゃく　　external pudendal artery
大腿深動脈 だいたいしんどうみゃく　　deep artery of thigh
下行膝動脈 かこうしつどうみゃく　　descending genicular artery
膝窩動脈 しっかどうみゃく　　popliteal artery
後脛骨動脈 こうけいこつどうみゃく　　posterior tibial artery
前脛骨動脈 ぜんけいこつどうみゃく　　anterior tibial artery
腓骨動脈 ひこつどうみゃく　　peroneal artery
内側足底動脈 ないそくそくていどうみゃく　　medial plantar artery
外側足底動脈 がいそくそくていどうみゃく　　lateral plantar artery
足背動脈 そくはいどうみゃく　　dorsalis pedis artery
足底動脈弓 そくていどうみゃくきゅう　　plantar arterial arch

● 静脈 Vein (V) ●

硬膜静脈洞 こうまくじょうみゃくどう　　sinuses of dura mater, dural sinuses
上矢状静脈洞 じょうしじょうじょうみゃくどう　　superior sagittal sinus
下矢状静脈洞 かしじょうじょうみゃくどう　　inferior sagittal sinus
横静脈洞 おうじょうみゃくどう　　transverse sinus
海綿静脈洞 かいめんじょうみゃくどう　　cavernous sinus
静脈洞交会 じょうみゃくどうこうかい　　confluence of sinuses
冠状静脈洞 かんじょうじょうみゃくどう　　coronary sinus (CS)
上大静脈 じょうだいじょうみゃく　　superior vena cava (SVC)
内頸静脈 ないけいじょうみゃく　　internal jugular vein
外頸静脈 がいけいじょうみゃく　　external jugular vein
顔面静脈 がんめんじょうみゃく　　facial vein
浅側頭静脈 せんそくとうじょうみゃく　　superficial temporal vein
鎖骨下静脈 さこつかじょうみゃく　　subclavian vein
肺静脈 はいじょうみゃく　　pulmonary vein
奇静脈 きじょうみゃく　　azygos vein
半奇静脈 はんきじょうみゃく　　hemiazygos vein
副半奇静脈 ふくはんきじょうみゃく　　accessory hemiazygos vein
腕頭静脈 わんとうじょうみゃく　　brachiocephalic vein
腋窩静脈 えきかじょうみゃく　　axillary vein
上腕静脈 じょうわんじょうみゃく　　brachial vein
橈骨静脈 とうこつじょうみゃく　　radial vein
尺骨静脈 しゃっこつじょうみゃく　　ulnar vein
橈側皮静脈 とうそくひじょうみゃく　　cephalic vein
尺側皮静脈 しゃくそくひじょうみゃく　　basilic vein
浅掌静脈弓 せんしょうじょうみゃくきゅう　　superficial palmar venous arch
深掌静脈弓 しんしょうじょうみゃくきゅう　　deep palmar venous arch

6. 循環器系　*477*

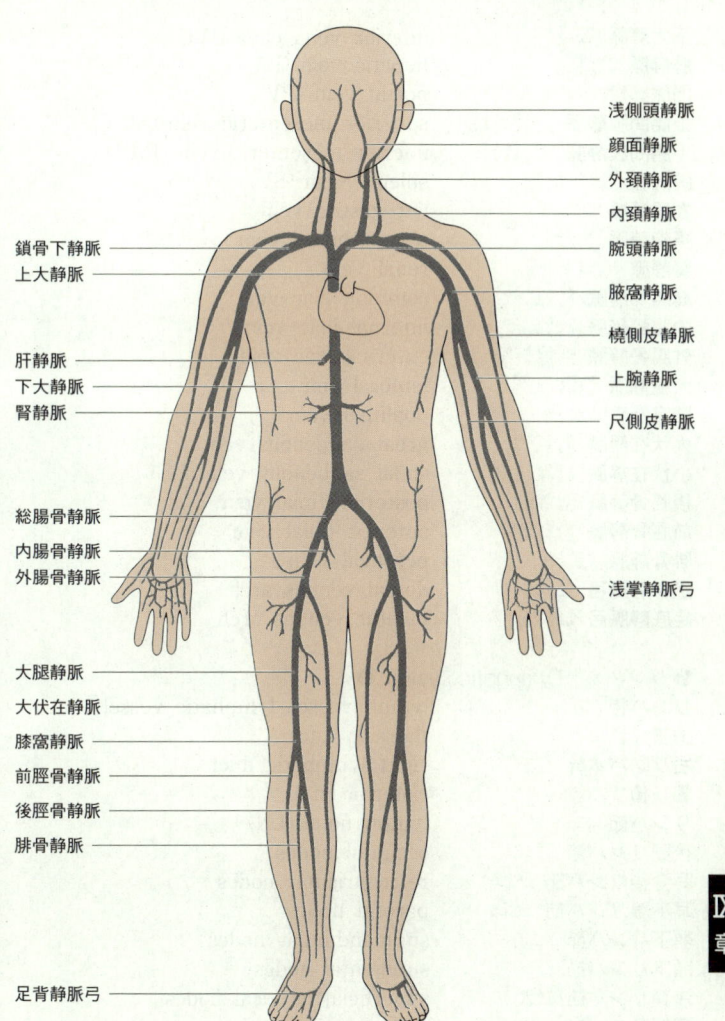

浅側頭静脈
顔面静脈
外頸静脈
内頸静脈
鎖骨下静脈
上大静脈
腕頭静脈
腋窩静脈
橈側皮静脈
肝静脈
下大静脈
腎静脈
上腕静脈
尺側皮静脈
総腸骨静脈
内腸骨静脈
外腸骨静脈
浅掌静脈弓
大腿静脈
大伏在静脈
膝窩静脈
前脛骨静脈
後脛骨静脈
腓骨静脈
足背静脈弓

静脈

IX章

下大静脈 かだいじょうみゃく	inferior vena cava (IVC)
肝静脈 かんじょうみゃく	hepatic vein (HV)
門脈 もんみゃく	portal vein (PV)
上腸間膜静脈 じょうちょうかんまくじょうみゃく	superior mesenteric vein (SMV)
下腸間膜静脈 かちょうかんまくじょうみゃく	inferior mesenteric vein (IMV)
脾静脈 ひじょうみゃく	splenic vein (SV)
左胃静脈 さいじょうみゃく	left gastric vein
臍傍静脈 さいぼうじょうみゃく	paraumbilical vein
腎静脈 じんじょうみゃく	renal vein
総腸骨静脈 そうちょうこつじょうみゃく	common iliac vein
内腸骨静脈 ないちょうこつじょうみゃく	internal iliac vein
外腸骨静脈 がいちょうこつじょうみゃく	external iliac vein
大腿静脈 だいたいじょうみゃく	femoral vein
膝窩静脈 しっかじょうみゃく	popliteal vein
大伏在静脈 だいふくざいじょうみゃく	great saphenous vein
小伏在静脈 しょうふくざいじょうみゃく	small saphenous vein
後脛骨静脈 こうけいこつじょうみゃく	posterior tibial vein
前脛骨静脈 ぜんけいこつじょうみゃく	anterior tibial vein
腓骨静脈 ひこつじょうみゃく	peroneal vein
足背静脈弓 そくはいじょうみゃくきゅう	dorsal venous arch
足底静脈弓 そくていじょうみゃくきゅう	plantar venous arch

● リンパ系　Lymphatic system ●

リンパ管 かん	lymph vessel, lymphatic vessel
胸管 きょうかん	thoracic duct
右リンパ本幹 うほんかん	right lymphatic duct
乳び槽 にゅうびそう	cisterna chyli
リンパ節 せつ	lymph node (LN)
後頭リンパ節 こうとうせつ	occipital nodes
耳介後リンパ節 じかいこうせつ	retroauricular nodes
耳下腺リンパ節 じかせんせつ	parotid nodes
顎下リンパ節 がくかせつ	submandibular nodes
頤下リンパ節 おとがいかせつ	submental nodes
浅頸リンパ節 せんけいせつ	superficial cervical nodes
深頸リンパ節 しんけいせつ	deep cervical nodes
鎖骨上窩リンパ節 さこつじょうかせつ	supraclavicular nodes
腋窩リンパ節 えきかせつ	axillary nodes
肘リンパ節 ちゅうせつ	cubital nodes, epitrochlear nodes
肺門リンパ節 はいもんせつ	hilar nodes
縦隔リンパ節 じゅうかくせつ	mediastinal nodes
腰リンパ節 ようせつ	lumbar nodes
幽門リンパ節 ゆうもんせつ	pyloric nodes

腸間膜リンパ節 ちょうかんまくせつ	mesenteric nodes
腸骨リンパ節 ちょうこつせつ	iliac nodes
仙骨リンパ節 せんこつせつ	sacral nodes
鼠径リンパ節 そけいせつ	inguinal nodes
膝窩リンパ節 しっかせつ	popliteal nodes

Tidbits

phlegmatic

phlegmatic（発音はフレグマティック）は，phlegm（「痰」，発音はフレム）の形容詞であるが，通常は「冷静な，沈着な」の意味で用いられる．本来 phlegm（ギリシャ語の phlegma）は「粘液」のことで，人の四体液 the four cardinal humors の一つである．かつて人の気質は，血液 blood，粘液 phlegm，黄胆汁 yellow bile (choler)，黒胆汁 black bile (melancholy) のバランスにより決まると考えられ（体液説 humoralism），粘液の多い粘液質 phlegmatic temperament の者は，無感動，不活発であるが粘り強いとされた．

医師に求められる冷静沈着な態度 imperturbability について Sir William Osler は，"Imperturbability means coolness and presence of mind under all circumstances, calmness amid storm, clearness of judgment in moments of grave peril, immobility, impassiveness, or, to use an old and expressive word, phlegm." と述べている．

7. 消化器系

● 消化器 Digestive organ ●

消化管 しょうかかん	digestive tract, gastrointestinal (GI) tract, alimentary canal
上部消化管 じょうぶしょうかかん	upper gastrointestinal tract
下部消化管 かぶしょうかかん	lower digestive tract
腸管 ちょうかん	intestinal tract

● 食道 Esophagus ●

上部食道括約筋 じょうぶしょくどうかつやくきん	upper esophageal sphincter (UES)
食道胃接合部 しょくどういせつごうぶ	esophagogastric junction (EGJ)
下部食道括約筋 かぶしょくどうかつやくきん	lower esophageal sphincter (LES)
扁平円柱上皮境界 へんぺいえんちゅうじょうひきょうかい	squamocolumnar junction (SCJ)

● 胃 Stomach ●

噴門 ふんもん	cardia, 〔形〕cardiac
胃底部 いていぶ	gastric fundus
円蓋 えんがい	fornix
胃体部 いたいぶ	gastric body
胃角 いかく	gastric angle
幽門洞 ゆうもんどう	pyloric antrum, gastric antrum
幽門 ゆうもん	pylorus, 〔形〕pyloric
大彎 だいわん	greater curvature
小彎 しょうわん	lesser curvature
胃腺 いせん	gastric gland
胃小窩 いしょうか	gastric pits, foveola gastricae
粘膜 ねんまく	mucosa (m), mucous membrane, tunica mucosa
粘膜筋板 ねんまくきんばん	muscularis mucosae (mm), lamina muscularis mucosae
粘膜下層 ねんまくかそう	submucosa (sm), submucous layer, tunica submucosa
固有筋層 こゆうきんそう	proper muscle layer (pm)
漿膜 しょうまく	serosa (s), serous layer, tunica serosa
壁細胞 へきさいぼう	parietal cell, oxyntic cell
主細胞 しゅさいぼう	chief cell

● 腸 Intestine, Bowel ●

小腸 しょうちょう	small intestine, small bowel

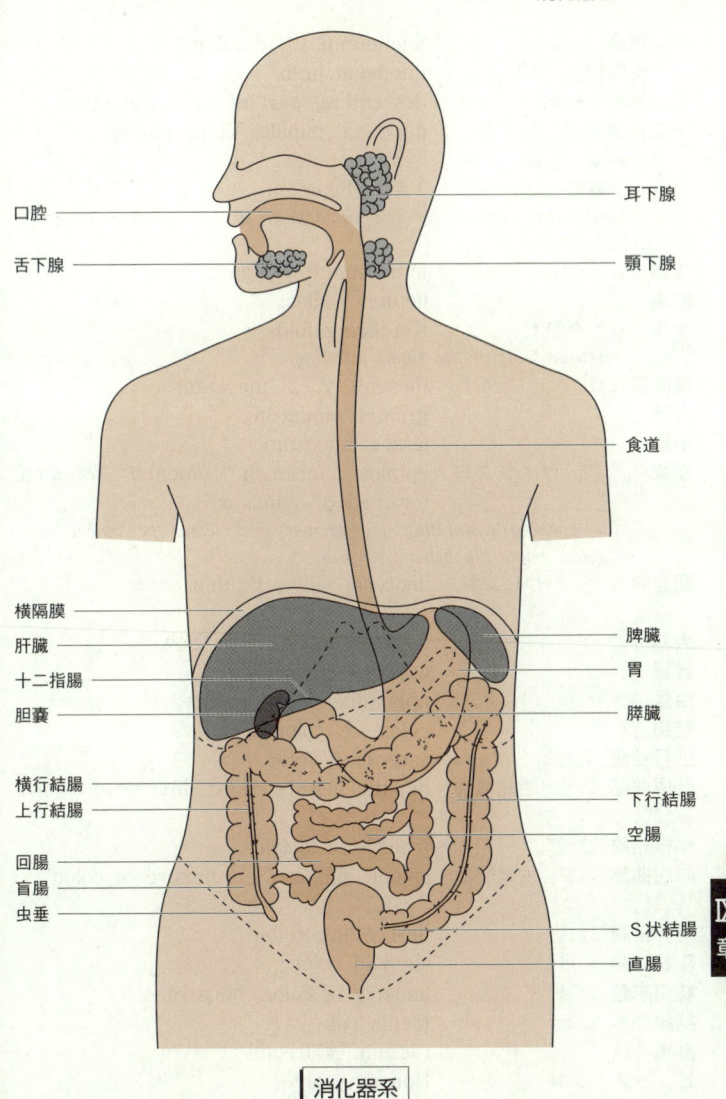

7. 消化器系

口腔	耳下腺
舌下腺	顎下腺
	食道
横隔膜	脾臓
肝臓	胃
十二指腸	膵臓
胆嚢	
横行結腸	下行結腸
上行結腸	空腸
回腸	
盲腸	S状結腸
虫垂	直腸

消化器系

十二指腸 じゅうにしちょう	duodenum, 〔形〕duodenal
十二指腸球部 じゅうにしちょうきゅうぶ	duodenal bulb
十二指腸下行部 じゅうにしちょうかこうぶ	descending part of the duodenum
十二指腸乳頭 じゅうにしちょうにゅうとう, ファーター乳頭 ーにゅうとう	duodenal papilla, Vater papilla
トライツ靱帯 ーじんたい	Treitz ligament

⟨*suspensory muscle of the duodenum at its junction with the jejunum*⟩

空腸 くうちょう	jejunum, 〔形〕jejunal
回腸 かいちょう	ileum, 〔形〕ileal
ケルクリングひだ	Kerckring folds

⟨*circular folds of the small intestine*⟩

腸間膜 ちょうかんまく	mesentery, 〔形〕mesenteric
大網 だいもう	greater omentum
小網 しょうもう	lesser omentum
網嚢孔 もうのうこう, ウインスロー孔 ーこう	epiploic foramen, omental foramen, foramen of Winslow

⟨*the opening connecting the greater and lesser peritoneal sacs, situated below the hepatic portal*⟩

回盲弁 かいもうべん, バウヒン弁 ーべん	ileocecal valve, Bauhin valve
大腸 だいちょう	large intestine, large bowel
盲腸 もうちょう	cecum, 〔形〕cecal
虫垂 ちゅうすい	appendix, 〔形〕appendiceal
結腸 けっちょう	colon, 〔形〕colonic
上行結腸 じょうこうけっちょう	ascending colon
肝屈曲部 かんくっきょくぶ, 右結腸曲 みぎけっちょうきょく	hepatic flexure, right flexure of colon
横行結腸 おうこうけっちょう	transverse colon
脾屈曲部 ひくっきょくぶ, 左結腸曲 ひだりけっちょうきょく	splenic flexure, left flexure of colon
下行結腸 かこうけっちょう	descending colon
S状結腸 ーじょうけっちょう	sigmoid colon
結腸膨起 けっちょうぼうき	haustra of colon, haustra coli
結腸ひも けっちょうー	taenia coli
直腸 ちょくちょう	rectum, 〔形〕rectal
ヒューストン弁 ーべん	Houston valves

⟨*three transverse folds, two on the left and one on the right, in the rectum*⟩

肛門 こうもん	anus, 〔形〕anal
肛門管 こうもんかん	anal canal
肛門括約筋 こうもんかつやくきん	anal sphincter

結腸間膜 (けっちょうかんまく)	mesocolon
腹膜 (ふくまく)	peritoneum, 〔形〕peritoneal
モリソン窩 (か)	Morison pouch

⟨*a deep pouch of peritoneum in the right subhepatic space; fluids drain here in the supine position*⟩

腸腺 (ちょうせん)	intestinal gland, Lieberkühn gland
ブルンネル腺 (せん)	Brunner gland

⟨*duodenal glands; found in the submucosa of the duodenum, secreting an alkaline mucoid substance that neutralizes gastric juice*⟩

パネート細胞 (いほう)	Paneth cell

⟨*pyramidal epithelial cells located at the base of small intestinal crypts, containing large eosinophilic granules that secrete lysozyme*⟩

アウエルバッハ神経叢 (しんけいそう)	Auerbach plexus

⟨*myenteric plexus; parasympathetic ganglion cells on connective tissue between muscle layers in the esophagus, jejunum, and ileum*⟩

マイスネル神経叢 (けいそう)	Meissner plexus

⟨*submucosal nervous plexus; termination of preganglion fibers of autonomic nervous system in GI tract*⟩

パイエル板 (ばん)	Peyer patches

⟨*aggregated lymphoid nodules of small intestine, found on the mucous membrane of the antimesenteric border*⟩

IX 章

● 肝臓　Liver ●

右葉 うよ	right lobe
左葉 さよ	left lobe
方形葉 ほうけいよう	quadrate lobe
尾状葉 びじょうよう	caudate lobe
肝門 かんもん	hepatic portal, porta hepatis
カロー三角 さんかく	Calot triangle

〈cystohepatic triangle; the triangle bounded by the cystic artery, the cystic duct, and the hepatic duct〉

肝鎌状間膜 かんかまじょうかんまく	falciform ligament of liver, ligamentum falciforme hepatis
肝円索 かんえんさく	round ligament of liver, ligamentum teres hepatis
肝小葉 かんしょうよう	hepatic lobule
類洞 るいどう	sinusoid
ディッセ腔 くう	Disse space

〈perisinusoidal spaces that store lymph of the liver〉

クッパー細胞 さいぼう　　Kupffer cells

〈stellate cells of liver; phagocytic cells on walls of hepatic sinusoids〉

● 胆道　Biliary tract ●

肝内胆管 かんないたんかん	intrahepatic bile duct
総肝管 そうかんかん	common hepatic duct
総胆管 そうたんかん	common bile duct (CBD)
オッディ括約筋 かつやくきん	sphincter of Oddi

〈sphincter of hepatopancreatic ampulla within the duodenal papilla〉

胆嚢 たんのう	gallbladder (GB)
胆嚢管 たんのうかん	cystic duct
ロキタンスキー・アショッフ洞 どう	Rokitansky-Aschoff sinus (RAS)

〈small outpouchings of the mucosa of the gallbladder extending through the muscular layer〉

● 膵臓　Pancreas ●

膵頭部 すいとうぶ	head of the pancreas
膵体部 すいたいぶ	body of the pancreas
膵尾部 すいびぶ	tail of the pancreas
主膵管 しゅすいかん, ウィルスング管 かん	main pancreatic duct, Wirsung duct
副膵管 ふくすいかん, サントリーニ管 かん	accessory pancreatic duct, Santorini duct

7. 消化器系　485

図：肝臓下面
- 胆嚢
- 右葉
- 下大静脈
- 方形葉
- 肝円索
- 肝門
- 左葉
- 尾状葉

肝臓下面

● 脾臓　Spleen ●

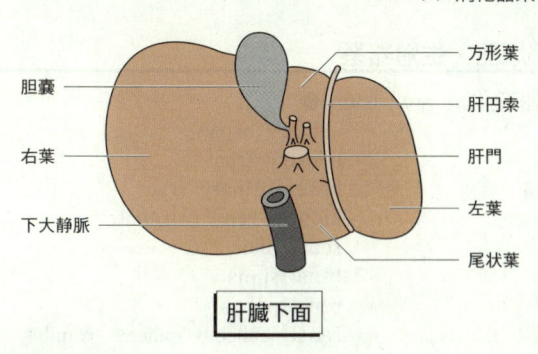

脾髄（ひず）　splenic pulp

Tidbits

double noun

可算，不可算両用の名詞（double nouns）では，動作，性質，状態，機能など抽象的概念を表すとき（抽象名詞）は不可算(U)で，具体的な行為，数値，個体などを意味するとき（普通名詞）は可算(C)となる．本来抽象名詞の size, strength, conductivity などが value(s) of ~（~の数値）という意味を含んでいるときには可算名詞として扱われる．物質名詞も状態，材料，食物，自然現象などは不可算で，種類，製品，個体を意味すれば可算となる．
(U)寒さ，寒気 the cold of winter, (C)かぜ have / catch a cold,
(U)病名 hay fever, scarlet fever, (C)発熱 have a high / low / slight fever
(U)感染 infection, (C)感染症；an ear infection

IX 章

8. 泌尿器・生殖器系

●泌尿器系 Urinary system●

泌尿器 ひにょうき	urinary organ
尿路 にょうろ	urinary tract
下部尿路 かぶにょうろ	lower urinary tract
腎臓 じんぞう	kidney, ren, [形]renal
腎門 じんもん	renal hilus
腎洞 じんどう	renal sinus
腎盂 じんう	renal pelvis
腎杯 じんぱい	renal calices, calices renales, kidney calices
大腎杯 だいじんぱい	major calyx
小腎杯 しょうじんぱい	minor calyx
腎柱 じんちゅう, ベルタン柱	renal columns, columnae renales, Bertin columns
腎乳頭 じんにゅうとう	renal papilla
腎小体 じんしょうたい, マルピギー小体	renal corpuscle, malpighian corpuscle

〈<*Marcello Malpighi; a glomerulus and the glomerular capsule*〉

ネフロン	nephron
糸球体 しきゅうたい	glomerulus, [形]glomerular
ボーマン嚢 のう	Bowman capsule

〈*glomerular capsule; the beginning of a nephron that is composed of two layers and surrounds the glomerulus*〉

メサンギウム	mesangium
糸球体基底膜 しきゅうたいきていまく	glomerular basement membrane (GBM)
傍糸球体装置 ぼうしきゅうたいそうち	juxtaglomerular apparatus (JGA)
尿細管 にょうさいかん	renal tubule
近位尿細管 きんいにょうさいかん	proximal tubule
中間尿細管 ちゅうかんにょうさいかん	intermediate tubule
遠位尿細管 えんいにょうさいかん	distal tubule
ヘンレループ	Henle loop, loop of Henle

〈*ansa nephroni; a long U-shaped part of the renal tubule*〉

集合管 しゅうごうかん	collecting duct
乳頭管 にゅうとうかん	papillary duct
尿管腎盂移行部 にょうかんじんういこうぶ	ureteropelvic junction (UPJ)
尿管 にょうかん	ureter, [形]ureteral
膀胱 ぼうこう	bladder, urinary bladder
膀胱三角 ぼうこうさんかく	trigone of the bladder, trigonum vesicae
尿管膀胱移行部 にょうかんぼうこういこうぶ	ureterovesical junction (UVJ)

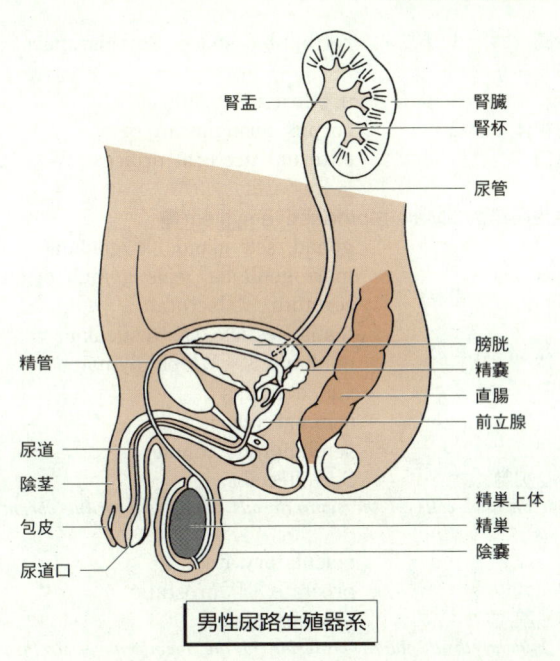

8. 泌尿器・生殖器系

男性尿路生殖器系

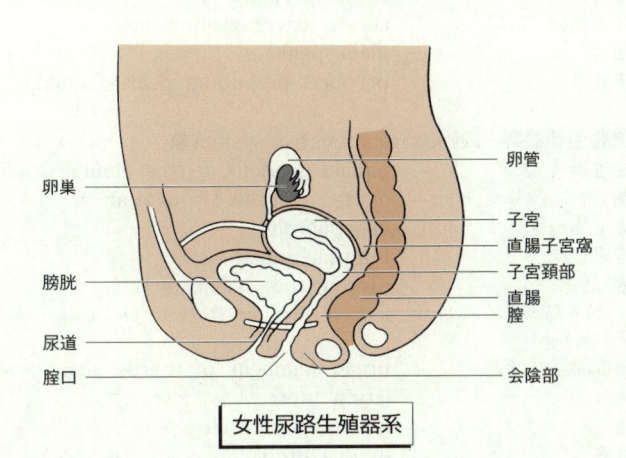

- 腎盂
- 腎臓
- 腎杯
- 尿管
- 膀胱
- 精嚢
- 直腸
- 前立腺
- 精管
- 尿道
- 陰茎
- 包皮
- 尿道口
- 精巣上体
- 精巣
- 陰嚢

女性尿路生殖器系

- 卵巣
- 卵管
- 子宮
- 直腸子宮窩
- 子宮頚部
- 直腸
- 膀胱
- 腟
- 尿道
- 腟口
- 会陰部

IX章 人体解剖図

恥骨後腔（ちこつこうくう），レチウス腔（くう）	retropubic space, Retzius space
尿道（にょうどう）	urethra, 〔形〕urethral
尿道海綿体（にょうどうかいめんたい）	corpus spongiosum penis
外尿道口（がいにょうどうこう）	external urethral orifice

● 男性生殖器系　Male reproductive system ●

性腺（せいせん）	gonad, sex gland, 〔形〕gonadal
男性性器（だんせいせいき）	male genitalia, male genital organ
陰嚢（いんのう）	scrotum, 〔形〕scrotal
精巣（せいそう）	testis, testicle, 〔形〕testicular
精巣上体（せいそうじょうたい）	epididymis, 〔形〕epididymal
精管（せいかん）	vas deferens
精嚢（せいのう）	seminal vesicle
精細管（せいさいかん）	seminiferous tubule
セルトリ細胞（ーさいぼう）	Sertoli cells

⟨*elongated cells in the seminiferous tubule, supporting spermiogenesis*⟩

射精管（しゃせいかん）	ejaculatory duct
前立腺（ぜんりつせん）	prostate, 〔形〕prostatic
カウパー腺（ーせん）	Cowper gland

⟨*bulbourethral gland; posterior to the membranous urethra above the bulb of the penis; mucoid secretion*⟩

陰茎（いんけい）	penis, 〔形〕penile
陰茎海綿体（いんけいかいめんたい）	corpus cavernosum penis
亀頭（きとう）	glans penis
包皮（ほうひ）	prepuce, preputium penis, foreskin

● 女性生殖器系　Female reproductive system ●

女性性器（じょせいせいき）	female genitalia, female genital organ
卵巣（らんそう）	ovary, ovarium, 〔形〕ovarian
卵巣上体（らんそうじょうたい）	epoophoron
卵管采（らんかんさい）	fimbriae tubae
卵管（らんかん）	uterine tube, fallopian tube

⟨<*Gabriele Fallopio; a tube from the ovary to the fundus of the uterus*⟩

子宮広間膜（しきゅうこうかんまく）	broad ligament of uterus, ligamentum latum uteri
子宮（しきゅう）	uterus, 〔形〕uterine
子宮底（しきゅうてい）	fundus uteri
子宮体（しきゅうたい）	corpus uteri
子宮峡（しきゅうきょう）	isthmus uteri

子宮頚 しきゅうけい	cervix uteri
子宮付属器 しきゅうふぞくき	adnexa uteri, uterine appendages
直腸子宮窩 ちょくちょうしきゅうか	rectouterine pouch, Douglas pouch, Douglas cul-de-sac
陰門 いんもん	vulva, 〔形〕vulval
腟 ちつ	vagina, 〔形〕vaginal
腟前庭 ちつぜんてい	vestibule of vagina
腟口 ちつこう	vaginal introitus, vaginal orifice
外尿道口 がいにょうどうこう	external urethral orifice
バルトリン腺 せん	Bartholin gland
〈*greater vestibular gland; mucoid-secreting tubulo-alveolar gland*〉	
前庭球 ぜんていきゅう	bulbus vestibuli
恥丘 ちきゅう	mons pubis
陰核 いんかく	clitoris, 〔形〕clitoral
大陰唇 だいいんしん	labium majus pudendi, labia majora
小陰唇 しょういんしん	labium minus pudendi, labia minora
陰唇小帯 いんしんしょうたい	fourchette, frenulum labiorum pudendi

9. 内分泌系

●内分泌臓器 Endocrine organ●

下垂体 かすいたい	pituitary gland, pituitary, hypophysis, 〔形〕pituitary, hypophysial
腺下垂体 せんかすいたい	adenohypophysis
神経下垂体 しんけいかすいたい	neurohypophysis
松果体 しょうかたい	pineal gland, pineal body
視床下部 ししょうかぶ	hypothalamus, 〔形〕hypothalamic
甲状腺 こうじょうせん	thyroid gland
副甲状腺 ふくこうじょうせん	parathyroid gland
胸腺 きょうせん	thymus, 〔形〕thymic
ハッサル小体 しょうたい	Hassall corpuscle

〈spherical bodies found in the medulla of the thymus, composed of concentric arrays of keratinized squamous epithelial cells〉

副腎 ふくじん	adrenal gland, suprarenal gland
副腎皮質 ふくじんひしつ	adrenal cortex
束状帯 そくじょうたい	fascicular zone, zona fasciculata
球状帯 きゅうじょうたい	glomerular zone, zona glomerulosa
網状帯 もうじょうたい	reticular zone, zona reticularis
副腎髄質 ふくじんずいしつ	adrenal medulla
膵臓 すいぞう	pancreas, 〔形〕pancreatic
ランゲルハンス島 とう	islets of Langerhans

〈pancreatic islets; endocrine portion of the pancreas〉

卵巣 らんそう	ovary, 〔形〕ovarian
精巣 せいそう	testis, 〔形〕testicular
ライディッヒ細胞 さいぼう	Leydig cells

〈interstitial cells; epithelioid cells secreting testosterone〉

9. 内分泌系　491

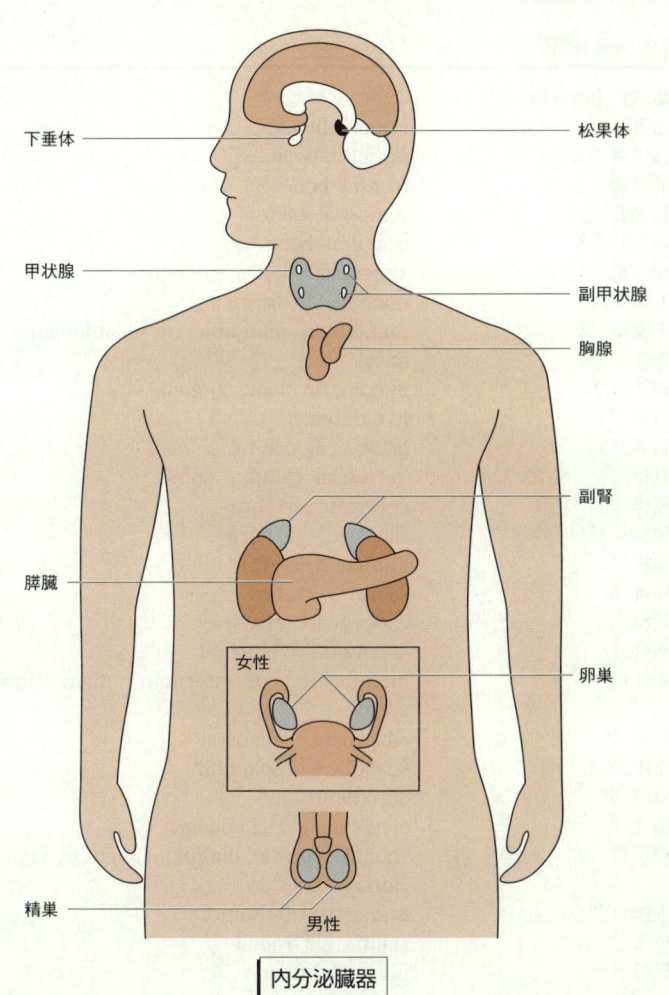

- 下垂体
- 松果体
- 甲状腺
- 副甲状腺
- 胸腺
- 副腎
- 膵臓
- 卵巣
- 女性
- 精巣
- 男性

内分泌臓器

10. 骨格系

● 骨　Bone ●

頭蓋骨 とうがいこつ	cranial bone
頭頂骨 とうちょうこつ	parietal bone
前頭骨 ぜんとうこつ	frontal bone
側頭骨 そくとうこつ	temporal bone
後頭骨 こうとうこつ	occipital bone
蝶形骨 ちょうけいこつ	sphenoid bone
上顎骨 じょうがくこつ	maxilla, 〔形〕maxillary
下顎骨 かがくこつ	mandibula, mandible, 〔形〕mandibular
鼻骨 びこつ	nasal bone
頬骨 きょうこつ	zygomatic bone, zygoma
舌骨 ぜっこつ	hyoid bone
眼窩 がんか	orbita, 〔形〕orbital
脊柱 せきちゅう, 脊椎 せきつい	vertebral column, spine
頚椎 けいつい	cervical vertebra
胸椎 きょうつい	thoracic vertebra
腰椎 ようつい	lumbar vertebra
仙椎 せんつい	sacral vertebra
尾椎 びつい	coccygeal vertebra
胸骨 きょうこつ	sternum, 〔形〕sternal
胸骨柄 きょうこつへい	manubrium of sternum, manubrium sterni
肋骨 ろっこつ	rib, costa, 〔形〕costal
肩甲骨 けんこうこつ	scapula, 〔形〕scapular
肩峰 けんぽう	acromion
鎖骨 さこつ	clavicula, 〔形〕clavicular
肩甲帯 けんこうたい, 上肢帯 じょうしたい	shoulder girdle, cingulum membri superioris
上腕骨 じょうわんこつ	humerus, 〔形〕humeral
橈骨 とうこつ	radius, 〔形〕radial
尺骨 しゃっこつ	ulna, 〔形〕ulnar
手根骨 しゅこんこつ	carpal bone
舟状骨 しゅうじょうこつ	scaphoid bone
月状骨 げつじょうこつ	lunate bone, semilunar bone
三角骨 さんかくこつ	triquetrum, triangular bone
豆状骨 とうじょうこつ	pisiform bone
大菱形骨 だいりょうけいこつ	trapezium bone
小菱形骨 しょうりょうけいこつ	trapezoid bone
有頭骨 ゆうとうこつ	capitate bone
有鉤骨 ゆうこうこつ	hamate bone

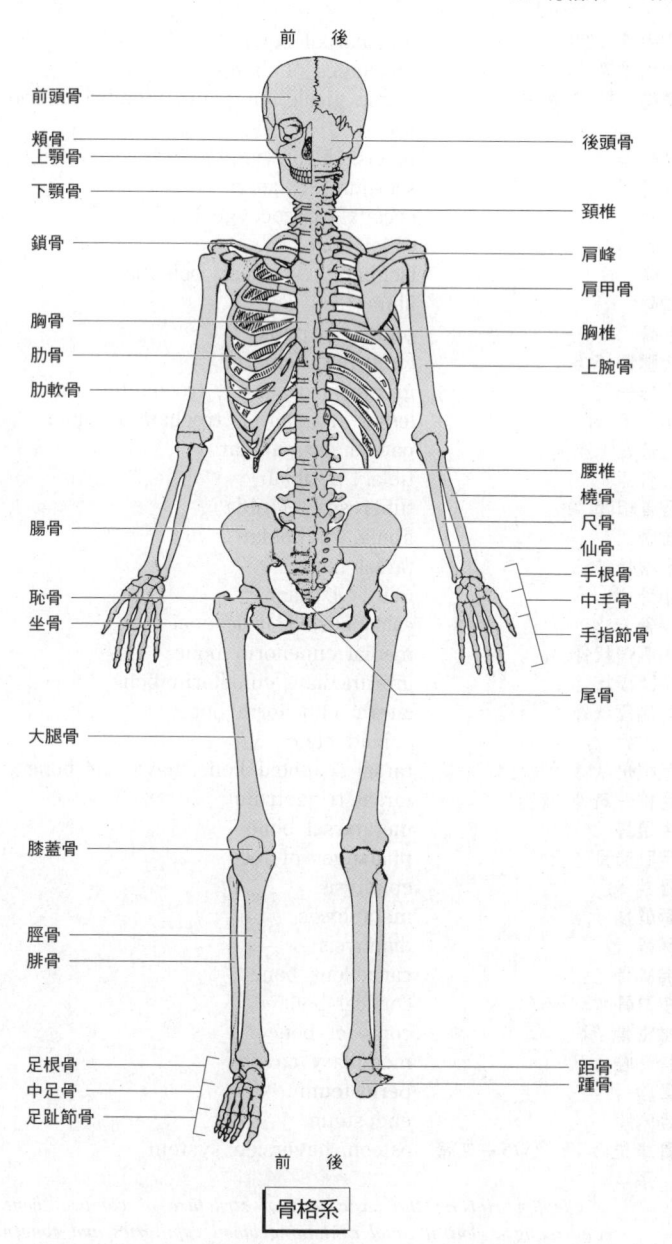

10. 骨格系

前　後

- 前頭骨
- 頬骨
- 上顎骨
- 下顎骨
- 鎖骨
- 胸骨
- 肋骨
- 肋軟骨
- 腸骨
- 恥骨
- 坐骨
- 大腿骨
- 膝蓋骨
- 脛骨
- 腓骨
- 足根骨
- 中足骨
- 足趾節骨

- 後頭骨
- 頚椎
- 肩峰
- 肩甲骨
- 胸椎
- 上腕骨
- 腰椎
- 橈骨
- 尺骨
- 仙骨
- 手根骨
- 中手骨
- 手指節骨
- 尾骨
- 距骨
- 踵骨

前　後

骨格系

中手骨 ちゅうしゅこつ	metacarpal bone
手指節骨 しゅしせっこつ	phalanges of fingers
腰帯 ようたい, 下肢帯 かしたい	pelvic girdle, cingulum membri inferioris
骨盤 こつばん	pelvis, 〔形〕pelvic
仙骨 せんこつ	sacrum, 〔形〕sacral
尾骨 びこつ	coccyx, 〔形〕coccygeal
寛骨 かんこつ	coxal bone
坐骨 ざこつ	ischium, 〔形〕ischial, ischiatic
腸骨 ちょうこつ	ilium, 〔形〕iliac
恥骨 ちこつ	pubis, 〔形〕pubic
大腿骨 だいたいこつ	femur, 〔形〕femoral
大転子 だいてんし	greater trochanter, trochanter major
小転子 しょうてんし	lesser trochanter, trochanter minor
膝蓋骨 しつがいこつ	patella, 〔形〕patellar
脛骨 けいこつ	tibia, 〔形〕tibial
脛骨粗面 けいこつそめん	tuberosity of tibia
腓骨 ひこつ	fibula, 〔形〕fibular
足根骨 そっこんこつ	tarsal bone
距骨 きょこつ	talus, 〔形〕talar
踵骨 しょうこつ	calcaneus, 〔形〕calcaneal
内側楔状骨 ないそくけつじょうこつ	medial cuneiform bone
中間楔状骨 ちゅうかんけつじょうこつ	intermediate cuneiform bone
外側楔状骨 がいそくけつじょうこつ	lateral cuneiform bone
立方骨 りっぽうこつ	cuboid bone
足根舟状骨 そっこんしゅうじょうこつ	tarsal scaphoid bone, navicular bone
足根三角骨 そっこんさんかくこつ	tarsal triquetrum
中足骨 ちゅうそくこつ	metatarsal bone
足趾節骨 そくしせっこつ	phalanges of toes
骨端 こつたん	epiphysis
骨幹端 こつかんたん	metaphysis
骨幹 こっかん	diaphysis
海綿骨 かいめんこつ	cancellous bone
皮質骨 ひしつこつ	cortical bone
緻密骨 ちみつこつ	compact bone
骨髄腔 こつずいくう	medullary cavity
骨膜 こつまく	periosteum
骨内膜 こつないまく	endosteum
骨単位 こつたんい, ハバース管系 はばーすかんけい	osteon, haversian system

⟨<*Clopton Havers; the basic unit of structure of compact bone, comprising a central canal containing blood capillaries and concen-*

tric osseous lamellae around it⟩

● 関節　Joint ●

環椎後頭関節 かんついこうとうかんせつ	atlantooccipital joint
環軸関節 かんじくかんせつ	atlantoaxial joint
顎関節 がくかんせつ	temporomandibular joint (TMJ)
肩関節 かたかんせつ	shoulder joint
胸鎖関節 きょうさかんせつ	sternoclavicular joint
肩鎖関節 けんさかんせつ	acromioclavicular (AC) joint
関節窩 かんせつか	glenoid cavity, glenoid fossa of scapula
肘関節 ちゅうかんせつ	elbow joint
手関節 しゅかんせつ	wrist joint
手根中手関節 しゅこんちゅうしゅかんせつ	carpometacarpal (CM) joint
中手指節関節 ちゅうしゅしせつかんせつ	metacarpophalangeal (MCP) joint
近位指節間関節 きんいしせつかんかんせつ	proximal interphalangeal (PIP) joint
遠位指節間関節 えんいしせつかんかんせつ	distal interphalangeal (DIP) joint
股関節 こかんせつ	hip joint
仙腸関節 せんちょうかんせつ	sacroiliac joint
膝関節 しつかんせつ	knee joint
脛腓関節 けいひかんせつ	tibiofibular joint
足関節 そくかんせつ	ankle joint
横足根関節 おうそくこんかんせつ, ショパール関節 _かんせつ	transverse tarsal joint, Chopart joint

⟨*transverse junction comprised of the calcaneocuboid and talocalcaneonavicular joints*⟩

足根中足関節 そくこんちゅうそくかんせつ, リスフラン関節 _かんせつ	tarsometatarsal (TM) joint, Lisfranc joint

⟨*articulation between the navicular, cuneiform, and cuboid bones and the metatarsals*⟩

中足趾節関節 ちゅうそくしせつかんせつ	metatarsophalangeal (MTP) joint

● 軟骨　Cartilage ●

耳介軟骨 じかいなんこつ	auricular cartilage
鼻軟骨 びなんこつ	nasal cartilages
甲状軟骨 こうじょうなんこつ	thyroid cartilage
輪状軟骨 りんじょうなんこつ	cricoid cartilage, annular cartilage
披裂軟骨 ひれつなんこつ	arytenoid cartilage
小角軟骨 しょうかくなんこつ	corniculate cartilage
楔状軟骨 くさびじょうなんこつ	cuneiform cartilage
喉頭軟骨 こうとうなんこつ	laryngeal cartilage
喉頭蓋軟骨 こうとうがいなんこつ	epiglottic cartilage
気管軟骨 きかんなんこつ	tracheal cartilage

IX章 人体解剖図

肋軟骨 ろくなんこつ	costal cartilage
関節軟骨 かんせつなんこつ	articular cartilage
関節間軟骨 かんせつかんなんこつ	interarticular cartilage
椎間軟骨 ついかんなんこつ	intervertebral cartilage
椎間板 ついかんばん	intervertebral disk
関節半月 かんせつはんげつ	semilunar cartilage, meniscus

● 靱帯 Ligament ●

烏口肩峰靱帯 うこうけんぽうじんたい	coracoacromial ligament (CAL)
烏口鎖骨靱帯 うこうさこつじんたい	coracoclavicular ligament (CCL)
横隔膜弓状靱帯 おうかくまくきゅうじょうじんたい	arcuate ligament of diaphragm
棘間靱帯 きょくかんじんたい	interspinal ligament
黄色靱帯 おうしょくじんたい	yellow ligaments, flaval ligaments
鼠径靱帯 そけいじんたい, プパール靱帯 ―じんたい	inguinal ligament, Poupart ligament
腸腰靱帯 ちょうようじんたい	iliolumbar ligament
腸骨大腿靱帯 ちょうこつだいたいじんたい	iliofemoral ligament
坐骨大腿靱帯 ざこつだいたいじんたい	ischiofemoral ligament
大腿骨円靱帯 だいたいこつえんじんたい	round ligament of femur
前十字靱帯 ぜんじゅうじじんたい	anterior cruciate ligament (ACL)
後十字靱帯 こうじゅうじじんたい	posterior cruciate ligament (PCL)
三角靱帯 さんかくじんたい	deltoid ligament

―Tidbits

funny bone

「おかしな骨」とは何だろうか．誰しも肘を机の角で打って，「ピリッとした」，「電気が走った」経験があることだろう．これが "funny bone" で "crazy bone" ともいうが，打ったところは olecranon 肘頭とよぶ尺骨の上の端である（前腕には尺骨 ulna と橈骨 radius という2本の骨がある）．もっとも実際に「ピリッとする」のは骨ではなく神経（尺骨神経 ulnar nerve）を打つからである．尺骨神経は，前腕と手の筋肉のほかに手掌と手背の内側半分の皮膚に分布している．さて痛みこそあれ「面白くもない」が，何故 "funny" なのか．一説によれば，打って痛いのは上腕骨 humerus の一部と誤認して，"humorous" つまり "funny" というようになったという．

11. 筋肉系

● 筋肉　Muscle ●

骨格筋 こっかくきん	skeletal muscle
横紋筋 おうもんきん	striated muscle
平滑筋 へいかつきん	smooth muscle
伸筋 しんきん	extensor
屈筋 くっきん	flexor
前頭筋 ぜんとうきん	frontal muscle
側頭筋 そくとうきん	temporal muscle
後頭筋 こうとうきん	occipital muscle
眼輪筋 がんりんきん	orbicularis oculi muscle
口輪筋 こうりんきん	orbicularis oris muscle
咬筋 こうきん	masseter muscle
表情筋 ひょうじょうきん	mimetic muscle
咀嚼筋 そしゃくきん	masticatory muscle
胸鎖乳突筋 きょうさにゅうとつきん	sternocleidomastoid muscle
僧帽筋 そうぼうきん	trapezius muscle
三角筋 さんかくきん	deltoid muscle
大胸筋 だいきょうきん	pectoralis major muscle
小胸筋 しょうきょうきん	pectoralis minor muscle
前鋸筋 ぜんきょきん	serratus anterior muscle
鎖骨下筋 さこつかきん	subclavian muscle
肋間筋 ろっかんきん	intercostal muscle
小円筋 しょうえんきん	teres minor muscle
大円筋 だいえんきん	teres major muscle
上腕二頭筋 じょうわんにとうきん	biceps brachii muscle
上腕三頭筋 じょうわんさんとうきん	triceps brachii muscle, triceps muscle of arm
上腕筋 じょうわんきん	brachial muscle
腕橈骨筋 わんとうこつきん	brachioradial muscle
円回内筋 えんかいないきん	pronator teres muscle
回外筋 かいがいきん	supinator muscle
指伸筋 ししんきん	extensor digitorum
尺側手根伸筋 しゃくそくしゅこんしんきん	extensor carpi ulnaris
尺側手根屈筋 しゃくそくしゅこんくっきん	flexor carpi ulnaris
橈側手根伸筋 とうそくしゅこんしんきん	extensor carpi radialis
橈側手根屈筋 とうそくしゅこんくっきん	flexor carpi radialis
伸筋支帯 しんきんしたい	extensor retinaculum
屈筋支帯 くっきんしたい	flexor retinaculum
手掌筋 しゅしょうきん	palmar muscles
腹直筋 ふくちょくきん	rectus abdominis muscle

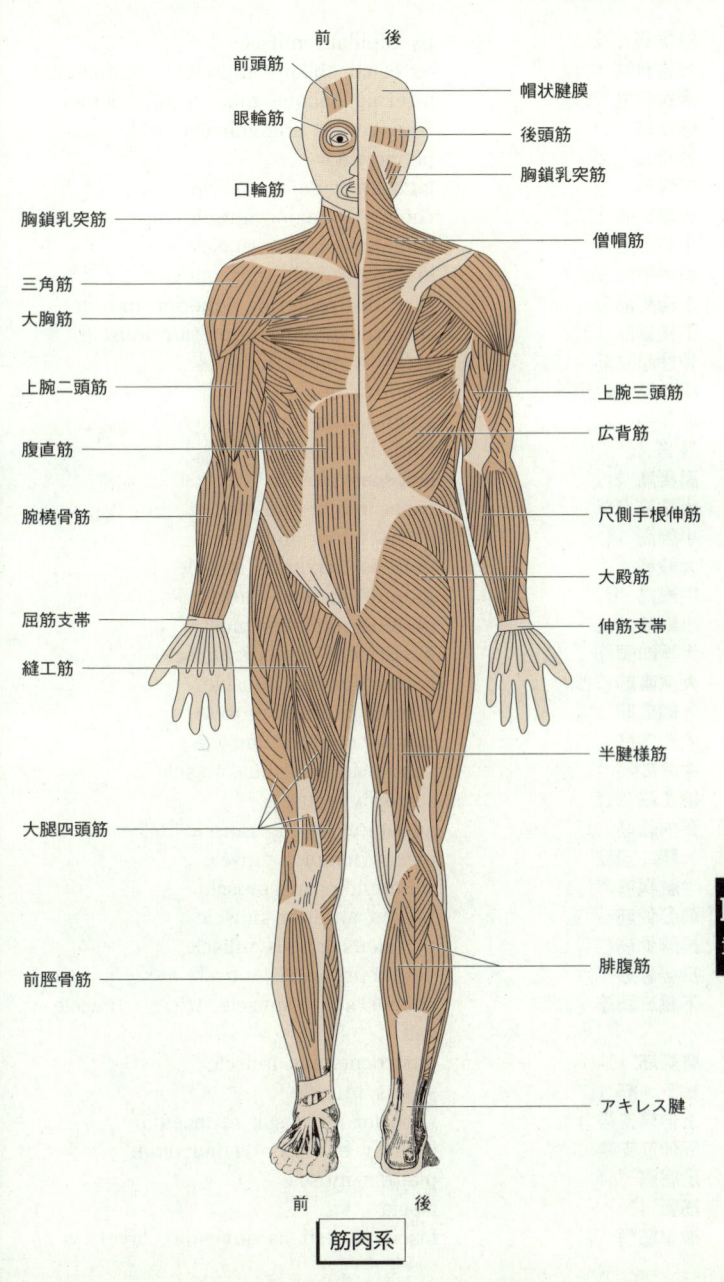

11. 筋肉系

筋肉系

前 / 後

- 前頭筋
- 眼輪筋
- 口輪筋
- 帽状腱膜
- 後頭筋
- 胸鎖乳突筋
- 胸鎖乳突筋
- 僧帽筋
- 三角筋
- 大胸筋
- 上腕二頭筋
- 腹直筋
- 腕橈骨筋
- 屈筋支帯
- 縫工筋
- 上腕三頭筋
- 広背筋
- 尺側手根伸筋
- 大殿筋
- 伸筋支帯
- 半腱様筋
- 大腿四頭筋
- 前脛骨筋
- 腓腹筋
- アキレス腱

前 / 後

IX章　人体解剖図

錐体筋 (すいたいきん)	pyramidalis muscle
外腹斜筋 (がいふくしゃきん)	external oblique muscle of abdomen
内腹斜筋 (ないふくしゃきん)	internal oblique muscle of abdomen
腹横筋 (ふくおうきん)	transversus abdominis muscle
骨盤底 (こつばんてい)	pelvic floor
広背筋 (こうはいきん)	latissimus dorsi muscle
大菱形筋 (だいりょうけいきん)	rhomboid major muscle
小菱形筋 (しょうりょうけいきん)	rhomboid minor muscle
肩甲挙筋 (けんこうきょきん)	levator muscle of scapula
上後鋸筋 (じょうこうきょきん)	serratus posterior superior muscle
下後鋸筋 (かこうきょきん)	serratus posterior inferior muscle
脊柱起立筋 (せきちゅうきりつきん)	erector spinae muscles
腸肋筋 (ちょうろくきん)	iliocostal muscle
最長筋 (さいちょうきん)	longissimus muscle
棘筋 (きょくきん)	spinalis muscle
腸腰筋 (ちょうようきん)	iliopsoas muscle
大腰筋 (だいようきん)	psoas major muscle
小腰筋 (しょうようきん)	psoas minor muscle
大殿筋 (だいでんきん)	gluteus maximus muscle
中殿筋 (ちゅうでんきん)	gluteus medius muscle
小殿筋 (しょうでんきん)	gluteus minimus muscle
大腿四頭筋 (だいたいとうきん)	quadriceps femoris muscle
大腿直筋 (だいたいちょくきん)	rectus femoris muscle
外側広筋 (がいそくこうきん)	vastus lateralis muscle
内側広筋 (ないそくこうきん)	vastus medialis muscle
中間広筋 (ちゅうかんこうきん)	vastus intermedius muscle
縫工筋 (ほうこうきん)	sartorius muscle
長内転筋 (ちょうないてんきん)	adductor longus muscle
大腿二頭筋 (だいたいにとうきん)	biceps femoris muscle
半腱様筋 (はんけんようきん)	semitendinosus muscle
前脛骨筋 (ぜんけいこつきん)	tibialis anterior muscle
長腓骨筋 (ちょうひこつきん)	peroneus longus muscle
短腓骨筋 (たんひこつきん)	peroneus brevis muscle
下腿三頭筋 (かたいさんとうきん)	triceps surae muscle, triceps muscle of calf
腓腹筋 (ひふくきん)	gastrocnemius muscle
ヒラメ筋 (きん)	soleus muscle
上伸筋支帯 (じょうしんきんしたい)	superior extensor retinaculum
下伸筋支帯 (かしんきんしたい)	inferior extensor retinaculum
足底筋 (そくていきん)	plantar muscle
筋膜 (きんまく)	fascia
被包筋膜 (ひほうきんまく)	fascia investiens, investing layer

11. 筋肉系　501

胸腰筋膜 きょうようきんまく	thoracolumbar fascia
腎筋膜 じんきんまく，ジェロタ筋膜	renal fascia, Gerota fascia
大腿筋膜 だいたいきんまく	fascia lata, deep fascia of thigh

● 腱　Tendon ●

腱膜 けんまく	aponeurosis
帽状腱膜 ぼうじょうけんまく	galea aponeurotica, epicranial aponeurosis
腹部腱膜 ふくぶけんまく	abdominal aponeurosis
白線 はくせん	linea alba
大腿部膝屈筋腱 だいたいぶしつくっきんけん	hamstring tendon
膝蓋腱 しつがいけん	patellar tendon
アキレス腱 けん	Achilles tendon
⟨*calcaneal tendon; triceps surae to calcaneal tuberosity*⟩	
伸筋腱 しんきんけん	extensor tendon
腱鞘 けんしょう	tendon sheath, vagina tendinis
滑液包 かつえきほう	synovial bursa

IX 章

12. 神経系

● 中枢神経系　Central nervous system (CNS) ●

大脳 だいのう	cerebrum, 〔形〕cerebral
大脳半球 だいのうはんきゅう	cerebral hemisphere
外套 がいとう	pallium, 〔形〕pallial
前頭葉 ぜんとうよう	frontal lobe
頭頂葉 とうちょうよう	parietal lobe
後頭葉 こうとうよう	occipital lobe
側頭葉 そくとうよう	temporal lobe
脳梁 のうりょう	corpus callosum
脳弓 のうきゅう	fornix, 〔形〕fornical
前交連 ぜんこうれん	anterior commissure
透明中隔 とうめいちゅうかく	septum pellucidum
嗅脳 きゅうのう	rhinencephalon
海馬 かいば	hippocampus, 〔形〕hippocampal
ライル島 とう	insula of Reil

〈*insula, insular lobe; oval region of the cerebral cortex lying deep in the lateral sulcus, and surrounded by the circular sulcus*〉

大脳回 だいのうかい	gyrus of cerebrum, 〔複〕gyri of cerebrum
大脳溝 だいのうこう	sulcus of cerebrum, 〔複〕sulci of cerebrum
ローランド溝 こう	rolandic fissure

〈*<Luigi Rolando; central sulcus; separating the frontal from the parietal lobe*〉

シルビウス溝 こう	sylvian fissure

〈*<Franciscus Sylvius; lateral sulcus; the deepest sulcus between the temporal and frontal lobes*〉

脳室 のうしつ	cerebral ventricle
側脳室 そくのうしつ	lateral ventricle
第三脳室 だいさんのうしつ	third ventricle
中脳水道 ちゅうのうすいどう, シルビウス水道 いどう	cerebral aqueduct, sylvian aqueduct

〈*<Franciscus Sylvius; the channel in the mesencephalon that connects the third and fourth ventricles*〉

第四脳室 だいよんのうしつ	fourth ventricle
菱形窩 りょうけいか	rhomboid fossa
青斑 せいはん	locus ceruleus
脳室周囲器官 のうしつしゅういきかん	circumventricular organs
最後野 さいこうや	area postrema
終板脈管器官 しゅうばんみゃっかんきかん	organum vasculosum of lamina terminalis (OVLT)

脳

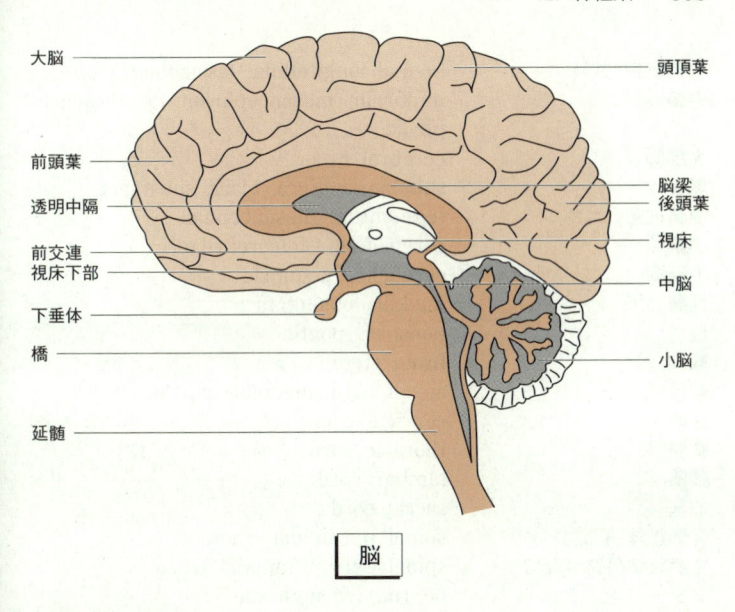

図の標識:
- 大脳
- 頭頂葉
- 前頭葉
- 透明中隔
- 脳梁
- 後頭葉
- 前交連
- 視床
- 視床下部
- 中脳
- 下垂体
- 橋
- 小脳
- 延髄

大脳皮質（だいのうひしつ）	cerebral cortex
運動野（うんどうや）	motor area
知覚野（しかくや）	sensory area
連合野（れんごうや）	association area
運動性言語中枢（うんどうせいげんごちゅうすう），ブローカ中枢（―ちゅうすう）	motor speech center, Broca center
感覚性言語中枢（かんかくせいげんごちゅうすう），ウェルニッケ中枢（―ちゅうすう）	sensory speech center, Wernicke center
大脳基底核（だいのうきていかく）	basal ganglia
尾状核（びじょうかく）	caudate nucleus
レンズ核（―かく）	lentiform nucleus
淡蒼球（たんそうきゅう）	globus pallidus
線条体（せんじょうたい）	corpus striatum
被殻（ひかく）	putamen
内包（ないほう）	internal capsule, capsula interna
間脳（かんのう）	diencephalon, 〔形〕diencephalic
視床（ししょう）	thalamus, 〔形〕thalamic
視床上部（ししょうじょうぶ）	epithalamus, 〔形〕epithalamic
視床下部（ししょうかぶ）	hypothalamus, 〔形〕hypothalamic
視床下核（ししょうかかく），リュイ体	subthalamic nucleus, Luys body

内側縦束 (ないそくじゅうそく)	medial longitudinal fasciculus (MLF)
中脳 (ちゅうのう)	midbrain, mesencephalon, 〔形〕mesencephalic
大脳脚 (だいのうきゃく)	cerebral crus
黒質 (こくしつ)	substantia nigra, black substance
中脳被蓋 (ちゅうのうひがい)	tegmentum mesencephali
小脳 (しょうのう)	cerebellum, 〔形〕cerebellar
小脳脚 (しょうのうきゃく)	cerebellar peduncle
延髄 (えんずい)	medulla oblongata
橋 (きょう)	pons, 〔形〕pontine
脳幹 (のうかん)	brain stem
脊髄 (せきずい)	spinal cord, medulla spinalis
頚髄 (けいずい)	cervical cord
胸髄 (きょうずい)	thoracic cord
腰髄 (ようずい)	lumbar cord
仙髄 (せんずい)	sacral cord
脊髄錐体路 (せきずいすいたいろ)	spinal pyramidal tract
脊髄錐体外路 (せきずいすいたいがいろ)	spinal extrapyramidal tract
ニューロン	neuron, 〔形〕neuronal
樹状突起 (じゅじょうとっき)	dendrite
軸索 (じくさく)	axon
神経細線維 (しんけいさいせんい)	neurofibril
ニッスル小体 (―しょうたい)	Nissl body

⟨*granular material found in the neuron cytoplasm, composed of rough endoplasmic reticulum and free ribosomes*⟩

遠心性ニューロン (えんしんせい―)	efferent neuron
求心性ニューロン (きゅうしんせい―)	afferent neuron
神経節 (しんけいせつ)	ganglion, 〔複〕ganglia, ganglions
髄膜 (ずいまく)	meninges, 〔形〕meningeal
硬膜 (こうまく)	dura mater
くも膜 (―まく)	arachnoid, 〔形〕arachnoidal
パッキオニ小体 (―しょうたい)	pacchionian body

⟨<*Antonio Pacchioni; arachnoid granulations; villous projections of subarachnoid tissue, effecting transfer of CSF to the venous system*⟩

軟膜 (なんまく)	pia mater
脈絡叢 (みゃくらくそう)	choroid plexus
硬膜下腔 (こうまくかくう)	subdural space
くも膜下腔 (―まくかくう)	subarachnoid space

●末梢神経系　Peripheral nervous system (PNS)●

脳神経 のうしんけい	cranial nerves (CN)
嗅神経 きゅうしんけい	olfactory nerve, the first cranial nerve (CN I)
視神経 ししんけい	optic nerve (CN II)
動眼神経 どうがんしんけい	oculomotor nerve (CN III)
滑車神経 かっしゃしんけい	trochlear nerve (CN IV)
三叉神経 さんさしんけい	trigeminal nerve (CN V)
三叉神経節 さんさしんけいせつ	trigeminal ganglion, gasserian ganglion

⟨<*Herbert Spencer Gasser; the sensory ganglion of the trigeminal nerve lying in a cleft within the dura mater on the anterior surface of the petrous part of the temporal bone*⟩

眼神経 がんしんけい	ophthalmic nerve
上顎神経 じょうがくしんけい	maxillary nerve
下顎神経 かがくしんけい	mandibular nerve
外転神経 がいてんしんけい	abducens nerve (CN VI)
顔面神経 がんめんしんけい	facial nerve (CN VII)
膝神経節 しつしんけいせつ	geniculate ganglion, ganglion geniculi nervi facialis
聴神経 ちょうしんけい	acoustic nerve (CN VIII)
蝸牛神経 かぎゅうしんけい	cochlear nerve
前庭神経 ぜんていしんけい	vestibular nerve
舌咽神経 ぜついんしんけい	glossopharyngeal nerve (CN IX)
迷走神経 めいそうしんけい	vagus nerve (CN X)
副神経 ふくしんけい	accessory nerve (CN XI)
舌下神経 ぜっかしんけい	hypoglossal nerve (CN XII)
脊髄神経 せきずいしんけい	spinal nerves
頚神経叢 けいしんけいそう	cervical plexus (C1-C4)
小後頭神経 しょうこうとうしんけい	lesser occipital nerve
鎖骨上神経 さこつじょうしんけい	supraclavicular nerve
腕神経叢 わんしんけいそう	brachial plexus (C5-Th1)
肩甲上神経 けんこうじょうしんけい	suprascapular nerve
胸筋神経 きょうきんしんけい	pectoral nerve
腋窩神経 えきかしんけい	axillary nerve
内側上腕皮神経 ないそくじょうわんひしんけい	medial brachial cutaneous nerve
内側前腕皮神経 ないそくぜんわひしんけい	medial antebrachial cutaneous nerve
正中神経 せいちゅうしんけい	median nerve
尺骨神経 しゃっこつしんけい	ulnar nerve
橈骨神経 とうこつしんけい	radial nerve
胸神経 きょうしんけい	thoracic nerve (Th1-Th12)
肋間神経 ろっかんしんけい	intercostal nerve
腰神経叢 ようしんけいそう	lumbar plexus (Th12-L4)

腸骨下腹神経 ちょうこつかふくしんけい	iliohypogastric nerve
腸骨鼠径神経 ちょうこつそけいしんけい	ilioinguinal nerve
陰部大腿神経 いんぶだいたいしんけい	genitofemoral nerve
閉鎖神経 へいさしんけい	obturator nerve
大腿神経 だいたいしんけい	femoral nerve
伏在神経 ふくざいしんけい	saphenous nerve
仙骨神経叢 せんこつしんけいそう	sacral plexus (L4-S3)
坐骨神経 ざこつしんけい	sciatic nerve
総腓骨神経 そうひこつしんけい	common peroneal nerve
浅腓骨神経 せんひこつしんけい	superficial peroneal nerve
深腓骨神経 しんひこつしんけい	deep peroneal nerve
脛骨神経 けいこつしんけい	tibial nerve
陰部神経叢 いんぶしんけいそう	pudendal plexus (S2-S4)
陰部神経 いんぶしんけい	pudendal nerve
尾骨神経叢 びこつしんけいそう	coccygeal plexus (S4-C0)
馬尾 ばび	cauda equina
自律神経系 じりつしんけいけい	autonomic nervous system
交感神経 こうかんしんけい	sympathetic nerve
副交感神経 ふくこうかんしんけい	parasympathetic nerve
神経線維鞘 しんけいせんいしょう, シュワン鞘 しょう	neurilemma, Schwann sheath
神経細線維 しんけいさいせんい	neurofibril

12. 神経系　507

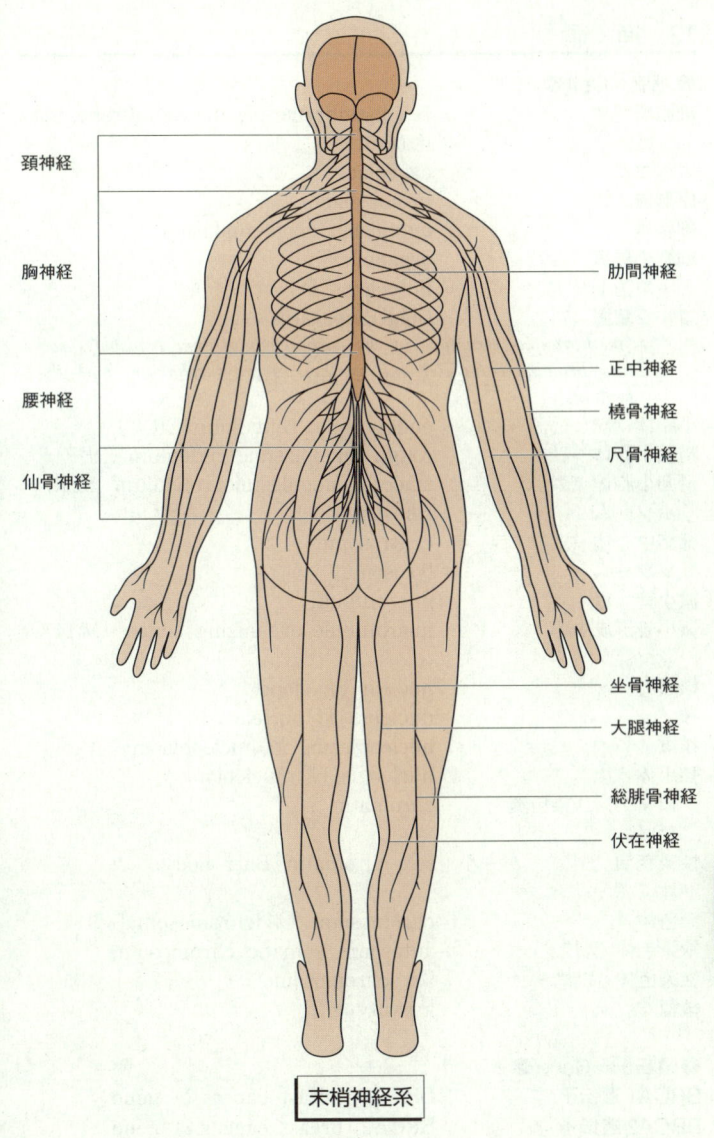

頸神経

胸神経

腰神経

仙骨神経

肋間神経

正中神経

橈骨神経

尺骨神経

坐骨神経

大腿神経

総腓骨神経

伏在神経

末梢神経系

13. 補遺

● 細胞 Cell ●

細胞膜 さいぼうまく	cell membrane, plasma membrane, plasmalemma
カベオラ	caveolae
原形質 げんけいしつ	protoplasm
細胞質 さいぼうしつ	cytoplasm, 〔形〕cytoplasmic
細胞小器官 さいぼうしょうきかん	organelle
ミトコンドリア	mitochondria
ゴルジ装置 —そうち	Golgi apparatus

⟨*membranous structure in the perinuclear region; transports secretory proteins from ER and synthesizes polysaccharides and glycoproteins*⟩

小胞体 しょうほうたい	endoplasmic reticulum (ER)
粗面小胞体 そめんしょうほうたい	rough endoplasmic reticulum (RER)
滑面小胞体 かつめんしょうほうたい	smooth endoplasmic reticulum (SER)
リボソーム	ribosome
細胞中心体 さいぼうちゅうしんたい	centrosome
リソソーム	lysosome
微小管 びしょうかん	microtubule
微小管形成中心 びしょうかんけいせいちゅうしん	microtubule organizing center (MTOC)
核膜 かくまく	nuclear envelope
核 かく	nucleus, 〔形〕nuclear
核質 かくしつ	nucleoplasm, 〔形〕nucleoplasmic
核小体 かくしょうたい	nucleolus, 〔形〕nucleolar
クロマチン, 染色質 せんしょくしつ	chromatin
性染色質 せいせんしょくしつ, バー小体 —しょうたい	sex chromatin, Barr body
染色体 せんしょくたい	chromosome, 〔形〕chromosomal
常染色体 じょうせんしょくたい	autosome, somatic chromosome
性染色体 せいせんしょくたい	sex chromosome
核型 かくがた	karyotype

● 遺伝子 Gene ●

BRCA1 遺伝子 —でんし	BRCA1 (breast cancer 1) gene
BRCA2 遺伝子 —でんし	BRCA2 (breast cancer 2) gene
c-kit 遺伝子 —でんし	c-kit gene
HOX 遺伝子 —でんし	HOX (homeobox) genes
K-ras 遺伝子 —でんし	K-ras gene

13. 補遺　509

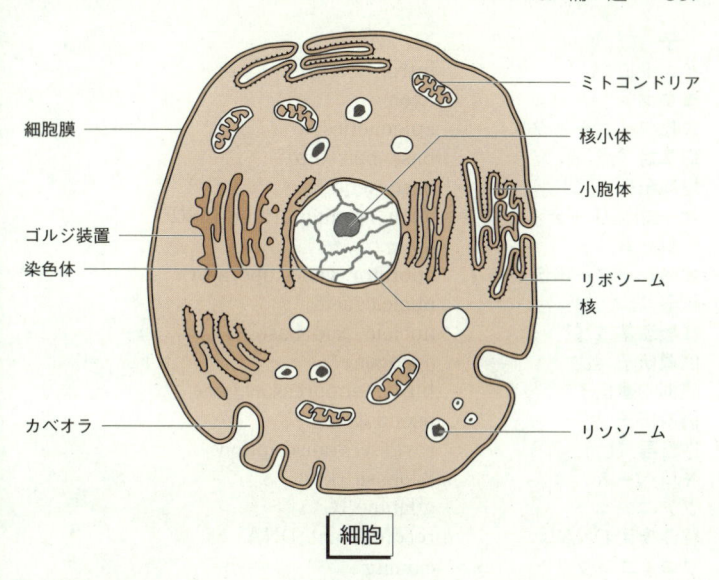

[図：細胞]

- 細胞膜
- ゴルジ装置
- 染色体
- カベオラ
- ミトコンドリア
- 核小体
- 小胞体
- リボソーム
- 核
- リソソーム

細胞

PAX 遺伝子	PAX (paired box) genes
X 染色体連鎖遺伝子	X-linked gene
Y 染色体連鎖遺伝子	Y-linked gene
アデニン	adenine (A)
一塩基多型	single nucleotide polymorphism (SNP)
一倍体	haploid
遺伝暗号	genetic code
遺伝子型	genotype
遺伝子欠損	gene deletion
遺伝子座	gene locus
遺伝子座調節領域	locus control region (LCR)
遺伝子増幅	gene amplification
遺伝子地図	gene map
遺伝子配列	gene arrangement
遺伝子発現	gene expression
遺伝子プール	gene pool
遺伝子変換	gene conversion
遺伝子融合	gene fusion
インターフェロン制御因	interferon regulatory factor (IRF)

IX 章

子（いんし）
イントロン	intron
エクソン	exon
エピジェネティクス	epigenetics
塩基対（ついき）	base pair (bp)
塩基配列（えんきはいれつ）	base sequence
オープンリーディングフレーム	open reading frame (ORF)
オペレーター遺伝子（いでんし）	operator gene, operator
核酸（かくさん）	nucleic acid
核酸塩基（かくさんえんき）	nucleic acid base
癌遺伝子（がんいでんし）	oncogene
癌抑制遺伝子（がんよくせいいでんし）	tumor suppressor gene
偽遺伝子（ぎいでんし）	pseudogene
逆転写（ぎゃくてんしゃ）	reverse transcription
キロベース	kilobase (kb)
グアニン	guanine (G)
組み換えDNA（くみかえ）	recombinant DNA
クローニング	cloning
ゲノミックス	genomics
ゲノム	genome
ゲノムインプリンティング	genomic imprinting (GI)
原癌遺伝子（げんがんいでんし）	proto-oncogene
構造遺伝子（こうぞういでんし）	structural gene
高変異反復列（こうへんいはんぷくれつ）	variable number tandem repeats (VNTR)
コドン	codon
シトシン	cytosine
スプライシング	splicing
制限酵素（せいげんこうそ）	restriction enzyme
制限酵素断片多型（せいげんこうそだんぺんたけい）	restriction fragment length polymorphism (RFLP)
染色体地図（せんしょくたいちず）	chromosome map
センチモルガン	centimorgan (cM)
セントロメア	centromere
相互転座（そうごてんざ）	reciprocal translocation (rcp)
相補DNA（そうほ）	complementary DNA (cDNA)
対立遺伝子（たいりついでんし）	allele, allelic gene
多倍数体（たばいすうたい）	polyploid
短縦列反復（たんじゅうれつはんぷく）	short tandem repeat (STR)
単純配列長多型	simple sequence length polymorphism

13. 補遺 511

たんじゅんはいれつちょうたけい	(SSLP)
チミン	thymine (T)
長端末反復 ちょうたんまつはんぷく	long terminal repeats (LTR)
デオキシリボ核酸 かくさん	deoxyribonucleic acid (DNA)
テロメア	telomere
テロメラーゼ	telomerase
転移RNA てんい	transfer RNA (tRNA)
転座 てんざ	translocation
転写 てんしゃ	transcription
突然変異遺伝子 とつぜんへんいいでんし	mutant gene
トランスクリプトーム	transcriptome
トランスポゾン	transposon
二重らせん にじゅう	double helix
二倍体 にばいたい	diploid
二本鎖DNA にほんさ	double-stranded DNA (dsDNA)
ヌクレオソーム	nucleosome
ヌクレオチド	nucleotide
ハウスキーピング遺伝子 いでんし	housekeeping gene
ハプロタイプ	haplotype
ヒストン	histone
表現型 ひょうげんがた	phenotype
複製 ふくせい	replication
プライマー	primer
プラスミド	plasmid
プレセニリン遺伝子 いでんし	presenilin (PSEN) gene
プロテオーム	proteome
変異 へんい	mutation
変更遺伝子 へんこういでんし	modifier gene
ホメオ遺伝子 いでんし	homeotic gene
翻訳 ほんやく	translation
マイクロアレイ	microarray
マイクロサテライト不安定性 ふあんていせい	microsatellite instability (MSI)
ミーム	meme
ミトコンドリアDNA	mitochondrial DNA (mtDNA)
ミニサテライト	minisatellite
メッセンジャーRNA	messenger RNA (mRNA)
優性遺伝子 ゆうせいいでんし	dominant gene
リボ核酸 かくさん	ribonucleic acid (RNA)
リボ核タンパク質 かくしつ	ribonucleoprotein (RNP)
リボソームRNA	ribosomal RNA (rRNA)

劣性遺伝子 れっせいいでんし　　　　　recessive gene
レプレッサー遺伝子 いでんし　　　repressor gene

● 組織　Tissue ●
上皮組織 じょうひそしき　　　　　epithelial tissue
腺組織 せんそしき　　　　　　　glandular tissue
支持組織 しじそしき　　　　　　supporting tissue
結合組織 けつごうそしき　　　　connective tissue
疎性結合組織 そせいけつごうそしき　loose connective tissue, areolar tissue, cribriform tissue
緻密性結合組織 ちみつせいけつごうそしき　dense connective tissue
線維組織 せんいそしき　　　　　fibrous tissue
膠様組織 こうようそしき　　　　gelatinous tissue
細網組織 さいもうそしき　　　　reticular tissue
弾性組織 だんせいそしき　　　　elastic tissue
脂肪組織 しぼうそしき　　　　　adipose tissue, fatty tissue
軟骨組織 なんこつそしき　　　　cartilaginous tissue
骨組織 こつそしき　　　　　　　osseous tissue, bony tissue
筋組織 きんそしき　　　　　　　muscular tissue
神経組織 しんけいそしき　　　　nervous tissue
間葉組織 かんようそしき　　　　mesenchymal tissue, mesenchyma

● 体液　Body fluid ●
細胞内液 さいぼうないえき　　　　intracellular fluid (ICF)
細胞外液 さいぼうがいえき　　　　extracellular fluid (ECF)
血液 けつえき　　　　　　　　　blood
血漿 けっしょう　　　　　　　　plasma
血管外液 けっかんがいえき　　　　extravascular fluid
細胞透過液 さいぼうとうかえき　　transcellular fluid
間質液 かんしつえき，組織液 そしきえき　interstitial fluid (ISF), tissue fluid
リンパ　　　　　　　　　　　lymph
漿液 しょうえき　　　　　　　　serous fluid
眼房水 がんぼうすい　　　　　　aqueous humor
心膜液 しんまくえき　　　　　　pericardial fluid
胸膜液 きょうまくえき　　　　　pleural fluid
腹水 ふくすい　　　　　　　　　ascitic fluid
汗 あせ　　　　　　　　　　　　sweat, sudor
唾液 だえき　　　　　　　　　　saliva
胃液 いえき　　　　　　　　　　gastric juice
十二指腸液 じゅうにしちょうえき　duodenal juice
胆汁 たんじゅう　　　　　　　　bile
膵液 すいえき　　　　　　　　　pancreatic juice

腸液 ちょうえき	intestinal juice
尿 にょう	urine
滑液 かつえき	synovial fluid
脳脊髄液 のうせきずいえき	cerebrospinal fluid (CSF)

X章

略語集

A

A	adenine	アデニン
A	ampere	アンペア
A	artery	動脈
AA	Alcoholics Anonymous	断酒会
AA	amino acid	アミノ酸
AA	amyloid A protein	アミロイドAタンパク質
AA	aplastic anemia	再生不良性貧血
$\overline{aa}$	ana	各々
AAA	abdominal aortic aneurysm	腹部大動脈瘤
AAC	antibiotic-associated colitis	抗生物質関連大腸炎
AAD	atlantoaxial dislocation	環軸関節脱臼
AAD	antibiotic-associated diarrhea	抗生物質関連下痢
AaDCO$_2$	alveolar-arterial carbon dioxide difference	肺胞気-動脈血二酸化炭素分圧較差
AaDN$_2$	alveolar-arterial nitrogen difference	肺胞気-動脈血窒素分圧較差
AaDO$_2$	alveolar-arterial oxygen difference	肺胞気-動脈血酸素分圧較差
AAE	annuloaortic ectasia	大動脈輪拡張
AAH	atypical adenomatous hyperplasia	非定型的腺腫様過形成
AAL	anterior axillary line	前腋窩線
AAR	antigen-antibody reaction	抗原抗体反応
AAS	aortic arch syndrome	大動脈弓症候群
AAS	atlantoaxial sublaxation	環軸関節亜脱臼
AAT	automatic atrial tachycardia	自動能性心房頻拍
AAV	adeno-associated virus	アデノ随伴ウイルス
Ab	antibody	抗体
Aβ	amyloid β-protein	アミロイドβタンパク質
ABC	aspiration biopsy cytology	吸引生検細胞診
ABC	aneurysmal bone cyst	動脈瘤性骨嚢胞
ABE	acute bacterial endocarditis	急性細菌性心内膜炎
ABG	arterial blood gas	動脈血ガス
ABI	ankle-brachial index	足関節上腕血圧比
ABK	arbekacin	アルベカシン
ABL	abetalipoproteinemia	無ベータリポタンパク血症
ABLB	alternate binaural loudness balance test	両耳音の大きさバランス検査
ABMT	autologous bone marrow transplantation	自己骨髄移植
ABO	ABO blood group system	ABO血液型
ABPA	allergic bronchopulmonary as-	アレルギー性気管支肺アス

	pergillosis	ペルギルス症
ABPC	ampicillin	アンピシリン
ABPC/MCIPC	ampicillin/cloxacillin	アンピシリン・クロキサシリン
ABPC/SBT	ampicillin/sulbactam	アンピシリン・スルバクタム
ABPM	ambulatory blood pressure monitoring	自由行動下血圧測定
ABR	auditory brainstem response	聴性脳幹反応
ABVD	Adriamycin, bleomycin, vinblastine, dacarbazine	アドリアマイシン（ドキソルビシン），ブレオマイシン，ビンブラスチン，ダカルバジン（化学療法）
AC	abdominal circumference	腹囲
AC	acromioclavicular (joint)	肩鎖（関節）
AC	Adriamycin, cyclophosphamide	アドリアマイシン（ドキソルビシン），シクロホスファミド（化学療法）
AC	air conduction	気導
AC	alternating current	交流
AC	anterior chamber	前房
AC	aortocoronary (bypass)	大動脈冠動脈（バイパス）
AC	asymptomatic carrier	無症候性キャリア
Ac	actinium	アクチニウム
a.c.	ante cibum	食前
ACA	anterior cerebral artery	前大脳動脈
ACA	anticentromere antibody	抗セントロメア抗体
ACC	adenoid cystic carcinoma	腺様嚢胞癌
ACCR	amylase creatinine clearance ratio	アミラーゼクレアチニンクリアランス比
ACD	anemia of chronic disease	慢性疾患に伴う貧血
ACDK	acquired cystic disease of kidney	後天性嚢胞性腎疾患
ACE	angiotensin-converting enzyme	アンギオテンシン変換酵素
ACEI	angiotensin-converting enzyme inhibitor	アンギオテンシン変換酵素阻害薬
ACG	angiocardiography	心血管造影法
ACG	apex cardiogram	心尖拍動図
ACGME	Accreditation Council for Graduate Medical Education	卒後医学教育認定協議会（米国）
ACh	acetylcholine	アセチルコリン
AChE	acetylcholine esterase	アセチルコリンエステラーゼ
ACL	anterior cruciate ligament	前十字靱帯

X章 略語集

ACL	anti-cardiolipin antibody	抗カルジオリピン抗体
ACLS	advanced cardiac life support	二次救命処置
ACMP	Adriamycin, cytarabine, 6-mercaptopurine, prednisolone	アドリアマイシン（ドキソルビシン），シタラビン，6-メルカプトプリン，プレドニゾロン（化学療法）
ACNU	nimustine	ニムスチン
ACP	acid phosphatase	酸性ホスファターゼ
ACPC	ciclacillin	シクラシリン
ACPS	acrocephalopolysyndactyly	尖頭多合指症
ACR	aclarubicin	アクラルビシン
ACS	abdominal compartment syndrome	腹部コンパートメント症候群
ACS	acute coronary syndrome	急性冠動脈症候群
ACS	American Cancer Society	米国対癌協会
ACT	activated clotting time	活性凝固時間
ACT	anticoagulant therapy	抗凝固療法
ACT-D	actinomycin D	アクチノマイシン D
ACTH	adrenocorticotropic hormone	副腎皮質刺激ホルモン
ACV	acyclovir	アシクロビル
AD	Alzheimer disease	アルツハイマー病
AD	atopic dermatitis	アトピー性皮膚炎
AD	auris dextra	右耳
ad lib.	ad libitum	随意に，適宜
ADA	adenosine deaminase	アデノシンデアミナーゼ
ADAS	Alzheimer disease assessment scale	アルツハイマー病評価スケール
ADCC	antibody-dependent cellular cytotoxicity	抗体依存性細胞傷害
ADD	attention deficit disorder	注意欠陥障害
ADEM	acute disseminated encephalomyelitis	急性散在性脳脊髄炎
ADH	antidiuretic hormone	抗利尿ホルモン
ADHD	attention-deficit hyperactivity disorder	注意欠陥多動障害
ADI	acceptable daily intake	1日摂取許容量
ADL	activities of daily living	日常生活動作
ADM	Adriamycin	アドリアマイシン，ドキソルビシン
ADP	adenosine diphosphate	アデノシン二リン酸
ADPKD	autosomal dominant polycystic kidney disease	常染色体優性多発嚢胞腎症
ADR	adverse drug reaction	有害薬物反応
ADR	alternative dispute resolution	裁判外紛争解決

ADS	antibody deficiency syndrome	抗体欠損症候群
ADT	androgen deprivation therapy	アンドロゲン欠損療法
A-E	above-elbow (amputation)	上腕(切断術)
AED	antiepileptic drug	抗てんかん薬
AED	automated external defibrillator	自動体外式除細動器
AEP	acute eosinophilic pneumonia	急性好酸球性肺炎
AEP	auditory evoked potential	聴覚誘発電位
AF	atrial fibrillation	心房細動
AF	atrial flutter	心房粗動
AFB	acid-fast bacillus	抗酸菌
AFD	appropriate-for-dates (infant)	在胎期間相当体重(児)
AFI	amniotic fluid index	羊水指数
AFIP	Armed Forces Institute of Pathology	米国軍病理研究所
AFLP	acute fatty liver in pregnancy	急性妊娠脂肪肝
AFO	ankle-foot orthosis	短下肢装具
AFP	alpha-fetoprotein	アルファフェトプロテイン
AFTN	autonomously functioning thyroid nodule	自律性機能性甲状腺結節
AFX	atypical fibroxanthoma	異型線維黄色腫
1,5-AG	1,5-anhydroglucitol	1,5-アンヒドログルシトール
AG	aminoglycoside	アミノ配糖体
AG	anion gap	陰イオンギャップ
Ag	antigen	抗原
Ag	argentum, silver	銀
A/G	albumin-globulin ratio	アルブミン・グロブリン比
AGA	allergic granulomatous angiitis	アレルギー性肉芽腫性血管炎
AGA	appropriate-for-gestational-age (infant)	在胎期間相当体重(児)
AGE	advanced glycation end product	最終糖化産物
AGML	acute gastric mucosal lesion	急性胃粘膜病変
AGN	acute glomerulonephritis	急性糸球体腎炎
AGS	adrenogenital syndrome	副腎性器症候群
AGT	antiglobulin test	抗グロブリン試験
AHA	acquired hemolytic anemia	後天性溶血性貧血
AHA	American Heart Association	米国心臓協会
AHC	acute hemorrhagic conjunctivitis	急性出血性結膜炎
AHC	acute hemorrhagic colitis	急性出血性大腸炎
AHF	antihemophilic factor	抗血友病因子

AHI	apnea-hypopnea index	無呼吸低換気指数
AHIP	America's Health Insurance Plans	アメリカ健康保険企画（米国）
AHL	artificial heart-lung	人工心肺
AHO	Albright hereditary osteodystrophy	オールブライト遺伝性骨形成異常症
AHP	acute hemorrhagic pancreatitis	急性出血性膵炎
AI	aortic insufficiency	大動脈弁閉鎖不全
AI	apnea index	無呼吸指数
AICA	anterior inferior cerebellar artery	前下小脳動脈
AICD	automatic implantable cardioverter-defibrillator	植え込み型自動除細動器
AID	artificial insemination by donor	非配偶者間人工授精
AIDP	acute inflammatory demyelinating polyneuropathy	急性炎症性脱髄性多発ニューロパチー
AIDS	acquired immunodeficiency syndrome	後天性免疫不全症候群，エイズ
AIE	acute infectious endocarditis	急性感染性心内膜炎
AIF	anterior interbody fusion	前方椎体間固定術
AIH	artificial insemination by husband	配偶者間人工授精
AIH	autoimmune hepatitis	自己免疫性肝炎
AIHA	autoimmune hemolytic anemia	自己免疫性溶血性貧血
AILD	angioimmunoblastic lymphadenopathy with dysproteinemia	異常タンパク血症を伴う血管免疫芽球性リンパ節症
AIN	acute interstitial nephritis	急性間質性腎炎
AION	anterior ischemic optic neuropathy	前部虚血性視神経症
AIP	acute intermittent porphyria	急性間欠性ポルフィリン症
AIP	acute interstitial pneumonia	急性間質性肺炎
AIP	autoimmune pancreatitis	自己免疫性膵炎
AIVR	accelerated idioventricular rhythm	促進心室固有調律
AJ	ankle jerk	アキレス腱反射
AK	artificial kidney	人工腎
AK	astigmatic keratectomy	乱視矯正角膜切開術
A-K	above-knee (amputation)	大腿（切断術）
AKBR	arterial ketone body ratio	動脈血中ケトン体比
AKI	acute kidney injury	急性腎障害
AKM	bekanamycin	ベカナマイシン

Al	aluminium	アルミニウム
ALA	aminolevulinic acid	アミノレブリン酸
ALA	antilymphocyte antibody	抗リンパ球抗体
ALD	adrenoleukodystrophy	副腎白質ジストロフィー
ALD	alcoholic liver disease	アルコール性肝疾患
ALDH	aldehyde dehydrogenase	アルデヒドデヒドロゲナーゼ
ALG	antilymphocyte globulin	抗リンパ球グロブリン
ALI	acute lung injury	急性肺損傷
ALL	acute lymphocytic leukemia	急性リンパ性白血病
ALP	alkaline phosphatase	アルカリホスファターゼ
ALPP	abdominal leak point pressure	腹圧下尿漏出圧
ALS	advanced life support	二次救命処置
ALS	amyotrophic lateral sclerosis	筋萎縮性側索硬化症
ALS	artificial liver support	人工肝補助療法
ALT	alanine aminotransferase	アラニンアミノトランスフェラーゼ
ALTA	aluminum potassium sulfate-tannnic acid	硫酸アルミニウムカリウム・タンニン酸
ALTE	apparent life-threatening event	乳幼児突発性危急事態
Am	americium	アメリシウム
a.m.	ante meridiem	午前
AMA	against medical advice	医療指示拒否
AMA	American Medical Association	米国医師会
AMA	antimitochondrial antibody	抗ミトコンドリア抗体
AMC	arthrogryposis multiplex congenita	先天性多発性関節拘縮症
AMD	age-related macular degeneration	加齢黄斑変性
AMI	acute myocardial infarction	急性心筋梗塞
AMK	amikacin	アミカシン
AML	acute myelogenous leukemia	急性骨髄性白血病
AMLR	autologous mixed lymphocyte reaction	自己由来混合リンパ球反応
AMMoL	acute myelomonocytic leukemia	急性骨髄単球性白血病
AMP	adenosine monophosphate	アデノシン一リン酸
amp.	ampulla	アンプル
AMPC	amoxicillin	アモキシシリン
AMPC/CVA	amoxicillin/clavulanic acid	アモキシシリン・クラブラン酸
AMPH	amphotericin B	アンホテリシン
AMR	amrubicin	アムルビシン
AMR	antibody-mediated rejection	抗体関連型拒絶反応

AN	acanthosis nigricans	黒色表皮腫
AN	anorexia nervosa	神経性食欲不振症
ANA	American Nurses Association	米国看護協会
ANA	anastrozole	アナストロゾール
ANA	antinuclear antibody	抗核抗体
ANCA	anti-neutrophil cytoplasmic antibody	抗好中球細胞質抗体
ANCOVA	analysis of covariance	共分散分析
ANF	antinuclear factor	抗核因子
ANLL	acute nonlymphocytic leukemia	急性非リンパ性白血病
ANOVA	analysis of variance	分散分析
ANP	acute necrotizing pancreatitis	急性壊死性膵炎
ANP	atrial natriuretic peptide	心房性ナトリウム利尿ペプチド
ANS	autonomic nervous system	自律神経系
ANUG	acute necrotizing ulcerative gingivitis	急性壊死性潰瘍性歯肉炎
AO	absorption ointment	吸水軟膏
AODM	adult-onset diabetes mellitus	成人発症型糖尿病
AOM	acute otitis media	急性中耳炎
AOSC	acute obstructive suppurative cholangitis	急性閉塞性化膿性胆管炎
AP	Adriamycin, cisplatin	アドリアマイシン（ドキソルビシン），シスプラチン（化学療法）
AP	angina pectoris	狭心症
AP	anteroposterior	前後
APA	aldosterone-producing adenoma	アルドステロン産生腺腫
APACHE	acute physiology and chronic health evaluation	急性生理慢性健康評価
APC	activated protein C	活性化プロテインC
APC	antigen-presenting cell	抗原提示細胞
APC	atrial premature complex (contraction)	心房性期外収縮
APD	automated peritoneal dialysis	自動腹膜透析
APDL	activities parallel to daily living	日常生活関連動作
APL	acute promyelocytic leukemia	急性前骨髄球性白血病
APMPPE	acute posterior multifocal placoid pigment epitheliopathy	急性後部多発性斑状色素上皮症
Apo	apolipoprotein	アポリボタンパク質
APP	amyloid precursor protein	アミロイド前駆体タンパク

		質
APR	acute phase reactant	急性相反応物質
APS	antiphospholipid antibody syndrome	抗リン脂質抗体症候群
APSGN	acute poststreptococcal glomerulonephritis	連鎖球菌感染後急性糸球体腎炎
APTT	activated partial thromboplastin time	活性化部分トロンボプラスチン時間
APUD	amine precursor uptake and decarboxylation (cell)	アプド（細胞）
aq.	aqua	水
AQP	aquaporin	水チャネル
AR	aortic regurgitation	大動脈弁逆流
Ar	argon	アルゴン
ARA	American Rheumatism Association	米国リウマチ協会
Ara-A	adenine arabinoside, vidarabine	ビダラビン
Ara-C	arabinosylcytosine, cytarabine	シタラビン
ARAS	ascending reticular activating system	上行性網様体賦活系
ARB	angiotensin II type I receptor blocker	I型アンギオテンシンII受容体拮抗薬
ARC	AIDS-related complex	エイズ関連症候群
ARC	anomalous retinal correspondence	網膜異常対応
ARDS	acute respiratory distress syndrome	急性呼吸促迫症候群
ARF	acute renal failure	急性腎不全
ARF	acute respiratory failure	急性呼吸不全
ARG	autoradiography	オートラジオグラフィー
ARMD	age-related macular degeneration	加齢黄斑変性
ARN	acute retinal necrosis	急性網膜壊死
ARPKD	autosomal recessive polycystic kidney disease	常染色体劣性多発囊胞腎症
ARR	aldosterone to renin activity ratio	アルドステロン・レニン活性比
ART	assisted reproductive technology	生殖補助医療
ARVD	arrhythmogenic right ventricular dysplasia	不整脈原性右室異形成
AS	acoustic shadow	音響陰影
AS	ankylosing spondylitis	強直性脊椎炎

X章 略語集

AS	aortic stenosis	大動脈弁狭窄
AS	auris sinistra	左耳
As	arsenic	ヒ素
ASA	acetylsalicylic acid	アセチルサリチル酸
ASC	anterior subcapsular cataract	前嚢下白内障
ASCO	American Society of Clinical Oncology	米国臨床腫瘍学会
ASCT	autologous stem cell transplantation	自己幹細胞移植
ASCVD	arteriosclerotic cardiovascular disease	動脈硬化性心血管疾患
ASD	atrial septal defect	心房中隔欠損
ASH	ankylosing spinal hyperostosis	強直性脊椎骨増殖症
ASHD	arteriosclerotic heart disease	動脈硬化性心疾患
ASK	antistreptokinase	抗ストレプトキナーゼ
ASLO, ASO	antistreptolysin O	抗ストレプトリジン O
ASMA	anti-smooth muscle antibody	抗平滑筋抗体
ASO	arteriosclerosis obliterans	閉塞性動脈硬化症
ASPC	aspoxicillin	アスポキシシリン
ASPD	anterior superior pancreaticoduodenal artery	前上膵十二指腸動脈
ASPD	antisocial personality disorder	反社会的人格障害
AST	aspartate aminotransferase	アスパラギン酸アミノトランスフェラーゼ
ASTM	astromicin	アストロマイシン
AT	Adriamycin, Taxotere	アドリアマイシン（ドキソルビシン），タキソテール（ドセタキセル）（化学療法）
AT	anaerobic threshold	無酸素閾値
AT	autogenic training	自律訓練法
At	astatine	アスタチン
AT-III	antithrombin III	アンチトロンビンIII
ATG	antithymocyte globulin	抗胸腺細胞グロブリン
ATL	adult T-cell leukemia	成人 T 細胞白血病
ATLL	adult T-cell leukemia/lymphoma	成人 T 細胞白血病リンパ腫
ATLV	adult T-cell leukemia virus	成人 T 細胞白血病ウイルス
ATN	acute tubular necrosis	急性尿細管壊死
ATNR	asymmetrical tonic neck reflex	非対称性緊張性頚反射
ATP	adenosine triphosphate	アデノシン三リン酸
ATP	atypical epithelium	異型上皮
ATR	Achilles tendon reflex	アキレス腱反射

ATRA	all-*trans*-retinoic acid, tretinoin	トレチノイン
ATTR	amyloidogenic transthyretin	アミロイド原性トランスサイレチン
ATV	atazanavir sulfate	アタザナビル硫酸塩
AU	aures unitas	両耳
AU	auris utreque	各耳
Au	aurum gold	金
AUC	area under the curve	血中濃度曲線下面積
AV	arteriovenous	動静脈の
AV	atrioventricular	房室の，房室間の
AVA	arteriovenous anastomosis	動静脈吻合
AVM	arteriovenous malformation	動静脈奇形
AVN	atrioventricular node	房室結節
AVNRT	atrioventricular nodal reentrant tachycardia	房室結節リエントリー頻拍
AVP	arginine vasopressin	アルギニンバゾプレシン
AVR	aortic valve replacement	大動脈弁置換術
AVRT	atrioventricular reciprocating tachycardia	房室回帰頻拍
AZM	azithromycin	アジスロマイシン
AZP	azathioprine	アザチオプリン
AZT	azidothymidine, zidovudine	アジドチミジン，ジドブジン
AZT	aztreonam	アズトレオナム

B

B	boron	ホウ素
BⅠ(Ⅱ)	Billroth Ⅰ (Ⅱ)	ビルロートⅠ法（Ⅱ法）
Ba	barium	バリウム
BA	basilar artery	脳底動脈
BA	bronchial asthma	気管支喘息
BAC	bronchioloalveolar cell carcinoma	細気管支肺胞上皮癌
BACOP	bleomycin, Adriamycin, cyclophosphamide, Oncovin, prednisolone	ブレオマイシン，アドリアマイシン（ドキソルビシン），シクロフォスファミド，オンコビン（ビンクリスチン），プレドニゾロン（化学療法）
BAE	bronchial arterial embolization	気管支動脈塞栓術
BAEP	brainstem auditory evoked potential	聴性脳幹反応
BAG	bronchial arteriography	気管支動脈造影法
BAI	bronchial arterial infusion	気管支動脈注入

BAL	bronchoalveolar lavage	気管支肺胞洗浄
BALF	bronchoalveolar lavage fluid	気管支肺胞洗浄液
BALT	bronchus-associated lymphoid tissue	気道系リンパ組織
BAO	basal acid output	基礎酸分泌量
BAPC	bacampicillin	バカンピシリン
BAR	BUdR-antimetabolie-continuous intraarterial infusion-radiation (therapy)	バー（療法）
BAS	balloon atrial septostomy	バルーン心房中隔裂開
BBB	blood-brain barrier	血液脳関門
BBB	bundle branch block	脚ブロック
BBBB	bilateral bundle branch block	両脚ブロック
BBT	basal body temperature	基礎体温
BC	bacitracin	バシトラシン
BC	bone conduction	骨伝導
BCAA	branched-chain amino acid	分枝鎖アミノ酸
BCC	basal cell carcinoma	基底細胞癌
BCG	bacille Calmette-Guérin	カルメット・ゲラン結核菌
BCG	ballistocardiogram	心弾動図
BCKA	branched-chain ketoacid	分枝鎖ケト酸
BCNU	1,3-bis(2-chloroethyl)-1-nitrosourea, carmustine	クロロエチルニトロソウレア，カルムスチン
BCOPS	board certified oncology pharmacy specialist	がん専門薬剤師
BCP	basic calcium phosphate	塩基性リン酸カルシウム
BCPOP	board certified pharmacist in oncology pharmacy	がん薬物療法認定薬剤師
BCR	biological clean room, bioclean room	無菌室
BCR	bulbocavernosus reflex	球海綿体反射
BDNF	brain-derived neurotrophic factor	脳由来神経栄養因子
BDP	beclomethasone dipropionate	ベクロメタゾンプロピオン酸エステル
BE	barium enema	バリウム注腸造影
BE	base excess	塩基過剰
Be	beryllium	ベリリウム
B-E	below-elbow (amputation)	前腕（切断術）
BECCT	benign epilepsy of childhood with centrotemporal spikes	中心・側頭部棘波をもつ良性小児てんかん
BEE	basal energy expenditure	基礎エネルギー消費量
BEIS	balloon-expandable intravascular stent	バルーン拡張式血管内ステント

BEMP	bleomycin, Endoxan, 6-mercaptopurine, prednisolone	ブレオマイシン，シクロホスファミド，6-メルカプトプリン，プレドニゾロン（化学療法）
BEP	bleomycin, etoposide, cisplatin	ブレオマイシン，エトポシド，シスプラチン（化学療法）
β_2-MG	β_2-microglobulin	β_2 ミクログロブリン
BF	biofeedback	バイオフィードバック
bFGF	basic fibroblast growth factor	塩基性線維芽細胞増殖因子
BFP	basic fetoprotein	塩基性胎児タンパク
BFP	biological false positive	生物学的偽陽性
BFU-E	burst-forming unit-erythroid	赤芽球バースト形成細胞
Bh	bohrium	ボーリウム
BH-AC	N-behenoyl-1-β-arabino-furanosyl-cytosine, enocitabine	エノシタビン
BH-ACDMP	enocitabine, daunorubicin, 6-mercaptopurien, predonisolone	エノシタビン，ダウノルビシン，6メルカプトプリン，プレドニゾロン（化学療法）
BHC	benzene hexachloride	ベンゼンヘキサクロリド
BHL	bilateral hilar lymphadenopathy	両側肺門リンパ節腫大
BI	Barthel index	バーセル指数
BI	Brinkman index	ブリンクマン指数
Bi	bismuth	ビスマス
b.i.d.	bis in die	1日2回
BIH	benign intracranial hypertension	良性頭蓋内圧亢進症
BiPAP	biphasic positive airway pressure	二相性陽性気道内圧
BIPM	biapenem	ビアペネム
BJP	Bence Jones protein	ベンスジョーンズタンパク質
Bk	berkelium	バークリウム
B-K	below-knee (amputation)	下腿（切断術）
BLM	bleomycin	ブレオマイシン
BLS	basic life support	一次救命処置
BM	bone marrow	骨髄
BM	bowel movement	便通
BMA	British Medical Association	英国医師会
BMD	bone mineral density	骨密度
BMG	benign monoclonal gammopathy	良性単クローン性免疫グロブリン症

BMI	body mass index	肥満指数
BMP	bone morphogenetic protein	骨形成因子
BMR	basal metabolic rate	基礎代謝率
BMT	bone marrow transplantation	骨髄移植
BNP	brain natriuretic peptide	脳性ナトリウム利尿ペプチド
BOA	behavioral observation audiometry	行動観察聴力検査
BOD	biochemical oxygen demand	生化学的酸素要求量
BOF	blow-out fracture	吹き抜け骨折
BOO	bladder outlet obstruction	膀胱下閉塞
BOOP	bronchiolitis obliterans with organizing pneumonia	器質化肺炎を伴う閉塞性細気管支炎
BOPP	bleomycin, Oncovin, procarbazine, prednisolone	ブレオマイシン,オンコビン(ビンクリスチン)プロカルバジン,プレドニゾロン(化学療法)
BOT	basal supported oral therapy	経口血糖降下剤と基礎インスリン注射併用
bp	base pair	塩基対
BP	bisphosphonate	ビスホスフォネート
BP	blood pressure	血圧
BP	bullous pemphigoid	水疱性類天疱瘡
BPD	biparietal diameter	大横径
BPD	borderline personality disorder	境界性人格障害
BPD	bronchopulmonary dysplasia	気管支肺異形成症
BPH	benign prostatic hypertrophy	良性前立腺肥大
BPN	brachial plexus neuropathy	腕神経叢障害
BPPV	benign paroxysmal positional vertigo	良性発作性頭位性めまい
BPS	biophysical profile score	胎児機能評価
BPSD	behavioral and psychological symptoms of dementia	認知症の行動・心理症状
Bq	becquerel	ベクレル
Br	bromine	臭素
BRAO	branch retinal artery occlusion	網膜動脈分枝閉塞症
BRCA1	breast cancer 1 (gene)	BRCA1遺伝子
BRCA2	breast cancer 2 (gene)	BRCA2遺伝子
BRM	biological response modifier	生体応答調節剤
BRP	bathroom privileges	トイレ許可
BRTO	balloon-occluded retrograde transvenous obliteration	バルーン閉塞下逆行性経静脈的塞栓術
BRVO	branch retinal vein occlusion	網膜静脈分枝閉塞症
BS	Bachelor of Science	理学士

BS	bowel sounds	腸雑音
BS	breath sounds	呼吸音
BSA	body surface area	体表面積
BSE	bovine spongiform encephalopathy	ウシ海綿状脳症
BSE	breast self-examination	乳房自己検診
BSL	bedside learning	臨床学習
BSR	blood sedimentation rate	赤血球沈降速度
BST	ubenimex, Bestatin	ウベニメクス（ベスタチン）
BT	bladder tumor	膀胱腫瘍
BT	bleeding time	出血時間
BT	body temperature	体温
BT	brain tumor	脳腫瘍
BT-PABA	N-benzoyl-L-tyrosyl-paraaminobenzoic acid	ベンゾイルチロシルパラアミノ安息香酸
BUD	budesonide	ブデソニド
BUdR	5-bromouridine-2'-deoxyrebose	5-ブロモウリジン-2'-デオキシリボース
BUN	blood urea nitrogen	血液尿素窒素
BUS	busulfan	ブスルファン
BUT	tear film breakup time	涙液層破壊時間
BV	binocular vision	両眼視
BV	blood volume	血液量
BVAD	biventricular assist device	両心室補助装置
BW	body weight	体重

C

C	carbon	炭素
C	cervical vertebra	頚椎
C	complement	補体
C	coulomb	クーロン
C	cytosine	シトシン
c̄	cum	と共に
°C	degree Celsius	摂氏
CA	cardiac arrest	心停止
CA	celiac artery	腹腔動脈
CA	cystic artery	胆嚢動脈
Ca	calcium	カルシウム
Ca	carcinoma, cancer	癌
ca.	circa	およそ
CA125	carbohydrate antigen 125	糖鎖抗原125
CA19-9	carbohydrate antigen 19-9	糖鎖抗原19-9
CAA	cerebral amyloid angiopathy	脳アミロイド血管症

CABG	coronary artery bypass graft	冠動脈バイパス移植片
CAD	cold agglutinin disease	寒冷凝集素症
CAD	coronary artery disease	冠動脈疾患
CAF	cyclophosphamide, Adriamycin, 5-fluorouracil	シクロホスファミド，アドリアマイシン（ドキソルビシン），フルオロウラシル（化学療法）
CAG	carotid angiography	頸動脈造影法
CAG	coronary angiography	冠血管造影法
CAH	chronic active hepatitis	慢性活動性肝炎
CAH	congenital adrenal hyperplasia	先天性副腎過形成
CAHS	central alveolar hypoventilation syndrome	中枢性肺胞低換気症候群
CAL	coracoacromial ligament	烏口肩峰靱帯
cal	calorie	カロリー
CALLA	common acute lymphoblastic leukemia antigen	急性リンパ芽球性白血病共通抗原
CAM	chorioamnionitis	絨毛膜羊膜炎
CAM	clarithromycin	クラリスロマイシン
CAM	complementary and alternative medicine	補完代替医療
cAMP	cyclic adenosine monophosphate	サイクリックアデノシン一リン酸
CAP	central arterial pressure of retina	網膜中心動脈圧
CAP	cyclophosphamide, Adriamycin, cisplatin	シクロホスファミド，アドリアマイシン（ドキソルビシン），シスプラチン（化学療法）
cap.	capsula	カプセル
CAPD	continuous ambulatory peritoneal dialysis	連続携行式腹膜透析
CAS	carotid artery stenting	頸動脈ステント留置術
CAT	choline acetyltransferase	コリンアセチルトランスフェラーゼ
CAT	computerized axial tomography	コンピュータ断層撮影
CAV	cyclophosphamide, Adriamycin, vincristine	シクロホスファミド，アドリアマイシン（ドキソルビシン），ビンクリスチン（化学療法）
CAVH	continuous arteriovenous hemofiltration	持続性動静脈血液濾過
CAVI	cardio-ankle vascular index	心臓足首血管指数

CAZ	ceftazidime	セフタジジム
CBA	congenital biliary atresia	先天性胆道閉鎖症
CBC	complete blood cell count	全血球計算
CBD	common bile duct	総胆管
CBDCA	carboplatin	カルボプラチン
CBF	cerebral blood flow	脳血流量
CBG	corticosteroid-binding globulin	コルチコステロイド結合グロブリン
CBPZ	cefbuperazone	セフブペラゾン
CBSCT	cord blood stem cell transplantation	臍帯血幹細胞移植
CBT	cognitive behavioral therapy	認知行動療法
CBT	computer-based testing	コンピュータ処理多岐選択試験
CBZ	carbamazepine	カルバマゼピン
CC	chief complaint	主訴
cc	cubic centimeter	立方センチメートル
CCA	common carotid artery	総頚動脈
CCAM	congenital cystic adenomatoid malformation of lung	先天性肺嚢胞性腺腫様奇形
CCB	calcium channel blocker	カルシウムチャネル遮断薬
CCC	cholangiocellular carcinoma	胆管細胞癌
CCD	charge-coupled device	電荷結合素子
CCF	carotid cavernous fistula	内頚動脈海綿静脈洞瘻
CCK	cholecystokinin	コレシストキニン
CCL	cefaclor	セファクロル
CCL	coracoclavicular ligament	烏口鎖骨靱帯
CCM	congestive cardiomyopathy	うっ血型心筋症
CCP	complement control protein	補体調節タンパク質
CCP	cyclic citrulinated peptide	環状シトルリン化ペプチド
CCPD	continuous cyclic peritoneal dialysis	連続サイクル式腹膜透析
Ccr	creatinine clearance	クレアチニンクリアランス
CCU	coronary care unit	冠疾患集中治療室
CCW	counterclockwise rotation	反時計方向回転
CD	choroidal detachment	脈絡膜剥離
CD	cluster of differentiation	CD 分類，分化抗原群
CD	contact dermatitis	接触皮膚炎
CD	Crohn disease	クローン病
CD	curative dose	治癒量
Cd	cadmium	カドミウム
cd	candela	カンデラ
C/D	cup-disk ratio	陥凹乳頭比

X章 略語集

CDA	congenital dyserythropoietic anemia	先天性赤血球生成不全性貧血
CDC	Centers for Disease Control and Prevention	米国疾病対策センター
CDCA	chenodeoxycholic acid	ケノデオキシコール酸
CDDP	*cis*-diamminedichloroplatinum, cisplatin	シスジアミンジクロロプラチナム，シスプラチン
CDGP	*cis*-diammineglycolatoplatinum, nedaplatin	シスジアミングリコレートプラチナム，ネダプラチン
CDH	congenital diaphragmatic hernia	先天性横隔膜ヘルニア
CDH	congenital dislocation of the hip	先天性股関節脱臼
cDNA	complementary DNA	相補 DNA
CDP	cytidine diphosphate	シチジンニリン酸
CDR	clinical dementia rating	臨床的認知症尺度
CDR	complementarity-determining region	相補性決定領域
CDTR-PI	cefditoren pivoxil	セフジトレンピボキシル
CDX	cefadroxil	セファドロキシル
Cdyn	dynamic lung compliance	動肺コンプライアンス
CDZM	cefodizime	セフォジジム
CE	contrast enhancement	造影剤増強
Ce	cerium	セリウム
CEA	carcinoembryonic antigen	癌胎児性抗原
CEA	carotid endarterectomy	頸動脈内膜切除術
CEF	cyclophosphamide, epirubicin, 5-fluorouracil	シクロホスファミド，エピルビシン，フルオロウラシル（化学療法）
CEP	chronic eosinophilic pneumonia	慢性好酸球性肺炎
CEP	congenital erythopoietic porphyria	先天性赤芽球性ポルフィリン症
CET	cephalothin	セファロチン
CETB	ceftibuten	セフチブテン
CETP	cholesterol ester transfer protein	コレステロールエステル転送タンパク質
CEX	cephalexin	セファレキシン
CEZ	cefazolin	セファゾリン
CF	complement fixation	補体結合反応
CF	counting fingers	指数弁
CF	cystic fibrosis	囊胞性線維症
Cf	californium	カリホルニウム
cf.	confero	参照せよ
CFA	complement-fixing antibody	補体結合抗体

CFAP	chronic functional abdominal pain	慢性機能性腹痛
CFDN	cefdinir	セフジニル
CFF	critical flicker frequency	限界フリッカー値
CFIX	cefixime	セフィキシム
CFPM	cefepime	セフェピム
CFPN-PI	cefcapene pivoxil	セフカペンピボキシル
CFS	cefsulodin	セフスロジン
CFS	chronic fatigue syndrome	慢性疲労症候群
CFT	cefatrizine	セファトリジン
CFT	complement fixation test	補体結合反応
CFTM-PI	cefteram pivoxil	セフテラムピボキシル
CFU	colony-forming unit	コロニー形成単位
CGA	comprehensive geriatric assessment	高齢者総合機能評価
CGD	chronic granulomatous disease	慢性肉芽腫病
CGH	comparative genomic hybridization	比較ゲノムハイブリダイゼーション
cGMP	cyclic guanosine monophosphate	サイクリックグアノシン一リン酸
CGN	chronic glomerulonephritis	慢性糸球体腎炎
CGRP	calcitonin gene-related peptide	カルシトニン遺伝子関連ペプチド
CH_{50}	50% hemolytic unit of complement	補体価（補体50％溶血単位）
CHA	common hepatic artery	総肝動脈
CHAI	continuous hepatic arterial infusion	肝動脈持続動注療法
CHARGE	coloboma, heart defects, atresia choanae, retarded growth and development, genital hypoplasia, ear anomalies (association)	チャージ（連合）
CHD	childhood disease	小児期疾患
CHD	congenital heart disease	先天性心疾患
CHD	coronary heart disease	冠動脈性心疾患
CHDF	continuous hemodiafiltration	持続性血液濾過透析
ChE	cholinesterase	コリンエステラーゼ
CHF	congestive heart failure	うっ血性心不全
CHF	continuous hemofiltration	持続性血液濾過
CHO	carbohydrate	炭水化物
CHOP	cyclophosphamide, hydroxydaunorubicin, Oncovin, prednisolone	シクロフォスファミド，塩酸ダウノルビシン（ドキソルビシン），オンコビン

		(ビンクリスチン), プレドニゾロン (化学療法)
CI	cardiac index	心係数
CI	cerebral infarction	脳梗塞
Ci	curie	キュリー
CIA	common iliac artery	総腸骨動脈
CIC	circulating immune complex	循環免疫複合体
CIC	clean intermittent catheterization	清潔間欠導尿
CIDP	chronic inflammatory demyelinating polyneuropathy	慢性炎症性脱髄性多発ニューロパチー
CIEP	counterimmunoelectrophoresis	対向流免疫電気泳動法
CIN	cervical intraepithelial neoplasia	子宮頚部上皮内腫瘍
CIN	chronic interstitial nephritis	慢性間質性腎炎
CINX	cinoxacin	シノキサシン
CIS	carcinoma in situ	上皮内癌
CISC	clean intermittent self-catheterization	清潔間欠自己導尿
CJD	Creutzfeldt-Jakob disease	クロイツフェルト・ヤコブ病
CK	clinical knowledge	臨床知識
CK	creatine kinase	クレアチンキナーゼ
CK-BB	creatine kinase isoenzyme BB	クレアチンキナーゼアイソザイム BB
CKD	chronic kidney disease	慢性腎臓病
CK-MB	creatine kinase isoenzyme MB	クレアチンキナーゼアイソザイム MB
CK-MM	creatine kinase isoenzyme MM	クレアチンキナーゼアイソザイム MM
CL	colistin	コリスチン
CL	contact lens	コンタクトレンズ
Cl	chlorine	塩素
CLBBB	complete left bundle branch block	完全左脚ブロック
CLDM	clindamycin	クリンダマイシン
CLE	cutaneous lupus erythematosus	皮膚エリテマトーデス
CLEIA	chemiluminescent enzyme immunoassay	化学発光酵素免疫測定法
CLIA	chemiluminescent immunoassay	化学発光免疫測定法
CLIP	corticotropin-like intermediate lobe peptide	コルチコトロピン様中葉ペプチド

CLL	chronic lymphocytic leukemia	慢性リンパ性白血病
CM	carpometacarpal (joint)	手根中手（関節）
CM	cervical mucus	頚管粘液
Cm	curium	キュリウム
cM	centimorgan	センチモルガン
cm	centimeter	センチメートル
CMAP	compound muscle action potential	複合筋活動電位
CMD	congenital muscular dystrophy	先天性筋ジストロフィー
CME	continuing medical education	医学生涯教育
CME	cystoid macular edema	囊胞様黄斑浮腫
CMF	cyclophosphamide, methotrexate, 5-fluorouracil	シクロホスファミド，メトトレキセート，フルオロウラシル（化学療法）
CMG	continuous glucose monitoring	持続血糖測定
CMI	cell-mediated immunity	細胞性免疫
CMI	Cornell Medical Index	コーネル医学指数
CMML	chronic myelomonocytic leukemia	慢性骨髄単球性白血病
CML	chronic myelogenous leukemia	慢性骨髄性白血病
CMNX	cefminox	セフミノクス
C-MOPP	cyclophosphamide, Oncovin, procarbazine, prednisolone	シクロホスファミド，オンコビン（ビンクリスチン），プロカルバジン，プレドニゾロン（化学療法）
CMP	cardiomyopathy	心筋症
CMP	cytidine monophosphate	シチジン一リン酸，シチジル酸
CMPD	chronic myeloproliferative disorders	慢性骨髄増殖性疾患
CMRO$_2$	cerebral metabolic rate of oxygen	脳酸素代謝率
CMS	Centers for Medicare and Medicaid Services	メディケア・メディケイドセンター（米国）
CMT	Charcot-Marie-Tooth disease	シャルコー・マリー・トゥース病
CMV	controlled mechanical ventilation	調節呼吸
CMV	cytomegalovirus	サイトメガロウイルス
CMX	cefmenoxime	セフメノキシム
CMZ	cefmetazole	セフメタゾール
CN	Certified Nurse	認定看護師
CN	cranial nerve	脳神経
Cn	copernicium	コペルニシウム

X章

CNL	chronic neutrophilic leukemia	慢性好中球性白血病
CNS	central nervous system	中枢神経系
CNS	Certified Nurse Specialist	専門看護師
CNS	coagulase-negative staphylococci	コアグラーゼ陰性ブドウ球菌
CNSDC	chronic nonsuppurative destructive cholangitis	慢性非化膿性破壊性胆管炎
CNV	choroidal neovascularization	脈絡膜新生血管
CO	carbon monoxide	一酸化炭素
CO	cardiac output	心拍出量
Co	cobalt	コバルト
COC	calcifying odontogenic cyst	石灰化歯原性嚢胞
COMT	catechol O-methyltransferase	カテコール・O メチル転移酵素
COP	colloid osmotic pressure	膠質浸透圧
COP	cryptogenic organizing pneumonitis	特発性器質化肺炎
COPD	chronic obstructive pulmonary disease	慢性閉塞性肺疾患
COPP	cyclophosphamide, Oncovin, procarbazine, prednisolone	シクロホスファミド，オンコビン（ビンクリスチン），プロカルバジン，プレドニゾロン（化学療法）
COX	cyclooxygenase	シクロオキシゲナーゼ
CP	cerebral palsy	脳性麻痺
CP	chloramphenicol	クロラムフェニコール
CP	clinical pathway	クリニカルパス
CP	cor pulmonale	肺性心
CPA	cardiopulmonary arrest	心肺停止
CPA	cyclophosphamide	シクロホスファミド
CPAOA	cardiopulmonary arrest on arrival	来院時心肺停止
CPAP	continuous positive airway pressure	持続気道陽圧呼吸
CPB	cardiopulmonary bypass	人工心肺
CPBA	competitive protein binding analysis	競合的タンパク結合分析法
CPC	clinical-pathological conference	臨床病理検討会
CPD	cephalopelvic disproportion	児頭骨盤不均衡
CPDX-PR	cefpodoxime proxetil	セフポドキシムプロキセチル
CPE	cytopathic effect	細胞変性効果
CPEO	chronic progressive external ophthalmoplegia	慢性進行性外眼筋麻痺

CPFX	ciprofloxacin	シプロフロキサシン
CPIP	chronic pulmonary insufficiency of prematurity	未熟児慢性呼吸不全
CPK	creatine phosphokinase	クレアチンリン酸酵素
CPM	cefpiramide	セフピラミド
CPM	central pontine myelinolysis	橋中心髄鞘崩壊症
CPM	cisplatin, pepleomycin, mitomycin-C	シスプラチン，ペプレオマイシン，マイトマイシンC（化学療法）
CPM	continuous passive motion	持続的他動運動
CPP	cerebral perfusion pressure	脳灌流圧
CPPB	continuous positive pressure breathing	持続陽圧呼吸
CPPD	calcium pyrophosphate dihydrate	ピロリン酸カルシウム
CPPV	continuous positive pressure ventilation	持続陽圧換気
CPR	cardiopulmonary resuscitation	心肺蘇生法
CPR	cefpirome	セフピロム
CPR	C-peptide immunoreactivity	免疫反応性Cペプチド
CPS	complex partial seizure	複雑部分発作
CPT-11	irinotecan	イリノテカン
CPZ	cefoperazone	セフォペラゾン
CR	complement receptor	補体受容体
CR	complete remission	完全寛解
Cr	chromium	クロム
Cr	creatinine	クレアチニン
CRA	central retinal artery	網膜中心動脈
CRAO	central retinal artery occlusion	網膜中心動脈閉塞症
CRBBB	complete right bundle branch block	完全右脚ブロック
CRBSI	catheter-related blood stream infection	カテーテル関連血流感染
CRC	clinical research coordinator	治験コーディネーター
CRC	concentrated red blood cells	濃厚赤血球
CREST	calcinosis cutis, Raynaud phenomenon, esophageal dysfunction, sclerodactyly, telangiectasia (syndrome)	クレスト（症候群）
CRF	chronic renal failure	慢性腎不全
CRH	corticotropin-releasing hormone	コルチコトロピン放出ホルモン
CRL	crown-rump length	頭殿長
CRMN	carumonam	カルモナム

CRP	C-reactive protein	C反応性タンパク
CRPS	complex regional pain sndrome	複合性局所疼痛症候群
CRS	congenital rubella syndrome	先天性風疹症候群
CRT	cardiac resynchronization therapy	心臓再同期療法
CRVO	central retinal vein occlusion	網膜中心静脈閉塞症
CS	cesarean section	帝王切開
CS	clinical skills	臨床技能
CS	coronary sinus	冠状静脈洞
CS	cycloserine	サイクロセリン
Cs	cesium	セシウム
C&S	culture and sensitivity	培養と感受性試験
CSCR	central serous chorioretinopathy	中心性漿液性脈絡網膜症
CsA	cyclosporin A	シクロスポリンA
CSF	cerebrospinal fluid	脳脊髄液
CSF	colony-stimulating factor	コロニー刺激因子
CSII	continuous subcutaneous insulin infusion	持続インスリン皮下注入療法
CSM	cervical spondylotic myelopathy	頚椎症性脊髄症
CSR	central supply room	中央材料室
CSR	cervical spondylotic radiculopathy	頚椎症性神経根症
CSSD	central sterile supply department	中央滅菌材料部門
CST	contraction stress test	収縮ストレステスト
CT	calcitonin	カルシトニン
CT	computed tomography	コンピュータ断層撮影法
CT	cover test	遮閉試験
CTA	CT angiography	CT血管造影法
CTCAE	Common Terminology Criteria for Adverse Events	有害事象共通用語基準
CTCL	cutaneous T-cell lymphoma	皮膚T細胞性リンパ腫
CTEPH	chronic thromboembolic pulmonary hypertension	慢性血栓塞栓性肺高血圧症
CTG	cardiotocography	胎児心拍陣痛図
CTL	cytotoxic T-lymphocyte	細胞傷害性Tリンパ球
CTM	cefotiam	セフォチアム
CTM-HE	cefotiam hexetil	セフォチアムヘキセチル
cTnI	cardiac troponin I	心筋トロポニンI
cTnT	cardiac troponin T	心筋トロポニンT
CTR	cardiothoracic ratio	心胸郭比
CTRX	ceftriaxone	セフトリアキソン

CTS	carpal tunnel syndrome	手根管症候群
CTX	cefotaxime	セフォタキシム
CTZ	chemoreceptor trigger zone	化学受容体ひきがね帯
Cu	cuprum, copper	銅
CUA	calcific uremic arteriolopathy	石灰化尿毒症性細動脈症
CUSA	Cavitron Ultrasonic Surgical Aspirator	キャビトロン超音波外科用吸収器
CUT	cover-uncover test	遮閉 – 遮閉除去試験
CV	curriculum vitae	履歴書
CVA	cerebral vascular accident	脳血管障害
CVA	costovertebral angle	肋骨脊柱角
CVD	cardiovascular disease	心血管疾患
CVD	cerebrovascular disease	脳血管疾患
CVD	combined valvular disease	連合弁膜症
CVID	common variable immuno-deficiency	分類不能型免疫不全症
CVP	central venous pressure	中心静脈圧
CVR	cerebral vascular resistance	脳血管抵抗
CVS	chorionic villi sampling	絨毛生検
CVVH	continuous venovenous hemofiltration	持続性静脈静脈血液濾過
CWP	cotton-wool patches	綿花様白斑
CWR	clockwise rotation	時計方向回転
CXD	cefroxadine	セフロキサジン
CXM-AX	cefuroxime axetil	セフロキシムアキセチル
CXR	chest x-ray, chest radiograph	胸部 X 線写真
CYA	cyclosporin A, cyclosporine	シクロスポリン A
CYFRA	cytokeratin 19 fragment	サイトケラチン19フラグメント
CZOP	cefozopran	セフォゾプラン
CZP	clonazepam	クロナゼパム
CZX	ceftizoxime	セフチゾキシム

D

D	decimal reduction time	死滅速度恒数
D	deuterium	重水素
D	diopter	ジオプトリー
DA	degenerative arthritis	変形性関節症
DA	dopamine	ドーパミン
Da	dalton	ダルトン
DAC	decitabine	デシタビン
DAC	docetaxel, doxorubicin, cyclophosphamide	ドセタキセル, ドキソルビシン, シクロホスファミド (化学療法)

DAD	diffuse alveolar damage	びまん性肺胞傷害
DALY	disability-adjusted life year	障害調整生存年
DASH	Dietary Approaches to Stop Hypertension	降圧食事療法（米国）
DAT	dementia of the Alzheimer type	アルツハイマー型認知症
DAT	direct antiglobulin test	直接抗グロブリン試験
Db	dubnium	ドブニウム
dB	decibel	デシベル
DBECPCG	benzylpenicillin benzathine	ベンジルペニシリンベンザチン
DBP	diastolic blood pressure	拡張期血圧
DBS	deep brain stimulation	深部脳刺激法
DC	direct current	直流
DC	discontinue	中止
DC	docetaxel, cisplatin	ドセタキセル，シスプラチン（化学療法）
D&C	dilatation and curettage	（子宮）頚管拡張術および掻爬術
DCA	directional coronary atherectomy	方向性冠動脈粥腫切除術
DCF	pentostatin	ペントスタチン
DCF	docetaxel, cisplatin, 5-fluorouracil	ドセタキセル，シスプラチン，フルオロウラシル（化学療法）
DCH	delayed cutaneous hypersensitivity	遅延型皮膚過敏症
DCIS	ductal carcinoma in situ	非浸潤性乳管癌
DCM	dilated cardiomyopathy	拡張型心筋症
DCP	des-γ-carboxy prothrombin	デスγカルボキシプロトロンビン
DCR	dacryocystorhinostomy	涙嚢鼻腔吻合術
3D-CRT	three-dimensional conformal radiotherapy	三次元原体放射線治療
DCT	direct Coombs test	直接クームス試験
DD	differential diagnosis	鑑別診断
DDAVP	1-deamino-8-D-arginine vasopressin	デスモプレシン酢酸塩
ddC	dideoxycytidine, zalcitabine	ジデオキシシチジン，ザルシタビン
DDH	developmental dysplasia of the hip	発育性股関節形成異常
ddI	dideoxyinosine, didanosine	ジデオキシイノシン，ジダノシン

DDR	diastolic descent rate	僧帽弁前尖弁後退速度
DDS	diaminodiphenylsulfone, dapsone	ジアミノジフェニルスルホン，ダプソン
DDS	drug delivery system	薬物送達システム
DDST	Denver Developmental Screening Test	デンバー式発達スクリーニング検査
DDT	dichlorodiphenyltrichloroethane	ジクロロジフェニルトリクロロエタン
DEA	Drug Enforcement Administration	米国麻薬取締局
DEEG	depth electroencephalogram	深部脳波
DES	diethylstilbestrol, fosfestrol	ジエチルスチルベストロール，ホスフェストロール
DES	drug-eluting stent	薬剤溶出性ステント
DET	diethyltryptamine	ジエチルトリプタミン
DEX	dexamethasone	デキサメタゾン
DEXA	dual-energy x-ray absorptiometry	二重エネルギーX線吸収法
DFA	direct fluorescent antibody technique	直接蛍光抗体法
DFO	deferoxamine	デフェロキサミン
DFPP	double-filtration plasmapheresis	二重濾過血漿分離交換法
DFS	disease-free survival	無病生存期間
5'-DFUR	5'-deoxy-5-fluorouridine, doxyfluridine	5'-デオキシ-5-フルオロウリジン，ドキシフルリジン
DHEA	dehydroepiandrosterone	デヒドロエピアンドロステロン
DHF	diastolic heart failure	拡張期心不全
DHHS	Department of Health and Human Services	米国保健社会福祉省
DHP	direct hemoperfusion	直接血液灌流
DHT	dihydrotestosterone	ジヒドロテストステロン
DI	diabetes insipidus	尿崩症
DIC	disseminated intravascular coagulation	播種性血管内凝固
DIC	drip infusion cholangiography	点滴静注胆管造影法
DID	double immunodiffusion	二重免疫拡散法
dieb. alt.	diebus alternis	隔日
dieb. tert.	diebus tertiis	三日目毎
DIHS	drug-induced hypersensitivity syndrome	薬剤性過敏症症候群
DIND	delayed ischemic neurological deficit	遅発性虚血性神経脱落症候

X章 略語集

DIP	desquamative interstitial pneumonia	剥離性間質性肺炎
DIP	distal interphalangeal (joint)	遠位指節間（関節）
DIP	drip infusion pyelography	点滴静注腎盂造影法
DISH	diffuse idiopathic skeletal hyperostosis	散在性特発性骨増殖症
DIT	diet-induced thermogenesis	食事性熱産生
DIT	diiodotyrosine	ジヨードチロシン
DJD	degenerative joint disease	変性関節疾患
DKA	diabetic ketoacidosis	糖尿病性ケトアシドーシス
DKB	dibekacin	ジベカシン
dl, dL	deciliter	デシリットル
DLco	diffusing capacity of the lung for carbon monoxide	一酸化炭素肺拡散能
DLB	dementia with Lewy bodies	レヴィ小体型認知症
DLBCL	diffuse large B cell lymphoma	びまん性大細胞B細胞リンパ腫
DLBD	diffuse Lewy body disease	びまん性レヴィー小体病
DLE	discoid lupus erythematosus	円板状エリテマトーデス
DLST	drug-induced lymphocyte stimulation test	薬剤誘発リンパ球刺激試験
DLT	dose-limiting toxicity	投与量制限毒性
DM	dermatomyositis	皮膚筋炎
DM	diabetes mellitus	糖尿病
DM	diastolic murmur	拡張期雑音
DMARD	disease-modifying antirheumatic drug	病態修飾性抗リウマチ薬
DMAT	disaster medical assistance team	災害派遣医療チーム
DMCTC	demethylchlortetracycline	デメチルクロルテトラサイクリン
DMSA	dimercaptosuccinic acid	ジメルカプトコハク酸
DMSO	dimethyl sulfoxide	ジメチルスルホキシド
DNA	deoxyribonucleic acid	デオキシリボ核酸
DNCB	dinitrochlorobenzene	ジニトロクロロベンゼン
DNR	daunorubicin	ダウノルビシン
DNR	do not resuscitate	蘇生拒否
DO	Doctor of Osteopathy	整骨療法士
do.	ditto	同上，同前
DOA	dead on arrival	来院時死亡
DOB	date of birth	生年月日
DOC	11-deoxycorticosterone	11-デオキシコルチコステロン
DOC	docetaxel	ドセタキセル
DOCA	deoxycorticosterone acetate	酢酸デオキシコルチコステ

		ロン
DOE	dyspnea on exertion	運動性呼吸困難
DOH	Department of Health	英国保健省
DOMP	diseases of medical practice	医原病
DOPA	dihydroxyphenylalanine	ジヒドロキシフェニルアラニン
DOPS	diffuse obstructive pulmonary syndrome	びまん性閉塞性肺症候群
DOXY	doxycycline	ドキシサイクリン
DPB	diffuse panbronchiolitis	びまん性汎細気管支炎
DPL	diagnostic peritoneal lavage	診断的腹腔洗浄
DPP	dipeptidyl peptidase	ジペプチジルペプチダーゼ
DPT	diphtheria and tetanus toxoids and pertussis vaccine	ジフテリア・破傷風・百日咳混合ワクチン
DQ	developmental quotient	発達指数
DR	diabetic retinopathy	糖尿病網膜症
DRE	digital rectal examination	直腸指診
DRG	diagnosis-related group	診断別疾患分類
DRPM	doripenem	ドリペネム
Ds	darmstadtium	ダームスタチウム
DSA	destructive spondyloarthropathy	破壊性脊椎関節症
DSA	digital subtraction angiography	ディジタル差分血管造影法
DSAP	disseminated superficial actinic porokeratosis	播種性表在性光線性汗孔角化症
DSCG	disodium cromoglycate	クロモグリク酸ナトリウム
DSD	detrusor-sphincter dyssynergia	排尿筋・括約筋協調不全
dsDNA	double-stranded DNA	二本鎖 DNA
DSM	Diagnostic and Statistical Manual of Mental Disorders	精神障害の診断と統計の手引き
DSPS	delayed sleep phase syndrome	睡眠相後退症候群
DST	dexamethasone suppression test	デキサメタゾン抑制試験
DT	delirium tremens	振戦せん妄
DTH	delayed-type hypersensitivity reaction	遅延型過敏反応
DTIC	dimethyl-triazeno-imidazolecarboxiamide, dacarbazine	ダカルバジン
DTP	diphtheria and tetanus toxoids and pertussis vaccine	ジフテリア・破傷風・百日咳混合ワクチン
DTPA	diethylenetriamine pentaacetic acid	ジエチレントリアミン五酢酸
DTR	deep tendon reflex	深部腱反射
dtr.	detur	与えよ
DU	duodenal ulcer	十二指腸潰瘍
DUB	dysfunctional uterine bleeding	機能不全性不正子宮出血

DVT	deep venous thrombosis	深部静脈血栓
D/W	dextrose in water	ブドウ糖液
Dx	diagnosis	診断
DXR	doxorubicin	ドキソルビシン
Dy	dysprosium	ジスプロシウム
dyn	dyne	ダイン
DZP	diazepam	ジアゼパム

E

E_1	estrone	エストロン
E_2	estradiol	エストラジオール
E_3	estriol	エストリオール
E_4	estetrol	エステトロール
EA	early antigen	早期抗原
EA	effort angina	労作性狭心症
EAA	essential amino acid	必須アミノ酸
EAC	external auditory canal	外耳道
EACA	epsilon-aminocaproic acid	イプシロン・アミノカプロン酸
EAEC	enteroadherent *Escherichia coli*	腸管付着性大腸菌
EAT	ectopic atrial tachycardia	異所性心房頻拍
EB	epidermolysis bullosa	表皮水疱症
EB	ethambutol hydrochloride	塩酸エタンブトール
EBD	endoscopic biliary drainage	内視鏡的胆道ドレナージ
EBF	erythroblastosis fetalis	胎児赤芽球症
EBL	estimated blood loss	推算出血量
EBM	evidence-based medicine	根拠に基づく医療
EBN	evidence-based nursing	根拠に基づく看護
EBNA	Epstein-Barr virus associated nuclear antigen	EBウイルス関連特異核抗原
EBP	epidural blood patch	硬膜外血液パッチ法
EBRT	external-beam radiation therapy	体外放射線照射療法
EBS	epidermolysis bullosa simplex	単純型先天表皮水疱症
EBUS	endobronchial ultrasonography	気管支内超音波断層法
EBV	Epstein-Barr virus	エプスタイン・バーウイルス
EC	enteric-coated (tablet)	腸溶（錠）
EC	epirubicin, cyclophosphamide	エピルビシン，シクロホスファミド（化学療法）
ECA	external carotid artery	外頚動脈
ECC	electrocorticogram	皮質脳波
ECC	extracorporeal circulation	体外循環
ECCE	extracapsular cataract extrac-	白内障囊外摘出術

	tion	
ECD	endocardial cushion defect	心内膜床欠損
ECF	extracellular fluid	細胞外液
ECFMG	Educational Commission for Foreign Medical Graduates	外国人医師卒後教育委員会（米国）
ECG	electrocardiogram	心電図
ECHO	enteric cytopathogenic human orphan virus	ECHO ウイルス
EC-IC	extracranial-intracranial (bypass)	頭蓋内外（バイパス）
ECLIA	electrochemiluminescent immunoassay	電気化学発光免疫測定法
ECM	external cardiac massage	体外心マッサージ
ECMO	extracorporeal membrane oxygenation	体外式膜型人工肺
ECP	eosinophilic cationic proteins	好酸球塩基性タンパク
ECT	electroconvulsive therapy	電気痙攣療法
ECT	emission computed tomography	放射型コンピュータ断層撮影
ECUM	extracorporeal ultrafiltration method	体外限外濾過法
ED	effective dose	有効量
ED	elemental diet	成分栄養
ED	emergency department	救急治療部
ED	erectile dysfunction	勃起不全
ED	erythema dose	紅斑線量
EDAS	encephaloduroarteriosynangiosis	脳硬膜動脈血管癒合術
EDC	expected date of confinement	分娩予定日
EDD	expected date of delivery	分娩予定日
EDG	electrodermogram	皮膚電位図
EDP	end-diastolic pressure	拡張末期圧
EDS	excessive daytime sleepiness	昼間過眠
EDTA	ethylenediaminetetraacetic acid	エチレンジアミン四酢酸
EDV	end-diastolic volume	拡張末期容量
EEG	electroencephalogram	脳波
EEM	erythema exudativum multiforme	多形滲出性紅斑
EF	ejection fraction	駆出率
EFL	English as a foreign language	外国語としての英語
EFV	efavirenz	エファビレンツ
e.g.	exempli gratia	たとえば
EGC	early gastric cancer	早期胃癌
EGD	esophagogastroduodenoscopy	食道胃十二指腸内視鏡検査

X章

EGF	epidermal growth factor	上皮細胞成長因子
EGFR	epidermal growth factor receptor	上皮細胞成長因子受容体
eGFR	estimated glomerular filtration rate	推算糸球体濾過量
EGJ	esophagogastric junction	食道胃接合部
EHEC	enterohemorrhagic *Escherichia coli*	腸管出血性大腸菌
EHL	electrohydraulic lithotripsy	電気水圧式砕石術
EHO	extrahepatic portal obstruction	肝外門脈閉塞症
EHR	electronic health record	電子保健医療記録
EIA	enzyme immunoassay	酵素免疫測定法
EIA	exercise-induced asthma	運動誘発喘息
EIA	external iliac artery	外腸骨動脈
EIEC	enteroinvasive *Escherichia coli*	腸管組織侵入性大腸菌
EIS	endoscopic injection sclerotherapy	内視鏡的(静脈瘤)硬化療法
EKC	epidemic keratoconjunctivitis	流行性角結膜炎
EKY	electrokymography	電気キモグラフィー
ELBW	extremely low birth weight	超低出生体重
ELCA	excimer laser coronary angioplasty	エキシマレーザー冠動脈形成術
ELISA	enzyme-linked immunosorbent assay	酵素免疫吸着法
EM	electron microscope	電子顕微鏡
EM	erythromycin	エリスロマイシン
EMA	epithelial membrane antigen	上皮細胞膜抗原
EMF	endomyocardial fibrosis	心内膜心筋線維症
EMG	electromyogram	筋電図
EMG	exomphalos-macroglossia-gigantism (syndrome)	臍帯ヘルニア・巨舌・巨大児(症候群)
EMIT	enzyme multiplied immunoassay technique	多元酵素免疫測定法
EMP	English for medical purposes	医学目的の英語
EMR	electronic medical record	電子カルテ
EMR	endoscopic mucosal resection	内視鏡的粘膜切除術
EMS	emergency medical service	救急医療
EMS	eosinophilia-myalgia syndrome	好酸球増多・筋痛症候群
EMS	expandable metallic stent	拡張性金属ステント
EMT	emergency medical technician	救急救命士
ENA	extractable nuclear antigen	抽出核抗原
ENBD	endoscopic nasobiliary drainage	内視鏡的経鼻胆道ドレナージ
ENG	electronystagmography	電気眼振検査法

ENT	ear, nose and throat	耳鼻咽喉科
ENX	enoxacin	エノキサシン
EOAE	evoked otoacoustic emission	誘発耳音響放射
EOG	electro-oculogram	眼電図
EOG	electro-olfactogram	嗅電図
EOG	ethylene oxide gas	エチレンオキサイドガス
EOM	extraocular movement	外眼運動
EOM	extraocular muscle	外眼筋
EP	esophoria	内斜位
EP	estramustine phosphate	エストラムスチン
EP	etoposide, cisplatin	エトポシド, シスプラチン (化学療法)
EPA	eicosapentaenoic acid	エイコサペンタエン酸
EPEC	enteropathogenic *Escherichia coli*	腸管病原性大腸菌
EPI	epirubicin	エピルビシン
EPO	erythropoietin	エリスロポエチン
EPOCH	etoposide, prednisolone, vincristine, cyclophosphamide, doxorubicin	エトポシド, プレドニゾロン, ビンクリスチン, シクロホスファミド, ドキソルビシン (化学療法)
EPP	erythropoietic protoporphyria	赤血球産生性プロトポルフィリン症
EPS	electrophysiologic study	電気生理学的検査
EPS	encapsulating peritoneal sclerosis	被包性腹膜硬化症
EPS	extrapyramidal syndrome	錐体外路症候群
EPSP	excitatory postsynaptic potential	興奮性シナプス後電位
EPT	endoscopic papillotomy	内視鏡的乳頭切開術
ER	emergency room	救急室
ER	endoplasmic reticulum	小胞体
ER	estrogen receptor	エストロゲン受容体
Er	erbium	エルビウム
ERA	electric response audiometry	皮膚電気反応聴力検査
ERBD	endoscopic retrograde biliary drainage	内視鏡的逆行性胆道ドレナージ
ERCP	endoscopic retrograde cholangiopancreatography	内視鏡的逆行性胆道膵管造影法
ERG	electroretinogram	網膜電図
ERM	epiretinal membrane	網膜上膜
ERV	expiratory reserve volume	予備呼気量
Es	einsteinium	アインスタイニウム
ESC	embryonic stem cell	胚性幹細胞

X章 略語集

ESD	endoscopic submucosal dissection	内視鏡的粘膜下層剥離術
ESL	English as a second language	第二言語としての英語
ESM	ethosuximide	エトスクシミド
ESP	end-systolic pressure	収縮末期圧
ESR	erythrocyte sedimentation rate	赤血球沈降速度
ESRD	end-stage renal disease	末期腎不全
EST	electric shock therapy, electroshock therapy	電気ショック療法
EST	endoscopic sphincterotomy	内視鏡的乳頭括約筋切開術
ESV	end-systolic volume	収縮末期容量
ESWL	extracorporeal shock-wave-lithotripsy	体外衝撃波砕石術
ET	esotropia	内斜視
ET	essential thrombocythemia	本態性血小板血症
et al.	et alii	およびその他
et seq.	et sequens	以下参照
etc.	et cetera	など，その他
ETEC	enterotoxigenic *Escherichia coli*	腸毒素産生性大腸菌
ETH	ethionamide	エチオナミド
EtOH	ethanol	エタノール
ETP	etoposide	エトポシド
ETT	endotracheal tube	気管チューブ
Eu	europium	ユウロピウム
EUS	endoscopic ultrasonography	超音波内視鏡検査
EVL	endoscopic variceal ligation	内視鏡的静脈瘤結紮術
EVM	enviomycin	エンビオマイシン
EVLW	extravascular lung water	血管外肺水分量
EVT	endovascular treatment	血管内治療

F

F	farad	ファラド
F	fluorine	フッ素
°F	degree Fahrenheit	華氏
FA	femoral artery	大腿動脈
FA	fluorescent antibody	蛍光抗体
FA	fusidic acid	フシジン酸
FAB	French-American-British (classification)	FAB（分類）
FAB	frontal assessment battery	前頭葉機能検査
Fab	antigen-binding fragment	抗原結合フラグメント
FAD	flavin adenine dinucleotide	フラビンアデニンヌクレオチド
FAG	fluorescein angiography	蛍光眼底撮影法

FAM	5-fluorouracil, doxorubicin, mitomycin C	フルオロウラシル,ドキソルビシン,マイトマイシン(化学療法)
FANA	fluorescent antinuclear antibody	蛍光抗核抗体
FAP	familial adenomatous polyposis	家族性腺腫性ポリポーシス
FAP	familial amyloid polyneuropathy	家族性アミロイド多発ニューロパチー
FAS	fetal alcohol syndrome	胎児性アルコール症候群
FAT	fluorescent antibody technique	蛍光抗体法
FB	fingerbreadth	横指
FB	foreign body	異物
FBS	fasting blood sugar	空腹時血糖
5-FC	5-fluorocytosine, flucytosine	5-フルオロシトシン,フルシトシン
Fc	crystallizable fragment	結晶形成フラグメント,Fcフラグメント
FCA	Freund complete adjuvant	フロイント完全アジュバント
FCHL	familial combined hyperlipidemia	家族性複合型高脂血症
FCM	flow cytometry	フローサイトメトリー
FCV	famcicrovir	ファムシクロビル
FD	faculty development	教員能力開発
FD	functional dyspepsia	機能性ディスペプシア
FDA	Food and Drug Administration	米国食品医薬品局
FDG	^{18}F-fluorodeoxyglucose	^{18}F標識フルオロデオキシグルコース
FDP	fibrin degradation product	フィブリン分解産物
Fe	iron	鉄
FEC	5-fluorouracil, epirubisin, cyclophosphamide	フルオロウラシル,エピルビシン,シクロホスファミド(化学療法)
FEIA	fluorescent enzyme immunoassay	蛍光酵素免疫測定法
FENa	fractional excretion of sodium	ナトリウム排泄分画
FES	fat embolism syndrome	脂肪塞栓症候群
FES	functional electrical stimulation	機能的電気刺激
FEV	forced expiratory volume	努力肺活量
FEV$_{1.0}$	forced expiratory volume in one second	1秒量
FEV$_{1.0\%}$	percent of one second forced	1秒率

	expiratory volume	
FF	filtration fraction	濾過分画
FFA	free fatty acid	遊離脂肪酸
F-FLCZ	fosfluconazole	ホスフルコナゾール
FFP	fresh frozen plasma	新鮮凍結血漿
FGF	fibroblast growth factor	線維芽細胞増殖因子
FGFR3	fibroblast growth factor receptor 3	線維芽細胞増殖因子受容体3
FGS	focal glomerulosclerosis	巣状糸球体硬化症
FH	family history	家族歴
FHR	fetal heart rate	胎児心拍数
FIA	fluorescent immunoassay	蛍光免疫測定法
FIA	Freund incomplete adjuvant	フロイント不完全アジュバント
FIM	functional independence measure	機能的自立度評価法
FIO$_2$	fraction of inspired oxygen	吸入酸素濃度
FISH	fluorescence in situ hybridization	蛍光インサイチュー・ハイブリダイゼーション
FITC	fluorescein isothiocyanate	フルオレセインイソチオシアネート
FL	femur length	大腿骨長
FL	follicular lymphoma	濾胞性リンパ腫
fl oz	fluid ounce	液量オンス
FLCZ	fluconazole	フルコナゾール
FLRX	fleroxacin	フレロキサシン
FLU	fludarabine	フルダラビン
Fm	fermium	フェルミウム
FM	fibromyalgia	線維筋痛症
FMD	fibromuscular dysplasia	線維筋異形成症
FMF	familial Mediterranean fever	家族性地中海熱
FMOX	flomoxef	フロモキセフ
FNA	fine needle aspiration	細針吸引
FND	functional neck dissection	機能的頚部リンパ節郭清術
FNH	focal nodular hyperplasia	限局性結節性過形成
FNS	functional neuromuscular stimulation	機能的神経筋刺激法
FOB	fecal occult blood	便潜血
FOLFIRI	5-fluorouracil/levofolinate, irinotecan	フルオロウラシル／レボホリナートカルシウム，イリノテカン（化学療法）
FOLFOX	5-fluorouracil/levofolinate, oxaliplatin	フルオロウラシル／レボホリナートカルシウム，オキサリプラチン（化学療法）

FOM	fosfomycin	ホスホマイシン
FOP	fibrodysplasia ossificans progressiva	進行性骨化性線維異形成症
FP	5-fluorouracil, cisplatin	フルオロウラシル，シスプラチン（化学療法）
FP	fluticasone propionate	フルチカゾンプロピオン酸エステル
FPC	familial polyposis coli	家族性大腸ポリポーシス
FPIA	fluorescence polarization immunoassay	蛍光偏光免疫検定法
FPU	fetoplacental unit	胎児胎盤系
FPV	fosamprenavir calcium	ホスアンプレナビルカルシウム
Fr	francium	フランシウム
FRC	functional residual capacity	機能的残気量
FRM	fradiomycin	フラジオマイシン
FRPM	faropenem	ファロペナム
FSH	follicle-stimulating hormone	卵胞刺激ホルモン
FT	tegafur	テガフール
FT_3	free triiodothyronine	遊離トリヨードサイロニン
FT_4	free thyroxin	遊離サイロキシン
ft	foot, feet	フィート
FTA	femorotibial angle	大腿脛骨角
FTA-ABS	fluorescent treponemal antibody absorption test	梅毒トレポネーマ蛍光抗体吸収試験
FTC	2'-deoxy-5-fluoro-3'-thiacytidine, emtricitabine	エムトリシタビン
FTD	frontotemporal dementia	前頭側頭型認知症
FTI	free thyroxin index	遊離サイロキシン指数
FTT	failure to thrive	発育不全
5-FU	5-fluorouracil	フルオロウラシル
FUB	functional uterine bleeding	機能性子宮出血
FUdR	5-fluorodeoxyuridine	5-フルオロデオキシウリジン
FUO	fever of unknown origin	不明熱
FUS	focused ultrasound surgery	集束超音波手術
FVC	forced vital capacity	努力性肺活量
Fx	fracture	骨折

G

G	gauss	ガウス
G	guanine	グアニン
g	gram	グラム
G6PD	glucose-6-phosphate dehydro-	グルコース-6-リン酸デヒ

	genase	ドロゲナーゼ
GA	glycoalbumin	グリコアルブミン
Ga	gallium	ガリウム
GABA	γ-aminobutyric acid	γアミノ酪酸
GAD	generalized anxiety disorder	全般性不安障害
GAD	glutamic acid decarboxylase	グルタミン酸デカルボキシラーゼ
GAF	Global Assessment of Functioning (scale)	包括的機能評価スケール
gal	gallon	ガロン
GALT	gut-associated lymphoid tissue	腸関連リンパ組織
GAVE	gastric antral vascular ectasia	胃前庭部毛細血管拡張症
γ-GT	γ-glutamyltransferase	γグルタミルトランスフェラーゼ
GB	gallbladder	胆嚢
GBM	glomerular basement membrane	糸球体基底膜
GBR	guided bone regeneration	骨再生誘導手術
GBS	Guillain-Barré syndrome	ギラン・バレー症候群
GC	gas chromatography	ガスクロマトグラフィー
GCA	giant cell arteritis	巨細胞動脈炎
GC-MS	gas chromatography-mass spectrometry	ガスクロマトグラフィー・質量分析法
GCP	good clinical practice	適正臨床試験実施基準
GCS	Glasgow Coma Scale	グラスゴー昏睡尺度
G-CSF	granulocyte colony-stimulating factor	顆粒球コロニー刺激因子
GCT	giant cell tumor	巨細胞腫
GCT	granular cell tumor	顆粒細胞腫
Gd	gadolinium	ガドリニウム
GDA	gastroduodenal artery	胃十二指腸動脈
GDM	gestational diabetes mellitus	妊娠糖尿病
GDP	guanosine diphosphate	グアノシンニリン酸
GE	glycerin enema	グリセリン浣腸
Ge	germanium	ゲルマニウム
GEM	gemcitabine	ゲムシタビン
GERD	gastroesophageal reflux disease	胃食道逆流症
GFAP	glial fibrillary acidic protein	グリア線維性酸性タンパク質
GFLX	gatifloxacin	ガチフロキサシン
GFP	green fluorescent protein	緑色蛍光タンパク質
GFR	glomerular filtration rate	糸球体濾過量
GH	growth hormone	成長ホルモン
GHB	γ-hydroxybutyric acid	γヒドロキシ酪酸

GHIH	growth hormone-inhibiting hormone	成長ホルモン分泌抑制ホルモン
GI	gastrointestinal	消化管の
GI	genomic imprinting	ゲノムインプリンティング
GI	glycemic index	血糖上昇指数
GIFT	gamete intrafallopian transfer	配偶子卵管内移植
GIO	general instructional objective	一般目標
GIP	gastric inhibitory polypeptide	胃抑制ポリペプチド
GIST	gastrointestinal stromal tumor	消化管間質腫瘍
GLC	gas-liquid chromatography	ガス液体クロマトグラフィー
GLP	glucagon-like peptide	グルカゴン様ペプチド
GLUT	glucose transporter	糖輸送体
GM	gentamicin	ゲンタマイシン
GMC	General Medical Council	英国医療管理評議会
GM-CSF	granulocyte-macrophage colony-stimulating factor	顆粒球マクロファージコロニー刺激因子
GMO	genetically modified organism	遺伝子改変生物
GMP	guanosine monophosphate	グアノシン一リン酸
GNB	gram-negative bacillus	グラム陰性桿菌
GnRH	gonadotropin-releasing hormone	ゴナドトロピン放出ホルモン
GOE	gas-oxygen-ether (anesthesia)	笑気・酸素・エーテル（麻酔）
GOF	gas-oxygen-fluothane (anesthesia)	笑気・酸素・フローセン（麻酔）
GOI	gas-oxygen-isoflurane (anesthesia)	笑気・酸素・イソフルレン（麻酔）
GOS	Glasgow Outcome Scale	グラスゴー転帰尺度
GOT	glutamic-oxaloacetic transaminase	グルタミン酸オキサロ酢酸トランスアミナーゼ
GP	gemcitabine, cisplatin	ゲムシタビン，シスプラチン（化学療法）
GP	general practitioner	一般（開業）医
GPC	giant papillary conjunctivitis	巨大乳頭結膜炎
GPC	gram-positive cocci	グラム陽性球菌
GPT	glutamic-pyruvic transaminase	グルタミン酸ピルビン酸トランスアミナーゼ
gr	grain	グレーン
GRA	glucocorticoid-remediable aldosteronism	グルココルチコイド反応性アルドステロン症
GRF	griseofulvin	グリセオフルビン
GRH	growth hormone-releasing hormone	成長ホルモン放出ホルモン

GRNX	garenoxacin	ガレノキサシン
GS	gestational sac	胎嚢
GSC	gas-solid chromatography	ガス固体クロマトグラフィー
GSH	reduced glutathione	還元型グルタチオン
GSL	goniosynechiolysis	隅角癒着解離術
GSR	galvanic skin reflex	皮膚電気反射
GSS	Gerstmann-Sträussler-Scheinker disease	ゲルストマン・ストロイスラー・シャインカー病
GSSG	glutathione disulfide	グルタチオンジスルフィド
GSW	gunshot wound	銃創
GTH	gonadotropic hormone	性腺刺激ホルモン
GTP	guanosine triphosphate	グアノシン三リン酸
GTR	guided tissue regeneration	歯周組織再生誘導手術
GTT	glucose tolerance test	ブドウ糖負荷試験
gtt.	guttae	滴
GU	gastric ulcer	胃潰瘍
GU	genitourinary	泌尿生殖器の
GVHD	graft-versus-host disease	移植片対宿主病
Gy	gray	グレイ

H

H	hydrogen	水素
H	henry	ヘンリー
h.	hora	時間
HA	hemagglutination	赤血球凝集反応
HA	hemagglutinin	赤血球凝集素
HAA	hepatitis-associated antigen	肝炎関連抗原
HA-Ab	anti-HAV antibody	A型肝炎ウイルス抗体
HAART	highly active antiretroviral therapy	高活性抗レトロウイルス療法
HACE	high-altitude cerebral edema	高地脳浮腫
HAE	hereditary angioedema	遺伝性血管浮腫
HALS	hand-assisted laparoscopic surgery	用手補助腹腔鏡手術
HAM	HTLV-1-associated myelopathy	HTLV-1関連脊髄障害
HANE	hereditary angioneurotic edema	遺伝性血管神経性浮腫
HAP	hospital-acquired pneumonia	院内肺炎
HAPE	high-altitude pulmonary edema	高地肺水腫
HAV	hepatitis A virus	A型肝炎ウイルス
Hb	hemoglobin	ヘモグロビン，血色素

HbA1c	hemoglobin A1c	ヘモグロビン A1c
HBcAg	hepatitis B core antigen	B 型肝炎コア抗原
HBE	His bundle electrogram	ヒス束心電図
HBeAg	hepatitis B envelope antigen	B 型肝炎 e 抗原
HBF	hepatic blood flow	肝血流量
HBIG	hepatitis B immune globulin	抗 HBs ヒト免疫グロブリン
HBP	high blood pressure	高血圧
HBsAg	hepatitis B surface antigen	B 型肝炎表面抗原
HBV	hepatitis B virus	B 型肝炎ウイルス
HC-Ab	anti-HCV antibody	C 型肝炎ウイルス抗体
HCC	hepatocellular carcinoma	肝細胞癌
HCD	heavy chain disease	重鎖病
HCFU	1-hexylcarbamoyl-5-fluorouracil, carmofur	カルモフール
HCG	human chorionic gonadotropin	ヒト絨毛性ゴナドトロピン
HCL	hairy cell leukemia	毛髪様細胞白血病
HCM	hypertrophic cardiomyopathy	肥大型心筋症
HCP	hereditary coproporphyria	遺伝性コプロポルフィリン症
Hct	hematocrit	ヘマトクリット
HCV	hepatitis C virus	C 型肝炎ウイルス
HD	hemodialysis	血液透析
HD	Hodgkin disease	ホジキン病
HD	Huntington disease	ハンチントン病
HDF	hemodiafiltration	血液濾過透析
HDG	hypotonic duodenography	低緊張性十二指腸造影
HDL	high-density lipoprotein	高比重リポタンパク
HDN	hemolytic disease of the newborn	新生児溶血性疾患
HDRS	Hamilton depression rating scale	ハミルトンうつ病評価尺度
HDV	hepatitis D virus	D 型肝炎ウイルス
He	helium	ヘリウム
H&E	hematoxylin and eosin stain	ヘマトキシリンエオジン染色
HELLP	hemolysis, elevated liver enzymes, low platelet count (syndrome)	HELLP 症候群
HEMPAS	hereditary erythroblastic multinuclearity associated with positive acidified serum	酸性化血清陽性を伴う遺伝性赤芽球多形核症
HEN	home enteral nutrition	在宅経腸栄養法
HER2	human epidermal growth fac-	ヒト上皮増殖因子受容体 2

	tor receptor type 2	型
HES	hypereosinophilic syndrome	好酸球増加症候群
HEV	hepatitis E virus	E 型肝炎ウイルス
HF	Hageman factor	ハーゲマン因子（血液凝固の第 12 因子）
HF	hemofiltration	血液濾過
Hf	hafnium	ハフニウム
H-FABP	heart-type fatty acid-binding protein	ヒト心臓由来脂肪酸結合タンパク
HFMD	hand-foot-and-mouth disease	手足口病
HFO	high-frequency oscillation	高頻度人工換気
HFV	high-frequency ventilation	高頻度換気
Hg	hydrargyrum, mercury	水銀
Hgb	hemoglobin	ヘモグロビン，血色素
HGF	hepatocyte growth factor	肝細胞増殖因子
HGH	human growth hormone	ヒト成長ホルモン
HGP	human genome project	ヒトゲノム計画
HGPRT	hypoxanthine-guanine phosphoribosyltransferase	ヒポキサンチングアニンホスホリボシルトランスフェラーゼ
HGV	hepatitis G virus	G 型肝炎ウイルス
HHD	hypertensive heart disease	高血圧性心疾患
HHM	humoral hypercalcemia of malignancy	腫瘍由来体液性高カルシウム血症
HHNKC	hyperglycemic hyperosmolar nonketotic coma	高血糖性高浸透圧性昏睡
HI	hemagglutination inhibition	赤血球凝集抑制反応
5-HIAA	5-hydroxyindoleacetic acid	5-ヒドロキシインドール酢酸
Hib	*Haemophilus influenzae* type b (vaccine)	インフルエンザ菌 b 型（ワクチン）
HiDAC	high-dose Ara-C	高用量シタラビン
HIE	hypoxic-ischemic encephalopathy	低酸素性虚血性脳症
HIFU	high-intensity focused ultrasound	高密度焦点式超音波療法
HIPAA	Health Insurance Portability and Accountability Act	医療保険の通算可能性と説明責任に関する法律（米国）
HIS	hospital information system	病院情報システム
HIT	heparin-induced thrombocytopenia	ヘパリン起因性血小板減少症
HIT	hysteroscopic insemination into tube	子宮鏡下卵管内精子注入法
HIV	human immunodeficiency vi-	ヒト免疫不全ウイルス

	rus	
HJR	hepatojugular reflux	肝頸静脈逆流
HL	Hodgkin lymphoma	ホジキンリンパ腫
HLA	human histocompatibility leukocyte antigen	ヒト組織適合白血球抗原
HLA	human leukocyte antigen	ヒト白血球抗原，HLA 抗原
HLH	hemophagocytic lymphohistiocytosis	血球貪食性リンパ組織球症
HLHS	hypoplastic left heart syndrome	左心低形成症候群
HM	hand movement	手動弁
HMBS	hydroxymethylbilane synthase	ヒドロキシメチルビレーン合成酵素
HMD	hyaline membrane disease	硝子膜症
hMG	human menopausal gonadotropin	ヒト閉経期ゴナドトロピン
HMG-CoA	hydroxymethylglutaryl‐Coenzyme A	ヒドロキシメチルグルタリル補酵素 A
HMO	health maintenance organization	健康維持機構（米国）
HMSN	hereditary motor and sensory neuropathy	遺伝性運動感覚ニューロパチー
HNCM	hypertrophic nonobstructive cardiomyopathy	肥大型非閉塞性心筋症
HNKC	hyperosmolar nonketotic coma	高浸透圧性非ケトン性昏睡
HNP	herniated nucleus pulposus	椎間板ヘルニア
HNPCC	hereditary nonpolyposis colorectal cancer	遺伝性非ポリポーシス大腸癌
HNSHA	hereditary nonspherocytic hemolytic anemia	遺伝性非球状赤血球性溶血性貧血
HO	hydrophilic ointment	親水軟膏
Ho	holmium	ホルミウム
HOCM	hypertrophic obstructive cardiomyopathy	肥大型閉塞性心筋症
HoLAP	holmium laser ablation of prostate	ホルミウムレーザー前立腺蒸散術
HoLEP	holmium laser enucleation of prostate	ホルミウムレーザー前立腺核出術
HOMA-R	homeostasis model assessment of insulin resistance	インスリン抵抗性指標
HONK	hyperosmolar nonketotic coma	高浸透圧性非ケトン性昏睡
HOS	hypo-osmotic swelling test	精子膨化試験
HOT	home oxygen therapy	在宅酸素療法

HP	*Helicobacter pylori*	ヘリコバクター・ピロリ
Hp	haptpglobin	ハプトグロビン
H&P	history and physical examination	病歴と身体的検査
HPA	hypothalamic-pituitary-adrenal axis	視床下部・下垂体・副腎系
HPD	histrionic personality disorder	演技性人格障害
HPF	high-power field	強拡大視野
HPI	history of present illness	現病歴
hPL	human placental lactogen	ヒト胎盤性乳腺刺激ホルモン
HPLC	high-performance liquid chromatography	高速液体クロマトグラフィー
HPN	home parenteral nutrition	在宅中心静脈栄養法
HPO	hypertrophic pulmonary osteoarthropathy	肺性肥厚性骨関節症
HPS	hemophagocytic syndrome	血球貪食症候群
HPT	hepaplastin test	ヘパプラスチンテスト
HPV	hypoxic pulmonary vasoconstriction	低酸素性肺血管収縮
HPV	*Human papillomavirus*	ヒトパピローマウイルス
HR	heart rate	心拍数
HRA	high right atrial (electrogram)	高右心房（心電図）
HRCT	high-resolution computed tomography	高分解能コンピュータ断層撮影法
HRT	hormone replacement therapy	ホルモン補充療法
HS	hereditary spherocytosis	遺伝性球状赤血球症
Hs	hassium	ハッシウム
h.s.	hora somni	眠前
HSA	human serum albumin	ヒト血清アルブミン
HSAN	hereditary sensory and autonomic neuropathy	遺伝性感覚自律性ニューロパチー
HSAP	heat-stable alkaline phosphatase	耐熱性アルカリホスファターゼ
HSCT	hematopoietic stem cell transplantation	造血幹細胞移植
HSE	hemorrhagic shock and encephalopathy syndrome	出血性ショック・脳症症候群
HSE	herpes simplex encephalitis	単純ヘルペス脳炎
HSG	hysterosalpingography	子宮卵管造影法
HSP	heat shock protein	熱ショックタンパク質
HSP	Henoch-Schönlein purpura	ヘノッホ・シェーンライン紫斑病
HSV	herpes simplex virus	単純ヘルペスウイルス

5-HT	5-hydroxytryptamine	5-ヒドロキシトリプタミン, セロトニン
ht	height	身長
HTL	human T-cell leukemia	ヒトT細胞白血病
HTLV-1	human T-lymphotropic virus 1	ヒトTリンパ球向性ウイルス1型
HTLV-2	human T-lymphotropic virus 2	ヒトTリンパ球向性ウイルス2型
HTN	hypertension	高血圧
HTO	high tibial osteotomy	高位脛骨骨切り術
HU	Hounsefield unit	ハンスフィールド単位
HU	hydroxycarbamide	ヒドロキシカルバミド
HUS	hemolytic uremic syndrome	溶血性尿毒症症候群
HV	hepatic vein	肝静脈
HVA	homovanillic acid	ホモバニル酸
HVS	hyperventilation syndrome	過換気症候群
HVS	hyperviscosity syndrome	過粘稠血症候群
Hx	history	病歴
Hyp	hydroxyproline	ヒドロキシプロリン
Hz	hertz	ヘルツ

I

I	iodine	ヨウ素
IABP	intra-aortic balloon pumping	大動脈内バルーン・パンピング
IADL	instrumental activities of daily living	手段的日常生活動作
IAHA	immune adherence hemagglutination	免疫粘着赤血球凝集反応
IAP	immunosuppressive acidic protein	免疫抑制性酸性タンパク
IAS	interatrial septum	心房中隔
IB	inclusion body	封入体
IBBB	incomplete bundle branch block	不完全脚ブロック
IBD	inflammatory bowel disease	炎症性腸疾患
ibid.	ibidem	同じ箇所(章, 節)に
IBL	inquiry-based learning	質問に基づく学習
IBM	inclusion body myositis	封入体筋炎
IBS	irritable bowel syndrome	過敏性腸症候群
IC	immune complex	免疫複合体
IC	informed consent	インフォームドコンセント
IC	inspiratory capacity	最大吸気量
ICA	internal carotid artery	内頚動脈
ICA	islet cell antibody	膵島細胞抗体

ICAM	intracellular adhesion molecule	細胞内接着分子
ICCE	intracapsular cataract extraction	白内障囊内摘出術
ICD	implantable cardioverter-defibrillator	植え込み型除細動器
ICD	International Classification of Diseases	国際疾病分類
ICD-10	International Statistical Classification of Diseases and Related Health Problems, Tenth Revision	疾病及び関連保健問題の国際統計分類第10回修正
ICF	International Classification of Functioning, Disbility, and Health	国際生活機能分類
ICF	intracellular fluid	細胞内液
ICG	indocyanine green (test)	インドシアニングリーン(試験)
ICGC	International Cancer Genome Consortium	国際癌ゲノムコンソーシアム
ICH	intracerebral hemorrhage	脳内出血
ICH	intracranial hematoma	頭蓋内血腫
ICH	intracranial hypertension	頭蓋内圧亢進
ICM	idiopathic cardiomyopathy	特発性心筋症
ICN	infection control nurse	感染管理看護師
ICN	International Council of Nurses	国際看護師協会
ICNP	International Classification for Nursing Practice	看護実践国際分類
ICP	intracranial pressure	頭蓋内圧
ICP-MS	inductively coupled plasma mass spectrometry	誘導結合プラズママススペクトロメトリー
ICS	intercostal space	肋間腔
ICSA	islet cell surface antibody	膵島細胞膜抗体
ICSH	interstitial cell-stimulating hormon	間質細胞刺激ホルモン
ICSI	intracytoplasmic sperm injection	卵細胞質内精子注入法
ICT	indirect Coombs test	間接クームス試験
ICT	infection control team	感染対策チーム
ICT	intracoronary thrombolysis	冠動脈内注入血栓溶解療法
ICT	intracranial tumor	頭蓋内腫瘍
ICU	intensive care unit	集中治療室
ID	identification	個人識別, 同定
id.	idem	同上, 同著者
I&D	incision and drainage	切開排膿

IDA	iron deficiency anemia	鉄欠乏性貧血
IDDM	insulin-dependent diabetes mellitus (type 1)	インスリン依存性糖尿病（1型）
IDK	internal derangement of the knee joint	膝内障
IDR	idarubicin	イダルビシン
IDUS	intraductal ultrasonography	管腔内超音波検査法
IDV	indinavir	インジナビル
IE	infectious endocarditis	感染性心内膜炎
i.e.	id est	すなわち，換言すれば
IEP	immunoelectrophoresis	免疫電気泳動法
IFA	indirect fluorescent antibody technique	間接蛍光抗体法
IFG	impaired fasting glucose	空腹時血糖異常
IFM	ifosfamide	イホスファミド
IFN	interferon	インターフェロン
IFX	infliximab	インフリキシマブ
Ig	immunoglobulin	免疫グロブリン
IgE	immunoglobulin E	免疫グロブリンE
IGF	insulinlike growth factor	インスリン様成長因子
IGF-I	insulinlike growth factor-I	インスリン様成長因子I
IGRA	interferon-gamma release assay	インターフェロンγ放出アッセイ
IGT	impaired glucose tolerance	耐糖能異常
IHA	idiopathic hyperaldosteronism	特発性高アルドステロン症
IHA	indirect hemagglutination	間接赤血球凝集法
IHD	ischemic heart disease	虚血性心疾患
IHSA	iodinated human serum albumin	ヨウ素標識ヒト血清アルブミン
IHSS	idiopathic hypertrophic subaortic stenosis	特発性肥大型大動脈弁下狭窄症
IIA	internal iliac artery	内腸骨動脈
IIP	idiopathic interstitial pneumonia	特発性間質性肺炎
IL	interleukin	インターロイキン
ILD	interstitial lung disease	間質性肺疾患
IM	infectious mononucleosis	伝染性単核球症
IM	intramuscular(ly)	筋肉内
IMA	inferior mesenteric artery	下腸間膜動脈
IMA	internal mammary artery	内胸動脈
IMF	intermaxillary fixation	顎間固定法
IMRT	intensity-modulated radiation therapy	強度変調放射線治療
IMT	intima-media thickness	内中膜複合体厚

X章 略語集

IMV	inferior mesenteric vein	下腸間膜静脈
IMV	intermittent mandatory ventilation	間欠的強制換気
In	indium	インジウム
in	inch	インチ
IND	investigational new drug	治験薬
INH	isonicotinic acid hydrazide, isoniazid	イソニコチン酸ヒドラジド, イソニアジド
INMS	isoniazid sodium methanesulfonate	イソニアジドメタンスルホン酸ナトリウム塩
INR	international normalized ratio	国際標準化比
I&O	intake and output	摂取量と排泄量
IOL	intraocular lens	眼内レンズ
ION	ischemic optic neuropathy	虚血性視神経障害
IOP	intraocular pressure	眼圧
IORT	intraoperative radiotherapy	術中放射線治療
IP	International Pharmacopeia	国際薬局方
IP	interphalangeal (joint)	指節間(関節)
IP	intraperitoneal	腹腔内
IP	irinotecan, cisplatin	イリノテカン, シスプラチン(化学療法)
IPA	icosapentaenoic acid	イコサペンタエン酸
IPD	intermittent peritoneal dialysis	間欠的腹膜透析
IPD	interpupillary distance	瞳孔間距離
IPF	idiopathic pulmonary fibrosis	特発性肺線維症
IPH	idiopathic portal hypertension	特発性門脈圧亢進症
IPI	International Prognostic Index	国際予後指標
IPM/CS	imipenem/cilastatin	イミペネム・シラスタチン
IPMN	intraductal papillary mucinous neoplasm	膵管内乳頭粘液新生物
IPPB	intermittent positive pressure breathing	間欠陽圧呼吸法
iPS	induced pluripotent stem (cell)	人工多分化能性幹(細胞)
IPSP	inhibitory postsynaptic potential	抑制性シナプス後電位
IPSS	international prostate symptom score	国際前立腺症状スコア
IPV	inactivated poliovirus vaccine	不活化ポリオウイルスワクチン
IQ	intelligence quotient	知能指数
Ir	iridium	イリジウム
IRB	institutional review board	施設内審査委員会
IRC	International Red Cross	国際赤十字社
IRDS	infant respiratory distress syn-	小児型呼吸促迫症候群

	drome	
IRF	interferon regulatory factor	インターフェロン制御因子
IRG	immunoreactive glucagon	免疫反応性グルカゴン
IRI	immunoreactive insulin	免疫反応性インスリン
IRMA	immunoradiometric assay	免疫放射定量測定
IRMA	intraretinal microvascular abnormality	網膜内細小血管異常
IRV	inspiratory reserve volume	予備吸気量
ISA	intrinsic sympathomimetic activity	内因性交感神経刺激作用
ISDN	isosorbide dinitrate	硝酸イソソルビド
ISDR	interferon sensitivity determining region	インターフェロン感受性領域
ISF	interstitial fluid	間質液
ISMN	isosorbide mononitrate	一硝酸イソソルビド
ISP	isepamicin	イセパミシン
ISS	injury severity score	外傷重症度スコア
IST	insulin shock therapy	インスリンショック療法
ISV	International Scientific Vocabulary	国際科学用語
IT	intrathecal	髄腔内
ITA	internal thoracic artery	内胸動脈
ITB	intrathecal baclofen	髄腔内バクロフェン投与
ITCZ	itraconazole	イトラコナゾール
ITP	idiopathic thrombocytopenic purpura	特発性血小板減少性紫斑病
ITT	insulin tolerance test	インスリン負荷試験
IU	International Unit	国際単位
IUCD	intrauterine contraceptive device	子宮内避妊器具
IUD	intrauterine device	子宮内器具
IUFD	intrauterine fetal death	子宮内胎児死亡
IUGR	intrauterine growth retardation	子宮内発育遅延
IV	intravenous(ly)	静脈内
IVC	inferior vena cava	下大静脈
IVCD	intraventricular conduction defect	心室内伝導障害
IVF	in vitro fertilization	体外受精
IVF-ET	in vitro fertilization and embryo transfer	体外受精胚移植
IVH	intravenous hyperalimentation	経静脈高カロリー輸液
IVH	intraventricular hemorrhage	脳室内出血
IVP	intravenous pyelography	静脈性腎盂造影法

IVR	interventional radiology	インターベンショナルラジオロジー，画像診断的介入治療
IVS	interventricular septum	心室中隔
IVUS	intravascular ultrasonography	血管内超音波検査法

J

J	joule	ジュール
JCAHO	Joint Commission on Accreditation of Healthcare Organizations	医療機関認定合同委員会（米国）
JCQHC	Japan Council for Quality Health Care	日本医療機能評価機構
JCI	Joint Commission International	国際病院評価機構
JCS	Japan Coma Scale	日本式昏睡尺度
JDDST	Japanese edition of Denver Developmental Screening Test	日本版デンバー式発達スクリーニング検査
JEV	Japanese encephalitis virus	日本脳炎ウイルス
JGA	juxtaglomerular apparatus	傍糸球体装置
JM	josamycin	ジョサマイシン
JMA	Japan Medical Association	日本医師会
JNA	Japanese Nursing Association	日本看護協会
JODM	juvenile-onset diabetes mellitus	若年型糖尿病
JP	Japanese Pharmacopoeia	日本薬局方
JPA	Japan Pharmaceutical Association	日本薬剤師会
JRA	juvenile rheumatoid arthritis	若年性関節リウマチ
JSHP	Japanese Society of Hospital Pharmacists	日本病院薬剤師会
JVD	jugular venous distention	頸静脈怒張

K

K	kalium, potassium	カリウム
K	kelvin	ケルヴィン
KAFO	knee-ankle-foot orthosis	長下肢装具
kb	kilobase	キロベース
KCS	keratoconjunctivitis sicca	乾性角結膜炎
KCZ	ketoconazole	ケトコナゾール
kg	kilogram	キログラム
KJ	knee jerk	膝蓋腱反射
KM	kanamycin	カナマイシン
km	kilometer	キロメートル
KP	keratic precipitates	角膜後面沈着物

KPE	Kelman phacoemulsification	ケルマン水晶体乳化術
Kr	krypton	クリプトン
17-KS	17-ketosteroid	17-ケトステロイド
KSS	Kearns-Sayer syndrome	カーンズ・セイヤー症候群
KTPP	keratodermia tylodes palmaris progressiva	進行性指掌角皮症
KUB	kidney, ureter, and bladder	腎・尿管・膀胱（単純X線撮影）
KW	Keith-Wagener (classification)	キース・ワグナー（分類）

L

L	left	左の
L	lumbar vertebra	腰椎
l, L	liter	リットル
La	lanthanum	ランタン
LA	latex agglutination	ラテックス凝集反応
LA	left atrium	左心房
LA	lupus anticoagulant	ループス抗凝固因子
lab	laboratory	検査室，実験室
LABA	long-acting inhaled $\beta2$-agonist	長時間作用型吸入 β_2 刺激薬
LABC	lymphadenosis benigna cutis	皮膚良性リンパ節症
LAC	laparoscopic-assisted colectomy	腹腔鏡補助下結腸切除術
LAD	left anterior descending branch	左前下行枝
LAD	left axis deviation	左軸偏位
LAE	left atrial enlargement	左房肥大
LAH	left anterior hemiblock	左脚前枝ブロック
LAK	lymphokine-activated killer cell	リンホカイン活性化キラー細胞
LAM	lymphangioleiomyomatosis	リンパ脈管筋腫症
LAO	left anterior oblique (position)	左前斜位，第2斜位
LAP	leucine aminopeptidase	ロイシンアミノペプチダーゼ
LAP	leukocyte alkaline phosphatase	白血球アルカリホスファターゼ
LAPC	lenampicillin	レナンピシリン
LAS	laparoscopy-assisted surgery	腹腔鏡補助下手術
LASER	light amplification by stimulated emission of radiation	レーザー
LASIK	laser-assisted in situ keratomileusis	レーザー角膜内切削形成術
L-ASP	L-asparaginase	L-アスパラギナーゼ
LATS	long-acting thyroid stimulator	持続性甲状腺刺激物質
LAVH	laparoscopically assisted vagi-	腹腔鏡補助下腟式子宮摘出

	nal hysterectomy	術
lb	pound	ポンド
LBBB	left bundle-branch block	左脚ブロック
LBM	lean body mass	除脂肪体重
LBP	low back pain	腰痛
LBW	low birth weight	出産時低体重
LC	laparoscopic cholecystectomy	腹腔鏡下胆嚢摘出術
LC	liver cirrhosis	肝硬変症
LC	lung cancer	肺癌
LCA	left colic artery	左結腸動脈
LCA	left coronary artery	左冠動脈
LCA	leukocyte common antigen	白血球関連抗原
LCAT	lecithin-cholesterol acyltransferase	レシチン・コレステロール・アシルトランスフェラーゼ
LCC	luxatio coxae congenita	先天性股関節脱臼
LCCA	late cortical cerebellar atrophy	晩発性小脳皮質萎縮症
LCH	Langerhans cell histiocytosis	ランゲルハンス細胞組織球症
LCIS	lobular carcinoma in situ	非浸潤性小葉癌
LCM	lincomycin	リンコマイシン
LCMV	lymphocytic choriomeningitis virus	リンパ球性脈絡髄膜炎ウイルス
LCP	Legg-Calvé-Perthes disease	レッグ・カルベ・ペルテス病
LCR	ligase chain reaction	リガーゼ連鎖反応
LCR	locus control region	遺伝子座調節領域
LCx	left circumflex branch	左回旋枝
LD	learning disability	学習障害
LD	lethal dose	致死量
LDA	low density area	低吸収域
LDH	lactate dehydrogenase	乳酸デヒドロゲナーゼ
LDL	low-density lipoprotein	低比重リポタンパク
LDXR	liposomal doxorubicin	リポソームルドキソルビシン
LE	lupus erythematosus	エリテマトーデス,紅斑性狼瘡
LEMS	Lambert-Eaton myasthenic syndrome	ランバート・イートン筋無力症候群
LEOPARD	lentigines, ECG abnormalities, ocular hypertension, pulmonary stenosis, abnormal genitalia, retardation of growth, and deafness	レオパード症候群

LES	lower esophageal sphincter	下部食道括約筋
LESP	lower esophageal sphincter pressure	下部食道括約筋圧
LFD	large-for-dates (infant)	在胎期間過大（児）
LFD	least fatal dose	最小致死量
LFLX	lomefloxacin	ロメフロキサシン
LFT	liver function test	肝機能検査
LGA	large-for-gestational-age (infant)	在胎期間過大（児）
LGA	left gastric artery	左胃動脈
LGB	laparoscopic gastric banding	腹腔鏡下胃緊縛術
LGL	large granular lymphocyte	大顆粒リンパ球
LGL	Lown-Ganong-Levine syndrome	ラウン・ギャノン・レバイン症候群
LGP	laser gonioplasty	レーザー隅角形成術
LH	luteinizing hormone	黄体形成ホルモン
LHA	left hepatic artery	左肝動脈
LHRH	luteinizing hormone-releasing hormone	黄体形成ホルモン放出ホルモン
LI	laser iridotomy	レーザー虹彩切開術
Li	lithium	リチウム
LIA	laser immunoassay	レーザー免疫測定法
LINAC	linear accelerator	直線加速器
LIP	lymphocytic interstitial pneumonia	リンパ球性間質性肺炎
Liq.	liquor	液
LLB	long leg brace	長下肢装具
LLL	left lower lobe	左下葉
LLQ	left lower quadrant	左下腹部
l-LV	levofolinate calcium	レボホリナートカルシウム
lm	lumen	ルーメン
LMDF	lupus miliaris disseminatus faciei	顔面播種状粟粒性狼瘡
LMN	lower motor neuron	下位運動ニューロン
LMOX	latamoxef	ラタモキセフ
LMP	last menstrual period	最終月経
LMT	left main trunk	左冠動脈主幹部
LMWH	low-molecular-weight heparin	低分子量ヘパリン
LN	lymph node	リンパ節
LNG	liquefied natural gas	液化天然ガス
LOA	left occipitoanterior	第1頭位第1分類(胎位)
LOC	loss of consciousness	意識消失
LOH	late-onset hypogonadism	加齢男性性腺機能低下
L-OHP	oxaliplatin	オキサリプラチン
LOP	left occipitoposterior	第1頭位第2分類(胎位)

X章 略語集

略語	英語	日本語
LOS	low output syndrome	低心拍出量症候群
lot.	lotio	ローション
LP	light perception	光覚弁
LP	lumbar puncture	腰椎穿刺
L-PAM	melphalan	メルファラン
LPCA	long posterior ciliary artery	長後毛様体動脈
LPF	low-power field	弱拡大視野
LPG	liquefied petroleum gas	液化石油ガス
LPH	left posterior hemiblock	左脚後枝ブロック
LPH	lipotropic hormone	リポトロピン
LPL	lipoprotein lipase	リポタンパク質リパーゼ
LPN	licensed practical nurse	実務看護師, 准看護師
LPS	lipopolysaccharide	リポ多糖
LPV	lopinavir	ロピナビル
LQTS	long QT syndrome	QT延長症候群
LR	likelihood ratio	尤度比
Lr	lawrencium	ローレンシウム
LRE	leukemic reticuloendotheliosis	白血病性細網内皮症
LSA	left sacroanterior	第1骨盤位第1分類（胎位）
LSA	lichen sclerosus et atrophicus	硬化性萎縮性苔癬
LSB	left sternal border	胸骨左縁
LScA	left scapuloanterior	第1横位第1分類（胎位）
LScP	left scapuloposterior	第1横位第2分類（胎位）
LSCS	lumbar spinal canal stenosis	腰部脊柱管狭窄症
LSD	lysergic acid diethylamide	リセルグ酸ジエチルアミド
LSO	lumbosacral orthosis	腰仙椎装具
LSP	left sacroposterior	第1骨盤位第2分類（胎位）
LST	lymphocyte stimulation test	リンパ球刺激試験
LT	leukotriene	ロイコトリエン
LTP	laser trabeculoplasty	レーザー線維柱帯形成術
LTR	long terminal repeats	長端末反復
Lu	lutetium	ルテチウム
LUFS	luteinized unruptured follicle syndrome	黄体化未破裂卵胞症候群
LUL	left upper lobe	左上葉
LUQ	left upper quadrant	左上腹部
LUTS	lower urinary tract symptoms	下部尿路症状
LV	calcium folinate	ホリナートカルシウム
LV	left ventricle	左心室
LVAD	left ventricular assist device	左室補助装置
LVEDP	left ventricular end-diastolic pressure	左室拡張終末期圧

LVEDV	left ventricular end-diastolic volume	左室拡張終末期容積
LVEF	left ventricular ejection fraction	左室駆出率
LVESP	left ventricular end-systolic pressure	左室収縮終末期圧
LVESV	left ventricular end-systolic volume	左室収縮終末期容積
LVFX	levofloxacin	レボフロキサシン
LVG	left ventriculography	左室造影法
LVH	left ventricular hypertrophy	左室肥大
LVRS	lung volume reduction surgery	肺容量減少術
lx	lux	ルクス
LZD	linezolid	リネゾリド

M

M.	misce	混和せよ
m	meter	メートル
m	mucosa	粘膜
MA	microaneurysm	小動脈瘤
MAA	macroaggregated albumin	大凝集アルブミン
MAB	maximum androgen blockade	最大アンドロゲン遮断
MAb	monoclonal antibody	モノクローナル抗体
MAC	membrane attack complex	膜侵襲複合体
MAC	mycobacterium avium complex	トリ型結核菌複合体
MAF	macrophage-activating factor	マクロファージ活性化因子
MALT	mucosa-associated lymphoid tissue	粘膜関連リンパ組織
MAO	maximal acid output	最高酸分泌量
MAO	monoamine oxidase	モノアミンオキシダーゼ
MAOI	monoamine oxidase inhibitor	モノアミンオキシダーゼ阻害薬
MAP	mannitol-adenine-phosphate (solution)	マンニトール・アデニン・リン酸（液）
MAP	mean arterial pressure	平均動脈圧
MAP	microtubule-associated protein	微小管結合タンパク質
MAP	muscle action potential	筋活動電位
MAPCA	major aortopulmonary collateral artery	主要大動脈肺動脈側副血行路
MAPK	mitogen-activated protein kinase	マイトジェン活性化プロテインキナーゼ
MARTA	multiacting receptor targeted	多元受容体標的化抗精神薬

	antipsychotic	
MAS	manifest anxiety scale	顕在性不安尺度
MAS	meconium aspiration syndrome	胎便吸引症候群
MAST	military antichock trousers	ショックパンツ
MAST	multiple antigen simultaneous test	多項目抗原同時検査
MAT	multifocal atrial tachycardia	多源性心房頻拍
MBD	minimal brain dysfunction	微細脳機能障害
MBP	major basic protein	主要塩基性タンパク
MBP	myelin basic protein	ミエリン塩基性タンパク
MCA	middle cerebral artery	中大脳動脈
MCA	middle colic artery	中結腸動脈
MCAT	Medical College Admission Test	医科大学入学共通試験（米国）
MCD	minimal change disease	微小変化群
MCE	myocardial contrast echocardiography	心筋コントラストエコー法
MCF	macrophage chemotactic factor	マクロファージ走化因子
MCFG	micafungin	ミカファンギン
MCH	mean corpuscular hemoglobin	平均赤血球ヘモグロビン量
MCHC	mean corpuscular hemoglobin concentration	平均赤血球ヘモグロビン濃度
MCL	midclavicular line	鎖骨中央線
MCLS	mucocutaneous lymph node syndrome	皮膚粘膜リンパ節症候群
MCNS	minimal change nephrotic syndrome	微小変化型ネフローゼ症候群
MCNU	methylchloroethyl nitrosourea, ranimustine	ラニムスチン
MCOS	mucocutaneous ocular syndrome	粘膜皮膚眼症候群
MCP	metacarpophalangeal (joint)	中手指節（関節）
MCQ	multiple-choice question	多肢選択式試問
MCR	micronomicin	ミクロノマイシン
MCTD	mixed connective tissue disease	混合性結合組織病
MCV	mean corpuscular volume	平均赤血球容積
MCZ	miconazole	ミコナゾール
MD	Medicinae Doctor, Doctor of Medicine	医学士
Md	mendelevium	メンデレビウム
MDA	metaphyseal-diaphyseal angle	骨幹端・骨幹角
MDCT	multidetector-row computed to-	多列検出器型コンピュータ

	mography	断層撮影法
MDI	metered-dose inhaler	定量吸入器
MDI	methylenediphenyl diisocyanate	メチレンジフェニルジイソシアナート
MDM	midecamycin	ミデカマイシン
MDMA	methylenedioxymethamphetamine	メチレンジオキシメタンフェタミン
MDR	multidrug-resistant	多剤耐性
MDRP	multidrug-resistant *Pseudomonas aeruginosa*	多剤耐性緑膿菌
MDR-TB	multidrug-resistant tuberculosis	多剤耐性結核
MDS	myelodysplastic syndrome	骨髄異形成症候群
ME	medical electronics	医用電子工学
ME	medical engineering	医用工学
MEA	multiple endocrine adenomatosis	多発性内分泌腺腫症
MED	minimal effective dose	最小有効量
MED	minimal erythema dose	最小紅斑量
MEDLARS	Medical Literature Analysis and Retrieval System	医学文献分析検索システム
MEG	magnetoencephalography	脳磁図法
MELAS	mitochondrial myopathy, encephalopathy, lactic acidosis, and stroke-like episodes	ミトコンドリア脳筋症・乳酸アシドーシス・脳卒中様発作
MEN	multiple endocrine neoplasia	多発性内分泌腫瘍
MEPM	meropenem	メロペネム
meq	milliequivalent	ミリグラム当量
MERRF	myoclonus epilepsy with ragged red fibers	赤ぼろ線維を伴うミオクローヌスてんかん
MESA	microsurgical epididymal sperm aspiration	精巣上体精子回収法
MeSH	Medical Subject Headings	医学件名標目集
MESS	mangled extremity severity score	切断四肢重症度スコア
MF	mycosis fungoides	菌状息肉症
MFH	malignant fibrous histiocytoma	悪性線維性組織球腫
MFLX	moxifloxacin	モキシフロキサシン
MG	myasthenia gravis	重症筋無力症
Mg	magnesium	マグネシウム
mg	milligram	ミリグラム
MGUS	monoclonal gammopathy of uncertain significance	意義不明の単クローングロブリン血症
MHA	microangiopathic hemolytic ane-	微小血管症性溶血性貧血

	mia	
MHC	major histocompatibility complex	主要組織適合複合体
MI	mitral insufficiency	僧帽弁閉鎖不全
MI	myocardial infarction	心筋梗塞
mi	mile	マイル
MIBG	metaiodobenzylguanidine	メタヨードベンジルグアニジン
MIC	minimum inhibitory concentration	最小発育阻止濃度
MICS	minimally invasive cardiac surgery	低侵襲心臓外科手術
μg	microgram	マイクログラム
min	minute	分
MINO	minocycline	ミノサイクリン
MIT	macrophage migration inhibition test	マクロファージ遊走阻止試験
MIT	mitoxantrone	ミトキサントロン
MIT	monoiodotyrosine	モノヨードチロシン
ML	malignant lymphoma	悪性リンパ腫
MLC	mixed lymphocyte culture	リンパ球混合培養
MLD	metachromatic leukodystrophy	異染性白質ジストロフィー
MLD	minimal lethal dose	最小致死量
MLF	medial longitudinal fasciculus	内側縦束
MLNS	mucocutaneous lymph node syndrome	皮膚粘膜リンパ節症候群
MLR	mixed lymphocyte reaction	リンパ球混合培養反応
MM	malignant melanoma	悪性黒色腫
MM	multiple myeloma	多発性骨髄腫
mm	millimeter	ミリメートル
mm	muscularis mucosae	粘膜筋板
m.m.	motus manus	手動弁
MMC	mitomycin C	マイトマイシンC
MMCP	MCNU (ranimustine), melphalan, cyclophosphamide, prednisolone	ラニムスチン，メルファラン，シクロホスファミド，プレドニゾロン（化学療法）
MMEFR	maximal mid-expiratory flow rate	最大中間呼気流量率
MMF	mycophenolate mofetil	ミコフェノール酸モフェチル
MMI	thiamazole	チアマゾール
MMN	multifocal motor neuropathy	多巣性運動ニューロパチー
MMP-3	matrix metalloproteinase-3	マトリックスメタロプロテ

イナーゼ3

MMPI	Minnesota Multiphasic Personality Inventory	ミネソタ多面的性格検査
MMR	measles-mumps-rubella (vaccine)	麻疹・流行性耳下腺炎・風疹混合ワクチン
MMSC	methylmethionine sulfonium chloride	メチルメチオニンスルホニウムクロライド
MMSE	Mini-Mental State Examination	簡易認知機能検査
MMT	manual muscle test	徒手筋力テスト
MN	membranous nephropathy	膜性腎症
Mn	manganese	マンガン
MNMS	myonephropathic metabolic syndrome	筋・腎障害性代謝異常症候群
Mo	molybdenum	モリブデン
MODS	multiple-organ dysfunction syndrome	多臓器不全症候群
MODY	maturity-onset diabetes of youth	若年性成人発症型糖尿病
MOF	multiple organ failure	多臓器不全
mol	mole	モル
MOM	milk of magnesia	マグネシア乳
MOPP	mechlorethamine, Oncovin, procarbazine, prednisolone	ナイトロジェンマスタード, オンコビン（ビンクリスチン），プロカルバジン，プレドニゾロン（化学療法）
MP	melphalan, prednisolone	メルファラン，プレドニゾロン（化学療法）
6-MP	6-mercaptopurine	6-メルカプトプリン
MPA	medroxyprogesterone	メドロキシプロゲステロン
MPA	microscopic polyangiitis	顕微鏡的多発血管炎
MPD	maximum permissible dose	最大許容線量
MPD	myeloproliferative disease	骨髄増殖性疾患
MPGN	membranoproliferative glomerulonephritis	膜性増殖性糸球体腎炎
MPHA	mixed passive hemagglutination	混合受身赤血球凝集反応
MPI	myocardial perfusion imaging	心筋血流イメージング
MPO	myeloperoxidase	ミエロペルオキシダーゼ
MPO-ANCA	antineutrophil cytoplasmic myeloperoxidase antibody	抗好中球細胞質ミエロペルオキシダーゼ抗体
MPS	mucopolysaccharide	ムコ多糖類
MPS	mucopolysaccharidosis	ムコ多糖症
MPT	mepitiostane	メピチオスタン
MR	medical representative	医薬情報担当者
MR	mental retardation	精神遅滞

MR	mitral regurgitation	僧帽弁逆流
MRA	magnetic resonance angiography	磁気共鳴血管撮影法
MRCP	magnetic resonance cholangiopancreatography	磁気共鳴胆道膵管撮影法
MRD	minimal residual disease	微少残存病変
MRI	magnetic resonance imaging	磁気共鳴画像検査
mRNA	messenger ribonucleic acid	メッセンジャーRNA
MRS	magnetic resonance spectroscopy	磁気共鳴分光法
MRSA	methicillin-resistant *Staphylococcus aureus*	メチシリン耐性黄色ブドウ球菌
MRSE	methicillin-resistant *Staphylococcus epidermidis*	メチシリン耐性表皮ブドウ球菌
MS	Master of Science	理学修士
MS	mitral stenosis	僧帽弁狭窄
MS	morphine sulfate	硫酸モルヒネ
MS	multiple sclerosis	多発性硬化症
MS.	manuscriptum	原稿
MSA	multiple system atrophy	多系統萎縮症
MSBP	Munchausen syndrome by proxy	代理人によるミュンヒハウゼン症候群
MSC	mesenchymal stem cell	間葉系幹細胞
MSCT	multislice computed tomography	マルチスライスコンピュータ断層撮影法
MSH	melanocyte-stimulating hormone	メラニン細胞刺激ホルモン
MSI	microsatellite instability	マイクロサテライト不安定性
MSL	midsternal line	胸骨中線
MSLT	multiple sleep latency test	睡眠潜時反復検査
MSSA	methicillin-sensitive *Staphylococcus aureus*	メチシリン感受性黄色ブドウ球菌
MSUD	maple syrup urine disease	メープルシロップ尿症
MSUM	monosodium urate monohydrate	痛風結晶
MSW	medical social worker	医療ソーシャルワーカー
MT	medical technologist	臨床検査技師
Mt	meitnerium	マイトネリウム
MTA	medical technology assessment	医療技術評価
MTD	maximum tolerated dose	最大耐量
mtDNA	mitochondrial deoxyribonucleic acid	ミトコンドリアDNA
MTOC	microtubule organizing center	微小管形成中心
MTP	metatarsophalangeal (joint)	中足趾節(関節)

MTX	methotrexate	メトトレキセート
MUGA	multiple-gated acquisition scan	多関門集積スキャン
MUP	mupirocin	ムピロシン
MUS	medically unexplained symptoms	医学的に説明困難な症状
M-VAC	methotrexate, vinblastine, Adriamycin, cisplatin	メトトレキセート，ビンブラスチン，アドリアマイシン（ドキソルビシン），シスプラチン（化学療法）
MVP	mitomycin C, vindesine, cisplatin	マイトマイシン，ビンデシン，シスプラチン（化学療法）
MVP	mitral valve prolapse	僧帽弁逸脱症
MVR	mitral valve replacement	僧帽弁置換術
MVV	maximal voluntary ventilation	最大換気量
MW	molecular weight	分子量

N

N	nerve	神経
N	newton	ニュートン
N	nitrogen	窒素
N	normal	規定（溶液）
NA	nalidixic acid	ナリジクス酸
NA	neuraminidase, sialidase	ノイラミニダーゼ，シアリダーゼ
Na	natrium, sodium	ナトリウム
NAC	N-acetylcysteine	N-アセチルシステイン
NAD	nicotinamide adenine dinucleotide	ニコチンアミドアデニンジヌクレオチド
NAD	no appreciable disease	特記すべき疾患なし
NADH	reduced nicotinamide adenine dinucleotide	還元ニコチンアミドアデニンジヌクレオチド
NAFLD	nonalcoholic fatty liver disease	非アルコール性脂肪性肝疾患
NAG	N-acetylglucosaminidase	N-アセチルグルコサミニダーゼ
NAIT	neonatal alloimmune thrombocytopenia	新生児同種免疫血小板減少症
NANDA	North American Nursing Diagnosis Association	北米看護診断協会
NAP	nerve action potential	神経活動電位
NAP	neutrophil alkaline phosphatase	好中球アルカリホスファターゼ
NASH	nonalcoholic steatohepatitis	非アルコール性脂肪性肝炎

NaSSA	noradrenergic and specific serotonergic antidepressant	ノルアドレナリン作動性・特異的セロトニン作動性抗うつ薬
NAT	nucleic acid amplification technique	核酸増幅法
NB	nota bene	よく注意せよ
Nb	niobium	ニオブ
NBTE	nonbacterial thrombotic endocarditis	非細菌性血栓性心内膜炎
NCA	neurocirculatory asthenia	神経循環無力症
NCF	neutrophil chemotactic factor	好中球遊走因子
NCI	National Cancer Institute	米国国立癌研究所
NCPAP	nasal continuous positive airway pressure	経鼻的持続気道陽圧呼吸
NCT	noncontact tonometer	非接触眼圧計
NCV	nerve conduction velocity	神経伝導速度
NCV	noncholera vibrios	非コレラビブリオ
Nd	neodymium	ネオジム
n.d.	numerus digitorum	指数弁
Nd: YAG	neodymium: yttrium-aluminum-garnet (laser)	ネオジム・ヤグレーザー
NDFX	nadifloxacin	ナジフロキサシン
NDRI	norepinephrine-dopamine reuptake inhibitor	ノルエピネフリン・ドーパミン再取り込み阻害薬
NE	norepinephrine	ノルエピネフリン
Ne	neon	ネオン
NEC	necrotizing enterocolitis	壊死性腸炎
NEFA	non-esterified fatty acid	非エステル結合型脂肪酸,遊離脂肪酸
NERD	non-erosive reflux disease	非びらん性食道逆流症
NET	nerve excitability test	神経興奮性検査
NF-AT	nuclear factor-activated T cell	T細胞活性化因子
NFLX	norfloxacin	ノルフロキサシン
NG	nasogastric (tube)	経鼻胃 (管)
ng	nanogram	ナノグラム
NGF	nerve growth factor	神経成長因子
NGFR	nerve growth factor receptor	神経成長因子受容体
NGT	nogitecan	ノギテカン
NHL	non-Hodgkin lymphoma	非ホジキンリンパ腫
NHS	National Health Service	国民保健サービス (英国)
Ni	nickel	ニッケル
NIC	Nursing Interventions Classification	看護介入分類
NICU	neonatal intensive care unit	新生児集中治療室

NIDDM	non-insulin-dependent diabetes mellitus (type 2)	インスリン非依存性糖尿病（2型）
NIH	National Institutes of Health	米国国立衛生研究所
NIHF	nonimmune hydrops fetalis	非免疫性胎児水腫
NIHSS	NIH Stroke Scale	NIH 脳卒中尺度
NIPPV	noninvasive positive pressure ventilation	非侵襲的陽圧換気
NK	natural killer (cell)	ナチュラルキラー（細胞）
NLA	neuroleptanesthesia	ニューロレプト麻酔
nm	nanometer	ナノメーター
NMR	nuclear magnetic resonance	核磁気共鳴
NMS	neurally mediated syncope	神経調節性失神
NMS	neuroleptic malignant syndrome	神経遮断薬による悪性症候群
NMJ	neuromuscular junction	神経筋接合部
NMU	neuromuscular unit	神経筋単位
NNRTI	nonnucleoside reverse transcriptase inhibitor	非ヌクレオシド系逆転写酵素阻害薬
No	nobelium	ノーベリウム
NOC	Nursing Outcomes Classification	看護成果分類
NOMI	nonocclusive mesenteric ischemia	非閉塞性腸管虚血症
NOS	nitric oxide synthase	一酸化窒素合成酵素
NP	nurse practitioner	ナースプラクティショナー
NP	vinorelbine, cisplatin	ビノレルビン，シスプラチン（化学療法）
Np	neptunium	ネプツニウム
NPD	narcissistic personality disorder	自己愛性人格障害
NPH	normal-pressure hydrocephalus	正常圧水頭症
NPO	nil per os, nothing by mouth	絶食
NPT	nocturnal penile tumescence	夜間勃起
NPV	negative predictive value	陰性反応適中度
NRC	normal retinal correspondence	網膜正常対応
NREM	non-rapid eye movement (sleep)	ノンレム（睡眠）
NRFS	nonreassuring fetal status	胎児機能不全
NRTI	nucleoside reverse transcriptase inhibitor	ヌクレオシド系逆転写酵素阻害薬
NS	normal saline	生理的食塩水
NSAID	nonsteroidal antiinflammatory drug	非ステロイド系抗炎症薬
NSCLC	non-small cell lung carcinoma	非小細胞肺癌
NSE	neuron-specific enolase	神経特異性エノラーゼ

NSIP	nonspecific interstitial pneumonia	非特異性間質性肺炎
NSR	normal sinus rhythm	正常洞調律
NST	non-stress test	ノンストレステスト
NSTEMI	non-ST-elevation myocardial infarction	非ST上昇型心筋梗塞
NT	neutralization test	中和試験
5'-NT	5'-nucleotidase	5'-ヌクレオチダーゼ
NTA	natural thymocytotoxic autoantibody	自然胸腺細胞傷害自己抗体
NTG	nitroglycerin	ニトログリセリン
NTG	normal-tension glaucoma	正常眼圧緑内障
NTL	netilmicin	ネチルマイシン
NTM	nontuberculous mycobacterium	非結核性抗酸菌
NT-proBNP	N-terminal pro-brain natriuretic peptide	脳性ナトリウム利尿ペプチド前駆体N端フラグメント
N&V	nausea and vomiting	悪心・嘔吐
NVAF	non-valvular atrial fibrillation	非弁膜症性心房細動
NVE	native valve endocarditis	自己弁心内膜炎
NYD	not yet diagnosed	診断未確定
NYHA	New York Heart Association (classification)	ニューヨーク心臓協会（分類）
NYS	nystatin	ナイスタチン

O

O	oxygen	酸素
OA	ocular albinism	眼型白皮症
OA	osteoarthritis	骨関節炎，変形性骨関節症
OAB	overactive bladder	過活動膀胱
OAE	otoacoustic emission	耳音響放射
OAF	osteoclast activating factor	破骨細胞活性化因子
OALL	ossification of the anterior longitudinal ligament	前縦靱帯骨化症
OASDHI	Old Age, Survivors, Disability, and Health Insurance	老齢・遺族・障害者年金および健康保険（米国）
OB-GYN	obstetrics and gynecology	産婦人科
OC	oral contraceptives	経口避妊薬
OCA	oculocutaneous albinism	眼皮膚型白皮症
OCD	obsessive-compulsive disorder	強迫性障害
OCD	osteochondritis dissecans	離断性骨軟骨炎
OCP	oral contraceptive pill	経口避妊薬
OCT	optical coherence tomography	光学的干渉断層検査

OCT	oxytocin challenge test	オキシトシン負荷試験
OCV	opacitas corporis vitrei	硝子体混濁
OD	oculus dexter	右眼
OD	orthostatic dysregulation	起立性調節障害
ODD	oppositional defiant disorder	反抗挑戦性障害
ODN	ophthalmodynamometry	眼底血圧測定法
ODT	occlusive dressing technique	密封包帯法
OFD	oral-facial-digital syndrome	口・顔・指症候群
OFLX	ofloxacin	オフロキサシン
OGTT	oral glucose tolerance test	経口ブドウ糖負荷試験
OH	ocular hypertension	高眼圧症
Ω	ohm	オーム
OHCA	out-of-hospital cardiac arrest	院外心停止
17-OHCS	17-hydroxycorticosteroid	17-ヒドロキシコルチコステロイド
OHP	oxygen under high pressure	高圧酸素療法
OHSS	ovarian hyperstimulation syndrome	卵巣過剰刺激症候群
OI	osteogenesis imperfecta	骨形成不全症
oint	ointment	軟膏剤
OK-432	picibanil	ピシバニール
OKN	optokinetic nystagmus	視運動性眼振
OLF	ossification of ligamentum flavum	黄色靱帯骨化症
OM	osteomalacia	骨軟化症
OME	otitis media with effusion	滲出性中耳炎
OMI	old myocardial infarction	陳旧性心筋梗塞
o.m.	omni mane	毎朝
o.n.	omni nocte	毎晩
op. cit.	opere citato	前掲（引用）書中に
OPCA	olivopontocerebellar atrophy	オリーブ橋小脳萎縮症
OPD	outpatient department	外来
OPLL	ossification of the posterior longitudinal ligament	後縦靱帯骨化症
OPSI	overwhelming postsplenectomy infection	脾摘後重症感染症
OR	operating room	手術室
ORF	open reading frame	オープンリーディングフレーム
ORIF	open reduction and internal fixation	観血的整復内固定術
ORT	oral rehydration therapy	経口補液療法
ORT	orthoptist	視能訓練士
OS	overall survival	全生存期間

580 X章 略語集

OS	oculus sinister	左眼
OS	opening snap	開放音
Os	osmium	オスミウム
OSAS	obstructive sleep apnea syndrome	閉塞性睡眠時無呼吸症候群
OSCE	objective structured clinical examination	客観的臨床能力試験
osmol	osmole	オスモル
OT	occupational therapist	作業療法士
OT	old tuberculin	旧ツベルクリン
OTC	over-the-counter (drugs)	一般用医薬品
OTC	oxytetracycline	オキシテトラサイクリン
OTD	organ tolerance dose	臓器許容量
OU	oculus unitas	両眼
OU	oculus utrisque	各眼
OVLT	organum vasculosum of lamina terminalis	終板脈管器官
OYL	ossification of yellow ligament	黄色靱帯骨化症
oz	ounce	オンス

P

P	phosphorus	リン
PA	particle agglutination	粒子凝集反応
PA	pernicious anemia	悪性貧血
PA	piromidic acid	ピロミド酸
PA	posteroanterior	後前の
PA	pulmonary artery	肺動脈
Pa	pascal	パスカル
Pa	protactinium	プロトアクチニウム
P&A	percussion and auscultation	打聴診
PAC	plasma aldosterone concentration	血漿アルドステロン濃度
PAC	premature atrial contraction	心房性期外収縮
PACG	primary angle-closure glaucoma	原発閉塞隅角緑内障
$PaCO_2$	arterial carbon dioxide tension	動脈血炭酸ガス分圧
PACS	picture archiving and communication system	画像保管伝送システム
PACU	postanesthesia care unit	全身麻酔後回復室
PAD	peripheral arterial disease	末梢動脈疾患
PAF	platelet-activating factor	血小板活性化因子
PAG	pelvic arteriography	骨盤動脈造影法
PAGE	polyacrylamide gel electrophoresis	ポリアクリルアミド・ゲル電気泳動法

PAH	p-aminohippuric acid	パラアミノ馬尿酸
PAI-1	plasminogen activator inhibitor-1	プラスミノーゲンアクチベーターインヒビター1
PAM	2-pyridine aldoxime methiodide, pralidoxime	プラリドキシム
PAO	peak acid output	最大刺激時酸分泌量
PaO$_2$	arterial oxygen tension	動脈血酸素分圧
PAL	posterior axillary line	後腋窩線
PAP	primary atypical pneumonia	原発性異型肺炎
PAP	prostatic acid phosphatase	前立腺酸性ホスファターゼ
PAP	pulmonary alveolar proteinosis	肺胞タンパク症
PAP	pulmonary artery pressure	肺動脈圧
Pap	Papanicolaou (smear test)	パパニコロー（スミア試験）
PAPM/BP	panipenem/betamipron	パニペネム・ベタミプロン
PAPP-A	pregnancy-associated plasma protein A	妊娠関連血漿タンパクA
PAPVR	partial anomalous pulmonary venous return	部分的肺静脈還流異常
PAS	p-aminosalicylic acid	パラアミノサリチル酸
PAS	periodic acid-Schiff (stain)	過ヨウ素酸シッフ(染色)
PAS	peripheral anterior synechia	周辺虹彩部癒着
PAS-Ca	calcium paraaminosalicylate	パラアミノサリチル酸カルシウム
PASG	pneumatic antichock garment	ショックパンツ
PAT	paroxysmal atrial tachycardia	発作性心房頻拍
PAT	platelet aggregation test	血小板凝集試験
PAVF	pulmonary arteriovenous fistula	肺動静脈瘻
PAX	paired box (genes)	PAX遺伝子
PB	phenobarbital	フェノバルビタール
Pb	plumbum, lead	鉛
PBC	primary biliary cirrhosis	原発性胆汁性肝硬変
PBG	porphobilinogen	ポルフォビリノーゲン
PBI	protein-bound iodine	タンパク結合ヨウ素
PBL	peripheral blood lymphocyte	末梢血リンパ球
PBL	problem-based learning	問題基盤型学習
PBP	progressive bulbar palsy	進行性球麻痺
PBSCT	peripheral blood stem cell transplantation	末梢血幹細胞移植
PC	penicillin	ペニシリン
PC	phosphatidylcholine, lecithin	ホスファチジルコリン, レシチン
PC	phosphocreatine	クレアチンリン酸

PC	photocoagulation	光凝固術
PC	platelet concentrate	血小板濃縮液
PC	posterior chamber	後房
PC	protein C	プロテインC
p.c.	post cibum	食後
PCA	passive cutaneous anaphylaxis	受動皮膚アナフィラキシー
PCA	patient controlled analgesia	自己調節鎮痛法
PCA	posterior cerebral artery	後大脳動脈
PCB	polychlorinated biphenyl	ポリ塩素化ビフェニル
PCD	paraneoplastic cerebellar degeneration	傍腫瘍性小脳変性症
PCD	primary ciliary dyskinesia	原発性線毛機能不全
PCG	benzylpenicillin	ベンジルペニシリン
PCG	phonocardiography	心音図検査
PCH	paroxysmal cold hemoglobinuria	発作性寒冷血色素尿症
PCI	percutaneous coronary intervention	経皮的冠動脈インターベンション
PCIA	particle counting immunoassay	微粒子計数免疫凝集測定法
PCL	posterior cruciate ligament	後十字靱帯
PCOS	polycystic ovary syndrome	多嚢胞性卵巣症候群
PCP	pneumocystis pneumonia	ニューモシスチス肺炎
PCPS	percutaneous cardiopulmonay support	経皮的心肺補助装置
PCR	polymerase chain reaction	ポリメラーゼ連鎖反応
PCR	protein catabolic rate	タンパク異化率
PCS	portacaval shunt	門脈下大静脈吻合術
PCT	porphyria cutanea tarda	晩発性皮膚ポルフィリン症
PCT	postcoital test	性交後試験
PCT	procalcitonin	プロカルシトニン
PCU	palliative care unit	緩和ケア病棟
PCV	polypoidal choroidal vasculopathy	ポリープ状脈絡膜血管症
PCWP	pulmonary capillary wedge pressure	肺動脈楔入圧
PCZ	procarbazine	プロカルバジン
PD	pancreaticoduodenectomy	膵頭十二指腸切除術
PD	Parkinson disease	パーキンソン病
PD	peritoneal dialysis	腹膜透析
PD	prism diopter	プリズム曲光度
Pd	palladium	パラジウム
PDA	patent ductus arteriosus	動脈管開存症
PDD	pervasive developmental disorder	広汎性発達障害

PDE	phosphodiesterase	ホスホジエステラーゼ
PDEI	phosphodiesterase inhibitor	ホスホジエステラーゼ阻害薬
PDGF	platelet-derived growth factor	血小板由来増殖因子
PDGFR	platelet-derived growth factor receptor	血小板由来増殖因子受容体
PDR	Physicians' Desk Reference	医療用医薬品情報集（米国）
PDR	proliferative diabetic retinopathy	増殖糖尿病網膜症
PDS	placental dysfunction syndrome	胎盤機能不全症候群
PDT	photodynamic therapy	光力学療法
PE	physical examination	身体的検査，診察
PE	plasma exchange	血漿交換
PE	pulmonary embolism	肺塞栓症
PEA	phacoemulsification and aspiration	水晶体超音波乳化吸引術
PEA	pulseless electrical activity	電導収縮解離
PEDF	pigment epithelium-derived factor	色素上皮由来因子
PEEP	positive end-expiratory pressure	呼気終末陽圧呼吸
PEF	peak expiratory flow	最大呼気流量
PEFR	peak expiratory flow rate	最大呼気速度
PEG	percutaneous endoscopic gastrostomy	経皮的内視鏡下胃瘻造設術
PEG	pneumoencephalography	気脳造影法
PEG	polyethylene glycol	ポリエチレングリコール
PEG-IFN	peginterferon	ペグインターフェロン
PEIT	percutaneous ethanol injection therapy	経皮的エタノール注入療法
PEO	progressive external ophthalmoplegia	進行性外眼筋麻痺
PEP	peplomycin	ペプロマイシン
PET	polyethylene terephthalate	ポリエチレンテレフタレート
PET	positron emission tomography	陽電子放出断層撮影法
PFC	persistent fetal circulation	胎児循環遺残
PFD	patellofemoral dysfunction	膝蓋大腿機能障害
PFD	pancreatic function diagnostant	膵機能診断薬
PFI	physical fitness index	体力指数
PFM	peak flow meter	最大呼気流量計
PFO	patent foramen ovale	卵円孔開存

PFS	progression-free survival	無増悪生存期間
PFT	pulmonary function test	肺機能検査
PG	phosphatidylglycerol	ホスファチジルグリセロール
PG	prostaglandin	プロスタグランジン
pg	picogram	ピコグラム
PG I	pepsinogen I	ペプシノーゲン I
PG II	pepsinogen II	ペプシノーゲン II
PGD	preimplantation genetic diagnosis	着床前遺伝子診断
PGE	prostaglandin E	プロスタグランジン E
PGF	prostaglandin F	プロスタグランジン F
PGM	phosphoglucomutase	ホスホグルコムターゼ
PH	past history	既往歴
PH	pulmonary hypertension	肺高血圧症
Ph	Philadelphia chromosome	フィラデルフィア染色体
pH	pondus hydrogenii, hydrogen ion exponent	水素イオン指数
PHA	passive hemagglutination	受身赤血球凝集反応
PHA	pseudohypoaldosteronism	偽性低アルドステロン症
PHC	primary health care	プライマリヘルスケア
PhD	Philosophiae Doctor, Doctor of Philosophy	博士号（医学博士）
PHN	postherpetic neuralgia	帯状疱疹後神経痛
PHN	public health nurse	保健師
PHT	phenytoin	フェニトイン
PI	present illness	現病歴
PICA	posterior inferior cerebellar artery	後下小脳動脈
PICU	pediatric intensive care unit	小児集中治療室
PID	pelvic inflammatory disease	骨盤内炎症性疾患
PIE	pulmonary infiltration with eosinophilia	肺好酸球浸潤
PIH	pregnancy-induced hypertension	妊娠高血圧症候群
PIH	prolactin-inhibiting hormone	プロラクチン抑制ホルモン
PIN	prostatic intraepithelial neoplasia	前立腺上皮内腫瘍
PIP	proximal interphalangeal (joint)	近位指節間（関節）
PIPC	piperacillin	ピペラシリン
PITR	plasma iron turnover rate	血漿鉄交代率
PIVKA	protein induced by vitamin K absence	ビタミン K 欠乏時産生タンパク
PKD	polycystic kidney disease	多発性嚢胞腎疾患

PKP	penetrating keratoplasty	全層角膜移植術
PK/PD	pharmacokinetics/pharmacodynamics	薬物動態学・薬力学
PKU	phenylketonuria	フェニルケトン尿症
PL	preferential looking	選択視法
PL-B	polymyxin B	ポリミキシンB
PLIF	posterior lumbar interbody fusion	後方進入腰椎椎体間固定術
PLS	primary lateral sclerosis	原発性側索硬化症
PM	polymyositis	多発性筋炎
Pm	promethium	プロメチウム
pm	proper muscle layer	固有筋層
p.m.	post meridiem	午後
PMB	postmenopausal bleeding	閉経後出血
PMC	pseudomembranous colitis	偽膜性大腸炎
PMCT	percutaneous microwave coagulation therapy	経皮的マイクロ波凝固療法
PMD	progressive muscular dystrophy	進行性筋ジストロフィー
PMDA	Pharmaceuticals and Medical Devices Agency	医薬品医療機器総合機構
PMDD	premenstrual dysphoric disorder	月経前神経不安障害
PMI	point of maximal impulse	最強拍動点
PML	progressive multifocal leukoencephalopathy	進行性多巣性白質脳症
PMN	polymorphonuclear neutrophil	多形核好中球
PMPC	pivmecillinam	ピブメシリナム
PMR	pimaricin	ピマリシン
PMR	polymyalgia rheumatica	リウマチ性多発筋痛症
PMR	proportionate mortality rate	特定死因死亡比
PMS	post-marketing surveillance	市販後調査
PMS	premenstrual syndrome	月経前症候群
PN	parenteral nutrition	非経口栄養
PN	percutaneous nucleotomy	経皮的髄核摘出術
PN	periarteritis nodosa	結節性動脈周囲炎
PN	polyarteritis nodosa	結節性多発動脈炎
PND	paroxysmal nocturnal dyspnea	発作性夜間呼吸困難
PND	postnasal drip	後鼻漏
PNET	primitive neuroectodermal tumor	原始神経外胚葉性腫瘍
PNF	proprioceptive neuromuscular facilitation	固有受容体神経筋促進法
PNH	paroxysmal nocturnal hemo-	発作性夜間血色素尿症

		globinuria
PNL	percutaneous nephrolithotomy	経皮的腎切石術
PNPV	positive negative pressure ventilation	陽陰圧換気
PNS	paraneoplastic neurological syndrome	傍腫瘍性神経症候群
PNS	percutaneous nephrostomy	経皮腎瘻造設術
PNS	peripheral nervous system	末梢神経系
PO	per os, by mouth	経口的
PO	postoperative	手術後
Po	polonium	ポロニウム
POA	pancreatic oncofetal antigen	膵癌胎児抗原
POAG	primary open-angle glaucoma	原発開放隅角緑内障
POCT	point-of-care testing	臨床現場即時検査
POEMS	polyneuropathy, organomegaly, endocrinopathy, M-proteins, and skin changes	多発ニューロパチー, 臓器腫大, 内分泌障害, Mタンパク, 皮膚病変 (POEMS症候群)
POF	premature ovarian failure	早期卵巣不全
POMP	prednisone, Oncovin, methotrexate, Purinethol	プレドニゾン, オンコビン (ビンクリスチン), メトトレキセート, プリンソール (6-メルカプトプリン) (化学療法)
POMR	problem-oriented medical record	問題志向型診療録
POS	problem-oriented system	問題志向型システム
POTS	postural orthostatic tachycardia syndrome	体位性起立性頻拍症候群
PP	postprandial	食後の
PⅢP	procollagen-3-peptide	プロコラーゲンⅢペプチド
PPA	pipemidic acid	ピペミド酸
PPBS	postprandial blood sugar	食後血糖
PPD	purified protein derivative (tuberculin)	精製ツベルクリン
PPF	plasma protein fraction	血漿タンパク質分画
PPH	primary pulmonary hypertension	原発性肺高血圧症
PPH	procedure for prolapse and hemorrhoids	直腸脱・内痔核手術
PPHN	persistent pulmonary hypertension of the newborn	新生児遷延性肺高血圧症
PPI	patient package insert	添付文書
PPI	proton pump inhibitor	プロトンポンプ阻害薬

PPIC	plasmin-α plasmin inhibitor complex	プラスミン・αプラスミンインヒビター複合体
PPLO	pleuropneumonia-like organism	牛肺疫菌様微生物
ppm	parts per million	百万分率
PPO	platelet peroxidase	血小板ペルオキシダーゼ
PPO	preferred providers organization	医療者選択会員制団体健康保険（米国）
PPP	pustulosis palmaris et plantaris	掌蹠膿疱症
PPV	positive predictive value	陽性反応適中度
PR	partial remission	部分寛解
PR	pulmonic regurgitation	肺動脈弁閉鎖不全
PR	pulse rate	脈拍数
Pr	praseodymium	プラセオジム
PRA	plasma renin activity	血漿レニン活性
PRCA	pure red cell aplasia	赤芽球癆
PRE	progressive resistance (resistive) exercise	漸増抵抗運動
PRH	prolactin-releasing hormon	プロラクチン放出ホルモン
PRK	photorefractive keratectomy	レーザー屈折矯正角膜切除術
PRL	prolactin	プロラクチン
PRM	primidone	プリミドン
p.r.n.	pro re nata	必要時
PROM	premature rupture of membranes	早期破水
PRP	panretinal photocoagulation	汎網膜光凝固術
PRP	platelet-rich plasma	多血小板血漿
PRPP	phosphoribosyl pyrophosphate	ホスホリボシルピロリン酸
PRSP	penicillin-resistant *Streptococcus pneumoniae*	ペニシリン耐性肺炎球菌
PS	performance status	行動状況
PS	phosphatidylserine	ホスファチジルセリン
PS	post scriptum	追伸
PS	protein S	プロテインS
PS	pulmonary stenosis	肺動脈弁狭窄
PSA	prostate-specific antigen	前立腺特異抗原
PSAGN	poststreptococcal acute glomerulonephritis	溶連菌感染後急性糸球体腎炎
PSC	posterior subcapsular cataract	後嚢下白内障
PSC	primary sclerosing cholangitis	原発性硬化性胆管炎
PSD	post-stroke depression	脳卒中後うつ状態
PSD	psychosomatic disease	心身症
PSE	partial splenic embolization	部分的脾動脈塞栓術

PSEN	presenilin	プレセニリン
PSG	polysomnography	ポリソムノグラフィー
PSK	krestin	クレスチン
PSL	prednisolone	プレドニゾロン
PSM	psychosomatic medicine	心身医学
PSMA	progressive spinal muscular atrophy	進行性脊髄性筋萎縮症
PSP	phenolsulfonphthalein (test)	フェノールスルホンフタレイン (試験)
PSP	progressive supranuclear palsy	進行性核上性麻痺
PSPD	posterior superior pancreaticoduodenal artery	後上膵十二指腸動脈
PSS	progressive systemic sclerosis	進行性全身性強皮症
PSTI	pancreatic secretory trypsin inhibitor	膵分泌性トリプシンインヒビター
PSTT	placental site trophoblastic tumor	胎盤部トロホブラスト腫瘍
PSV	pressure-supported ventilation	圧補助換気
PSW	psychiatric social worker	精神科ソーシャルワーカー
PT	physical therapist	理学療法士
PT	physical therapy	理学療法
PT	prothrombin time	プロトロンビン時間
Pt	patient	患者
Pt	platinum	白金
pt	pint	パイント
PTA	percutaneous transluminal angioplasty	経皮経管血管形成術
PTA	peritonsillar abscess	扁桃周囲膿瘍
PTA	prior to admission	入院前
PTB	patellar tendon bearing	膝蓋腱支持
PTBD	percutaneous transhepatic biliary drainage	経皮経肝胆汁ドレナージ
PTC	percutaneous transhepatic cholangiography	経皮経肝胆管造影法
PTC	plasma thromboplastin component	血漿トロンボプラスチン成分
PTCA	percutaneous transluminal coronary angioplasty	経皮経管的冠動脈形成術
PTCR	percutaneous transluminal coronary recanalization	経皮経管的冠動脈再開通術
PTCS	percutaneous transhepatic cholangioscopy	経皮経肝胆道鏡検査
PTE	pulmonary thromboembolism	肺塞栓血栓症

PTGBD	percutaneous transhepatic gallbladder drainage	経皮経肝胆嚢ドレナージ
PTH	parathyroid hormone	副甲状腺ホルモン
PTH	post-transfusion hepatitis	輸血後肝炎
PTHrP	parathyroid hormone-related hormone	副甲状腺ホルモン関連タンパク質
PTK	phototherapeutic keratectomy	治療的レーザー角膜切除術
PTMC	percutaneous transvenous mitral commissurotomy	経皮経静脈的僧帽弁交連切開術
PTO	percutaneous transhepatic obliteration (of esophageal varices)	経皮経肝食道静脈瘤塞栓術
PTP	percutaneous transhepatic portography	経皮経肝門脈造影法
PTP	press through package	圧迫包装
PTR	patellar tendon reflex	膝蓋腱反射
PTRA	percutaneous transluminal renal angioplasty	経皮経管的腎動脈形成術
PTS	permanent threshold shift	永久閾値上昇
PTSD	posttraumatic stress disorder	心的外傷後ストレス障害
PTT	partial thromboplastin time	部分トロンボプラスチン時間
PTU	propylthiouracil	プロピルチオウラシル
PTX	paclitaxel	パクリタキセル
Pu	plutonium	プルトニウム
PUD	peptic ulcer disease	消化性潰瘍
PUFA	polyunsaturated fatty acid	多価不飽和脂肪酸
PUFX	prulifloxacin	プルリフロキサシン
pulv.	pulvis	散剤
PUVA	psoralen-ultraviolet A (therapy)	ソラレン長波長紫外線（療法）
PV	peritoneovenous (shunt)	腹腔・静脈（短絡術）
PV	polycythemia vera	真性多血症
PV	portal vein	門脈
PVB	cisplatin, vincristine, bleomycin	シスプラチン，ビンクリスチン，ブレオマイシン（化学療法）
PVC	polyvinyl chloride	ポリ塩化ビニル
PVC	premature ventricular contraction	心室性期外収縮
PVD	peripheral vascular disease	末梢血管疾患
PVD	posterior vitreous detachment	後部硝子体剥離
PVE	prosthetic valve endocarditis	人工弁心内膜炎
PVL	periventricular leukomalacia	脳室周囲白質軟化症

PVL	periventricular lucency	脳室周囲低吸収域
PWM	pokeweed mitogen	ポークウィードマイトジェン, アメリカヤマゴボウ有糸分裂原物質
PWS	Prader-Willi syndrome	プラダー・ウィリ症候群
PVP	polyvinylpyrroridone, povidone	ポリビニルピロリドン, ポビドン
PVP-I	povidone-iodine	ポビドンヨード
PVR	pressure-volume relation	圧容積関係
PVR	proliferative vitreoretinopathy	増殖硝子体網膜症
PVR	pulmonary vascular resistance	肺血管抵抗
PVS	persistent vegetative state	持続性植物状態
PVS	pigmented villonodular synovitis	色素性絨毛結節性滑膜炎
PWP	pulmonary wedge pressure	肺動脈楔入圧
PXE	pseudoxanthoma elasticum	弾力線維性仮性黄色腫
PZA	pyrazinamide	ピラジナミド
PZFX	pazufloxacin	パズフロキサシン

Q

q.	quaque	毎
QC	quality control	品質管理
QCT	quantitative computed tomography	定量的CT
q.d.	quaque die	毎日
QFT	QuantiFERON-TB (test)	クオンティフェロンTB (試験)
q.h.	quaque hora	毎時
q.i.d.	quater in die	1日4回
q.l.	quantum libet	所要量
QNS	quantity not sufficient	量不足
QOL	quality of life	生活の質
QPR/DPR	quinupristin/dalfopristin	キヌプリスチン・ダルホプリスチン
q.q.h.	quaque quarta hora	4時間毎
q.s.	quantum satis	十分量
q.s.	quantum sufficit	十分量
qt	quart	クオート
q.v.	quod vide	その項を見よ

R

R	right	右の
R	roentgen	レントゲン
RA	refractory anemia	不応性貧血

RA	rheumatoid arthritis	関節リウマチ
RA	right atrium	右心房
Ra	radium	ラジウム
RAD	right axis deviation	右軸偏位
rad	radian	ラジアン
RAE	right atrial enlargement	右房肥大
RAEB	refractory anemia with excess blasts	芽球増加性不応性貧血
RAHA	rheumatoid arthritis hemagglutination test	関節リウマチ赤血球凝集試験
RAI	radioactive iodine	放射性ヨウ素
RAIU	radioactive iodine uptake (test)	放射性ヨウ素摂取（試験）
RALS	remote-controlled afterloading system	遠隔操作後充填方式
RAO	right anterior oblique (position)	右前斜位，第1斜位
RAP	retinal arterial pressure	網膜動脈圧
RAPD	relative afferent pupillary defect	相対的瞳孔求心路障害
RAS	renal artery stenosis	腎動脈狭窄
RAS	renin-angiotensin system	レニン・アンギオテンシン系
RAS	Rokitansky-Aschoff sinus	ロキタンスキー・アショッフ洞
RAST	radioallergosorbent test	放射性アレルゲン吸着試験
Rb	rubidium	ルビジウム
RBBB	right bundle-branch block	右脚ブロック
RBC	red blood cell (count)	赤血球（数）
RBD	REM sleep behavior disorder	レム睡眠時行動障害
RBE	relative biological effectiveness	生物学的効果比
RBF	renal blood flow	腎血流量
RB-ILD	respiratory bronchiolitis-associated interstitial lung disease	呼吸細気管支炎関連間質性肺疾患
RBP	retinol-binding protein	レチノール結合タンパク質
RBT	rifabutin	リファブチン
RCA	right colic artery	右結腸動脈
RCA	right coronary artery	右冠動脈
RCC	renal cell carcinoma	腎細胞癌
RCC	rituximab, cladribine, cyclophosphamide	リツキシマブ，クラドリビン，シクロホスファミド（化学療法）
RCF	root canal filling	根管充填
R-CHOP	rituximab, cyclophosphamide, hydroxydaunorubicin, Oncovin,	リツキシマブ，シクロフォスファミド，塩酸ダウノル

	prednisone	ビシン（ドキソルビシン），オンコビン（ビンクリスチン），プレドニゾン（化学療法）
RCM	restrictive cardiomyopathy	拘束型心筋症
rcp	reciprocal translocation	相互転座
RCT	randomized controlled trial	ランダム化比較試験
RCT	root canal treatment	根管治療
RCU	red cell iron utilization	赤血球鉄利用率
R-CVP	rituximab, cyclophosphamide, vincristine, prednisolone	リツキシマブ，シクロホスファミド，ビンクリスチン，プレドニゾロン（化学療法）
RD	retinal detachment	網膜剥離
RDA	recommended dietary allowance	栄養基準量
RDS	respiratory distress syndrome	呼吸窮迫症候群
RDW	red cell distribution width	赤血球容積分布幅
Re	rhenium	レニウム
REA	radioenzymatic assay	放射酵素測定法
REM	rapid eye movement (sleep)	急速眼球運動（睡眠），レム（睡眠）
rem	roentgen-equivalent-man	レム
Rep.	repetatur	反復せよ
rep	roentgen-equivalent-physical	レプ
RER	rough endoplasmic reticulum	粗面小胞体
RES	reticuloendothelial system	細網内皮系
RF	rheumatic fever	リウマチ熱
RF	rheumatoid factor	リウマトイド因子
RF	rituximab, fludarabine	リツキシマブ，フルダラビン（化学療法）
Rf	rutherfordium	ラザホージウム
RFA	radiofrequency ablation	ラジオ波焼灼療法
RFLP	restriction fragment length polymorphism	制限酵素断片多型
RFP	rifampicin	リファンピシン
RFS	relapse-free survival	無再発生存期間
Rg	roentgenium	レントゲニウム
RGA	right gastric artery	右胃動脈
Rh	rhesus factor	Rh因子
Rh	rhodium	ロジウム
RHA	right hepatic artery	右肝動脈
RHD	rheumatic heart disease	リウマチ性心疾患
r-HuEPO	recombinant human erythro-	遺伝子組み換えヒトエリス

	poietin	ロポエチン
RI	radioisotope	放射性同位元素
RIA	radioimmunoassay	放射免疫測定法
RIBA	recombinant immunoblot assay	組み換え免疫ブロット法
RICE	rest, ice, compression, elevation	安静, 氷冷, 圧迫, 挙上
RIND	reversible ischemic neurological deficit	回復性虚血性神経脱落症候
RISA	radioiodinated human serum albumin	放射性ヨウ素標識ヒト血清アルブミン
RIST	radioimmunosorbent test	放射免疫吸着試験
RK	radial keratotomy	放射状角膜切開術
RKM	rokitamycin	ロキタマイシン
RLF	retrolental fibroplasia	後水晶体線維増殖症
RLL	right lower lobe	右下葉
RLQ	right lower quadrant	右下腹部
RLS	restless legs syndrome	下肢むずむず症候群
RML	right middle lobe	右中葉
RMSF	Rocky Mountain spotted fever	ロッキー山紅斑熱
RN	registered nurse	登録看護師, 看護師
Rn	radon	ラドン
RNA	ribonucleic acid	リボ核酸
RND	radical neck dissection	根治的頸部リンパ節郭清術
RNP	ribonucleoprotein	リボ核タンパク質
R/O	rule out	除外せよ
ROA	right occipitoanterior	第2頭位第1分類(胎位)
ROD	renal osteodystrophy	腎性骨異栄養症
ROI	region of interest	関心領域
ROM	range of motion	関節可動域
ROP	retinopathy of prematurity	未熟児網膜症
ROP	right occipitoposterior	第2頭位第2分類(胎位)
ROS	review of systems	系統別病歴
RP	relapsing polychondritis	再発性多発軟骨炎
RP	retinitis pigmentosa	網膜色素変性症
RP	retrograde pyelography	逆行性腎盂造影法
RPF	renal plasma flow	腎血漿流量
RPGN	rapidly progressive glomerulonephritis	急速進行性糸球体腎炎
RPHA	reversed passive hemagglutination	逆受身赤血球凝集反応
RPLND	retroperitoneal lymph node dissection	後腹膜リンパ節郭清
rpm	revolutions per min	毎分回転数

RPR	rapid plasma reagin (test)	血漿レアギン迅速試験
RQ	respiratory quotient	呼吸商
RR	recovery room	回復室
RR	respiratory rate	呼吸数
rRNA	ribosomal ribonucleic acid	リボソーム RNA
RSA	right sacroanterior	第2骨盤位第1分類（胎位）
RSB	right sternal border	胸骨右縁
RScA	right scapuloanterior	第2横位第1分類（胎位）
RScP	right scapuloposterior	第2横位第2分類（胎位）
RSD	reflex sympathetic dystrophy	反射性交感神経性ジストロフィー
RSI	repetitive strain (stress) injury	反復運動過多損傷
RSM	ribostamycin	リボスタマイシン
RSP	right sacroposterior	第2骨盤位第2分類（胎位）
RSU	resin sponge uptake	レジンスポンジ摂取率
RSV	respiratory syncytial virus	呼吸器合胞体ウイルス
RT	radiation therapy, radiotherapy	放射線治療
RTA	renal tubular acidosis	尿細管性アシドーシス
RTC	return to clinic	外来再診
RTF	resistance transfer factor	耐性伝達因子
rt-PA	recombinant tissue plasminogen activator	遺伝子組み換え組織プラスミノーゲン活性化因子
RT-PCR	reverse transcriptase-polymerase chain reaction	逆転写酵素・ポリメラーゼ連鎖反応
RTV	ritonavir	リトナビル
Ru	ruthenium	ルテニウム
RUG	Resource Utilization Groups	医療資源利用群（米国）
RUL	right upper lobe	右上葉
RUQ	right upper quadrant	右上腹部
RUT	rapid urease test	迅速ウレアーゼ試験
RV	residual volume	残気量
RV	right ventricle	右心室
RVAD	right ventricular assist device	右室補助装置
RVH	renovascular hypertension	腎血管性高血圧
RVH	right ventricular hypertrophy	右室肥大
RVP	right ventricular pressure	右室圧
RVT	renal vein thrombosis	腎静脈血栓症
Rx	recipe (take; prescription, treatment)	服用（処方, 治療）
RXM	roxithromycin	ロキシスロマイシン

S

S	sacral vertebra	仙椎
S	siemens	ジーメンス
S	sulfur	硫黄
S_1	first heart sound	第1心音
S_2	second heart sound	第2心音
S_3	third heart sound	第3心音
S_4	fourth heart sound	第4心音
s	second	秒
s	serosa	漿膜
s̄	sine	なしに
SA	sinoatrial	洞房の
SA	splenic artery	脾動脈
s.a.	secundum artem	常法に従って
SAA	serum amyloid A protein	血清アミロイドAタンパク質
SAB	selective aldosterone blocker	選択的アルドステロンブロッカー
SABA	short-acting inhaled β_2-agonist	短時間作用型吸入 β_2 刺激薬
SACT	sinoatrial conduction time	洞房伝導時間
SAD	seasonal affective disorder	季節的の感情障害
SADBE	squaric acid dibutylester	スクアラン酸ジブチルエステル
SADS	Schedule for Affective Disorders and Schizophrenia	感情障害ならびに統合失調症面接基準
SAH	subarachnoid hemorrhage	くも膜下出血
SALT	skin-associated lymphoid tissue	皮膚関連リンパ組織
SAM	systolic anterior motion	収縮期前方運動
SaO_2	arterial oxygen saturation	動脈血酸素飽和度
SARS	severe acute respiratory syndrome	重症急性呼吸器症候群
SAS	sleep apnea syndrome	睡眠時無呼吸症候群
SASP	salazosulfapyridine	サラゾスルファピリジン
Sb	stibium, antimony	アンチモン
SB	Sengstaken-Blakemore (tube)	ゼンクスターケン・ブレークモア（管）
SBE	subacute bacterial endocarditis	亜急性細菌性心内膜炎
SBMA	spinobulbar muscular atrophy	球脊髄性筋萎縮症
SBO	specific behavioral objective	行動目標
SBP	spontaneous bacterial peritonitis	特発性細菌性腹膜炎

SBP	systolic blood pressure	収縮期血圧
SBS	sinobronchial syndrome	副鼻腔気管支症候群
SBT/CPZ	sulbactam/cefoperazone	スルバクタム・セフォペラゾン
SBTPC	sultamicillin	スルタミシリン
Sc	scandium	スカンジウム
sc	subcutaneous	皮下
SCA	selective celiac angiography	選択的腹腔動脈造影法
SCA	superior cerebellar artery	上小脳動脈
SCC	squamous cell carcinoma	扁平上皮癌
SCD	spinocerebellar degeneration	脊髄小脳変性症
SCD	sudden cardiac death	心原性突然死
SCFE	slipped capital femoral epiphysis	大腿骨頭すべり症
SCI	spinal cord injury	脊髄損傷
SCID	severe combined immunodeficiency	重症複合免疫不全症
SCJ	squamocolumnar junction	扁平円柱上皮境界
SCLC	small cell lung carcinoma	小細胞肺癌
SCS	spinal cord stimulation	脊髄電気刺激法
SCT	sentence completion test	文章完成法検査
SCU	self-care unit	セルフケア・ユニット
SD	standard deviation	標準偏差
SDA	serotonin-dopamine antagonist	セロトニン・ドーパミン拮抗薬
SDA	specific dynamic action	特異動の作用
SDB	sleep-disordered breathing	睡眠時呼吸障害
SDH	subdural hematoma	硬膜下血腫
SDS	self-rating depression scale	自己評定抑うつ尺度
SE	standard error	標準誤差
Se	selenium	セレン
SEM	scanning electron microscope	走査型電子顕微鏡
SEM	systolic ejection murmur	収縮期駆出性雑音
SEP	somatosensory evoked potential	体性感覚誘発電位
SER	smooth endoplasmic reticulum	滑面小胞体
SERM	selective estrogen receptor modulator	選択的エストロゲン受容体修飾薬
SFA	superficial femoral artery	浅大腿動脈
SFD	small-for-dates (infant)	在胎期間軽小(児)
SFEMG	single fiber electromyogram	単一筋線維筋電図
SG	Swan-Ganz (catheter)	スワン・ガンツ（カテーテル）
Sg	seaborgium	シーボーギウム

SGA	small-for-gestational-age (infant)	在胎期間軽小(児)
SGB	stellate ganglion block	星状神経節ブロック
SH	social history	社会歴
SHBG	sex hormone-binding globulin	性ホルモン結合グロブリン
SHR	spontaneously hypertensive rat	高血圧自然発症ラット
SHS	supine hypotensive syndrome	仰臥位低血圧症候群
SI	Système International d'Unités	国際単位系
Si	silicon	ケイ素
SIADH	syndrome of inappropriate secretion of antidiuretic hormone	抗利尿ホルモン不適切分泌症候群
SIAS	Stroke Impairment Assessment Set	脳卒中障害評価法
SIDS	sudden infant death syndrome	乳児突然死症候群
Sig.	signetur	表示せよ
SIL	squamous intraepithelial lesion	扁平上皮内病変
SIMV	synchronized intermittent mandatory ventilation	同期式間欠的強制換気
SIRS	systemic inflammatory response syndrome	全身性炎症反応症候群
SISI	short increment sensitivity index	短時間増強感覚指数
SISO	sisomicin	シソマイシン
SjS	Sjögren syndrome	シェーグレン症候群
SKSD	streptokinase-streptodornase	ストレプトキナーゼ・ストレプトドルナーゼ
SL	sublingual	舌下の
s.l.	sensus luminis	光覚弁
SLB	short leg brace	短下肢装具
SLE	systemic lupus erythematosus	全身性エリテマトーデス
SLK	superior limbic keratoconjunctivitis	上輪部角結膜炎
SLO	scanning laser ophthalmoscope	走査レーザー検眼鏡
SLR	straight leg raising test	下肢伸展挙上テスト
SLTA	standard language test of aphasia	標準失語症検査
SM	streptomycin	ストレプトマイシン
Sm	samarium	サマリウム
sm	submucosa	粘膜下層
SMA	Sequential Multiple Analyzer	連続多項目分析装置
SMA	smooth muscle antibody	平滑筋抗体
SMA	spinal muscular atrophy	脊髄性筋萎縮症
SMA	superior mesenteric artery	上腸間膜動脈
SMBG	self-monitoring of blood glu-	血糖自己測定

	cose	
SMI	silent myocardial ischemia	無症候性心筋虚血
SMON	subacute myelo-opticoneuropathy	スモン，亜急性脊髄視神経障害
SMR	standardized mortality rate	標準化死亡比
SMV	superior mesenteric vein	上腸間膜静脈
SMX	sulfamethoxazole	スルファメトキサゾール
Sn	stannum, tin	スズ
SNAP	sensory nerve action potential	感覚神経活動電位
SND	striatonigral degeneration	線条体黒質変性症
SNE	subacute necrotizing encephalomyelopathy	亜急性壊死性脳脊髄症
SNGFR	single nephron glomerular filtration rate	単一ネフロン糸球体濾過量
SNOMED	Systematized Nomenclature of Medicine	国際医学用語コード
SNOP	Systematized Nomenclature of Pathology	国際病理学用語コード
SNP	single nucleotide polymorphism	一塩基多型
SNP	sodium nitroprusside	ニトロプルシドナトリウム
SNRI	serotonin-noradrenaline reuptake inhibitor	セロトニン・ノルアドレナリン再取り込み阻害薬
SNRT	sinus nodal reentry tachycardia	洞結節リエントリー頻拍
SNRT	sinus node recovery time	洞結節機能回復時間
SOAP	subjective data, objective data, assessment, plan	主観的データ，客観的データ，評価，計画
SOB	shortness of breath	息切れ
SOD	superoxide dismutase	スーパーオキシドジスムターゼ，活性酸素分解酵素
S-OIV	swine-origin influenza A virus	ブタ由来インフルエンザウイルスA型
SOL	space-occupying lesion	占拠性病変
SOMI	sternal-occipital-mandibular immobilizer	胸骨・後頭骨・下顎骨固定用装具
s.o.s.	si opus sit	必要時
SP	simulated patient	模擬患者
SP	simultaneous perception	同時視
SP	standardized patient	標準模擬患者
sp gr	specific gravity	比重
SP-A	surfactant protein A	サーファクタントプロテインA
SPAC	cytarabine ocfosfate	シタラビンオクホスファート

SPCA	serum prothrombin conversion accelerator	血清プロトロンビン転化促進因子
SPCM	spectinomicin	スペクチノマイシン
SP-D	surfactant protein D	サーファクタントプロテインD
SPE	streptococcal pyrogenic exotoxin	連鎖球菌発熱外毒素
SPECT	single photon emission computed tomography	単光子放出コンピュータ断層撮影法
SPEP	serum protein electrophoresis	血清タンパク電気泳動
SPF	specific pathogen-free (animal)	特定病原体不在（動物）
SPF	sun protection factor	日焼け止め指数
SPFX	sparfloxacin	スパルフロキサシン
SPG	sizofiran	シゾフィラン
SPI	serine protease inhibitor	セリンプロテアーゼインヒビター
SPK	superficial punctate keratitis	点状表層角膜炎
SPM	spiramycin	スピラマイシン
SpO_2	oxygen saturation by pulse oximetry	経皮の動脈血酸素飽和度
SQUID	superconducting quantum interference device	超伝導量子干渉素子
Sr	strontium	ストロンチウム
SRA	superior rectal artery	上直腸動脈
SRC	scleroderma renal crisis	強皮症腎クリーゼ
SRID	single radial immunodiffusion	一元放射免疫拡散法
SRS	stereotactic radiosurgery	定位手術的照射
SRS-A	slow reacting substance of anaphylaxis	遅反応性アナフィラキシー物質
SRT	speech reception threshold test	語音聴取閾値検査
SRT	stereotactic radiotherapy	定位放射線治療
ss.	semis	半分
SSCP	single-strand conformational polymorphism	単一鎖形体的多型
SSD	source-skin distance	線源皮膚間距離
SSE	soapsuds enema	石鹸浣腸
SSI	surgical site infection	手術部位感染
SSKI	saturated solution of potassium iodide	ヨウ化カリウム溶液
SSLP	simple sequence length polymorphism	単純配列長多型
SSPE	subacute sclerosing panencephalitis	亜急性硬化性全脳炎
SSRI	selective serotonin reuptake	選択的セロトニン再取り込

600　X章　略語集

	inhibitor		み阻害薬
SSS	sick sinus syndrome		洞機能不全症候群
SSSS	staphylococcal scalded skin syndrome		ブドウ球菌性熱傷様皮膚症候群
SST	social skills training		社会生活技能訓練
ST	speech therapist		言語療法士
ST	sulfamethoxazole/trimethoprim		スルファメトキサゾール・トリメトプリム
STA	superficial temporal artery		浅側頭動脈
STA-MCA	superficial temporal artery – middle cerebral artery (anastomosis)		浅側頭動脈・中大脳動脈（吻合術）
stat.	statim		直ちに
STD	sexually transmitted disease		性感染症
STEMI	ST-elevation myocardial infarction		ST上昇型心筋梗塞
STFX	sitafloxacin		シタフロキサシン
STI	stereotactic irradiation		定位放射線照射
STI	systolic time intervals		収縮時間
STR	short tandem repeat		短縦列反復
STS	serologic test for syphilis		梅毒血清検査
SU	sulfonylurea		スルホニルウレア
SUD	sudden unexplained death		原因不明突然死
SUZI	subzonal insemination		囲卵腔内精子注入法
SV	selective vagotomy		選択的迷走神経切離術
SV	splenic vein		脾静脈
SV	stroke volume		1回心拍出量
Sv	sievert		シーベルト
SVC	superior vena cava		上大静脈
SVCS	superior vena cava syndrome		上大静脈症候群
SVI	slow virus infection		遅発性ウイルス感染症
SVR	sustained virological response		持続性ウイルス陰性化
SVR	systemic vascular resistance		体血管抵抗
SVT	supraventricular tachycardia		上室性頻拍
SWS	slow wave sleep		徐波睡眠
Sx	symptom		症状
syr.	syrupus		シロップ

T

T	tesla		テスラ
T	thoracic vertebra		胸椎
T	thymine		チミン
T_3	triiodothyronine		トリヨードサイロニン
T_4	thyroxine		サイロキシン

TA	temporal arteritis	側頭動脈炎
TA	transactional analysis	交流分析
TA	tricuspid atresia	三尖弁閉鎖症
Ta	tantalum	タンタル
T&A	tonsillectomy and adenoidectomy	扁桃アデノイド手術
TAA	thoracic aortic aneurysm	胸部大動脈瘤
TAA	tumor-associated antigen	腫瘍関連抗原
TAC	docetaxel, doxorubicin, cyclophosphamide	ドセタキセル，ドキソルビシン，シクロホスファミド（化学療法）
TACE	transcatheter arterial chemoembolization	経カテーテル動脈化学塞栓術
TACO	transfusion-associated circulatory overload	輸血関連循環過負荷
TAE	transcatheter arterial embolization	経カテーテル動脈塞栓術
TAH	total abdominal hysterectomy	腹式子宮全摘術
TAH	total artificial heart	完全置換型人工心臓
TAI	transhepatic arterial infusion	肝動脈注入療法
TAM	tamoxifen	タモキシフェン
TAM	transient abnormal myelopoiesis	一過性異常骨髄造血
TAO	thromboangiitis obliterans	閉塞性血栓血管炎
TAP	paclitaxel, doxorubicin, cisplatin	パクリタキセル，ドキソルビシン，シスプラチン（化学療法）
TAPC	talampicillin	タランピシリン
TAPVR	total anomalous pulmonary venous return	全肺静脈還流異常
TARC	thymus and activation-regulated chemokine	白血球走化性ケモカイン
TAT	thrombin-antithrombin Ⅲ complex	トロンビン・アンチトロンビンⅢ複合体
TAZ/PIPC	tazobactam/piperacillin	タゾバクタム・ピペラシリン
TB	tuberculosis	結核
Tb	terbium	テルビウム
TBA	total bile acid	総胆汁酸
TBAB	transbronchial aspiration biopsy	経気管支吸引生検
TBB	transbronchial biopsy	経気管支生検
TBG	thyroxin-binding globulin	サイロキシン結合グロブリン

X章　略語集

TBI	total body irradiation	全身放射線照射
TBI	traumatic brain injury	外傷性脳損傷
TBII	thyrotropin-binding inhibitory immunoglobulin	甲状腺刺激ホルモン結合阻害免疫グロブリン
TBLB	transbronchial lung biopsy	経気管支肺生検
TBPM-PI	tebipenem pivoxil	テビペネムピボキシル
TBV	total blood volume	全血液量
TBW	total body water	体内総水分量
TC	paclitaxel, carboplatin	パクリタキセル，カルボプラチン（化学療法）
TC	tetracycline	テトラサイクリン
TC	total cholesterol	総コレステロール
Tc	technetium	テクネチウム
T&C	type and cross-match	血液型と交差適合試験
TCA	tricarboxylic acid (cycle)	トリカルボン酸（回路），TCA回路
TCA	tricyclic antidepressant	三環系抗うつ薬
TCD	transcranial Doppler ultrasonography	経頭蓋ドプラ超音波診断法
TCGF	T-cell growth factor	T細胞増殖因子
TCP	transcutaneous pacing	経皮的ペーシング
TDF	tenofovir disoproxil fumarate	テノホビルジソプロキシルフマル酸
TDI	toluene diisocyanate	トルエンジイソシアネート
TDM	therapeutic drug monitoring	治療薬濃度測定
TDP	torsade de pointes	トルサードドポアンツ
TDS	thiamine disulfide	チアミンジスルフィド
TdT	terminal deoxynucleotidyl transferase	末端デオキシヌクレオチド転移酵素
Te	tellurium	テルル
TEA	thromboendarterectomy	血栓内膜切除術
TEE	transesophageal echocardiography	経食道心エコー検査
TEF	tracheoesophageal fistula	気管食道瘻
TEG	thromboelastogram	トロンボエラストグラム，血栓弾性描写図
TEIC	teicoplanin	テイコプラニン
TEL	telithromycin	テリスロマイシン
TEN	toxic epidermal necrolysis	中毒性表皮壊死症
TENS	transcutaneous electrical nerve stimulation	経皮的電気神経刺激法
TERMS	Thalidomide Education and Risk Management System	サリドマイド製剤安全管理手順
TESE	testicular sperm extraction	精巣内精子回収法

TESPA	triethylenethiophosphoramide, thiotepa	チオテパ
TEV	talipes equinovarus	内反足
TEVAR	thoracic endovascular aortic repair	胸部大動脈瘤ステントグラフト内挿術
TEWL	transepidermal water loss	経表皮水分喪失
Tf	transferrin	トランスフェリン
TFCC	triangular fibrocartilage complex	三角線維軟骨複合体
TFLX	tosufloxacin	トスフロキサシン
TFT	thyroid function test	甲状腺機能検査
TG	triglyceride	トリグリセリド
Tg	thyroglobulin	サイログロブリン
TGA	transient global amnesia	一過性全健忘
TgAb	antithyroglobulin antibody	抗サイログロブリン抗体
TGF	tegafur	テガフール
TGF	therapeutic gain factor	治療利得係数
TGF	transforming growth factor	形質転換成長因子
Th	thorium	トリウム
THA	total hip arthroplasty	股関節全置換術
THC	tetrahydrocannabinol	テトラヒドロカンナビノール
THP	4'-O-tetrahydropyranyldoxorubicin, pirarubicin	ピラルビシン
THR	total hip replacement	股関節全置換術
Ti	titanium	チタン
TIA	transient ischemic attack	一過性脳虚血発作
TIA	turbidimetric immunoassay	免疫比濁法
TIBC	total iron-binding capacity	総鉄結合能
t.i.d.	ter in die	1日3回
TIG	tetanus immune globulin	破傷風免疫グロブリン
TIL	tumor-infiltrating lymphocyte	腫瘍浸潤リンパ球
TIN	tubulointerstitial nephritis	尿細管間質性腎炎
TIPS	transjugular intrahepatic portosystemic shunt	経頸静脈性肝内門脈体循環短絡
TKA	total knee arthroplasty	膝関節全置換術
TKD	tokodynamometer	陣痛計
TKR	total knee replacement	膝関節全置換術
Tl	thallium	タリウム
TLC	thin-layer chromatography	薄層クロマトグラフィー
TLC	total lung capacity	全肺気量
TLC	total lymphocyte count	総リンパ球数
Tm	thulium	ツリウム
TM	thrombomodulin	トロンボモジュリン

TMA	thrombotic microangiopathy	血栓性微小血管症
TMJ	temporomandibular joint	顎関節
TMP	trimethoprim	トリメトプリム
TNF	tumor necrosis factor	腫瘍壊死因子
TNI	total nodal irradiation	全リンパ節照射
TNM	tumor, node, metastasis (classification)	腫瘍, リンパ節, 転移 (悪性腫瘍臨床国際分類)
TNR	tonic neck reflex	緊張性頚反射
TOB	tobramycin	トブラマイシン
TOEFL	Test of English as a Foreign Language	外国語としての英語テスト
TOEIC	Test of English for International Communication	国際コミュニケーション英語能力テスト
TOF	tetralogy of Fallot	ファロー四徴症
TOR	toremifene	トレミフェン
TORCH	toxoplasmosis, other agents, rubella, cytomegalovirus, herpes simplex (syndrome)	トーチ (症候群)
torr	torricelli	トール
TOS	thoracic outlet syndrome	胸郭出口症候群
TP	paclitaxel, cisplatin	パクリタキセル, シスプラチン (化学療法)
TP	thiamphenicol	チアンフェニコール
TP	total protein	総タンパク
TPA	tissue polypeptide antigen	組織ポリペプチド抗原
t-PA	tissue plasminogen activator	組織プラスミノーゲン活性化因子
TPHA	*Treponema pallidum* hemagglutination	梅毒トレポネーマ赤血球凝集 (試験)
TPI	*Treponema pallidum* immobilization	梅毒トレポネーマ運動制御 (試験)
TPN	total parenteral nutrition	完全静脈栄養
TPOAb	anti-thyroid peroxidase antibody	抗甲状腺ペルオキシダーゼ抗体
TPR	temperature, pulse, respiration	体温, 脈拍, 呼吸
TPR	total peripheral resistance	全末梢血管抵抗
TR	tricuspid regurgitation	三尖弁閉鎖不全
TRAb	thyroid-stimulating hormone receptor antibody	甲状腺刺激ホルモン受容体抗体
TRALI	transfusion-related acute lung injury	輸血関連急性肺傷害
TRAPS	TNF-receptor-associated periodic syndrome	腫瘍壊死因子受容体関連周期熱症候群
TRH	thyrotropin-releasing hormone	甲状腺刺激ホルモン放出ホ

		ルモン
TRIC	trachoma-inclusion conjunctivitis	トラコーマ封入体結膜炎
tRNA	transfer ribonucleic acid	転移 RNA
TRT	tinnitus retraining therapy	耳鳴再訓練療法
TRUS	transrectal ultrasonography	経直腸的超音波検査
TS	tricuspid stenosis	三尖弁狭窄
TSA	tumor-specific antigen	腫瘍特異抗原
TSD	Tay-Sachs disease	テイ・サックス病
TSF	triceps skinfold	上腕三頭筋皮下脂肪
TSH	thyroid stimulating hormone	甲状腺刺激ホルモン
TSI	thyroid stimulating immunoglobulin	甲状腺刺激免疫グロブリン
TSLS	toxic shock-like syndrome	毒素性ショック様症候群
TSS	toxic shock syndrome	毒素性ショック症候群
TSS	transsphenoidal surgery	経蝶形骨洞手術
TSST	toxic shock syndrome toxin	毒素性ショック症候群毒素
TSTA	tumor-specific transplantation antigen	腫瘍特異移植抗原
TT	thrombin time	トロンビン時間
TT	thrombotest	トロンボテスト
TTAB	transtracheal aspiration biopsy	経気管吸引生検
TTD	temporary threshold decay test	一過性閾値減衰試験
TTD	trichothiodystrophy	裂毛症
TTN	transient tachypnea of the newborn	新生児一過性多呼吸
TTP	thrombotic thrombocytopenic purpura	血栓性血小板減少性紫斑病
TTS	temporary threshold shift	一過性閾値変動
TTT	thymol turbidity test	チモール混濁試験
TTTS	twin-twin transfusion syndrome	双胎間輸血症候群
TUL	transurethral lithotripsy	経尿道的砕石術
TULIP	transurethral laser-induced prostatectomy	経尿道的レーザー前立腺切除術
TUMT	transurethral microwave thermotherapy	経尿道的極超短波温熱療法
TUNA	transurethral needle ablation	経尿道的針焼灼療法
TUR	transurethral resection	経尿道的切除術
TURBT	transurethral resection of bladder tumor	経尿道的膀胱腫瘍切除術
TURP	transurethral resection of the prostate	経尿道的前立腺切除術
TUVP	transurethral vaporization of	経尿道的前立腺蒸散術

	the prostate	
TV	tidal volume	1回換気量
TVH	total vaginal hysterectomy	膣式子宮全摘術
TVM	tension-free vaginal mesh	テンションフリー腟メッシュ
TX	thromboxane	トロンボキサン
TXT	Taxotere, docetaxel	ドセタキセル
TZD	thiazolidinedione	チアゾリジンジオン

U

U	uranium	ウラン
u	atomic mass unit	原子質量単位
UA	uric acid	尿酸
UA	urinalysis	検尿
UBM	ultrasound biomicroscopy	超音波生体顕微鏡
UBT	urea breath test	尿素呼気試験
UC	ulcerative colitis	潰瘍性大腸炎
UCG	ultrasonic cardiography	心エコー検査
UCHD	usual childhood diseases	通常の小児期疾患
UDCA	ursodeoxycholic acid	ウルソデオキシコール酸
UDP	uridine diphosphate	ウリジンニリン酸
UDS	urodynamic study	尿流動態検査法
UES	upper esophageal sphincter	上部食道括約筋
UFR	ultrafiltration rate	限外濾過率
UFT	tegafur-uracil	テガフール・ウラシル
UGIS	upper gastrointestinal series	上部消化管造影法
UIBC	unsaturated iron-binding capacity	不飽和鉄結合能
UIC	uninhibited contraction	無抑制収縮
UICC	Unio Internationalis Contra Cancrum	国際対癌連合
UIP	usual interstitial pneumonia	通常型間質性肺炎
UK	urokinase	ウロキナーゼ
UMLS	Unified Medical Language System	統合医学用語システム
UMN	upper motor neuron	上位運動ニューロン
UMP	uridine monophosphate	ウリジン一リン酸
ung.	unguentum	軟膏
UPI	uteroplacental insufficiency	子宮胎盤機能不全
UPJ	ureteropelvic junction	尿管腎盂移行部
UPPP	uvulopalatopharyngoplasty	口蓋垂軟口蓋咽頭形成術
URI	upper respiratory tract infection	上気道感染症
US	ultrasonography, ultrasound	超音波検査法

USMLE	United States Medical Licensing Examination	米国医師免許試験
USP	United States Pharmacopeia	米国薬局方
ut dict.	ut dictum	指示通り
UTI	urinary tract infection	尿路感染症
UTP	uridine triphosphate	ウリジン三リン酸
UV	ultraviolet	紫外線
UVA	ultraviolet A	長波長紫外線
UVB	ultraviolet B	中波長紫外線
UVC	ultraviolet C	短波長紫外線
UVJ	ureterovesical junction	尿管膀胱移行部

V

V	vanadium	バナジウム
V	volt	ボルト
V	vein	静脈
v.	vide	見よ，参照せよ
VA	vertebral artery	椎骨動脈
VA	visual acuity	視力
VAB	veno-arterial bypass	静動脈バイパス
VAC	vincristine, actinomycin D, cyclophosphamide	ビンクリスチン，アクチノマイシンD，シクロホスファミド(化学療法)
VACV	valacyclovir hydrochloride	バラシクロビル塩酸塩
VAD	ventricular assist device	心室補助装置，補助人工心臓
VAD	vincristine, doxorubicin, dexamethasone	ビンクリスチン，ドキソルビシン，デキサメタゾン(化学療法)
VAG	vertebral angiography	椎骨動脈造影法
VAHS	virus-associated hemophagocytic syndrome	ウイルス関連血球貪食症候群
VAMP	vincristine, amethopterin, 6-mercaptopurine, prednisolone	ビンクリスチン，アメトプテリン(メトトレキサート)，6-メルカプトプリン，プレドニゾロン(化学療法)
VAP	variant angina pectoris	異型狭心症
VAP	ventilator-associated pneumonia	人工呼吸器関連肺炎
VAPP	vaccine-associated paralytic poliomyelitis	ワクチン関連麻痺性ポリオ
VAS	ventricular assist system	補助人工心臓システム
VAS	visual analog scale	視覚的評価尺度
VAT	ventricular activation time	心室興奮時間

VATS	video-assisted thoracoscopic surgery	ビデオ下胸腔鏡手術
VBAC	vaginal birth after cesarean section	帝王切開後経腟分娩
VBG	vertical banded gastroplasty	垂直遮断式胃形成術
VBI	vertebrobasilar insufficiency	椎骨脳底動脈循環不全
VBMCP	vincristine, BCNU, melphalan, cyclophosphamide, prednisolone	ビンクリスチン，カルムスチン，メルファラン，シクロホスファミド，プレドニゾロン(化学療法)
VC	vital capacity	肺活量
VCA	viral capsid antigen	ウイルスカプシド抗原
VCG	vectorcardiogram	ベクトル心電図
VCM	vancomycin	バンコマイシン
VCR	vincristine	ビンクリスチン
VCUG	voiding cystourethrography	排尿時膀胱尿道造影法
VD	venereal disease	性病
VDDR	vitamin D-dependent rickets	ビタミンD依存性くる病
VDRL	Venereal Disease Research Laboratory (test)	性病研究所梅毒血清反応
VDS	vindesine	ビンデシン
VDT	visual display terminal	端末表示装置
VEE	Venezuelan equine encephalitis	ベネズエラウマ脳炎
VEGF	vascular endothelial growth factor	血管内皮増殖因子
VEMP	vincristine, Endoxan, 6-mercaptopurine, prednisolone	ビンクリスチン，シクロホスファミド，6-メルカプトプリン，プレドニゾロン(化学療法)
VEP	visual evoked potential	視覚誘発電位
VEPA	vincristine, Endoxan, prednisolone, adriamycin	ビンクリスチン，シクロホスファミド，プレドニゾロン，ドキソルビシン(化学療法)
VF	ventricular fibrillation	心室細動
VF	visual field	視野
VFP	vitreous fluorophotometry	硝子体蛍光測定法
VHDL	very-high-density lipoprotein	超高比重リポタンパク
VHL	von Hippel-Lindau disease	フォンヒッペル・リンダウ病
VIG	vaccinia immune globulin	ワクシニア免疫グロブリン
VIP	vasoactive intestinal polypeptide	血管作動性腸管ポリペプチド

viz.	videlicet	すなわち
VLAP	visual laser ablation of prostate	直視下レーザー前立腺切除術
VLB	vinblastine	ビンブラスチン
VLBW	very low birth weight	極低出生体重
VLCD	very low calorie diet	超低カロリー食
VLDL	very-low-density lipoprotein	超低比重リポタンパク
VMA	vanillylmandelic acid	バニリルマンデル酸
VNR	vinorelbine	ビノレルビン
VNS	vagal nerve stimulation	迷走神経刺激法
VNTR	variable number tandem repeats	高変異反復列
VO	verbal order	口頭指示
VOD	veno-occlusive disease	肝静脈閉塞性疾患
VP	variegate porphyria	異型ポルフィリン症
VP	ventriculoperitoneal (shunt)	脳室腹腔（シャント）
VP-16	etoposide	エトポシド
VPA	valproic acid	バルプロ酸
VPC	ventricular premature complex (contraction)	心室性期外収縮
VPF	vascular permeability factor	血管透過性因子
VRCZ	voriconazole	ボリコナゾール
VRE	vancomycin-resistant *Enterococcus*	バンコマイシン耐性腸球菌
VRSA	vancomycin-resistant *Staphylococcus aureus*	バンコマイシン耐性黄色ブドウ球菌
VS	vital signs	生命徴候
vs.	versus	対
VSA	vasospastic angina	血管攣縮性狭心症
VSD	ventricular septal defect	心室中隔欠損
VT	ventricular tachycardia	心室性頻拍
VT	verotoxin	ベロ毒素
VTEC	Verotoxin-producing *Escherichia coli*	ベロ毒素産生性大腸菌
VUR	vesicoureteral reflux	膀胱尿管逆流
VVR	vasovagal reflex	血管迷走神経反射
vWD	von Willebrand disease	フォンウィルブランド病
vWF	von Willebrand factor	フォンウィルブランド因子
VZIG	varicella-zoster immune globulin	水痘帯状疱疹免疫グロブリン
VZV	varicella-zoster virus	水痘帯状疱疹ウイルス

W

W	wolfram, tungsten	タングステン
W	watt	ワット
WAD	whiplash-associated disorders	むち打ち損傷関連障害
WAIS	Wechsler Adult Intelligence Scale	ウェクスラー成人用知能検査
WaR	Wassermann reaction	ワッセルマン反応
WAS	Wiskott-Aldrich syndrome	ウィスコット・アルドリッチ症候群
Wb	weber	ウェーバー
WB	Western blotting	ウェスタンブロット法
WB	whole blood	全血
WBC	white blood cell	白血球
WBGT	wet-bulb globe temperature index	湿球黒球温度指数
WD	well-developed	発育良好な
WDHA	watery diarrhea-hypokalemia-achlorhydria syndrome	WDHA症候群
WEE	Western equine encephalitis	西部ウマ脳炎
WHO	World Health Organization	世界保健機関
WHO	wrist-hand orthosis	手関節手指装具
WISC	Wechsler Intelligence Scale for Children	ウェクスラー児童用知能検査
WLRT	well leg raising test	交叉下肢伸展挙上試験
WN	well-nourished	栄養良好な
WNL	within normal limits	正常範囲内
WPW	Wolff-Parkinson-White (syndrome)	ウォルフ-パーキンソン-ホワイト(症候群)
wt	weight	体重

X

X	xanthosine	キサントシン
Xe	xenon	キセノン
XLP	X-linked lymphoproliferative syndrome	伴性リンパ増殖症候群
XP	exophoria	外斜位
XP	xeroderma pigmentosum	色素性乾皮症
XT	exotropia	外斜視

Y

Y	yttrium	イットリウム
YAM	young adult mean	若年成人平均値
Yb	ytterbium	イッテルビウム

yd	yard	ヤード
Y-G	Yatabe-Guilford (Personality Inventory)	矢田部・ギルフォード（性格検査）

Z

ZES	Zollinger-Ellison syndrome	ゾリンジャー・エリソン症候群
ZIFT	zygote intrafallopian transfer	受精卵卵管内移植
ZIG	zoster immune globulin	帯状ヘルペス免疫グロブリン
Zn	zinc	亜鉛
ZNS	zonisamide	ゾニサミド
Zr	zirconium	ジルコニウム
ZST	zinc sulfate turbidity test	硫酸亜鉛混濁試験

索引

- 日本語索引……………614
- 英語索引………………701
- 冠名用語索引…………825
- 薬剤商品索引…………833

日本語索引

項目	ページ
1回換気量	162, 606
1回心拍出量	181, 600
1型糖尿病	255
1日3回	24, 603
1日摂取許容量	518
1日2回	23, 527
1日4回	3, 590
1秒率	162, 550
1秒量	162, 549
I型アンギオテンシンII受容体拮抗薬	188, 523
1,5-アンヒドログルシトール	247, 519
2型糖尿病	255
4時間毎	23, 590
5'-デオキシ-5-フルオロウリジン	541
5'-ヌクレオチダーゼ	578
5年生存率	92
5-ヒドロキシインドール酢酸	250, 556
5-ヒドロキシトリプタミン	559
5-フルオロシトシン	549
5-フルオロデオキシウリジン	551
5-ブロモウリジン-2'-デオキシリボース	529
6-メルカプトプリン	573
9の法則	320
11-デオキシコルチコステロン	249, 542
17-ケトステロイド	249, 565
17-ヒドロキシコルチコステロイド	249, 579
^{18}F標識フルオロデオキシグルコース	80, 549
24時間尿検体	218
A型肝炎	107, 207
A型肝炎ウイルス	200, 554
A型肝炎ウイルス抗体	200, 554
A型ボツリヌス毒素	315
A群溶血性連鎖球菌咽頭炎	109
ABO血液型	267, 516
ADH分泌異常症	114
αグルコシダーゼ阻害薬	258
α受容体遮断薬	188
αフェトプロテイン	29, 201, 519
Bウイルス病	108
B型肝炎	207
B型肝炎e抗原	200, 555
B型肝炎ウイルス	200, 555
B型肝炎ウイルスDNA定量	201
B型肝炎コア抗原	200, 555
B型肝炎表面抗原	200, 555
Bモード超音波法	80
BCGワクチン	344
β遮断薬	188
β_2ミクログロブリン	219, 527
β溶血性連鎖球菌	334
BRCA1遺伝子	508, 528
BRCA2遺伝子	508, 528
BT-PABA試験	202
C型肝炎	207
C型肝炎ウイルス	200, 555
C型肝炎ウイルス核酸増幅定性	201
C型肝炎ウイルス群別判定	201
C型肝炎ウイルス抗体	201, 555
C反応性タンパク	538
Cペプチド	247
CD分類	531
c-kit遺伝子	508
COMT阻害薬	315
CREST症候群	111, 328
CT血管造影法	79, 538
D型肝炎	207
D型肝炎ウイルス	200, 555
Dダイマー	159, 266
E型肝炎	107, 207
E型肝炎ウイルス	200, 556
EBウイルス関連特異核抗原	544
ECHOウイルス	545
EMG症候群	339
FAB分類	262, 548
Fcフラグメント	549
G型肝炎ウイルス	200, 556
γアミノ酪酸	552
γグルタミルトランスフェラーゼ	199, 552
γヒドロキシ酪酸	553
H_1受容体拮抗薬	145
H_2受容体拮抗薬	210
HBc抗体	200
HBe抗体	200
HBs抗体	200
HELLP症候群	238, 555
HER2タンパク	234
HLA抗原	557
HOX遺伝子	508
HTLV-1関連脊髄障害	116, 309, 554
IgA腎症	115, 221
IgM型HA抗体	201
IgM型HBc抗体	201
K-ras遺伝子	508
L-アスパラギナーゼ	565
LE細胞	321
LH-RHアゴニスト	224
Mモード心エコー法	181
MR唾液腺造影法	150
MRC息切れスケール	158
N-アセチルグルコサミニダーゼ	219, 575
N-アセチルシステイン	575

日本語索引　615

NIH 脳卒中尺度	298, 577	アインスタイニウム		悪性線維性組織球腫	571
O 脚	279		436, 547	悪性貧血	269, 580
PAX 遺伝子	509, 581	アウエルバッハ神経叢		悪性リンパ腫	272, 572
PIVKA-Ⅱ	201		483	アクチニウム	436, 517
POEMS 症候群	273, 586	アウゲ	29	アクチノマイシン D	518
PR 時間延長	178	アウス	29	アクチン	34
PR 時間短縮	178	アウスピッツ徴候	321	悪魔恐怖症	296
Q 熱	108	アウフネーメン	29	悪夢	104
QRS 群	179	あえぎ	154	アクラルビシン	518
QT 延長症候群		亜鉛	434, 611	握力	278
	113, 183, 568	亜鉛華軟膏	328	握力計	283
REAL 分類	263	青あざ	261, 318	顎	442
Rh 因子	592	赤あざ	318	あご先	442
Rh 血液型	267	アーガイルロバートソン		顎鬚	442
RS ウイルス感染症	109	瞳孔	129	アザチオプリン	525
S 状結腸	482	あかぎれ	318	脚	446
S 状結腸動脈	474	暁現象	246	足	5, 446
S 状結腸内視鏡検査	204	赤ぼろ線維を伴うミオク		足首	446
SOAP 形式	96	ローヌスてんかん		足クローヌス	301
SOAPIE 形式	96		311, 571	アシクロビル	329, 518
ST 下降	179	アカラシア	205	アジスロマイシン	525
ST 上昇	179	アカルボース	258	アジソン病	115, 254
ST 上昇型心筋梗塞		亜急性	91	足治療医	37
	185, 600	亜急性壊死性脳脊髄症		アジドチミジン	275, 525
T 細胞活性化因子	576		307, 598	足の裏	446
T 細胞増殖因子	602	亜急性肝炎	207	足の親指	446
TCA 回路	602	亜急性硬化性全脳炎		足の甲	446
WDHA 症候群	255, 610		112, 307, 599	足の指	446
WHO 疼痛緩和ラダー		亜急性甲状腺炎	251	アシャール・チール症候	
	122	亜急性細菌性心内膜炎		群	254
X 脚	280		186, 595	亜硝酸アミル	189
X 線検査	78	亜急性脊髄視神経障害		アショッフ・田原結節	
X 線検査室	54		309, 598		470
X 線写真	79	亜急性連合性脊髄変性症		アスタチン	436, 524
X 染色体連鎖遺伝子	509		308	アズトレオナム	525
X 染色体連鎖性遺伝	74	アキレス腱	501	アストロマイシン	524
X 染色体連鎖優性	74	アキレス腱断裂	285	アスパラギン酸アミノト	
X 染色体連鎖劣性	74	アキレス腱反射		ランスフェラーゼ	
X 線診断	84		300, 520, 524		199, 524
X 線造影剤	79	悪液質	76	アスピリン	190
X 線パノラマ撮影法	150	悪性	82	アスベスト曝露	156
Y 染色体連鎖遺伝子	509	悪性関節リウマチ	114	アスペルガー症候群	313
		悪性胸膜中皮腫	167	アスポキシシリン	524
あ		悪性高体温症	105	アズレンスルホン酸ナト	
アイエルザ症候群	186	悪性黒色腫	327, 572	リウム	152
アイゼンメンゲル複合		悪性疾患	106	汗	512
	183	悪性腫瘍	106	アセタゾラミド	136, 188
アイテル	29	悪性腫瘍臨床国際分類	85	アセチルコリン	517
アイバンク	138	悪性症候群	314	アセチルコリンエステラ	

ーゼ	517	アドソン試験	282	アミロイド原性トランス	
アセチルサリチル酸		アドヒアランス	86	サイレチン	525
	122, 288, 524	アトピー性皮膚炎		アミロイドーシス	
アセチルシステイン	167		324, 518		114, 257
アセトアミノフェン	122	アドリアマイシン	518	アミロイド前駆体タンパ	
アセトヘキサミド	258	アドレナリン	189, 250	ク質	305, 522
アセトン臭	148	アナストロゾール	522	アミロイドβタンパク質	
あせも	318, 330	アナムネ	29		305, 516
与えよ	543	アニサキス	199	アムスラーチャート	132
アタザナビル硫酸塩	525	アーノルド・キアリ奇形		アムルビシン	521
アダパレン	329		306	アムロジピンベシル酸塩	
頭	5, 442	アフェレシス	315		188
アダムス・ストークス症		アプガースコア	331	アメーバ赤痢	109
候群	176	アフタ	147	アメリカ健康保険企画	
アダリムマブ	289	アフタ性口内炎	150		50, 520
悪化	91	アブド(細胞)	523	アメリカヤマゴボウ有糸	
暑がり	244	あぶみ骨	459	分裂原物質	590
厚着	244	あぶみ骨形成術	145	アメリシウム	436, 521
圧痕浮腫	177	あぶみ骨摘除術	145	アモキシシリン	521
圧挫症候群	222	あぶみ骨板開窓術	145	アモキシシリン・クラブ	
アッシャー症候群	150	アブラ	29	ラン酸	521
アッシャーマン症候群		アペール症候群	341	アーユルヴェーダ	118
	239	アヘン	122	アラニンアミノトランス	
圧痛	121, 197	アヘンアルカロイド塩酸		フェラーゼ	199, 521
圧迫	289, 593	塩	122	アリピプラゾール	316
圧迫骨折	282	アポ	29	アルカリホスファターゼ	
圧迫痛	172	アポクリン腺	462		199, 521
圧迫包装	86, 589	アポトーシス	82	アルカローシス	34
圧迫包帯	289	アポリポタンパク質		アルギニンバゾプレシン	
アッペ	29		250, 522		249, 525
圧平眼圧計	131	アマルガム修復	152	アルコール依存	296
圧補助換気	170, 588	アマンタジン塩酸塩		アルコール依存症	17, 296
圧容積関係	182, 590		168, 315	アルコール性肝疾患	
圧力計	304	アミオダロン塩酸塩	189		207, 521
アディー症候群	129	アミカシン	521	アルゴン	434, 523
アディポネクチン	250	アミトロ	29	アルサス反応	323
アテトーシス	299	アミノ酸	516	アルツハイマー型認知症	
アデニン	509, 516	アミノ酸尿	218		311, 540
アデノイド切除術	146	アミノ配糖体	519	アルツハイマー病	
アデノウイルス	160	アミノフィリン	167		308, 518
アデノシン一リン酸	521	アミノレブリン酸	521	アルツハイマー病評価ス	
アデノシン三リン酸	524	アミラーゼ	2, 202	ケール	303, 518
アデノシンデアミナーゼ		アミラーゼアイソザイム		アルデヒドデヒドロゲナ	
	518		202	ーゼ	521
アデノシン二リン酸	518	アミラーゼクレアチニン		アルテプラーゼ	189, 315
アデノ随伴ウイルス	516	クリアランス比		アルドステロン	249
アデホビルピボキシル			202, 517	アルドステロン産生腺腫	
	211	アミロイドAタンパク質			253, 522
アテレク	29		516	アルドステロン・レニン	

日本語索引 617

活性比	249, 523	アンドロゲン	12	医学物理士	57
アルドラーゼ	283	アンドロゲン欠損療法	224, 519	医学文献分析検索システム	571
アルバート縫合	88	アンドロゲン不応症候群	240	医学目的の英語	2, 546
アルフェト	29			医学用語	2
アルブミン・グロブリン比	200, 519	鞍鼻	141	異化作用	10
アルブミン尿	19	アンピシリン	517	以下参照	548
アルベカシン	516	アンピシリン・クロキサシリン	517	胃下垂	18, 205
アルホス	29	アンピシリン・スルバクタム	517	医科大学	62
アルポート症候群	222			医科大学職名	62
アルミニウム	434, 521	アンビュー	190	医科大学入学共通試験	570
亜鈴	40	アンプタ	29		
アレルギー科	53	アンプル	34, 521	胃癌	205
アレルギー学	63	アンペア	438, 516	息切れ	154, 172, 261, 519
アレルギー性気管支肺アスペルギルス症	165, 516	アンホテリシン	521	意気消沈	295
		あん摩マッサージ指圧師	57	意義不明の単クローングロブリン血症	273, 571
アレルギー性結膜炎	133	アンモニア	200	医業停止処分	42
アレルギー性通年性鼻炎	144	安楽死	26, 93	胃空腸吻合	14
アレルギー性肉芽腫性血管炎	111, 114, 519	**い**		胃空腸吻合術	214
アレルギー性鼻炎	25, 144	胃	5, 480	育児	330
アレルギー専門医	59	胃亜全摘術	214	イクテルス	29
アレルゲン	17	医員	59	イクテロメータ	333
アレン試験	176	イェーガー視力検査文字	131	異型	82
アレンドロン酸ナトリウム水和物	289			異型狭心症	185, 607
アロプリノール	259	胃液	512	異型上皮	205, 524
アロマセラピー	118	胃液検査	201	異形成	18
アンギオ	29	胃炎	14	異型赤血球	15
アンギオテンシン		イエンドラシック操作	300	異型赤血球増加	264
アンギオテンシン変換酵素	517	イオウ(硫黄)	38, 434, 595	異型線維黄色腫	327, 519
アンギオテンシン変換酵素阻害薬	188, 517	胃潰瘍	205, 554	異型ポルフィリン症	257, 609
		胃角	480		
安産	230	医学英語	2	異型リンパ球	265
暗視野顕微鏡検査	236	医学教育学	63	医原性	14
安静	289, 593	医学教育用語	66	医原病	106, 543
安静時狭心症	185	医学件名標目集	3, 571	移行期	91
安静時呼吸困難	154	医学士	66, 570	イコサペンタエン酸	562
安全ピン	78	医学生涯教育	66, 535	イコサペント酸エチル	259
アンダーソン病	257	医学的に説明困難な症状	104, 575		
アンチトロンビンⅢ	266, 275, 524	医学的問題	96	胃固定術	18
		医学博士	66, 584	胃酸過多	26, 195
アンチモン	435, 595	医学部	62	医師	57
安定狭心症	185	医学部教育	66	医師間通用語	2
暗点	132	医学部教授会	62	意識	293
アントラサイクリン	274	医学部長	62	意識混濁	293
				意識消失	28, 567
				意識のある	35
				意識不明	76, 293
				意識明瞭	76

意識レベル	76, 297	胃洗浄	211	一酸化窒素合成酵素	577
医師国家試験	66	異染性白質ジストロフィー		一側性	12
医事裁判	42		307, 572	一側性腎腫瘤	217
医師賠償責任保険	42	胃前庭部毛細血管拡張症		イッテルビウム	435, 610
医事紛争	42		205, 552	イットリウム	435, 610
医事紛争処理委員会	42	胃全摘術	214	一般医	57, 553
医師法	46	位相差顕微鏡	79	一般外科	53
医事法	46	異側半盲	132	一般外科医	59
医師免許交付	66	イソニアジド	168, 562	一般名	36, 86
胃十二指腸動脈	474, 552	イソニアジドメタンスルホン酸ナトリウム塩		一般目標	66, 553
萎縮	19, 82			一般用医薬品	85, 580
萎縮腎	223		562	溢流性尿失禁	217
萎縮性鼻炎	144	イソニコチン酸ヒドラジド		胃底部	480
異種抗体	14		562	遺伝暗号	509
異種親和性	14	胃体部	480	遺伝医学	63
胃小窩	480	イダルビシン	561	遺伝学	63
異状死	93	一塩基多型	509, 598	遺伝子	508
胃症状	194	位置覚	302	遺伝子改変生物	553
異常タンパク血症を伴う血管免疫芽球性リンパ節症		位置覚低下	262	遺伝子型	509
		一元放射免疫拡散法		遺伝子組み換え組織プラスミノーゲン活性化因子	
	272, 520		80, 599		
異常の	10	いちご舌	148		315, 594
異常分娩	230	いちご状動脈瘤	307	遺伝子組み換えヒトエリスロポエチン	
移植	12	一次救命処置	527		
異食	261	一時的問題	96		224, 274, 593
移植外科	53	一次縫合	88	遺伝子欠損	509
移植外科学	63	一硝酸イソソルビド		遺伝子工学	63
移植コーディネーター	57		189, 563	遺伝子座	509
胃食道逆流症	204, 552	一倍体	509	遺伝子座調節領域	
移植片	9	胃腸科	53		509, 566
移植片対宿主病	274, 554	一類感染症	107	遺伝子増幅	509
異所性	10, 36, 82	一連の出来事	96	遺伝子地図	509
異所性 ACTH 産生症候群		異痛	120, 294	遺伝子治療	117
	253	一過性閾値減衰試験		遺伝子配列	509
異所性心房頻拍	174, 544		142, 605	遺伝子発現	509
異所性膵	210	一過性閾値変動	142, 605	遺伝子プール	509
維持療法	118	一過性異常骨髄造血		遺伝子変換	509
石綿肺	165		336, 601	遺伝子融合	509
医真菌学	63	一過性黒内障	134	遺伝性運動感覚ニューロパチー	
遺精	228	一過性視力障害	125		309, 557
異性恐怖症	296	一過性全健忘	302, 603	遺伝性感覚自律性ニューロパチー	
胃生検	204	一過性脳虚血発作			309, 558
胃石	5, 209		306, 603	遺伝性球状赤血球症	
胃切除	17	一過性脳卒中	294		269, 558
胃切除後症候群	206	一酸化炭素	536	遺伝性血管神経性浮腫	
胃切除術	214	一酸化炭素肺拡散能			324, 554
イセパミシン	563		162, 542	遺伝性血管浮腫	324, 554
胃腺	480	一酸化炭素ヘモグロビン		遺伝性コプロポルフィリン症	
胃腺腫	205		267		257, 555

日本語索引

遺伝性疾患	73, 106	胃抑制ポリペプチド		医療保険の通算可能性と	
遺伝性出血性末梢血管拡			247, 553	説明責任に関する法律	
張症	274	囲卵腔内精子注入法			50, 556
遺伝性進行性関節眼症			242, 600	医療補助者	59
	341	イリジウム	436, 562	医療面接	66
遺伝性楕円赤血球症	269	イリノテカン	537	医療用医薬品情報集	583
遺伝性非球状赤血球性溶		医療	42	医療倫理	43
血性貧血	269, 557	医療科学大学	62	医療倫理学	64
遺伝性非ポリポーシス大		医療過誤	42	医療連携	43
腸癌	207, 557	医療過誤訴訟	42	イルベサルタン	188
遺伝の	36	医療過誤保険	48	イレウス	206
医道審議会	42	医療関係職種	57	いれずみ	321
移動性ペースメーカー		医療監査	42	入れ歯	148
	179	医療監視	42	違和感	104
医動物学	63	医療機関認定合同委員会		陰イオンギャップ	
イトラコナゾール			42, 564		159, 219, 519
	329, 563	医療技術評価	42, 574	陰イオン交換樹脂	259
胃内視鏡検査	203	医療機能評価	42	陰影欠損	203
犬恐怖症	296	医療行政	42	インオベ	29
イヌリード	220	医療計画	42	院外心停止	176, 579
イヌリンクリアランス		医療系教育機関	62	陰核	489
	220	医療経済学	63	印環	40
居眠り	104	医療行為	42	印環細胞	82
胃粘膜下腫瘍	205	医療資源利用群	42, 594	いんきんたむし	318
胃の	5	医療事故	42	インクレチン	247
胃バイパス術	260	医療指示拒否	521	陰茎	488
いびき	140	医療施設	52	陰茎海綿体	488
易疲労感	104	医療社会学	63	隠語	2
イプシロン・アミノカプ		医療者選択会員制団体健		インジウム	435, 562
ロン酸	544	康保険	50, 587	インジナビル	561
異物	127, 549	医療情報	42	飲酒	74
イブプロフェン	122	医療情報学	63	陰唇小帯	489
疣(いぼ)	28, 318	医療水準	42	インスリノーマ	255
違法な	35	医療制度	42	インスリン依存性糖尿病	
イホスファミド	561	医療センター	52		255, 561
胃ポリープ	205	医療ソーシャルワーカー		インスリン感受性試験	
イミダフェナシン	224		57, 574		250
イミプラミン塩酸塩	314	医療訴訟	42	インスリングラルギン	
イミペネム・シラスタチ		医療チーム	95		258
ン	562	医療廃棄物	42	インスリングルリジン	
イムラッド	29	医療費	42		258
医薬情報担当者	57, 573	医療費控除	48	インスリン抗体	247
医薬食品局	42	医療費適正化計画	42	インスリンショック療法	
医薬品医療機器総合機構		医療福祉大学	62		563
	42, 585	医療扶助	42	インスリン抵抗性	247
医薬分業	42	医療法	46	インスリン抵抗性指標	
医用工学	571	医療法人	43		247, 557
医用生体工学	63	医療保険	48	インスリン非依存性糖尿	
医用電子工学	571	医療保険制度	48	病	255, 577

インスリン負荷試験	陰部大腿神経 506	ウィルヒョウ三徴 177
250, 563	陰部の 37	ウィルヒョウリンパ節
インスリン様成長因子	インプラント義歯 152	198
249, 561	インフリキシマブ	ウィルムス腫瘍 342
インスリン様成長因子I	211, 289, 561	ウインスロー孔 482
249, 561	インフルエンザ	ウェクスラー児童用知能
陰性冠性T波 179	26, 109, 155	検査 334, 610
陰性逆転T波 179	インフルエンザウイルス	ウェクスラー成人用知能
陰性反応適中度 577	A型 160	検査 303, 610
インターフェロン	インフルエンザウイルス	ウェゲナー肉芽腫症
211, 561	抗原 160	111, 114, 165
インターフェロン感受性	インフルエンザウイルス	植え込み型自動除細動器
領域 201, 563	B型 160	190, 520
インターフェロンγ放出	インフルエンザ菌 159	植え込み型除細動器
アッセイ 160, 561	インフルエンザ菌b型ワ	190, 560
インターフェロン制御因	クチン 344, 556	植え込み型ペースメーカ
子 509, 563	インフルエンザ定点 109	ー 190
インターベンショナルラ	インフルエンザワクチン	ウェスターマーク徴候
ジオロジー 117, 564	344	180
インターロイキン 561	インポテンス 228	ウェスタンブロット法
インチ 438, 562	陰毛 444	610
院長 59	陰門 489	ウエスト 444
咽頭 465	引用書中に 22, 579	ウエストナイル熱 108
咽頭異物感 140	インレー修復 152	ウェストファール徴候
咽頭炎 144		300
咽頭結膜熱 109	う	ウェーバー 439, 610
咽頭充血 141	ヴァンサン口峡炎 151	ウェーバー試験 142
咽頭切除術 146	ウィスコット・アルドリ	ウェーバー症候群 299
咽頭痛 120, 140	ッチ症候群 339, 610	ウェルドニッヒ・ホフマ
咽頭反射 141, 301	右胃大網動脈 474	ン病 341
咽頭扁桃 465	ヴィダール苔癬 325	ウェルニッケ失語症 302
インドシアニングリーン	ウィッカム線条 320	ウェルニッケ中枢 503
試験 200, 560	ウィップル三徴 246	ウェルニッケ脳症 311
インドメタシン 122	ウィップル手術 215	ウェルマー症候群 255
イントロン 510	ウィップル病 206	ウェンケバッハ型ブロッ
院内感染 105	右胃動脈 474, 592	ク 179
院内肺炎 163, 554	ウィリアムソン徴候 158	ウォーターズ撮影法 150
陰嚢 488	ウィリス動脈輪 471	ウォーターハウス・フリ
陰嚢腫脹 217	ウィリス動脈輪閉塞症	ーデリクセン症候群
陰嚢腫瘤 217	111	340
陰嚢水瘤 237	ウイルス 28	うおのめ 318
インピンジメント症候群	ウイルスカプシド抗原	ウォルフ・パーキンソ
284	608	ン・ホワイト症候群
陰部 444	ウイルス感染 106	179, 610
インフォームドコンセン	ウイルス関連血球貪食症	ウォルフラム症候群 336
ト 95, 559	候群 607	ウォールマン病 256
陰部潰瘍 231	ウイルス性肝炎 109, 207	うがい 147
陰部神経 506	ウィルスング管 484	うがい薬 147
陰部神経叢 506	ウィルソン病 209	右下葉 466, 593

右眼	23, 579	ウリジンニリン酸	606	栄養大学	62
右冠動脈	471, 591	右リンパ本幹	478	栄養士	54
右肝動脈	472, 592	ウルソデオキシコール酸		栄養不良	11, 76, 244
右脚ブロック	179, 591		211, 606	栄養良好な	76, 610
右胸心	13, 183	ウロ	29	会陰切開	243
受付	54	ウロキナーゼ	189, 606	会陰痛	216, 228
右結腸動脈	474, 591	ウロビリノーゲン尿	218	会陰の	37
受身赤血球凝集反応		上顎	442	会陰部	452
	80, 584	上唇	442	会陰縫合	18
烏口肩峰靱帯	496, 530	ウンウンオクチウム	437	エヴァンス症候群	273
烏口鎖骨靱帯	496, 531	ウンウンクアジウム	436	液	23, 567
う歯	149	ウンウンセプチウム	437	腋窩	450
右耳	22, 518	ウンウントリウム	437	腋窩温	75
ウシ海綿状脳症	307, 529	ウンウンヘキシウム	437	疫学	63
右室圧	181, 594	ウンウンペンチウム	436	腋窩静脈	476
右室肥大	175, 594	運動覚	302	腋窩神経	505
右室補助装置	192, 594	運動緩慢	299	液化石油ガス	568
右上葉	466, 594	運動器官系	278	腋窩中央線	454
う食窩	149	運動器官症候群	278	液化天然ガス	567
右心室	470, 594	運動失調	299	腋窩動脈	472
右心不全	186	運動失調性歩行	298	腋窩の	34
右心房	470, 591	運動性言語中枢	503	腋窩部	450
薄着	244	運動性呼吸困難	154, 543	腋窩リンパ節	478
打ち身	261, 318	運動性失語症	302	腋窩リンパ節郭清	243
宇宙医学	64	運動負荷試験	180	エキシマレーザー冠動脈	
右中葉	466, 593	運動野	503	形成術	190, 546
うっ血	82	運動誘発喘息	163, 546	液体窒素	329
うっ血型心筋症	187, 531	運動療法	117, 290	エキノコックス	199
うっ血性心不全	185, 533			エキノコックス症	108
うっ乳頭	130	え		腋毛欠如	245
うつ状態	295	エアゾール	169	液量オンス	438, 550
ウッド灯	322	エアゾール剤	86	エクソン	510
うつ病	25	鋭角三角形	39	えくぼ	442
腕	5, 444	永久閾値上昇	142, 589	エクリン腺	462
腕の	5	永久歯	147	壊死	82
うなじ	444	英国医師会	527	壊死性腸炎	576
右肺	466	英国医療管理評議会	553	エスエス	29
右肺下葉	468	英国保健省	50, 543	エステトロール	234, 544
右肺上葉	468	エイコサペンタエン酸		エストラジオール	
右肺中葉	468		547		234, 241, 544
ウベニメクス	529	エイズ	237, 520	エストラムスチン	547
右房肥大	179, 591	エイズ関連症候群	523	エストリオール	234, 544
膿む	319	エイズ治療拠点病院	52	エストロゲン	234
埋め込み型インスリンポ		衛生学	63	エストロゲン受容体	234
ンプ	258	英米の医療保険	50	エストロゲン代償療法	
右葉	484	栄養	76, 90		241
ウラン	436, 606	栄養学	35, 64	エストロン	234, 544
ウリジン一リン酸	606	栄養基準量	592	エストロゲン受容体	547
ウリジン三リン酸	607	栄養士	57	エゼチミブ	259

壊疽性口内炎	151	エリスロマイシン	268, 547	遠心性ニューロン	504
エタネルセプト	288	エリスロマイシン	546	円錐	40
エタノール	548	エリテマトーデス	566	延髄	504
エダラボン	315	エリトロ	30	円錐角膜	128
エタンブトール塩酸塩		エルケー	30	円錐切除診	78
	168	エルスワース・ハワード		塩素	434, 534
エチオナミド	168, 548	試験	250	エンタカポン	315
エチレンオキサイドガス		エルビウム	435, 547	円柱	40
	547	エルプ・デュシェンヌ麻		円柱尿	218
エチレンジアミン四酢酸		痺	335	エンテカビル水和物	211
負荷試験	250	エルブレ	30	エント	30
エチレンジアミン四酢酸		エルロチニブ	168	円板状エリテマトーデス	
	545	エワート徴候	176		327, 542
エッセン	29	遠位	448	エンビオマイシン	548
エデーム	29	遠位指節間関節	495, 542	エンボリ	30
エトスクシミド	316, 548	遠位尿細管	486	延命	92
エトポシド	548, 609	円蓋	480	遠用眼鏡	126
エドワーズ症候群	336	円回内筋	498		
エナメル質	464	塩化エドロホニウム試験		**お**	
エナメル上皮腫	148		305	横位	232, 233
エノキサシン	547	遠隔医療	43	横隔膜	444, 455, 466
エノシタビン	527	遠隔操作後充填方式	591	横隔膜弓状靱帯	496
エバスチン	145	遠隔転移	82	横隔膜ヘルニア	25, 204
エパルレスタット	258	塩基過剰	159, 526	横行結腸	482
エピ	29	演技性人格障害	313, 558	横行膵動脈	474
エピジェネティクス	510	塩基性線維芽細胞増殖因		横指	549
エピジオ	29	子	527	横静脈洞	476
エピネフリン	189	塩基性胎児タンパク		黄色	39
エピルビシン	547		201, 527	黄色腫	245
エファビレンツ	275, 545	塩基性リン酸カルシウム		黄色腫症	256
エプシュタイン真珠	332		284, 526	黄色靱帯	496
エプスタイン奇形	183	塩基対	510, 528	黄色靱帯骨化症	
エプスタイン・バーウイ		塩基配列	510		112, 287, 579, 580
ルス	267, 544	遠近両用眼鏡	126	黄色ブドウ球菌	202
エプーリス	149	嚥下	195	横切開	88
エプリー法	145	円形	40	凹足	280
エプレレノン	188	円形陰影	161	横足根関節	495
エポエチンアルファ	274	円形脱毛症	326	黄体	5
エポエチンベータ	274	嚥下困難	195	黄体化未破裂卵胞症候群	
エボラ出血熱	107	嚥下障害	35		239, 568
エムケー	30	嚥下不能	34	黄体形成ホルモン	
エムトリシタビン		塩酸エタンブトール	544		234, 249, 567
	275, 551	塩酸ピロカルピン	136	黄体形成ホルモン放出ホ	
エラスターゼ1	202	遠視	125	ルモン	249, 567
エーラス・ダンロー症候		炎症	82	黄体形成ホルモン放出ホ	
群	337	炎症細胞	82	ルモン試験	234
鰓の	34	炎症性腸疾患	206, 559	黄体嚢胞	238
エリキシル剤	86	遠心咬合	149	黄疸	26, 36, 196, 197, 262
エリスロポエチン		遠心性	34	嘔吐	195

黄熱	108	頤	5, 442	温度覚	301
黄斑	130, 458	頤下リンパ節	478	温度覚消失	301
黄斑円孔	130	頤形成術	5	温度眼振試験	143
黄斑上膜	130	頤舌骨筋	5	温度計	16
黄斑浮腫	130	頤の	36	温熱療法	11
往復雑音	175	頤部	450	温パック	289
オウム病	108	オートラジオグラフィー	523		
横紋筋	498			**か**	
横紋筋肉腫	288	同じ箇所に	21, 559	果	36
横紋筋融解症	285	同じ章に	21, 559	窩	35
太田母斑	326	同じ節に	21, 559	臥位	76
悪寒	105	おねしょ	331	外陰炎	238
悪寒戦慄	105	各々	21, 516	外陰掻痒症	229
オキサリプラチン	567	オピオイド	123	外陰部	444
オキシコドン塩酸塩	122	オプソクロヌス	332	外陰部動脈	476
オキシテトラサイクリン	580	汚物恐怖症	296	下位運動ニューロン	567
オキシトシン	241, 249	オフロキサシン	579	回外	279
オキシトシン負荷試験	235, 579	オープンリーディングフレーム	510, 579	回外筋	498
オギルヴィー症候群	199	オーベー	30	外眼運動	129, 547
小口病	135	オペ	30	外眼角	456
オクトレオチド酢酸塩	258	オペレーター遺伝子	510	外眼筋	458, 547
奥歯	147, 442	オーベン	30	回帰熱	108
おくび	26, 195	オマリズマブ	167	開業医	57, 553
汚言	300	オーム	439, 579	開胸術	16, 170
オージオメータ	141	オムスク出血熱	108	会計	54
悪心	195	おむつかぶれ	318, 330	外頚静脈	476
悪心・嘔吐	578	オメプラゾール	211	外頚動脈	471, 544
オスキー	30	親	73	解決済み問題	96
オスグッド・シュラッター病	287	親知らず	147	回結腸動脈	474
オースティン・フリント雑音	175	親の	37	開口障害	148
オステオカルシン	283	親指	444	外向性の人	296
オスミウム	435, 580	およそ	21, 529	外国語としての英語	66, 545
オスモル	439, 580	およびその他	21, 548	外国語としての英語テスト	66, 604
オスラー結節	177	オリエ病	288	外国人医師卒後教育委員会	66, 545
オセルタミビルリン酸塩	168	オリバー徴候	177	介護支援専門員	57
悪阻	229	オリーブ橋小脳萎縮症	310, 579	介護施設	55
おたふくかぜ	330	オルト	30	外骨格	6
オッカムの剃刀	19	オルトラニ徴候	333	介護福祉士	57
オッディ括約筋	484	オールブライト遺伝性骨形成異常症	252, 520	介護保険	48
オッペンハイム反射	301	音楽療法士	57	介護保険施設	55
オーディット	95	音響陰影	523	介護療養型医療施設	55
おでき	318	音叉	78	介護老人保健施設	55
オト	30	音叉検査	142	カイザー	30
		オンス	439, 580	カイザー・フライシャー輪	197
		温泉療法	118		
		温存	87	開始	36

外耳	458	灰白髄炎	15	楓糖尿症	336
外耳炎	143	灰白脳炎	15	顔	5, 442
外耳道	458, 544	外反膝	26, 280	下顎顔面異形成症	341
外斜位	128, 610	外反肘	280	下顎後退症	149
外斜視	11, 35, 128, 610	外反母趾	280	下顎骨	492
外傷	73	外皮	462	化学受容体ひきがね帯	
外傷重症度スコア	76, 563	開腹	19		539
外傷性鼓膜穿孔	143	回復	92	下顎神経	505
外傷性脳損傷	306, 602	回復期	92	下顎前突症	149
灰色	39	回復室	54, 594	化学走性	13
回診	66	外腹斜筋	500	化学的除去	328
開心術	191	開腹術	14, 214	化学発光酵素免疫測定法	
ガイスベック症候群	271	回復性虚血性神経脱落症			80, 534
疥癬	27, 325	候	306, 593	化学発光免疫測定法	
改善	91	外分泌	11		80, 534
外旋	279	外方	448	下顎半切除術	3
開窓	87	開放音	175, 580	下顎部	450
咳嗽	28	解剖学	63	化学療法	13, 118
開創鉤	89	解剖学的肢位	448	過活動膀胱	223, 578
開窓術	291	解剖学的診断	84	踵	34, 446
外側	448	開放型質問	66	かかりつけ医	57
外側楔状骨	494	開放骨折	281	過換気症候群	166, 559
外側広筋	500	開放式病院	52	下眼瞼	456
外側足底動脈	476	開放貼布試験	323	蝸牛	459
外側中葉区	468	解剖の	34	蝸牛管	459
外側直筋	458	蓋膜	459	蝸牛神経	460, 505
外側肺底区	468	海綿骨	494	芽球増加性不応性貧血	
外側半規管	460	海綿状の	34		270, 591
回虫	199	海綿静脈洞	476	蝸牛内直流電位	142
懐中電灯	77	回盲弁	482	蝸牛マイクロホン電位	
回腸	36, 482	潰瘍	28, 320		142
外腸骨静脈	478	潰瘍性大腸炎		掻く	319
外腸骨動脈	474, 546		113, 206, 606	核	508
回腸動脈	474	外来	54, 579	学位	66
回腸の	36	外来血圧	75	額位	232
外転	34, 279	外来再診	594	核医学	64
回転試験	143	外来受診日	93	核医学科	53
外転神経	505	解離性障害	312	核医学検査	79
回転性粥腫切除術	191	解離性動脈瘤	187	学位論文	66
開頭	8	カイロプラクティック		核黄疸	335
外套	502		118	角化	320
開頭クリッピング	317	カイロミクロン	250	角化症	14, 36, 320
開頭術	317	下咽頭癌	145	顎下腺	464
回内	279	ガウス	438, 551	顎下腺管	464
概日リズム睡眠障害	312	カウデン病	207	核家族	73
外尿道口	488, 489	カウパー腺	488	核型	508
海馬	502	カウプ指数	331	核型分類	14
外胚葉	10	カウフマン療法	241	顎下リンパ節	478
灰白便	196	カウンセリング	316	各眼	23, 580

顎間固定法	290, 561	核崩壊	18	下伸筋支帯	500
顎関節	495, 604	角膜	456	過伸展	279
顎関節症	152	核膜	508	下垂手	298
顎後退症	149	角膜移植術	137	下膵十二指腸動脈	474
学際的	66	角膜異物	128	下垂体	490
核左方移動	264	角膜炎	14, 36	下垂体窩	461
核酸	510	角膜潰瘍	128	下垂体機能亢進症	252
核酸塩基	510	角膜矯正術	137	下垂体機能低下症	
核酸増幅法	80, 576	角膜血管新殖	128		116, 252
各耳	23, 525	角膜後面沈着物	128, 565	下垂体性巨人症	253
核磁気共鳴	577	角膜混濁	128	下垂体性小人症	253
学士号	66	角膜知覚	128	下垂体切除術	259
核質	508	角膜白斑	128	下垂体腺腫	252, 313
隔日	23, 541	角膜剥離	128	下垂体ブロック	123
角質層	462	角膜反射	301	ガス液体クロマトグラフ	
学習障害	302, 566	角膜びらん	128	ィー	80, 553
核出	87	核融解	14	ガスクロマトグラフィー	
核上	38	隔離病院	52		80, 552
核小体	508	学歴社会	66	ガスクロマトグラフィ	
角錐	40	家系図	73	ー・質量分析法	80, 552
郭清	87	過形成	18, 82	ガス固体クロマトグラフ	
覚せい剤取締法	46	下後鋸筋	500	ィー	80, 554
顎前突症	149, 245	下行結腸	482	かすり傷	318
拡大家族	73	下行膝動脈	476	ガスリー試験	333
拡大鏡	78	鵞口瘡	150	かぜ	155
額帯鏡	77	下行大動脈	472	ガーゼ	89
喀痰	155	過誤腫	83	化生	83
喀痰培養	159	かごベッド	330	仮性半陰陽	240
拡張	87	カサバッハ・メリット症		かぜ症候群	163
学長	62	候群	326	下舌区	468
拡張型心筋症		かさぶた	318	画像診断	84
	115, 187, 540	華氏	438, 548	画像診断学	64
拡張期血圧	75, 540	下肢	446	画像診断の介入治療	564
拡張期雑音	175, 542	かじかむ	295	画像保管伝送システム	
拡張期心不全	186, 541	下矢状静脈洞	476		580
拡張初期	16	下肢静脈瘤	187	家族	73
拡張性金属ステント		下肢伸展挙上テスト		家族看護学	65
	213, 546		281, 597	家族支援	60
拡張早期雑音	175	下肢帯	494	家族性	35
拡張中期雑音	175	下肢浮腫	177	家族性アミロイド多発ニ	
拡張末期圧	182, 545	下肢むずむず症候群		ューロパチー	309, 549
拡張末期容量	182, 545		279, 593	家族性大腸腺腫性ポリポーシ	
確定拠出年金	48	下斜筋	458	ス	207, 549
確定診断	84	荷重関節	278	家族性大腸ポリポーシス	
学童	330	歌手結節	140		207, 551
顎動脈	472	過少月経	228	家族性地中海熱	550
角度計	283	過剰歯	149	家族性突然死症候群	113
角皮症	321	過食	18, 194	家族性複合型高脂血症	
核分裂の	37	頭文字語	56		256, 549

家族病	106	転移酵素	536	カポジ肉腫	272
加速歩行	298	カテーテル関連血流感染		カマ	30
家族歴	70, 73, 95, 397, 550		537	カマグ	30
肩	444	カテーテル焼灼術	191	がま腫	148
下腿	446	カテーテル尿	218	鎌状赤血球貧血	269
下腿圧痕浮腫	217	蝸電図法	142	過眠症	312
下腿三頭筋	500	過度〜	71	カムラチ・エンゲルマン	
下大静脈	478, 563	ガードナー症候群	207	症候群	341
下肢切断術	292, 527	ガードネレラ・バジナリ		仮面高血圧	173
カタカナ用語	29	ス	235	痒み	319
肩関節	495	カドミウム	435, 531	過ヨウ素酸シッフ(染色)	
肩関節周囲炎	284	ガドリニウム	79, 435, 552		581
過多月経	228	ガードルストーン手術		空えずき	195
肩腱板損傷	284		292	ガラクトース血症	333
肩こり	278	カナー症候群	343	ガラス圧診法	319
ガチフロキサシン	552	カナマイシン	564	空咳	155
下腸間膜静脈	478, 562	カーニー複合	188	体	5
下腸間膜動脈	474, 561	過粘稠度症候群	559	空巣症候群	229
下直筋	458	化膿性関節炎	286	ガーランド三角	157
滑液	513	化膿性脊椎炎	287	カリウム	434, 564
滑液分析	284	ガバペンチン	316	ガリウム	434, 552
滑液包	501	痂皮	320	仮診断	84
滑液包炎	285	下鼻甲介	460	カリパス	34
喀血	155	下鼻道	460	カーリーB線	180
学校医	57	過敏性腸症候群	206, 559	カリフラワー	40
学校保健法	46	過敏性肺炎	163	カリホルニウム	436, 532
滑車神経	505	カフェオレ斑点	298	顆粒	83
褐色	39	ガフキー号数	160	顆粒円柱	218
褐色細胞腫	254	下腹壁動脈	474	顆粒球	17, 264
活性化部分トロンボプラ		下部消化管	480	顆粒球減少	265
スチン時間	265, 523	下部食道括約筋	480, 567	顆粒球コロニー刺激因子	
活性化プロテインC		下部食道括約筋圧			552
	266, 522		201, 567	顆粒球マクロファージコ	
活性凝固時間	265, 518	カプセル	23, 86, 530	ロニー刺激因子	
活性酸素分解酵素	598	カプセル内視鏡検査	204		276, 553
活動性問題	96	カプトプリル	188	顆粒球輸血	276
合併症	93	下部尿路	486	顆粒剤	86
滑膜切除術	291	下部尿路症状	216, 568	顆粒細胞腫	552
滑面小胞体	508, 596	カプラン症候群	165	顆粒層	462
割礼	242	カプラン・マイヤー生存		カーリング潰瘍	205
カテ	30	曲線	92	カルシウム	434, 529
家庭医	57	かぶれる	319	カルシウム拮抗薬	188
家庭医学	64	花粉症	27, 140, 144	カルシウムチャネル遮断	
家庭血圧	75	カベオラ	508	薬	188, 531
家庭的問題	96	下壁心筋梗塞	185	カルシトニン	248, 289
家族療法	118	カベルゴリン	315	カルシトニン遺伝子関連	
カテコールアミン		カーペンター症候群	341	ペプチド	533, 538
	189, 250	下方	448	カルタゲナー症候群	183
カテコール・Oメチル		下膀胱動脈	474	カルチ	30

カルチノイド症候群	255	肝外門脈閉塞症		間欠的強制換気	170, 562
カルテオロール塩酸塩			113, 208, 546	観血的整復	291
	136	眼窩縁	127	観血的整復内固定術	
カルノフスキースケール		眼科学	64		291, 579
	92	がん化学療法看護	61	間欠的腹膜透析	225, 562
カルバマゼピン	315, 531	眼窩下の	11	間欠熱	105
カルボプラチン	531	眼窩下部	450	間欠陽圧呼吸	170
カルマン症候群	240	眼角	456	間欠陽圧呼吸法	562
カルムスチン	526	感覚神経活動電位		肝血流量	201, 555
カルメット・ゲラン結核			304, 598	緩下薬	27
菌	526	感覚性言語中枢	503	眼瞼	126, 456
カルモナム	537	眼窩周囲部	450	眼瞼炎	133
カルモフール	555	眼窩上部	450	眼瞼黄色腫	245
加齢黄斑変性		眼型白皮症	134, 578	眼瞼外反	127
	113, 135, 521	眼科定点	110	眼瞼下垂	2, 18, 127
加齢男性性腺機能低下		眼窩底吹き抜け骨折	135	還元型グルタチオン	554
	237, 567	眼窩部	450	眼瞼痙攣	127
ガレノキサシン	554	肝鎌状間膜	484	眼瞼結膜	456
カレン徴候	198	がん看護	60	眼瞼結膜露出	127
下肋部	36	宦官症	231	眼瞼後退	127
カロー三角	484	がんがんする	121	眼瞼縮小	127
カロリー	438, 530	眼乾燥症	133	換気すれば	21, 561
カロリ病	209	眼間代	332	眼瞼遅滞	127
ガロン	438, 552	換気血流スキャン	161	眼瞼内反	127
川崎病	111, 340	肝機能検査	199, 567	還元ニコチンアミドアデ	
ガワース徴候	299	眼球	442, 456	ニンジヌクレオチド	
環	40	眼球陥凹	128		575
〜感	71	眼球結膜	456	眼瞼の	37
癌	18, 34, 83, 529	眼球斜位	128	眼瞼反転	127
眼圧	129, 562	肝吸虫	199	眼瞼皮膚弛緩症	127
眼圧測定法	131	眼球沈下運動	298	眼瞼浮腫	217
顔位	232	眼球摘出術	137	看護	89
肝移植	215	眼球突出	26, 128, 246	肝硬変	35
癌遺伝子	510	眼球突出性眼筋麻痺	135	肝硬変症	208, 566
簡易認知機能検査		眼球内容除去術	137	看護疫学	65
	303, 573	環境医学	64	看護介入	89
眼位不同	128	環境基本法	46	看護介入分類	89, 576
癌ウイルス	15	癌恐怖症	296	看護学	65
肝炎	2, 26	環境保健学	62	看護学校	62
眼炎	9	眼筋麻痺	15, 135	看護過程	89
肝炎ウイルスマーカー		管腔内超音波検査法		看護監査	89
	200		204, 561	看護管理学	65
肝炎関連抗原	200, 554	肝屈曲部	482	看護技術	89
肝円索	484	ガングリオン	285	看護基準	89
陥凹乳頭比	130, 531	肝頚静脈逆流	175, 557	看護教育学	65
感音性難聴	142	間隙	149	看護業務	89
眼科	53	冠血管造影法	182, 530	看護記録	89
眼窩	456, 492	間欠性水腎症	339	看護ケア	89
眼科医	59	間欠性跛行	173	看護計画	89

看護師	57	感情線	446	関節置換術	291
看護師長	59	環状鉄芽球	267	関節痛	17, 120, 278
看護実践国際分類	4, 560	肝静脈	478, 559	関節内注射	86
看護助手	59	肝静脈閉塞性疾患		関節軟骨	496
看護診断	84		208, 609	関節ねずみ	280
看護成果分類	89, 577	冠状面	448	関節半月	496
看護大学	62	肝小葉	484	関節半月板切除術	291
寛骨	494	間食	194	間接ビリルビン	199
看護手順	89	緩徐呼吸	13	関節変形	278
看護部	54	汗疹	27, 36, 320	関節傍の	14
看護福祉大学	62	眼振	129	関節リウマチ	
看護部長	59	眼神経	505		110, 286, 591
看護倫理	65	肝腎症候群	222	関節リウマチ赤血球凝集	
監査	96	関心領域	593	試験	283, 591
幹細胞移植	276	カーンズ・セイヤー症候		関節離断術	10
肝細胞癌	208, 555	群	342, 565	関節裂隙狭細	284
肝細胞性	14	乾性角結膜炎	133, 564	感染	105
肝細胞増殖因子	200, 556	肝生検	204	汗腺	462
カンサシー抗酸菌	160	肝性口臭	148, 197	完全右脚ブロック	
監察医	57	がん性疼痛看護	61		179, 537
間擦疹	320	癌性の	34	完全寛解	92, 537
鉗子	88	肝性脳症	208	感染管理	61
眼脂	127	眼精疲労	126	感染管理看護師	560
環軸関節	495	関節	5, 495	感染経路	106
環軸関節亜脱臼	287, 516	関節炎	5, 17, 278	完全骨折	281
環軸関節脱臼	287, 516	関節窩	495	完全左脚ブロック	
カンジダ・アルビカンス		関節覚	302		179, 534
	235	関節可動域	280, 593	感染症	106, 107
間質液	512, 563	関節可動域訓練	290	感染症科	53
冠疾患集中治療室	54, 531	関節可動性	280	感染症看護	60
間質細胞刺激ホルモン		関節間軟骨	496	完全静脈栄養	91, 604
	249, 560	関節鏡	5	感染症予防法	46
間質性肺炎	164	関節鏡検査	13, 284	感染性胃腸炎	110
間質性肺疾患	164, 561	間接クームス試験		感染性関節炎	286
鉗子分娩	230		267, 560	乾癬性関節炎	286
患者	588	間接蛍光抗体法	80, 561	感染性眼内炎	133
患者識別情報	70	関節形成術	13, 291	感染性心内膜炎	186, 561
患者紹介	392	関節血症	280	感染性腸炎	206
患者像	95, 394	間接抗グロブリン試験		がんセンター	52
患者中心の医療	95		267	感染対策チーム	560
癌腫症	13	関節拘縮	281	完全置換人工心臓	
肝腫大	5, 14, 198, 262	関節固定術	291		192, 601
杆状核好中球	264	関節腫脹	278	がん専門薬剤師	58, 526
環状シトルリン化ペプチ		肝切除術	215	肝臓	5, 484
ド	531	関節水症	280	肝臓科	53
感情障害ならびに統合失		間接赤血球凝集法	80, 561	肝臓学	64
調症面接基準	304, 595	関節穿刺	284	乾燥甲状腺	258
冠状静脈洞	476, 538	関節造影法	284	含嗽剤	86
環状切除	242	間接鼠径ヘルニア	210	肝臓病医	59

含嗽薬	152
間代	300
眼帯	136
癌胎児性抗原	201, 532
肝濁音界	198
間置	87
灌注法	289
浣腸	90
浣腸器	90
環椎後頭関節	495
貫通	87
眼痛	120, 125
眼底	458
眼底鏡	77
眼底血圧測定法	132, 579
眼底検査法	15, 131
カンデサルタンシレキセチル	188
カンデラ	438, 531
眼電図	132, 547
冠動脈	471
眼動脈	472
冠動脈硬化症	184
肝動脈持続動注療法	213, 533
冠動脈疾患	184, 530
冠動脈性心疾患	184, 533
冠動脈造影法	530
肝動脈注入療法	213, 601
冠動脈内注入血栓溶解療法	190, 560
冠動脈バイパス	191
冠動脈バイパス移植片	191, 530
嵌頓	9
嵌頓ヘルニア	198
眼内異物感	126
肝内結石症	114, 209
肝内胆管	484
肝内胆汁うっ滞	208
眼内レンズ	137, 562
眼内レンズ挿入眼	137
嵌入骨折	282
陥入爪	281
肝の	5
間脳	503
還納性ヘルニア	198
肝膿瘍	208
肝斑	319

肝脾腫	3
乾皮症	35, 321
眼皮膚型白皮症	326, 578
カンピロバクター・ジェジュニ	202
カンファレンス室	54
肝不全	208
貫壁性心筋梗塞	185
鑑別診断	85, 540
漢方	118
汗疱	324
眼房	456
がん放射線療法看護	61
眼房水	512
がん保険	48
陥没骨折	282
陥凹した	197
ガンマナイフ	317
冠名用語	38
顔面紅潮	262
顔面静脈	476
顔面神経	505
顔面神経麻痺	5, 294
顔面痛	120
顔面動脈	472
顔面の	5, 35
顔面播種状粟粒性狼瘡	328, 567
肝門	484
がん薬物療法認定薬剤師	58, 526
間葉系幹細胞	574
間葉組織	512
癌抑制遺伝子	510
管理医療	48
管理栄養士	58
眼輪筋	498
寒冷凝集素症	270, 530
寒冷赤血球凝集素	268
肝レンズ核変性症	209
関連痛	121
関連病院	52
緩和ケア	61
緩和ケア病棟	54, 582

き

キアリ・フロンメル症候群	253
奇異性尿失禁	217
偽遺伝子	510
既往症	73
既往歴	70, 73, 95, 396, 584
記憶	295
記憶力減退	295
機械的換気	169
機械的歯面清掃	152
気管	5, 28, 466
義眼	126
気管呼吸音	157
気管支	5, 466
気管支炎	17, 163
気管支拡張症	17, 164
気管支拡張薬	13, 167
気管支含気像	161
気管支鏡検査	163
気管支呼吸音	157
気管支声	157
気管支喘息	163, 525
気管支造影	5
気管支造影法	161
気管支動脈	472
気管支動脈造影法	161, 525
気管支動脈塞栓術	170, 525
気管支動脈注入	170, 525
気管支内超音波断層法	163, 544
気管支の	5, 34
気管支肺異形成症	336, 528
気管支肺炎	13
気管支肺洗浄	169
気管支肺胞呼吸音	157
気管支肺胞洗浄	163, 526
気管支肺胞洗浄液	163, 526
気管食道瘻	338, 602
偽関節	282
気管切開	5, 19, 170
気管支炎	25
気管チューブ	168, 548
基幹定点	110

用語	ページ
気管内吸引	168
気管内挿管	168
気管軟骨	495
気管の	5
気管分岐部	466
気管偏位	156
気胸	15, 167
木靴心	180
奇形	11, 83
奇形学	63
奇形腫	83
機嫌	295
既婚	74
起座呼吸	15, 18, 154
キサンチン誘導体	167
キサントクロミー	305
キサントシン	610
義歯	148
義肢	279
義肢学	64
既視感	293
義肢装具士	58
技師長	59
気質	295
器質化肺炎を伴う閉塞性細気管支炎	164, 528
器質性雑音	175
器質性疾患	106
義手	279
気性	295
気象医学	64
奇静脈	476
疑診	85
偽陣痛	121
キース・ワグナー分類	131, 565
偽性球麻痺	308
寄生虫学	63
寄生虫卵	199
偽性低アルドステロン症	115, 254, 584
偽性肥大性筋ジストロフィー	308
偽性副甲状腺機能低下症	12, 115, 252
気絶	293
季節性インフルエンザ	155
季節的感情障害	595

用語	ページ
キセノン	435, 610
キーセルバッハ部位	141, 460
基礎医学	63
基礎エネルギー消費量	526
基礎看護学	65
規則	46
義足	279
基礎血圧	75
基礎酸分泌量	201, 526
基礎食	90
基礎体温	231, 526
基礎代謝率	246, 528
気体縦隔造影法	161
偽痛風	286
喫煙	74
喫煙指数	156
吃逆	28
ぎっくり腰	279
規定(溶液)	575
基底細胞癌	327, 526
基底層	462
ギテルマン症候群	254
亀頭	36, 488
気道	466
気導	517
亀頭炎	237
気道可逆性試験	162
気道過敏性試験	162
気道系リンパ組織	526
気道閉塞	156
危篤状態	76
希突起膠細胞	15
きぬた骨	459
キヌプリスチン・ダルホプリスチン	590
ギネ	30
機能性雑音	175
機能性子宮出血	239, 551
機能性疾患	106
機能性ディスペプシア	204, 549
気脳造影法	305, 583
機能装具	289
機能的頚部リンパ節郭清術	146, 550
機能的残気量	162, 551

用語	ページ
機能的自立度評価法	92, 550
機能的神経筋刺激法	316, 550
機能的電気刺激	291, 549
機能不全性不正子宮出血	239, 544
希発月経	228
義父	73
ギプス	279
ギプス固定法	289
気分	76, 295
気分障害	312
気分変調	35
気分変調性障害	312
義母	73
偽膜	12, 141
偽膜性大腸炎	206, 585
奇脈	173
脚	37
偽薬	85
逆受身赤血球凝集反応	81, 593
逆成語	407
虐待	38
逆転写	510
逆転写酵素・ポリメラーゼ連鎖反応	81, 594
脚ブロック	526
逆流	195
逆流性食道炎	204
キャサヌル森林病	108
客観的データ	96, 598
客観的臨床能力試験	66, 580
逆行性射精	228
逆行性腎盂造影法	220, 593
逆行性尿道造影法	221
逆行性尿路造影法	220
キャッスルマン病	272
キャビトロン超音波外科用吸収器	539
キャフィー病	340
吸引細胞診	78
吸引生検	78
吸引生検細胞診	78, 516
臼蓋形成術	292
球海綿体反射	231, 526

嗅覚	140		271	急性閉塞性化膿性胆管炎		209, 522
嗅覚異常	140	急性好酸球性肺炎		急性網膜壊死		135, 523
嗅覚器	460		164, 519	急性リンパ芽球性白血病		
嗅覚検査	143	急性好酸球性白血病	271	共通抗原		268, 530
嗅覚減退	140	急性甲状腺炎	251	急性リンパ性白血病		
嗅覚認知域のにおい	143	急性喉頭蓋炎	340			270, 521
吸気	154	急性喉頭気管気管支炎		球脊髄性筋萎縮症		
吸気時痛	156		340		112, 309, 595	
救急医学	64	急性後部多発性斑状色素		急速眼球運動(睡眠)		592
救急医療	546	上皮症	135, 522	急速進行性糸球体腎炎		
救急看護	60	急性呼吸促迫症候群			115, 221, 593	
救急救命士	58, 546		166, 523	球体		40
救急室	54, 547	急性呼吸不全	166, 523	吸着		34
救急車	34	急性骨髄性白血病		旧ツベルクリン		580
救急治療部	54, 545		270, 521	嗅電図		143, 547
救急病院	52	急性骨髄単球性白血病		吸入器		169
球形嚢	460		270, 521	吸入酸素濃度		162, 550
灸師	58	急性細菌性心内膜炎		吸入ステロイド・長時間		
吸収	34		186, 516	作用型吸入β₂刺激薬合		
吸収不良症候群	206	急性散在性脳脊髄炎		剤		169
球状赤血球	264		307, 518	吸入ステロイド薬		169
球状赤血球症	264	急性糸球体腎炎	221, 519	吸入麻酔		87
球状帯	490	急性・重症患者看護	60	吸入療法		169
丘疹	319	急性出血性結膜炎		嗅脳		502
嗅神経	505		110, 133, 519	牛肺疫菌様微生物		587
求心性	34	急性出血性膵炎	209, 520	給付金		48
求心性ニューロン	504	急性出血性大腸炎		救命救急センター		52
求心路遮断性疼痛	121		206, 519	灸療法		118
吸水軟膏	328, 522	急性小脳性失調症	339	キュリー		534
急性	91	急性心筋梗塞	185, 521	キュリウム		436, 535
急性胃炎	205	急性腎障害	222, 522	ギュンター病		335
急性胃粘膜病変	205, 519	急性腎不全	222, 523	橋		504
急性壊死性潰瘍性歯肉炎		急性膵炎	209	共圧陣痛		121
	151, 522	急性生理慢性健康評価		教育		74
急性壊死性膵炎	210, 522		92, 522	教育学		66
急性炎症性脱髄性多発ニ		急性脊髄前角炎	25	教育的計画		96
ューロパチー	309, 520	急性前骨髄球性白血病		教育病院		52
急性灰白髄炎	107		270, 522	教育目標		66
急性肝炎	207	急性相反応物質	523	教育目標分類体系		66
急性間欠性ポルフィリン		急性単球性白血病	270	教員能力開発		66, 549
症	257, 520	急性中耳炎	143, 522	境界域高血圧		184
急性間質性腎炎	222, 520	急性動脈閉塞疾患	187	境界性人格障害		313, 528
急性間質性肺炎	164, 520	急性尿細管壊死	222, 524	仰臥位低血圧症候群		
急性感染性心内膜炎		急性妊娠脂肪肝	207, 519			231, 597
	186, 520	急性脳炎	109	胸郭		5, 156, 444
急性冠動脈症候群		急性肺損傷	166, 521	胸郭形成術		5, 170
	184, 518	急性非リンパ性白血病		強拡大視野		558
急性巨核球性白血病	270		270, 522	胸郭出口症候群		284, 604
急性好塩基球性白血病		急性腹症	210			

胸管	478	強心薬	189	強膜	456
共感覚	301	胸水	158, 217	胸膜	468
共感性対光反射	129	胸髄	504	胸膜液	512
橋義歯術	152	胸声	157	強膜炎	133
胸筋神経	505	強制経管栄養	212	胸膜炎	37, 167
胸腔	455	矯正歯科	53	胸膜腔	468
胸腔鏡下生検	163	矯正歯科医	59	強膜虹彩炎	16
胸腔鏡下肺全摘	170	矯正歯科学	64	胸膜痛	17, 120, 156
胸腔鏡下肺嚢胞切除	170	矯正視力	126	強膜内陥術	137
胸腔鏡検査	16, 163	胸腺	490	胸膜の	9, 37
胸腔穿刺	17, 163	胸腺摘除術	259, 317	胸膜剥離術	170
胸腔洗浄	169	共存疾患	106	胸膜摩擦音	158
胸腔ドレーン	169	兄弟	73	胸膜癒着術	170
凝血塊	262	蟯虫	199	共鳴音	156
狂犬病	108	橋中心髄鞘崩壊症		希用薬	85
凝固因子	265		309, 537	胸腰筋膜	501
競合的タンパク結合分析		協調運動障害	300	共用試験	66
法	81, 536	強直	34	巨核芽球	267
凝固時間	265	強直性脊椎炎	287, 523	巨核球	11, 266
胸骨	5, 492	強直性脊椎骨増殖症		棘間靱帯	496
頬骨	492		287, 524	棘筋	500
胸骨・後頭骨・下顎骨固		胸椎	492, 600	局所解剖学	68
定用装具	290	胸痛	120, 155, 172	局所性	38
胸骨右縁	175, 594	共同介護	43	局所麻酔	87
胸骨下痛	120	強度変調放射線治療		局所麻酔薬	123
胸骨・後頭骨・下顎骨固			117, 561	局所用ベータ遮断薬	136
定用装具	598	強迫神経症	312	極低出生体重	609
胸骨左縁	175, 568	強迫性障害	578	極低出生体重児	331
胸骨切開	5	強皮症	111, 114	虚血	83
胸骨線	454	強皮症腎クリーゼ		虚血性拘縮	281
胸骨中線	454, 574		328, 599	虚血性視神経障害	
胸骨の	5	胸部	450		134, 562
胸骨部	450	頬部	450	虚血性心疾患	184, 561
頬骨部	450	胸部Ｘ線写真		虚血性大腸炎	206
胸骨柄	492		161, 180, 539	距骨	494
凝固能	262	胸部外科	53	巨細胞腫	288, 552
凝固能亢進	266	胸部外科医	59	巨細胞動脈炎	187, 552
凝固能低下	266	胸部外科学	64	鋸歯	40
共済組合健康保険	48	恐怖症	35, 296	虚弱な	104
胸鎖関節	495	胸部大動脈	472	巨手症	8
狭窄	198	胸部大動脈瘤	187, 601	挙上	289, 593
胸鎖乳突筋	498	胸部大動脈瘤ステントグ		鋸状縁	458
胸鎖乳突筋部	450	ラフト内挿術	192, 603	巨人症	245
胸式呼吸	154	胸部単純撮影法	161	巨赤芽球性貧血	269
教授	62	胸部不快感	172	巨大血小板症候群	273
狭小頭蓋	14	胸部誘導	178	巨大結腸	11
胸神経	505	胸部理学療法	169	巨大舌	11, 148, 245
狭心症	185, 522	共分散分析	522	巨大乳頭結膜炎	133, 553
狭心症発作	172	恐糞症	296	巨大リンパ節増殖症	272

虚脱脈	173	候群	187, 573	空洞音	157
去痰薬	167	銀親和性細胞腫	255	空洞音性共鳴	156
虚脈	173	筋生検	284	空腹	194
魚鱗癬	320	金製剤	288	空腹時血糖	246, 549
魚類恐怖症	296	筋性防御	198	空腹時血糖異常	247, 561
ギラン・バレー症候群		筋線維腫	15	空腹痛	195
	112, 310, 552	筋組織	512	クエッケンシュテット試	
キリアン手術	146	筋脱力	278	験	305
切り傷	318	巾着縫合	88	クエン酸塩添加血	275
きりきりする	121	緊張	37, 295	クオート	439, 590
起立性	15	緊張性頚反射	333, 604	クオンティフェロンTB	
起立性調節障害	341, 579	緊張性頭痛	120	試験	160, 590
起立性低血圧	184, 262	緊張性尿失禁	217	クーゲルベルク・ウェラ	
キリップ分類	177	筋電図	14, 283, 546	ンダー病	342
亀裂骨折	282	キント	30	楔状椎	284
亀裂舌	148	筋肉	498	楔状軟骨	495
キレート療法	118	筋肉圧痛	278	くしゃみ	139, 154
キログラム	438, 564	筋肉痛	120, 278	駆出音	175
キロベース	510, 564	筋肉内	561	駆出性雑音	175
キロメートル	438, 564	筋肉内注射	86	駆出率	182, 545
筋	5	筋の	5	駆出率正常心不全	186
金	436, 525	キーンベック病	285	くすぶり白血病	271
銀	435, 519	筋膜	500	クスマウル呼吸	246
近位	448	筋膜の	35	薬指	444
近位咬合	36, 149	勤務医	57	口	6, 37, 442
近位指節間関節	495, 584	キンメルスチール・ウィ		口呼吸	140
筋萎縮	278, 294	ルソン症候群	222	口対口人工呼吸	190
筋萎縮性側索硬化症		筋力計	283	口とがらせ反射	301
	112, 308, 521	筋力低下	261	口の	34
近位尿細管	486			口髭	442
筋炎	285	く		唇	6, 442
禁煙外来	169	クアゼパム	314	唇形成術	152
筋活動電位	304, 569	グアニン	510, 551	唇の	6, 36
近眼	125	グアノシン一リン酸	553	駆虫薬	211
禁忌	10	グアノシン三リン酸	554	屈曲	279
緊急時連絡	71	グアノシン二リン酸	552	屈曲拘縮	281
緊急避妊薬	241	区域気管支	466	屈曲変形	279
筋拘縮	281	クインケ浮腫	320	屈筋	498
均衡食	90	隅角検査	131	屈筋支帯	498
筋硬直	198	隅角後退緑内障	134	クッシング潰瘍	205
筋骨格系	75	隅角癒着解離術	137, 554	クッシング三主徴	298
筋骨格系疾患	278	空気液面	203	クッシング症候群	253
近視	125	空気嚥下症	18	クッシング病	116, 252
筋弛緩薬	289	空気感染	105	屈折異常	125
近視性	37	空気伝導	142	屈折検査	131
均質性	36	空虚トルコ鞍症候群	313	屈側	448
筋腫	5, 83	空腸	482	グッドパスチャー症候群	
菌状息肉症	272, 327, 571	空腸動脈	474		221
筋・腎障害性代謝異常症		空洞	161	クッパー細胞	484

クナイプ式療法	118	クリスマス病	274	グルタミン酸ピルビン酸トランスアミナーゼ	553
クーパーネイル徴候	233	グリセオフルビン	329, 553	クルドスコピー	236
首	442	グリセリン浣腸	90, 552	くる病	337
クベイム試験	323	グリソンスコア	221	くる病じゅず	156
クボステック徴候	246	クリック	175	踝(くるぶし)	36, 278
組合管掌健康保険	48	グリッペ	30	クループ症候群	340
組み換えDNA	510	クリッペル・フェール症候群	341	グループ診療	43
組み換え免疫ブロット法	593	クリティカルケア看護学	65	クールボアジエ徴候	198
クームス試験	267	クリニカルパス	89, 536	車椅子	90
くも恐怖症	296	クーリー貧血	269	クルンプケ麻痺	335
くも状血管腫	197	クリプトスポリジウム症	109	クレアチニン	537
くも状指	17			クレアチニンクリアランス	219, 531
くも膜	504	クリプトン	434, 565		
くも膜下腔	504	グリベンクラミド	258	クレアチンキナーゼ	178, 283, 534
くも膜下出血	307, 595	クリミア・コンゴ出血熱	107	クレアチンキナーゼアイソザイム MM	534
くも膜下ブロック	123	クリーム剤	86		
くも指症	9	グリメピリド	258	クレアチンキナーゼアイソザイム MB	178, 534
クライネ・レヴィン症候群	312	クリュヴェイエ・バウムガルテン症候群	198	クレアチンキナーゼアイソザイム BB	534
クラインフェルター症候群	240	クリューバー・ビューシー症候群	312	クレアチンリン酸	582
グラヴィッツ腫瘍	223	クリンダマイシン	534	クレアチンリン酸酵素	178, 537
グラスゴー昏睡尺度	297, 552	クール	30, 35	グレアム・スティール雑音	176
グラスゴー転帰尺度	92, 553	グル音	196	グレイ	438, 554
クラッツキン腫瘍	209	グルカゴン様ペプチド	247, 553	グレイターナー徴候	198
クラッベ病	337	クルーケンベルク腫瘍	233	グレーヴス病	251
グラデニゴー症候群	143	グリコアルブミン	552	クレオラ体	159
グラニセトロン塩酸塩	211	グルココルチコイド抵抗症	115	クレスチン	588
クラミジア尿道炎	237			クレスト(症候群)	537
クラミジア肺炎	110	グルココルチコイド反応性アルドステロン症	254, 553	クレチン病	251, 336
クラミジア封入体	235			グレーフェ徴候	246
グラム	438, 551	グルコース-6-リン酸デヒドロゲナーゼ	552	クレブス	30
グラム陰性桿菌	202, 553			グレーン	438, 553
グラム陽性球菌	553	クルシュマンらせん体	159	クロイツフェルト・ヤコブ病	109, 112, 311, 534
暗闇恐怖症	296	グルタチオンジスルフィド	554		
クラリスロマイシン	530			クロウ・深瀬症候群	112, 273
クランケ	30	グルタミン酸オキサロ酢酸トランスアミナーゼ	553		
グランツマン病	273			クロザピン	316
グリア線維性酸性タンパク質	305, 552	グルタミン酸デカルボキシラーゼ	552	黒そこひ	125
クリグラー・ナジャール症候群	335			グロッコ三角	157
				クロナゼパム	316, 539
グリコアルブミン	247			クローニング	510
クリスチャンサイエンス	118			クローヌス	300
				クローバー	40

クロピドグレル硫酸塩	315	
クロマチン	508	
クロミフェンクエン酸塩	241	
クロム	434, 537	
クロモグリク酸ナトリウム	167, 543	
クロラムフェニコール	536	
クロルフェニラミンマレイン酸塩	145	
クロロエチルニトロソウレア	526	
クーロン	438, 529	
クロンカイト・カナダ症候群	207	
クローン病	113, 206, 531	
群集恐怖症	296	
群発頭痛	120

け

毛	6, 462
ケアハウス	55
茎	40
経過	91
経過記録	70, 91, 95, 96
計画	70, 96, 403, 598
経カテーテル動脈化学塞栓術	213, 601
経カテーテル動脈塞栓術	213, 601
鶏眼	25
経管栄養	212
頚管拡張術および掻爬術	242
頚管粘液	235, 535
経気管吸引生検	163, 605
経気管支吸引生検	163, 601
経気管支生検	163, 601
経気管支肺生検	163, 602
経頚静脈性肝内門脈体循環短絡	213, 603
軽減	91
経験的治療	118
蛍光インサイチュー・ハイブリダイゼーション	81, 550

蛍光眼底撮影法	132, 549
経口血糖降下剤と基礎インスリン注射併用	258, 528
経口血糖降下薬	258
蛍光顕微鏡	79
蛍光抗核抗体	549
蛍光酵素免疫測定法	81, 549
蛍光抗体	548
蛍光抗体法	81, 549
経口的	6, 11, 586
経口内視鏡検査	78
経口避妊薬	230, 241, 578
経口ブドウ糖負荷試験	247, 579
蛍光偏光免疫検定法	81, 551
経口補液療法	117, 579
蛍光免疫測定法	81, 550
脛骨	6, 27, 494
脛骨神経	506
脛骨粗面	494
脛骨痛	6
脛骨の	6
警察医	57
経産	232
計算障害	302
経産の	37
経産婦	11, 230
憩室炎	205
形質細胞	265
形質転換成長因子	603
形状	39
経静脈高カロリー輸液	91, 212, 563
頚静脈怒張	174, 564
頚静脈波	180
経食道心エコー検査	181, 602
頚神経叢	505
頚髄	504
痙性クループ	340
形成外科	53
形成外科医	59
形成外科学	64
痙性歩行	298
痙性麻痺	298
痙性両麻痺	306

ケイ素	434, 597
脛側	448
経腟超音波検査	236
経腸栄養	91, 212
経蝶形骨洞手術	317, 605
経直腸的の超音波検査	220, 605
頚椎	492, 529
頚椎牽引	291
頚椎症性神経根症	287, 538
頚椎症性脊髄症	287, 538
頚椎装具	290
系統	37
経頭蓋ドプラ超音波診断法	305, 602
経瞳孔温熱療法	136
系統別病歴	70, 75, 95, 593
頚動脈雑音	176
頚動脈ステント留置術	316, 530
頚動脈造影法	305, 530
頚動脈洞症候群	184
頚動脈内膜切除術	316, 532
頚動脈波	180
経尿道の極超短波温熱療法	226, 605
経尿道の砕石術	225, 605
経尿道の生検	221
経尿道の切除術	226, 605
経尿道の前立腺蒸散術	226, 606
経尿道の前立腺切除術	226, 605
経尿道の尿管砕石術	226
経尿道の針焼灼療法	226, 605
経尿道の膀胱腫瘍切除術	226, 605
経尿道のレーザー前立腺切除術	226, 605
経妊婦	229
珪肺症	165
経皮	11
経鼻胃管	211, 576
脛腓関節	495
経鼻気管吸引	169
経皮経管血管形成術	

	317, 588	
経皮経肝食道静脈瘤塞栓術	213, 589	
経皮経肝胆管造影法	203, 588	
経皮経肝胆汁ドレナージ	213, 588	
経皮経肝胆道鏡検査	204, 588	
経皮経肝胆嚢ドレナージ	213, 589	
経皮経管的冠動脈形成術	190, 588	
経皮経管的冠動脈再開通術	190, 588	
経皮経管的腎動脈形成術	225, 589	
経皮経肝門脈造影法	589	
経皮経静脈的僧帽弁交連切開術	191, 588	
経皮腎尿管切石術	225	
経皮腎瘻造設術	225, 586	
経皮のエタノール注入療法	213, 583	
経皮の冠動脈インターベンション	190, 582	
経鼻の持続気道陽圧呼吸	170, 576	
経皮的腎切石術	225, 586	
経皮的心肺補助装置	192, 582	
経皮的髄核摘出術	291, 585	
経皮的電気神経刺激法	123, 602	
経皮的動脈血酸素飽和度	159, 599	
経皮的内視鏡下胃瘻造設術	213, 583	
経皮的バルーン大動脈弁形成術	192	
経皮的ペーシング	190, 602	
経皮的マイクロ波凝固療法	213, 585	
経表皮水分喪失	322, 603	
軽費老人ホーム	55	
頸部	75, 450	
鶏歩	298	

傾眠	297	
稽留熱	105	
稽留流産	238	
痙攣	35, 293	
痙攣重積	331	
痙攣発作	25	
頸腕症候群	285	
外科	53	
外科医	59	
外科学	64	
外科療法	118	
下痢	34, 231	
劇症1型糖尿病	255	
劇症型溶血性連鎖球菌感染症	109	
劇症肝炎	113, 207	
下血	195	
下剤	211	
血圧	172, 173, 528	
血圧計	77	
血液	6, 512	
血液科	53	
血液化学検査	78	
血液学	2, 64	
血液学的検査	78	
血液型	267	
血液型と交差適合試験	602	
血液型不適合	267	
血液凝固	262	
血液銀行	275	
血液検査	78	
血液疾患	261	
血液浄化法	225	
血液透析	6, 225, 555	
血液尿素窒素	219, 529	
血液脳関門	526	
血液病医	59	
血液量	529	
血液濾過	225, 555	
血液濾過透析	225, 555	
血縁	73	
結核	18, 28, 107, 601	
結核菌	160	
結核性	38	
結核性脊椎炎	287	
結核病院	52	
結核予防法	46	
結核療養所	52	

血管	6	
血管運動	16	
血管外液	512	
血管外肺水分量	162, 548	
血管外遊出	11	
血管拡張	6	
血管拡張薬	189	
血管形成術	18	
血管外科	53	
血管外科医	59	
血管外科学	64	
血管雑音	198	
血管作動性腸管ポリペプチド	608	
血管腫	83, 326	
血管周囲性	11	
血管収縮	16	
血管収縮薬	189	
血管神経性	12	
血管造影法	6, 12, 17, 79	
血管透過性因子	609	
血管内超音波検査法	182, 564	
血管内治療	192, 548	
血管内皮増殖因子	608	
血管迷走神経反射	176, 609	
血管攣縮性狭心症	185, 609	
血球計算器	263	
血球除去療法	212, 276	
血球貪食症候群	272, 558	
血球貪食性リンパ組織球症	272, 557	
血胸	14, 36, 167	
決疑論	35	
月経	27, 228	
月経間出血	229	
月経間の	11	
月経困難	10, 228	
月経前症候群	228, 585	
月経前神経不安障害	237, 585	
月経中間疼痛	228	
月経痛	121, 228	
月経不順	228	
月経抑制	15	
結合組織	512	
結婚恐怖症	296	

結婚歴	74	結節性硬化症	116, 326	ケトアシドーシス	247
結紮	87	結節性紅斑	326	ケトコナゾール	329, 564
血色素	263, 555	結節性多発動脈炎		ケトチフェンフマル酸塩	
血腫	261		111, 114, 585		145
血漿	512	結節性動脈周囲炎	585	ケトン体	247
血漿アルドステロン濃度		結節の	38	ケトン尿	218
	249, 580	結節縫合	88	原因不明突然死	600
結晶形成フラグメント		血栓除去術	191	解熱処置	117
	549	血栓性血小板減少性紫斑		解熱薬	117
血漿交換	225, 276, 583	病	115, 273, 605	ケノデオキシコール酸	
月状骨	492	血栓性静脈炎	187		211, 532
結晶性関節炎	286	血栓性微小血管症		ゲノミックス	510
血漿タンパク質分画	586		273, 604	ゲノム	510
血漿鉄交代率	269, 584	血栓塞栓	16	ゲノムインプリンティン	
血漿トロンボプラスチン		血栓弾性描写図	602	グ	510, 553
成分	588	血栓内膜切除術	191, 602	ゲフィチニブ	168
結晶尿	218	血栓溶解	16, 17	毛深い	319
血小板活性化因子		血栓溶解薬	189	ケブナー現象	321
	265, 580	血族結婚	74	ゲブルト	30
血小板凝集試験	265, 581	欠損歯	149	ゲムシタビン	552
血小板凝集抑制薬	189	結滞	172	ゲムシタビン塩酸塩	168
血小板減少	18, 265	血痰	155	ケモ	30
血小板数	263	血中濃度曲線下面積	525	下痢	196
血小板増加	265	結腸	6, 482	ケルヴィン	438, 564
血小板濃縮液	276, 582	結腸癌	207	ケルクリングひだ	482
血小板ペルオキシダーゼ		結腸間膜	11, 483	ゲルストマン症候群	302
	268, 587	結腸切除術	214	ゲルストマン・ストロイ	
血小板由来増殖因子	583	結腸内視鏡	6	スラー・シャインカー	
血小板由来増殖因子受容		結腸の	6, 35	病	112, 311, 554
体	583	結腸ひも	482	ケール徴候	262
血漿レアギン迅速試験		結腸膨起	482	ケルニヒ徴候	298
	236, 594	血糖自己測定	257, 598	ゲルマニウム	434, 552
血漿レニン活性	219, 587	血糖上昇指数		ケルマン水晶体乳化術	
欠神てんかん	297		244, 247, 553		136, 565
血性	261	血尿	216	腱	6, 501
血清アミロイドAタンパ		げっぷ	195	減圧	87
ク質	595	血餅収縮	265	牽引	87
血清学	63	血便	196	原因不明突然死	176
血清学的陰性	16	欠乏性疾患	106	牽引療法	290
血清学的検査	78	結膜	456	原因療法	117
血清クレアチニン	219	結膜溢血	262	検影法	131
血清診断	84	結膜炎	25	検疫法	46
血清タンパク電気泳動		結膜下出血	128	減塩食	90
	599	結膜弛緩症	133	限界フリッカー値	
血清鉄	268	結膜充血	127		131, 533
血清プロトロンビン転化		結膜蒼白	262	限外濾過	12, 225
促進因子	599	結膜浮腫	127	限外濾過率	606
結石症	15	血友病	14, 26, 274	幻覚	293
結節	40, 83	血友病関節炎	286	原癌遺伝子	510

項目	ページ
検眼法	131
嫌気症	296
研究員	62
研究機関	62
研究者	57
研究助手	62
限局性結節性過形成	550
限局性の	10
原形質	16, 508
献血	262
顕血便	195
原稿	22, 574
健康維持機構	50, 557
肩甲下部	452
肩甲間部	452
健康管理手帳	43
肩甲挙筋	500
肩甲骨	444, 492
肩甲骨中央線	454
肩甲上神経	505
健康状態	104
肩甲上部	452
健康食品	194
健康診査	72
健康診断書	67
健康政策局	43
健康増進法	46
肩甲帯	492
健康な	104
肩甲部	452
健康保険	48, 71
健康保険組合	48
健康保険適用	48
健康保険による払い戻し	48
健康保険被保険者証	48
言語障害	294
言語聴覚士	58
腱固定	6
言語療法	145, 316
言語療法士	600
肩鎖(関節)	517
顕在性不安尺度	303, 570
肩鎖関節	495
腱索	470
検査室	54, 565
検査室診断	84
検査所見	70, 95, 400
検査法	78

項目	ページ
犬歯	464
原子質量単位	439, 606
原始神経外胚葉性腫瘍	342, 585
幻肢痛	121
研修医	59
現住所	71
腱鞘	501
～減少	71
腱鞘炎	6, 285
腱鞘滑膜切除術	291
剣状突起	450
県条例	46
懸垂牽引	291
減数分裂	37
ゲンズレン徴候	281
ゲンタマイシン	553
幻聴	293
限定基礎データ	96
見当識	76
ケント束	179
検尿	78, 217, 606
原発開放隅角緑内障	133, 586
原発性アルドステロン症	115, 253
原発性異型肺炎	163, 581
原発性硬化性胆管炎	114, 208, 587
原発性高脂血症	113
原発性線毛機能不全	164, 582
原発性側索硬化症	116, 308, 585
原発性胆汁性肝硬変	113, 208, 581
原発性肺高血圧症	116, 166, 586
原発性免疫不全症候群	114
原発閉塞隅角緑内障	133, 580
瞼板	38, 456
腱反射	300
瞼板腺	456
顕微鏡	11
顕微鏡的血尿	218
顕微鏡的診断	84
顕微鏡的多発血管炎	111, 573

項目	ページ
現病歴	70, 72, 95, 395, 558, 584
検便	78
肩峰	492
健忘	295
腱膜	501
原理	37
県立病院	52
減量食	91
瞼裂斑	127

こ

項目	ページ
コア・カリキュラム	67
コアグラ	30
コアグラーゼ陰性ブドウ球菌	536
コイル塞栓術	317
抗SS-A/Ro抗体	149
抗SS-B/La抗体	150
抗アセチルコリン受容体抗体	303
高圧医学	64
高圧酸素療法	579
降圧食事療法	540
降圧薬	188, 224
抗ENA抗体	322
高位脛骨骨切り術	292, 559
抗EBNA抗体	267
抗EBV-EA抗体	267
抗EBV-VCA抗体	267
抗インフルエンザウイルス抗体	160
抗ウイルス薬	117, 314
高右心房心電図	180, 558
抗うつ薬	314
抗HBsヒト免疫グロブリン	555
後腋窩線	454, 581
抗Sm抗体	322
好塩基球	264
好塩基性斑点	264
構音障害	302
公害	43
口蓋	464
口蓋形成術	152
口蓋垂	464
口蓋垂炎	150

口蓋垂軟口蓋咽頭形成術	146, 606	抗胸腺細胞グロブリン	276, 524	抗好中球細胞質抗体	219, 522
後外側の	15	咬筋	498	抗好中球細胞質ミエロペルオキシダーゼ抗体	219, 573
口蓋披裂	150	抗菌物質	117	後交通動脈	471
口蓋扁桃	465	航空医学	64	交互切開	88
口蓋隆起	150	口腔衛生	147	交互脈	173
口蓋裂	332	口腔温	75	抗コリン作動薬	315
高額医療	48	口腔カンジダ症	27	抗コリン薬	210
抗核因子	522	口腔外科	53	高コレステロール血症	256
口角炎	150	口腔外科医	59	虹彩	456
光学顕微鏡	78	口腔外科学	64	虹彩異色症	128
抗核抗体	283, 321, 522	口腔内装具	168	虹彩炎	134
光学的干渉断層検査	132, 579	口腔病学	64	虹彩学	118
		後屈	12	虹彩血管新生	129
口角びらん	150, 262	抗グルタミン酸デカルボキシラーゼ抗体	247	虹彩毛様体炎	134
光覚弁	127, 568, 597	抗グロブリン試験	519	抗サイログロブリン抗体	248, 603
高額療養費	48	口径	34		
膠芽腫	313	後脛骨静脈	478	交叉下肢伸展挙上試験	281, 610
後下小脳動脈	472, 584	後脛骨動脈	476		
硬化性萎縮性苔癬	114, 325, 568	後脛骨動脈拍動	176	交差適合試験	267
硬化像	161	後頚三角部	450	好酸球	264
後下腿部	453	抗 Ku 抗体	283	好酸球塩基性タンパク	159, 545
口渇	244	抗痙攣薬	314	好酸球性筋膜炎	114, 285
高活性抗レトロウイルス療法	275, 554	高血圧	11, 217, 555, 559	好酸球増加	18, 265
		高血圧自然発症ラット	597	好酸球増加症候群	271, 556
抗ガラクトース欠損 IgG 抗体	283	高血圧症	184	好酸球増多・筋痛症候群	286, 546
高カリウム血症	219, 251	高血圧性心疾患	184, 556		
高カルシウム血症	251	高血圧網膜症	135	好酸球尿	218
抗カルジオリピン抗体	322, 518	抗結核薬	117	抗酸菌	519
		抗血小板薬	314	講師	62
高カロリー食	90	硬結性紅斑	325	抗 Jo-1 抗体	283
強姦	229	高血糖	26, 246	後耳介動脈	472
高眼圧症	133, 579	高血糖性高浸透圧性昏睡	256, 556	高色素血	263
口・顔・指症候群	338, 579			抗糸球体基底膜腎炎	221
		抗血友病因子	519	高脂血症	3, 256
抗環状シトルリン化ペプチド抗体	283	抗原	17, 519	光視症	126
		抗原結合フラグメント	548	合指症	333
交感神経	506			膠質浸透圧	536
交感神経切除術	123	抗原抗体反応	516	後膝部	453
交感神経ブロック	123	抗原提示細胞	522	口臭	26, 147
交換輸血	343	膠原病	106, 110	口周囲部	450
広基	40	硬膏	328	公衆衛生学	63
講義	67	硬口蓋	464	公衆衛生行政	43
後期高齢者医療制度	48	硬膏剤	86	後縦隔	468
講義時間割	67	抗甲状腺ペルオキシダーゼ抗体	248, 604		
抗凝固薬	189				
抗凝固療法	189, 518	抗甲状腺薬	258		

後十字靱帯	496, 582	
後縦靱帯骨化症		
	112, 287, 579	
拘縮	278	
甲状頚動脈	472	
後上膵十二指腸動脈		
	474, 588	
恒常性	14, 36	
甲状腺	490	
甲状腺癌	252	
甲状腺機能検査	247, 603	
甲状腺機能亢進症	2, 251	
甲状腺機能正常の	10	
甲状腺機能低下症	11, 251	
甲状腺結節	246	
甲状腺刺激ホルモン		
	248, 605	
甲状腺刺激ホルモン結合阻害免疫グロブリン		
	248, 602	
甲状腺刺激ホルモン受容体異常症	115	
甲状腺刺激ホルモン受容体抗体	248, 604	
甲状腺刺激ホルモン放出ホルモン	605	
甲状腺刺激免疫グロブリン		
	248, 605	
甲状腺腫大	246	
甲状腺切除術	259	
甲状腺中毒症	251	
甲状腺ホルモン不応症		
	115	
甲状軟骨	495	
後上葉区	468	
後上腕部	452	
高所恐怖症	18, 296	
紅色陰癬	325	
口唇	464	
口唇炎	6, 150	
抗真菌薬	117	
向神経性	15	
高身長	245	
高浸透圧性非ケトン性昏睡		
	256, 557	
口唇ヘルペス	150	
口唇裂	150, 332	
光錐	458	
後水晶体線維増殖症		
	134, 593	
抗水痘帯状疱疹ウイルス抗体	322	
抗ストレプトキナーゼ		
	524	
抗ストレプトリジンO		
	283, 524	
合成	12	
硬性癌	37	
硬性癌の	37	
抗精神病薬	314	
後正中線	454	
厚生年金保険	48	
硬性白斑	130	
硬性皮膚	11	
抗生物質	10, 117	
抗生物質関連下痢		
	196, 516	
抗生物質関連大腸炎		
	206, 516	
抗生物質療法	117	
厚生労働省	43	
高線維食	90	
光線過敏試験	323	
光線過敏症	320	
光線性	34	
光線貼布試験	323	
抗セントロメア抗体		
	322, 517	
後前	15, 580	
光線力学療法	136, 170	
光線療法	343	
後前腕部	452	
酵素	10	
構造遺伝子	510	
梗塞	83	
口側	448	
高速液体クロマトグラフィー	81, 558	
拘束型心筋症		
	113, 187, 592	
拘束性肺疾患	163	
高ソマトトロピン分泌症		
	253	
酵素免疫吸着法	81, 546	
酵素免疫測定法	81, 546	
抗体	10, 516	
抗体依存性細胞傷害	518	
高体温	11	
抗体関連型拒絶反応	521	
抗体欠損症候群	519	
交代遮閉試験	128	
交代性片麻痺	299	
後大腿部	453	
後大脳動脈	471, 582	
高炭酸ガス血症	159	
抗単純ヘルペスウイルス抗体	322	
高タンパク食	90	
高窒素血症	219	
高地脳浮腫	306, 554	
高地肺水腫	166, 554	
鉤虫	199	
好中球	264	
好中球アルカリホスファターゼ	265, 575	
好中球減少	18, 265	
好中球遊走因子	576	
後肘部	452	
抗DNA抗体	321	
口底蜂巣炎	151	
公的健康保険	48	
公的年金	48	
抗てんかん薬	315, 519	
後天性嚢胞性腎疾患		
	222, 517	
後天性免疫不全症候群		
	109, 270, 520	
後天性溶血性貧血		
	270, 519	
咽頭	465	
喉頭	6, 466	
喉頭炎	144	
喉頭蓋	466	
喉頭蓋炎	144	
喉頭蓋軟骨	495	
行動科学	63	
喉頭癌	145	
行動観察聴力検査		
	334, 528	
喉頭鏡検査	6, 143	
後頭筋	498	
喉頭形成術	146	
喉頭痙攣	144	
後頭骨	492	
口頭指示	609	
口頭試問	67	
行動状況	92, 587	

口頭症例提示	392
喉頭ストロボスコープ	143
喉頭切開術	146
喉頭摘出術	146
後頭動脈	472
喉頭軟骨	495
喉頭の	6
後頭部	442, 450
行動目標	67, 595
後頭葉	502
後頭リンパ節	478
高度先進医療	48
抗トポイソメラーゼ I 抗体	322
高トリグリセリド血症	256
口内炎	6, 150
口内乾燥症	151
高ナトリウム血症	251
抗二本鎖 DNA 抗体	322
高尿酸血症	250
高熱	105
更年期	229
更年期障害	229
後囊下白内障	587
広背筋	500
後肺底区	468
高拍出性心不全	186
後発医薬品	85
後発白内障	134
紅斑	319
後半規管	460
広汎性子宮全摘術	243
広汎性発達障害	313, 582
紅斑性狼瘡	566
広範脊柱管狭窄症	112
紅斑線量	545
後鼻鏡検査	143
高比重リポタンパク	555
高比重リポタンパクコレステロール	250
紅皮症	14, 17, 319
硬皮症	16, 17
抗ヒスタミン薬	145
抗ヒトリンパ球向性ウイルス 1 型抗体	268
高非抱合型ビリルビン血症	268

後鼻漏	139, 585
高頻度換気	556
高頻度人工換気	170, 556
口部	450
項部	452
抗不安薬	314
抗風疹ウイルス抗体	334
後腹膜線維症	224
後腹膜リンパ節郭清	226, 593
項部固縮	298
後部硝子体剥離	134, 589
抗不整脈薬	189
高プロラクチン血症	253
興奮	295
高分解能コンピュータ断層撮影法	79, 558
高分子	11
興奮性シナプス後電位	547
抗平滑筋抗体	524
後壁心筋梗塞	185
抗ヘリコバクター・ピロリ抗体	201
硬便	196
高変異反復列	510, 609
後方	448
後房	456, 582
後方進入腰椎椎体間固定術	291, 585
硬膜	504
硬膜炎	307
硬膜外	10
硬膜外腔鏡	123
硬膜外血液パッチ法	316, 544
硬膜外血腫	307
硬膜外出血	307
硬膜外ブロック	123
硬膜外麻酔	87
硬膜下腔	504
硬膜下血腫	307, 596
硬膜静脈洞	476
高マグネシウム血症	251
抗麻疹ウイルス抗体	334
抗ミクロソーム抗体	248
高密度焦点式超音波療法	226, 556
抗ミトコンドリア抗体	201, 521

硬脈	173
抗ムスカリン薬	224
抗ムンプス抗体	334
後迷路性難聴	143
咬耗症	149
肛門	482
肛門括約筋	482
肛門括約筋緊張	198
肛門管	482
肛門出血	195
肛門側	448
肛門病学	65
肛門部	452
絞扼性ニューロパチー	282, 285
絞扼痛	172
膠様組織	512
高用量シタラビン	556
咬翼撮影法	150
公立病院	52
合理的	37
抗利尿ホルモン	249, 518
抗利尿ホルモン不適切分泌症候群	253, 597
高リポタンパク血症	256
交流	517
交流分析	316, 601
口輪筋	498
高リン酸血症	251
光輪視	126
抗リン脂質抗体	322
抗リン脂質抗体症候群	111, 114, 523
抗リンパ球グロブリン	276, 521
抗リンパ球抗体	521
高齢化社会	43
高齢者総合機能評価	533
声変わり	244
誤嚥性肺炎	163
氷パック	289
鼓音性	38
語音聴取閾値検査	142, 599
語音聴力検査	142
語音弁別検査	142
コカイン	25
コカイン塩酸塩	122

五角形	39	国際看護師協会看護師の倫理綱領	44	鼓室形成術	145
コーガン症候群	141	国際コミュニケーション英語能力テスト	67, 604	鼓室	458
股関節	495	国際疾病分類	85, 560	鼓室岬角	458
股関節全置換術	291, 603	国際助産師連盟助産師の倫理綱領	44	鼓室性	38
股関節痛歩行	279	国際生活機能分類	92, 560	五十肩	278
呼気	154	国際赤十字社	562	誤診	85
呼気悪臭	148	国際前立腺症状スコア	217, 562	個人衛生	77
呼気延長	157	国際対癌連合	606	個人健康保険	48
呼気終末陽圧呼吸	170, 583	国際単位	563	個人識別	560
呼気炭酸ガス分圧	162	国際単位系	597	個人歴	96
呼気中一酸化炭素濃度	162	国際病院評価機構	43, 564	コステン症候群	141
呼気中一酸化窒素濃度	162	国際標準化比	562	ゴセレリン酢酸塩	224
呼気分析	162	国際病理学用語コード	4, 598	午前	22, 521
呼吸	75, 154, 604	国際薬局方	85, 562	枯草熱	144
呼吸音	157, 529	国際予後指標	263, 562	姑息の療法	118
呼吸音減弱	157	コクシジオイデス症	108	誇大妄想	293
呼吸器科	53	黒質	504	鼓腸	26, 196, 197
呼吸器系	75	黒色	39	骨	6, 37, 492
呼吸器合胞体ウイルス	334, 594	黒色腫	15	骨移植	292
呼吸器症状	154	黒色舌	148	骨延長術	291
呼吸器内科学	64	黒色表皮腫	327, 522	骨化	6
呼吸窮迫症候群	592	黒色便	195	国家医療	43
呼吸筋トレーニング	169	黒内障	125	骨格	6
呼吸訓練	169	黒皮症	319	骨学	63
呼吸困難	18, 154, 172	国保	48	骨格筋	498
呼吸細気管支	466	国民皆保険	48	骨格の	6
呼吸細気管支炎関連間質性肺疾患	164, 591	国民健康保険	48	骨芽細胞	17
呼吸商	594	国民年金保険	48	骨化性筋炎	285
呼吸数	75, 594	国民保健サービス	50, 576	骨型アルカリホスファターゼ	283
呼吸性アシドーシス	159	国民保健サービス・地域医療法	50	骨幹	494
呼吸性移動	156	黒毛舌	148	骨関節炎	285, 578
呼吸性洞不整脈	174	国立病院	52	骨幹端	494
呼吸促進薬	167	国立病院機構	52	骨幹端・骨幹角	280, 570
呼吸リハビリテーション	169	固形食	90	骨棘	284
呼吸療法	167	固形物	194	骨切り術	291
呼吸療法認定士	58	固形便	196	コッククロフト・ゴールト式	220
呼吸予備量	162	語形変化	2	骨形成因子	528
国際医学用語コード	3, 598	語源	2	骨形成不全症	288, 579
国際科学用語	4, 563	午後	23, 585	骨減少	284
国際癌ゲノムコンソーシアム	44, 560	語根	2	骨再生誘導手術	153, 552
国際看護師協会	560	腰	38, 444	骨再造形	282
		ゴーシェ病	257	骨産道	232
		鼓室階	459	骨腫	83
				骨シンチグラフィー	284
				骨髄	527
				骨髄異形成症候群	115, 270, 571

日本語索引

骨髄移植	276, 528	骨膜	494	コリンアセチルトランスフェラーゼ	530
骨髄炎	15	骨密度	527	コリンエステラーゼ	200, 533
骨髄芽球	266	骨密度検査	283	ゴーリン症候群	327
骨髄球	266	骨迷路	459	五類感染症	109
骨髄腔	494	固定	87	コルサコフ症候群	302
骨髄生検	266	固定橋義歯	152	ゴルジ装置	508
骨髄線維症	15, 115, 271	コデインリン酸塩	122	コールターカウンター	263
骨髄穿刺	266	コート	31		
骨髄穿刺液	266	毎	23, 590	コルチ器	459
骨髄造血	15	孤独恐怖症	296	コルチコステロイド結合グロブリン	531
骨髄増殖性疾患	270, 573	コドマン体操	290		
骨髄抑制	266	子供	73	コルチコトロピン	248
骨髄抑制療法	276	コドン	510	コルチコトロピン放出ホルモン	248, 537
骨性	6	ゴードン症候群	254		
骨生検	251, 284	ゴードン反射	301	コルチコトロピン放出ホルモン試験	249
骨折	278, 551	ゴナドトロピン分泌異常症	113		
骨接合術	291			コルチコトロピン様中葉ペプチド	248, 534
骨折評価ツール	278	ゴナドトロピン放出ホルモン	553		
骨組織	512			コルチゾール	249
骨粗鬆症	255, 288	コーネル医学指数	303, 535	ゴールドマン視野計	132
骨端	494			コルヒチン	259
骨単位	494	ゴノ	31	コルポスコピー	236
骨直達牽引	291	後嚢下白内障	134	コレシストキニン	531
骨痛	120	語の原形	2	コレス骨折	282
骨伝導	142, 526	コバルト	434, 536	コレスチラミン	259
ゴットロン徴候	321	コープ徴候	197	コレステリン腫	143
骨内膜	494	股部白癬	27, 325	コレステロールエステル転送タンパク質	532
骨軟化症	17, 255, 288, 579	コプリック斑	148		
骨軟骨症	286	個別化医療	118	コレラ	107
骨肉腫	288	コペルニクシウム	436	コレラ菌	202
骨パジェット病	286	鼓膜	139, 458	コロイド	35
骨盤	6, 494	鼓膜炎	143	コロトコフ音	75
骨盤位	232, 233	鼓膜形成術	145	コロナウイルス	160
骨盤位分娩	230	鼓膜硬化	143	コロニー形成単位	533
骨盤下口	232	鼓膜切開術	145	コロニー刺激因子	538
骨盤腔	455	鼓膜穿孔	140	コロボーマ	131
骨盤傾斜	279	ゴム手袋	77	根管充填	152, 591
骨盤計測	6, 234	こむらがえり	279	根管治療	152, 592
骨盤上口	232	こめかみ	442	根拠に基づく医療	67, 544
骨盤痛	228	固有感覚	302	根拠に基づく看護	67, 544
骨盤底	231, 500	固有肝動脈	472	混合受身赤血球凝集反応	81, 573
骨盤動脈造影法	236, 580	固有筋層	480, 585		
骨盤内炎症性疾患	238, 584	固有受容体神経筋促進法	290, 585	混合静脈血酸素分圧	182
				混合性結合組織病	111, 116, 328, 570
骨盤の	6	小指	444		
骨盤腹膜炎	238	雇用主	71	コン症候群	253
コーツ病	134	コリガン脈	173	昏睡	76, 297
コッヘル鉗子	89	コリスチン	534		
コッヘル切開	88	コーリー病	257		

コンタクトレンズ	126, 534	サイクロセリン	168, 538		201, 581
混濁尿	216	細隙灯顕微鏡検査	131	最大耐量	574
コンタミ	31	再建	87	最大中間呼気流量率	
根治的	37	鰓溝	34		162, 572
根治的頸部リンパ節郭清術	146, 593	再興感染症	106	最大尿流率	220
		在郷軍人病	165	臍帯ヘルニア	6, 339
根治的乳房切除術	243	最高酸分泌量	201, 569	臍帯ヘルニア・巨舌・巨大児(症候群)	546
昆虫恐怖症	296	最後野	502		
根治療法	118	臍周囲部	450	左胃大網動脈	474
コンドーム	230	最終月経	228, 567	在宅医療	43
コントラ	31	最終診断	84	在宅介護	43
～困難	71	最終糖化産物	247, 568	在宅経腸栄養法	91, 555
コンピュータ処理多岐選択試験	67, 531	再手術	12	在宅酸素療法	169, 558
		最小可聴域	141	在宅中心静脈栄養法	
コンピュータ断層撮影	530	最小可聴閾値	142		91, 558
		最小血圧	75	最長筋	500
コンピュータ断層撮影法	79, 538	最小紅斑量	324, 571	最低点	91
		最小致死量	567, 572	細動脈	8
金平糖状赤血球	264	最小発育阻止濃度	572	左胃動脈	474, 567
昏迷	297	左胃静脈	478	臍動脈	474
混和せよ	23, 569	最小有効量	571	サイトケラチン19フラグメント	539
		菜食主義	261		
## さ		菜食主義者	261	サイトメガロウイルス	535
		細針吸引	78, 550		
ザー	31	細針生検	78	催乳反射	232
臍	6	再生	83	臍の	6
サイアザイド	188	再生医療	118	再発	91
在院日数	93	再生不良性貧血		再発性多発軟骨炎	144, 593
災害医療センター	52		115, 269, 516		
災害派遣医療チーム	43, 542	砕石位	77	裁判外紛争解決	43, 518
		砕石術	15, 19	臍部	450
再感染	12	臍帯	232	臍ヘルニア	210
細気管支	466	最大アンドロゲン遮断	224, 569	細胞	508
細気管支肺胞上皮癌	166, 525			細胞遺伝学	63
		最大換気量	575	細胞外	11
最強拍動点	175, 585	在胎期間過大児	331, 567	細胞外液	512, 545
細菌円柱	218	在胎期間軽小児		細胞化学	268
細菌学	63		331, 596, 597	細胞学	35
細菌学的検査	78	在胎期間相当体重児		細胞学的診断	84
細菌感染	106		331, 519	細胞質	13, 508
細菌恐怖症	296	最大吸気量	162, 559	細胞傷害性Tリンパ球	538
細菌性髄膜炎	110	最大許容線量	573		
細菌性赤痢	107	最大血圧	75	細胞小器官	508
細菌性腟症	238	臍帯血幹細胞移植		臍傍静脈	478
細菌尿	218		276, 531	細胞診	78
サイクリックアデノシン一リン酸	530	最大呼気速度	162, 583	細胞性免疫	535
		最大呼気流量	162, 583	細胞中心体	508
サイクリックグアノシン一リン酸	178, 533	最大呼気流量計	162, 583	細胞透過液	512
		最大刺激時酸分泌量		細胞毒性	13

細胞内	11	鎖骨上	12	左方視	14
細胞内液	512, 560	鎖骨上窩	450	左房肥大	179, 565
細胞内接着分子	560	鎖骨上窩リンパ節	478	サマリウム	435, 597
細胞変性効果	536	鎖骨上神経	505	寒がり	244
細胞マーカー	267	坐骨神経	506	さめ皮様皮膚	319
細胞膜	508	坐骨神経痛	121	サーモグラフィー	182, 322
催眠薬	117, 314	鎖骨大腿靱帯	496	左葉	484
催眠療法	118	鎖骨中央線	454, 570	座浴	89
サイム切断術	292	鎖骨の	6	サラゾスルファピリジン	211, 288, 595
細網細胞	267	鎖骨離断術	6	サリドマイド	274
細網組織	512	坐剤	86	サリドマイド製剤安全管	
細網内皮系	265, 592	左耳	22, 524	理手順	274, 602
サイロキシン	247, 601	左軸偏位	178, 565	サルコイド	16
サイロキシン結合グロブ		匙状爪	262, 321	サルコイドーシス	113, 165
リン	248, 601	左室拡張終末期圧	182, 568	ザルシタビン	275, 540
サイログロブリン	248, 603	左室拡張終末期容積	182, 569	猿手	298
サウナ	118	左室駆出率	182, 569	サル痘	108
逆子出産	230	左室収縮終末期圧	182, 569	サルファ(剤)	38
さかまつげ	127	左室収縮終末期容積	182, 569	サルメテロール	169
左下葉	466, 567	左室造影法	182, 569	サルモネラ	202
左眼	23, 580	左室肥大	175, 569	サルモネラ症	206
左肝動脈	474, 567	左室補助装置	192, 568	産院	52
左冠動脈	471, 566	挫傷	25, 37	産科医	59
左冠動脈主幹部	471, 567	左上葉	466	産科学	64
左脚後枝ブロック	179, 568	左心室	470, 568	三角窩	458
左脚前枝ブロック	179, 565	左心低形成症候群	338, 557	三角巾	289
左脚ブロック	179, 566	左心不全	185	三角筋	498
左胸心	14	左心房	470, 565	三角筋部	452
作業療法	117	サーズ	31	三角形	39
作業療法士	58, 580	刺すような	121	三角骨	492
索	35	嗄声	140, 244	三角靱帯	496
酢酸デオキシコルチコス		左前斜位	565	三角線維軟骨複合体	280, 603
テロン	542	痤瘡	245	三角柱	40
酢酸の	34	錯覚	36	産科病院	52
錯味覚	147	擦過傷	320	産科病棟	54
裂くような	121	ザナミビル水和物	168	三環系抗うつ薬	314, 602
錯乱	297	左肺	466	産休	230
作話	302	左肺下葉	468	産業医	57
左結腸動脈	474, 566	左肺上葉	468	産業医学	64
鎖肛	338	さび色	39	残気量	162, 594
鎖骨	6, 25, 492	サーファクタントプロテ		サングラス	126
坐骨	494	イン A	159, 598	塹壕口内炎	151
鎖骨下筋	498	サーファクタントプロテ		サンゴ状結石	219
鎖骨下静脈	476	イン D	159, 599	散剤	86, 589
鎖骨下動脈	472			散在性特発性骨増殖症	
鎖骨下部	450				

項目	ページ
	287, 542
三叉神経	505
三叉神経節	505
三叉神経痛	121
三次元原体放射線治療	117, 540
三次元コンピュータ断層撮影法	79
三次元心エコー法	181
三枝ブロック	179
三重焦点眼鏡	135
三種混合ワクチン	343
参照せよ	532, 607
産褥	230
産褥熱	230
産褥敗血症	27
酸性化血清陽性を伴う遺伝性赤芽球多形核症	269, 555
酸性ホスファターゼ	219, 518
三尖弁	470
三尖弁狭窄	184, 605
三尖弁の	12
三尖弁閉鎖症	183, 601
三尖弁閉鎖不全	184, 604
酸素	434, 578
酸素テント	168
酸素マスク	168
酸素療法	168
三段脈	12, 173
暫定診断	84
散瞳	129
産道	232
三頭筋反射	300
散瞳薬	136
サントリーニ管	484
残尿	220
残尿感	216
産婦	230
産婦人科	53, 578
産婦人科学	64
産瘤	332
霰粒腫	133
三類感染症	107

し

項目	ページ
趾	446
ジアゼパム	314, 544
ジアゾキシド	258
指圧痕	177
指圧痕のない	177
指圧痕のない浮腫	246
指圧療法	118
ジアテルミー療法	10
ジアノッティ・クロスティ症候群	339
ジアミノジフェニルスルホン	541
シアリダーゼ	575
ジアルジア症	109
自慰	228
死因	74
ジーヴ症候群	208
視運動性眼振	129, 579
シェーグレン症候群	111, 114, 151, 597
ジエチルスチルベストロール	541
ジエチルトリプタミン	541
ジエチレントリアミン五酢酸	543
シェッツ眼圧計	131
シェディアック・東症候群	272
ジェロタ筋膜	501
ジオプトリー	539
耳音響放射	142, 578
歯科	53
歯科医	57, 59
耳介	458
耳介結節	140
耳介後部	450
耳介後リンパ節	478
歯科医師法	46
歯牙移植	153
紫外線	607
紫外線角膜炎	133
紫外線の	34
耳介前部	450
紫外線分光光度法	81
耳介軟骨	495
耳介変形	140
歯科衛生士	58
歯科学	64
歯科技工士	58
視覚	37, 125

項目	ページ
痔核	26, 207
視覚障害	125
痔核切除術	215
視覚的評価尺度	122, 607
歯学部	62
知覚野	503
視覚誘発電位	133, 608
歯牙再植	153
歯牙腫	148
耳下腺	464
耳下腺管	464
耳下腺リンパ節	478
歯科大学	62
歯牙動揺	149
歯科補綴術	152
子癇	238
歯冠	148, 464
耳管	458
時間	554
耳管炎	143
時間外診療	43
耳管開放症	144
耳管鏡検査	143
耳管狭窄	143
弛緩歯	149
歯冠周囲炎	151
歯冠修復	152
弛緩性麻痺	298
子癇前症	238
耳管通気法	143, 145
歯間ブラシ	147
耳管閉塞	144
視器	456
色覚	125
色覚異常	125
色覚検査	131
磁気共鳴画像検査	79, 574
磁気共鳴血管撮影法	79, 574
磁気共鳴胆道膵管撮影法	203, 574
磁気共鳴分光法	574
色彩	39
色情狂	18
色素嫌性	13
色素上皮由来因子	583
色素性乾皮症	116, 325, 610
色素性絨毛結節性滑膜炎	

	286, 590	子宮内胎児死亡	232, 563	耳甲介	458
色素性蕁麻疹	324	子宮内発育遅延	232, 563	耳硬化症	144
色素沈着	245, 319	子宮内避妊器具	241, 563	持効型インスリン	258
色素斑	319	子宮内膜炎	238	視交叉	458
ジギタリス	189	子宮内膜癌	239	耳垢栓塞	140
ジギタリス投与	189	子宮内膜症	239	自己幹細胞移植	276, 524
ジギタリス飽和	189	子宮内膜生検	236	嗄語胸声	157
子宮	6, 28, 488	子宮の	6	自己恐怖症	296
子宮外妊娠	237	子宮破裂	18	自己骨髄移植	276, 516
子宮癌	239	子宮付属器	489	事故死	74
子宮鏡	14	子宮付属器圧痛	231	自己調節硬膜外鎮痛法	
子宮峡	488	子宮傍の	37		123
子宮鏡下選択的卵管通水		子宮卵管切除術	243	自己調節鎮痛法	123, 582
法	242	子宮卵管造影法		篩骨洞	460
子宮鏡下卵管内精子注入			3, 236, 558	篩骨洞炎	144
法	242, 556	子宮留血症	239	死後の	12
子宮鏡検査	236	耳鏡	77	自己評定抑うつ尺度	596
子宮筋弛緩薬	241	耳鏡検査	141	自己負担額	48
子宮筋刺激薬	241	死恐怖症	94	自己負担限度額	48
子宮筋腫	239	死去した	35	自己負担率	48
子宮筋腫摘出術	243	軸索	504	自己弁心内膜炎	186, 578
子宮腔癒着	239	しくしくする	121	自己免疫	10
子宮頚	489	じくじくする	319	自己免疫疾患	106
子宮頚癌	239	軸捻	338	自己免疫性肝炎	
子宮頚管炎	238	軸偏位	178		113, 207, 520
(子宮)頚管拡張術および		シクラシリン	518	自己免疫性膵炎	210, 520
掻爬術	540	シクロオキシゲナーゼ		自己免疫性溶血性貧血	
子宮頚管ポリープ	239		536		270, 520
子宮頚管裂傷	239	シクロオキシゲナーゼ抑		自己融解	83
子宮頚癌ワクチン	242	制薬	122	自己輸血	275
子宮頚部上皮内腫瘍		シクロスポリン	276	自己由来混合リンパ球反	
	239, 534	シクロスポリンA		応	521
子宮頚部びらん	239		538, 539	歯根	464
子宮広間膜	488	ジクロフェナクナトリウ		歯根管	464
子宮後傾	239	ム	122	歯根尖切除術	152
子宮固定術	6, 14, 243	ジクロロジフェニルトリ		歯根嚢胞	151
子宮出血	229	クロロエタン	541	歯根膜	465
糸球体	486	刺激薬	27	視索	458
子宮体	488	止血	19, 36, 87, 262	自殺	74
子宮体癌	239	止血鉗子	89	自殺企図	296
糸球体基底膜	486, 552	試験開腹術	214	自殺行為	296
糸球体腎炎	26	歯原性	8	自殺念慮	296
子宮胎盤機能不全		歯原性嚢胞	151	自殺未遂	296
	237, 606	試験切開	87	指示	70
糸球体濾過量	219, 552	事故	73	示指	444
子宮脱	239	自己愛性人格障害		歯式	149
子宮底	488		313, 577	支持組織	512
子宮摘出	17	歯垢	147	脂質	250
子宮内器具	241, 563	耳垢	25, 139	脂質異常症	256

脂質蓄積症	256	シスプラチン	532	下顎	442
指示通り	24, 607	ジスプロシウム	435, 544	死体愛	18
四肢麻痺	299	自声強調	139	死体解剖保存法	46
止瀉薬	211	歯性上顎洞炎	152	死体恐怖症	296
耳珠	458	歯石	147	死体腎	226
歯周炎	151	耳石	460	下唇	442
歯周症	152	耳石器	460	シタグリプチン	258
歯周組織再生誘導手術		歯石除去	152	下敷きギプス包帯	289
	152, 554	施設	36	舌の	7
四肢誘導	178	指節間(関節)	562	ジダノシン	275, 540
歯周ポケット	149	指節骨	446	シタフロキサシン	600
思春期	244, 330	施設内審査委員会	43, 562	シタラビン	523
思春期早発症	254, 343	指尖	444	シタラビンオクホスファート	
視床	503	脂腺	462		598
視床下核	503	自然胸腺細胞傷害自己抗		肢端腫大	245
視床下部	490, 503	体	578	肢端疼痛症	12, 18
視床下部・下垂体・副腎		自然死	93	シチジル酸	535
系	558	自然食品	194	シチジン一リン酸	535
耳小骨	459	自然療法	118	シチジンニリン酸	532
耳小骨形成術	145	シゾ	31	市中感染	105
耳小骨摘出術	145	歯槽	465	市中肺炎	163
死傷者	35	歯槽膿瘍	151	弛張熱	105
視床上部	503	歯槽膿漏	151	膝	7
視床痛	294	持続インスリン皮下注入		歯痛	120, 147
糸状乳頭	464	療法	258, 538	耳痛	120, 139
矢状面	448	持続気道陽圧呼吸		膝窩	453
市条例	46		170, 536	膝蓋	27
紫色	39	持続血糖測定	258, 535	膝蓋腱	501
支持療法	118	持続牽引	291	膝蓋腱支持	290, 588
視診	77	持続性ウイルス陰性化		膝蓋腱反射	300, 564, 589
持針器	89		201, 600	膝蓋骨	494
指伸筋	498	持続性血液濾過	533	膝蓋大腿機能障害	
耳真菌症	144	持続性血液濾過透析			279, 583
視神経	458, 505		225, 533	膝蓋跳動	280
視神経萎縮	130	持続性甲状腺刺激物質		膝蓋部	453
視神経炎	134		248, 565	膝窩静脈	478
視神経交叉	458	持続性静脈静脈血液濾過		膝窩動脈	476
視神経脊髄炎	308		225, 539	膝窩動脈拍動	176
視神経乳頭	130, 458	持続性植物状態	590	膝窩リンパ節	479
歯髄	464	持続性動静脈血液濾過		膝関節	495
耳垂	458		225, 530	膝関節炎	286
歯髄炎	151	持続的他動運動	290, 537	膝関節腫	7
指数弁	127, 532, 576	持続熱	105	膝関節全置換術	291, 603
シスジアミングリコレートプラチナム		持続勃起	228	膝関節痛	278
	532	持続陽圧換気	170, 537	膝関節の	7
シスジアミンジクロロプラチナム		持続陽圧呼吸	170, 537	湿球黒球温度指数	610
	532	シゾフィラン	599	失業	74
シスタチンC	219	シソマイシン	597	膝胸位	77
シスチン結石	218	舌	7	失業保険	48

失禁	11	耳内	10	シーベルト	439, 600
膝クローヌス	301	歯内療法	152	四辺形	39
実験医学	63	歯肉	7, 147, 464	死亡	74
実験室	565	歯肉炎	7, 151	脂肪円柱	218
実験動物学	63	歯肉出血	149, 261	死亡学	94
失行	300	歯肉の	7	脂肪過多	12, 245
失語症	18, 34, 302	歯肉肥大	262	脂肪肝	207
失算	302	歯肉皮弁術	152	脂肪織炎	245
実習	67	ジニトロクロロベンゼン		脂肪腫	14, 83
湿潤剤	328		542	死亡診断書	84
失書	302	ジニトロクロロベンゼン		脂肪性肝炎	16
失神	293	試験	323	死亡前診断	84
湿疹	319	ジニトロフェニルヒドラ		脂肪塞栓症候群	549
膝神経節	505	ジン試験	333	脂肪組織	512
失声症	18, 140, 302	シーネ	31	脂肪の	12
膝内障	286, 561	指嚢	77	脂肪便	16, 197
室内便器	90	視能訓練	136	死亡率	93
失認	302	視能訓練士	58, 579	シーボーギウム	436, 597
失敗恐怖症	296	シノキサシン	534	姉妹	73
シップル症候群	255	自発的運動練習	290	嗜眠	297
疾病及び関連保健問題の		紫斑	261, 319	シムズ体位	77
国際統計分類第10回修		市販後調査	585	事務部	54
正	3, 560	シーハン症候群	252	事務部長	59
疾病恐怖症	296	耳鼻咽喉	75	氏名	71
疾病特徴的	84	耳鼻咽喉科	53	耳鳴	28, 139
実脈	173	耳鼻咽喉科医	59	耳鳴検査	142
実務看護師	57, 568	耳鼻咽喉科学	3, 64	耳鳴再訓練療法	145, 605
失明	125	耳鼻咽喉科	547	シメチジン	210
質問に基づく学習	67, 559	自費診療費	48	ジメチルスルホキシド	
指定介護老人福祉施設	55	ジヒドロキシフェニルア			542
ジデオキシイノシン		ラニン	543	死滅速度恒数	539
	275, 540	ジヒドロテストステロン		ジメルカプトコハク酸	
ジデオキシシチジン			234, 541		542
	275, 540	しびれ感	294	ジーメンス	439, 595
シデナム舞踏病	310	しびれる	295	しもやけ	318, 331
自転車エルゴメーター		しびん	38, 90	指紋	444
	180	ジフェンヒドラミン塩酸		視野	132, 608
指導医	57	塩	145	シャイ・ドレーガー症候	
児頭骨盤不均衡	232, 536	ジフテリア	107	群	111, 310
自動視野計	132	ジフテリア・破傷風・百		社会医学	64
児童性的虐待	343	日咳混合ワクチン	543	社会医療	43
自動体外式除細動器		しぶり腹	196	社会生活技能訓練	
	190, 519	シプロフロキサシン	537		316, 600
自動能性心房頻拍		耳閉感	139	社会福祉士	58
	174, 516	自閉症	296	社会福祉大学	62
児童福祉法	46	自閉性障害	313, 343	社会保険	48
自動腹膜透析	225, 522	ジベカシン	542	社会保険庁	49
シトシン	510, 529	ジペプチジルペプチダー		社会保障	49
ジドブジン	275, 525	ゼ	543	社会歴	70, 74, 597

シャーカステン	31	獣医学部	62	舟状頭蓋症	332
シャーガス病	340	縦隔	468	重症複合免疫不全症	596
視野狭窄	132	縦隔炎	167	重水素	539
弱拡大視野	568	縦隔気腫	167	臭素	434, 528
弱視	125	縦隔鏡検査	163	銃創	554
弱視視能矯正	136	縦隔腫瘍	167	集束超音波手術	551
尺側	448	集学的治療	118	重態	76
尺側手根屈筋	498	縦隔リンパ節	478	集団検診	72
尺側手根伸筋	498	習慣	74	重炭酸イオン濃度	158
尺側皮静脈	476	臭汗症	321	集中ケア	61
ジャクソン型てんかん		重感染	12	集中治療室	54, 560
	297	習慣流産	238	充塡	87
灼熱痛	121	周期性四肢麻痺	311	柔道整復師	58
若年型糖尿病	255, 564	宗教	74	十二指腸	482
若年性関節リウマチ		周径	10	十二指腸液	512
	340, 564	充血	83	十二指腸炎	205
若年成人平均値	283, 610	住血吸虫	199	十二指腸潰瘍	205, 543
若年性成人発症型糖尿病		充血除去薬	145	十二指腸下行部	482
	255, 573	集合管	486	十二指腸球部	482
若年性肺気腫	114	自由行動下血圧測定		十二指腸憩室	205
雀卵斑	26, 319		75, 517	十二指腸内視鏡検査	203
斜頚	28, 285, 332	重鎮病	273, 555	十二指腸乳頭	482
視野計測法	132	シュウ酸塩	218	終板脈管器官	502, 580
瀉血	276	シュウ酸カルシウム結石		臭鼻症	144
視野欠損	132		218	重病	73
社交的な	296	周産期	230	修復	87
斜視	27, 36, 125	周産期医学	64	重複腎盂	223
射精	228	修士号	67	十分量	590
射精管	488	収縮期駆出性雑音	596	周辺虹彩切除術	137
シャッキー輪	203	収縮期血圧	75, 596	周辺虹彩部癒着	129, 581
しゃっくり	27, 155	収縮期雑音	175	周辺視	132
尺骨	492	収縮期前方運動	181, 595	終末細気管支	466
尺骨静脈	476	収縮時間	182, 600	充満欠損	203
尺骨神経	505	収縮ストレステスト		差明	127
尺骨動脈	472		235, 538	絨毛	38, 40
シャッテン	31	収縮性心膜炎	186	絨毛癌	239
遮閉 - 遮閉除去試験		収縮早期雑音	175	絨毛生検	235, 539
	128, 539	収縮中期雑音	175	絨毛膜	232
遮閉試験	128, 538	収縮末期圧	182, 548	絨毛膜羊膜炎	238, 530
車輪付き担架	90	収縮末期容量	182, 548	重粒子線治療	117
シャルコー関節	280	舟状窩	458	手関節	495
シャルコー三主徴		重症急性呼吸器症候群		手関節指装具	290
	196, 298		107, 166, 595	手関節背屈副子	290
シャルコー・マリー・トゥス病		重症急性膵炎	114	手関節指装具	610
	310, 535	重症筋無力症		主観的データ	96, 598
斜裂	466		111, 310, 571	縮小	71
シャンバーグ病	327	舟状骨	492	粥状硬化	18, 34
ジャンパー膝	279	重症多形滲出性紅斑(急性期)		宿題	67
獣医	57		116	縮瞳	37, 129

日本語索引

縮瞳の	37
縮瞳薬	136
手根管症候群	285, 539
手根骨	492
手根中手関節	495, 535
主細胞	480
酒皶鼻	141
手指	444
主治医	57
手指節骨	494
踵膝試験	300
手術	73, 86
手術看護	61
手術記録	87
手術後	586
手術室	54, 579
手術室看護師	59
手術部位感染	599
手術名	93
手術用器具	88
手掌	444, 452
手掌筋	498
手掌紅斑	197
手掌線	446
樹状突起	40, 504
手掌白癬	325
手掌皮膚蒼白	262
主膵管	484
受精卵卵管内移植	242, 611
酒石酸エルゴタミン	122
主訴	70, 71, 95, 531
受胎調節	241
シュタイン・レーベンタール症候群	238
手段的日常生活動作	92, 559
出血	83, 261
出血傾向	261
出血時間	265, 529
出血性ショック・脳症候群	339, 558
出血性素因	261
術語	2
術後	12
出産	230
出産時低体重	566
出産予定日	230
出生地	74

出生証明書	74
出生前	230
出生前検査	236
出生前診断	85
術前診断	84
術前貯血式自己血輸血	275
術中胆管造影法	203
術中放射線治療	117, 562
シュテルワーグ徴候	246
授動	87
受動運動	290
受動失禁	217
受動皮膚アナフィラキシー	324, 582
手動弁	127, 557, 572
授乳	343
主任看護師	59
手背	444, 452
守秘義務	43
守秘義務違反	43
趣味	74
シュミット症候群	255
事務員	59
シュモール結節	284
腫瘍	11, 83, 604
腫瘍壊死因子	604
腫瘍壊死因子受容体関連周期熱症候群	604
主要塩基性タンパク	570
腫瘍科	53
腫瘍学	64
腫瘍関連抗原	601
腫瘍浸潤リンパ球	603
主要診断	84
腫瘍性骨軟化症	255
受容性失語症	302
腫瘍切除術	243
腫瘍専門医	59
主要組織適合複合体	572
主要大動脈肺動脈側副血行路	183, 569
腫瘍特異移植抗原	605
腫瘍特異抗原	605
主要な	37
腫瘍マーカー	201
腫瘍由来体液性高カルシウム血症	251, 556
腫瘤触知	198

ジュール	438, 564
シュルマン症候群	285
シュレム管	456
手話通訳士	58
シュワン細胞腫	313
シュワン鞘	506
純音聴力検査	142
潤滑剤	78
循環	173
循環器科	53
循環器系	75
循環器病医	59
准看護師	57, 568
循環免疫複合体	322, 534
春季カタル	133
准教授	62
順行性	10
ショイエルマン病	287
昇圧薬	189
上位運動ニューロン	606
小陰唇	489
小円筋	498
上横隔動脈	472
消化	194
紹介	73
紹介医	71
紹介状	418
紹介状返答	419
障害調整生存年	540
障害年金	49
傷害保険	49
紹介率	73
消化管	26, 480
消化管間質腫瘍	205, 553
消化管内視鏡検査	203
消化管の	553
消化器	480
消化器科	53
消化器系	75
消化器症状	194
消化器病医	59
消化器病学	64
上顎後退症	149
上顎骨	492
小顎症	149, 332
上顎神経	505
上顎前突症	149
上顎洞	460

上顎洞炎	144		132, 608	小頭症	332
上顎洞癌	144	硝子体混濁	129, 579	情動脱力発作	10
小角軟骨	495	硝子体手術	137	情動不安	295
上顎部	450	硝子体出血	129	静脈バイパス	192, 607
消化性潰瘍	205, 589	硝子体切除術	137	小動脈瘤	130, 569
松果体	490	硝子体浮遊物	129	消毒	10
消化不良	10, 26, 194	〜消失	71	小児科	53
上・下葉区	468	上室性頻拍	174, 600	小児科医	37, 60
上眼瞼	456	硝子膜症	334, 557	小児科学	64
笑気・酸素・イソフルレン麻酔	87, 553	上斜筋	458	小児型呼吸促迫症候群	339, 563
笑気・酸素・エーテル麻酔	87, 553	焼灼	87	小児科定点	109
		上縦隔	468	小児看護	60
笑気・酸素・フローセン麻酔	87, 553	症状	72, 120, 600	小児看護学	65
		床上安静	89	小児期疾患	73, 533
上気道	466	症例検討	392	小児虐待	343
上気道炎	28	上小脳動脈	472, 596	小児救急看護	61
上気道感染症	163, 606	上伸筋支帯	500	小児外科	53
上気道症状	154	小腎杯	486	小児外科医	60
小臼歯	464	小水疱	28, 38, 320	小児外科学	64
小球性貧血	263	掌蹠膿疱症	327, 587	小児健康保険制度	50
小胸筋	498	上舌区	468	小児交代性片麻痺	342
上強膜炎	133	常染色体	508	小児呼吸	157
小結節	40, 83	常染色体優性遺伝	73	小児歯科学	15
上行咽頭動脈	472	常染色体優性多発嚢胞腎症	222, 518	小児集中治療室	343, 584
上後鋸筋	500			小児性愛	15
症候群	12	常染色体劣性遺伝	74	小児病院	52
上行結腸	482	常染色体劣性多発嚢胞腎症	222, 523	小児麻痺	294, 331
上甲状腺動脈	472			静脈切開術	15
症候診断学	84	小泉門	332	鞘の	35
上行性網様体賦活系	523	踵足	280	小脳	7, 35, 504
上行大動脈	471	消息子	89	小脳脚	504
小後頭神経	505	消退出血	234	小脳橋の	7
猩紅熱	330	上大静脈	476, 600	小脳の	7
踵骨	494	上大静脈症候群	166, 600	上皮	10
踵骨隆起関節角	280	条虫	38	上皮円柱	218
冗語法	371	小腸	480	上鼻甲介	460
小根	37	上腸間膜静脈	478, 598	上皮細胞成長因子	546
錠剤	86	上腸間膜動脈	474, 597	上皮細胞成長因子受容体	546
小細胞肺癌	166, 596	小腸結膜炎			
硝酸イソソルビド	189, 563	小腸コレステロールトランスポーター阻害薬	259	上皮細胞膜抗原	546
				上皮真珠	332
上肢	444	小腸内視鏡検査	203	上皮組織	512
硝子円柱	218	上直筋	458	上鼻道	460
小耳症	332	上直腸動脈	474, 599	上皮内癌	534
上矢状静脈洞	476	情緒不安定	295	商標名	86
硝子体	456	小殿筋	500	踵部	453
上肢帯	492	小転子	494	小伏在静脈	478
硝子体蛍光測定法		焦点性てんかん	297	上部消化管	480

上部消化管出血	204	除外診断	85	食欲	194
上部消化管造影法		除外せよ	593	食欲不振	194
	203, 606	初期	91	食料切符支給計画	50
上部食道括約筋	480, 606	初期計画	95, 96	初経	228
上方	448	初期症状	72	書痙	293
情報源	70, 71	助教	62	除細動器	190
情報源別診療録	95	食塊	34	ジョサマイシン	564
小胞体	508, 547	職業	71, 74	助産学	65
常法に従って	24, 595	職業病	106	助産師	58
小発作てんかん	297	食後	23, 582	助産師手位	298
漿膜	480, 595	食後血糖	586	助産所	52
漿膜炎	16	食後愁訴症候群	195	初産婦	230
静脈	7, 476, 607	食後痛	195	除脂肪体重	245, 566
静脈炎	7, 15	食後の	586	叙述式記録	96
静脈雑音	176	食細胞	265	女性化	244
静脈性	7	食事	90, 194	女性化症候群	240
静脈性腎盂造影法		食事介助	89	女性化乳房	14, 197, 246
	220, 564	食事指導	93	女性恐怖症	296
静脈洞交会	476	食事性熱産生	105, 542	女性性器	488
静脈内	11, 563	食習慣	74	女性生殖器系	488
静脈内注射	86	食事療法	117, 194	処置室	54
静脈麻酔	87	触診	77	初潮	228
静脈瘤抜去	192	食前	517	触覚器	462
静脈瘤抜去兼筋膜下交通		褥瘡	318, 324	触覚振盪音	156
枝結紮	192	褥瘡性潰瘍	25	ショックパンツ	
小網	482	触知可能の	37		290, 570, 581
絨毛状	38	食中毒	196	ジョードチロシン	
睫毛乱生	127	食堂	54		248, 542
小腰筋	500	食道	7, 26, 480	初乳	343
小菱形筋	500	食道胃十二指腸内視鏡検		初妊婦	229
小菱形骨	492	査	203, 546	除脳	10
上輪部角結膜炎	133, 597	食道胃接合部	480, 546	除脳硬直	298
省令	46	食道炎	7	徐波睡眠	600
症例検討会	392	食道癌	205	ショパール関節	495
症例提示	392, 405	食道憩室	204	ジョフロイ徴候	246
症例報告	392	食道静脈瘤	204	処方する	37
小彎	480	食道切除術	214	処方箋薬	85
上腕	444	食道動脈	472	処方薬	85
上腕筋	498	食道内圧	201	徐脈	13, 172
上腕骨	492	食道内圧検査	202	徐脈頻脈症候群	174
上腕三頭筋	498	食道の	7	所要量	590
上腕三頭筋皮下脂肪	605	食道発声	145	白髪	319
上腕三頭筋皮下脂肪厚		植皮術	329	しらくも	318
	245	食品衛生法	46	シラミ	37, 318
上腕静脈	476	食品交換表	258	シラミ症	325
上腕切断術	292, 519	植物状態	297	シーラント	152
上腕動脈	472	食毛症	6	尻	444
上腕二頭筋	498	食物	194	自律訓練法	316, 524
除外食	90	食物恐怖症	296	自律神経系	506, 522

自律性	10	心窩部痛症候群	195	神経性食欲不振症	
自律性機能性甲状腺結節		心悸亢進	172		312, 522
	251, 519	心機図	180	神経性大食症	312
市立病院	52	心気的	36	神経成長因子	576
私立病院	52	腎機能検査	219	神経成長因子受容体	576
視力	125, 607	心胸郭比	180, 538	神経節	504
視力検査	131	心筋	470	神経線維腫症	313
視力検査表	131	伸筋	498	神経線維腫症Ⅰ型	116
視力減退	125	真菌	36	神経線維腫症Ⅱ型	116
耳輪	458	心筋炎	15, 186	神経線維鞘	506
シリング試験	268	心筋血流イメージング		神経組織	512
耳輪結節性軟骨皮膚炎			181, 573	神経調節性失神	184, 577
	140	心筋腱	501	神経痛	17, 120, 294
ジルコニウム	435, 611	心筋梗塞	27, 185, 572	神経伝導速度	
シルデナフィルクエン酸塩	242	心筋コントラストエコー法	181, 570		283, 304, 576
ジルドラトゥレット症候群	310	伸筋支帯	498	神経特異性エノラーゼ	578
シルビウス溝	502	心筋症	186, 535	神経内科	53
シルビウス水道	502	真菌性肺疾患	165	神経内科医	60
ジルベール症候群	208	心筋トロポニンⅠ		神経内科学	64
シルマー試験	128		178, 538	神経の	7
歯列	149	心筋トロポニンT		神経梅毒	308
歯列矯正	152		178, 538	深頚部膿瘍	144
痔瘻	207	真菌の	36	神経ブロック	123
耳漏	9, 139	腎筋膜	501	深頚リンパ節	478
脂漏症	325	神経	7, 575	腎血管筋脂肪腫	223
脂漏性角化症	324	神経因性疼痛	294	心血管外科	53
脂漏性皮膚炎	324	神経因性膀胱	223	腎血管雑音	217
シロスタゾール	315	神経芽腫	15, 342	心血管疾患	184, 539
シロップ	24, 600	神経下垂体	490	腎血管性	16
シロップ剤	86	神経活動電位	304, 575	腎血管性高血圧	
腎移植	226	神経筋接合部	577		184, 222, 594
心イベント記録計	180	神経筋単位	283, 577	心血管造影法	182, 517
腎盂	486	神経近傍の	10	心血管動画撮影法	182
腎盂腎炎	223	神経系	75, 293	心血管の	13
心エコー検査	181, 606	神経膠腫	313	腎血漿流量	220, 593
心エコー図	181	神経興奮性検査	304, 576	腎結石	223
腎炎	7	神経根痛	121	腎血流量	220, 591
心音	175	神経細線維	504, 506	心原性ショック	176
心音図検査	180, 582	神経耳科学	64	心原性突然死	176, 596
心音の分裂	175	神経質	295	信仰	74
心外膜	470	神経遮断薬	314	進行	91
唇顎口蓋披裂	150	神経遮断薬による悪性症候群	314, 577	人工栄養	343
唇顎口蓋裂	338			腎硬化	223
人格障害	313	神経腫	83	人口学	35
腎下垂	223	神経循環無力症	187, 576	人工関節	292
心窩部	450	神経鞘腫	313	新興感染症	106
心窩部痛	120	神経衰弱	295	人工肝補助療法	212, 521
		心係数	181, 534	進行期	91

語	ページ	語	ページ
人工血管	192	心室興奮時間	608
人工肛門造設	19	心室細動	174, 608
人工肛門造設術	215	心室期外収縮	174
人工呼吸	169	心室性期外収縮	589, 609
人工呼吸器	169	心室性頻拍	174, 609
人工呼吸器関連肺炎	164, 607	心室造影法	16
人工授精	242	心室中隔	470, 564
人工授精児	25	心室中隔欠損	183, 609
深紅色	39	心室内伝導障害	563
人工腎	225, 520	心室補助装置	192, 607
人工心臓	192	心室瘤	185
人工心肺	192, 520, 536	伸縮反復筋力増強法	290
人工膵臓	259	真珠腫	143
進行性外眼筋麻痺	135, 583	滲出	83
進行性核上性麻痺	112, 308, 588	滲出液	26
進行性球麻痺	308, 581	滲出する	319
進行性筋ジストロフィー	308, 585	滲出性中耳炎	143, 579
進行性骨化性線維異形成症	116, 341, 551	滲出性網膜炎	134
進行性骨幹異形成症	341	浸潤	83
進行性色素失調性皮膚症	327	浸潤像	161
進行性指掌角皮症	324, 565	浸潤麻酔	87
進行性脊髄性筋萎縮症	309, 588	腎症	18
進行性全身性強皮症	328, 588	腎症候性出血熱	108
進行性多巣性白質脳症	112, 307, 585	深掌静脈弓	476
人工多分化能性幹(細胞)	562	尋常性乾癬	327
人工透析	225	尋常性魚鱗癬	325
人工内耳	146	尋常性痤瘡	25, 324
人工肺	171	尋常性天疱瘡	327
人工弁心内膜炎	186, 589	尋常性白斑	326
人工流産	229	尋常性毛瘡	27
人工涙液	136	腎小体	486
腎固定術	15, 226	深掌動脈弓	472
腎細胞癌	223, 591	腎静脈	478
診察	70, 583	腎静脈血栓症	222, 594
心雑音	175	腎触知	217
診察室	54	心身医学	64, 588
診察的診断	84	心身症	312, 587
診察用具	77	心身症的	16
心室	470	じんじんする	295
		腎シンチグラフィー	221
		心腎貧血症候群	222
		振水音	198
		親水軟膏	328, 557
		新生血管	130
		針生検	78
		腎生検	221
		腎性骨異栄養症	223, 593
		新生児	330
		新生児一過性多呼吸	334, 605
		新生児壊死性腸炎	336
		新生児黄疸	335
		新生児仮死	334
		新生児高ビリルビン血症	335
		新生児呼吸窮迫症候群	334
		新生児室	54
		新生児集中ケア	61
		新生児集中治療	343
		新生児集中治療室	55, 343, 577
		新生児遷延性肺高血圧症	336, 586
		新生児同種免疫血小板減少症	335, 575
		新生児の	11
		新生児膿漏眼	336
		新生児溶血性疾患	335, 555
		真性多血症	271, 589
		新生物	11
		振戦	175, 245
		振戦せん妄	25, 308, 543
		腎仙痛	216
		新鮮凍結血漿	276, 550
		心尖拍動	175
		心尖拍動図	180, 517
		心臓	7, 470
		腎臓	7, 486
		心臓足首血管指数	180, 530
		心臓移植	192
		腎臓科	53
		心臓カテーテル法	182
		心臓外科	53
		心臓外科医	60
		心臓外科学	64
		心臓再同期療法	190, 538
		心臓除細動	190
		腎臓の	7, 37
		心臓の雑音	173
		腎臓病	216
		腎臓病医	60
		心臓病学	7, 64
		腎臓病学	64
		心臓ペーシング	190
		心臓ペースメーカー	190

心臓弁膜症	28, 183	親等	73	心房中隔欠損	183, 524
心臓発作	172	腎洞	486	心房粘液腫	188
心臓麻痺	172	浸透圧脆弱性試験	266	心嚢	11, 470
心臓リハビリテーション	190	浸透圧性利尿薬	136	心膜液	512
親族	73	振動覚	302	心膜炎	186
迅速ウレアーゼ試験	201, 594	振動覚消失	262	心膜滲出液	186
靱帯	496	腎動脈	474	心膜タンポナーデ	186
靱帯骨棘形成	284	腎動脈狭窄	222, 591	心膜摩擦音	176
身体障害者福祉法	46	腎動脈血栓症	222	蕁麻疹	28, 318, 320
身体所見	398	腎動脈造影法	221	蕁麻疹誘発	320
身体の診断	84	腎毒性	15	腎門	486
身体の検査	70, 75, 583	心内注射	86	信頼性	71
身体の所見	95	心内膜	470	心理の問題	96
身体表現性障害	312	心内膜炎	186	診療医	59
身体部位	5	心内膜下心筋梗塞	185	診療科	53
心濁音界	175	心内膜床欠損	183, 545	診療ガイドライン	43
診断	70, 84, 401, 544	心内膜心筋線維症	187, 546	診療圏	43
診断医	57	腎乳頭	486	診療参加型臨床実習	67
診断印象	84	腎・尿管・膀胱（単純X線撮影）	565	診療所	52
診断基準	84	腎杯	486	診療情報開示	43
診断群分類別包括評価	49	塵肺	34, 486	診療情報学	64
診断書	43	心配事	165	診療情報管理士	58
診断的計画	96	心肺蘇生法	71	心療内科	53
診断的腹腔洗浄	204, 543	心肺停止	190, 537	診療部長	59
心弾道図	181, 526	心肺の	176, 536	診療放射線技師	58
診断別関連群	49	心拍	13	診療報酬	49
診断別疾患分類	543	心拍出量	172	診療報酬点数	49
診断未確定	578	心拍数	181, 536	診療録	70
人畜共通感染症	106	真皮	75, 558		
シンチグラフィー	80	深腓骨神経	462	**す**	
シンチスキャン	80	心肥大	506	随意に	518
腎柱	486	深部感覚	175	髄液	512
身長	38, 76, 559	深部感覚消失	302	髄液圧	304
深腸骨回旋動脈	474	深部腱反射	302	髄液細胞増加	305
陣痛	121, 230	深部静脈血栓	300, 543	髄液タンパク	305
陣痛計	235, 603	心不全	177, 544	膵炎	7
陣痛抑制	230	深部痛	185	水癌	151
陣痛抑制薬	241	深部脳刺激法	120	膵管	210
心停止	176, 529	深部脳波	316, 540	膵管空腸吻合	19
心的外傷後ストレス障害	312, 589	心房	304, 541	膵癌胎児抗原	201, 586
腎摘除術	226	心房期外収縮	470	膵管内乳頭粘液新生物	562
伸展	279	心房細動	174	膵偽性嚢胞	210
伸展拘縮	281	心房性期外収縮	174, 519	膵機能検査	202
心電図	17, 178, 545	心房性ナトリウム利尿ペプチド	522, 580	膵機能診断薬	202, 583
心電図検査	17, 178	心房粗動	178, 522	水胸	167
伸展側	448	心房中隔	174, 519	水銀	436, 556
			470, 559	膵空腸吻合術	215
				髄腔内	563

髄腔内注射	86	随伴	72	候群	342
髄腔内バクロフェン投与		膵尾部	484	スタチン系薬	259
	315, 563	膵分泌性トリプシンイン		スチーブンス・ジョンソン症候群	326
推算糸球体濾過量		ヒビター	202, 588		
	219, 546	水平	448	頭痛	120, 244
推算出血量	544	水平感染	106	スティックラー症候群	341
衰弱	104	水平半盲	132		
水晶体	456	水平面	448	スティル病	111, 286
水晶体混濁	129	水平裂	466	スティール・リチャードソン・オルゼウスキー症候群	308
水晶体超音波乳化吸引術		水疱	320		
	136, 583	水泡音	157		
水腎症	223	水疱性	34	ステト	31
膵石症	210	水疱性口峡炎	339	ステる	31
膵切除術	259	水疱性類天疱瘡	327, 528	ステンセン管	464
水素	14, 434, 554	髄膜	504	ストップウォッチ	77
水素イオン指数	584	髄膜炎	307	ストファー症候群	223
水素イオン濃度	158	髄膜炎菌	15	ストーマケア	212
膵臓	7, 484, 490	髄膜炎菌性髄膜炎	109	ストルビット結石	218
膵臓の	7	髄膜腫	313	ストレス心エコー法	181
錐体外路症候群	299, 547	髄膜出血	15	ストレプトキナーゼ・ストレプトドルナーゼ	
錐体筋	500	髄膜瘤	342		
膵体尾部切除術	215	睡眠	74, 104		597
膵体部	484	睡眠時呼吸障害	167, 596	ストレプトマイシン	597
水中運動	290	睡眠時随伴症	104	ストロンチウム	435, 599
垂直	448	睡眠時無呼吸	140	すなわち	561, 609
垂直感染	106	睡眠時無呼吸症候群		スネレン表	131
垂直遮断式胃形成術			167, 595	頭脳線	446
	260, 608	睡眠潜時反復検査		スパイロ	31
垂直面	448		163, 304, 574	スパイロメータ呼吸訓練	
水治療法	289	睡眠相後退症候群			169
推定診断	84		104, 543	スーパーオキシドジスムターゼ	
水痘	28, 110, 325, 330	睡眠ポリグラフ計	304		598
膵島移植	259	水薬	86	スパルフロキサシン	599
膵島細胞抗体	247, 560	髄様癌	252	スピラマイシン	599
膵島細胞腫瘍	210	水様便	196	スピロノラクトン	188
膵島細胞腺腫	255	スウィート病	327	ズブアラ	31
膵島細胞膜抗体	247, 560	スカルパ三角	452	スプライシング	510
膵頭十二指腸切除術		スカンジウム	434, 596	スペクチノマイシン	599
	215, 582	ずきずきする	121	スペクトル	37
水頭症	14, 306, 332	空き腹	194	ズポ	31
水痘帯状疱疹ウイルス		スキルス胃癌	205	スポーツ医学	64
	322, 609	スクアラン酸ジブチルエステル		スポロトリキン試験	323
水痘帯状疱疹免疫グロブリン			329, 595	スマトリプタンコハク酸塩	
	328, 609	スクラルファート水和物			122
膵頭部	484		210	スミス骨折	282
水痘ワクチン	344	スコダ共鳴音	157	スモン	116, 309, 598
髄内釘固定法	291	筋違い	278	すり足	294
膵嚢胞	210	スズ	435, 598	スリガラス様陰影	161
膵嚢胞線維症	114, 210	スタージ・ウェーバー症		スルタミシリン	596

鋭い	121	清潔採取尿	218	精神看護学	66
スルバクタム・セフォペラゾン	596	生検	13, 138	成人看護学	66
		制限酵素	510	精神刺激薬	314
スルファメトキサゾール	598	制限酵素断片多型	510, 592	精神障害の診断と統計の手引き	303, 543
スルファメトキサゾール・トリメトプリム	600	性交	228	精神神経症	27
		性交後試験	235, 582	成人スティル病	114
スルホニルウレア	600	性交疼痛	229	精神遅滞	303, 574
スルホニルウレア薬	258	性交不能症	228	成人T細胞白血病ウイルス	524
スワイヤ・ジェームス症候群	161	整骨医学	65	成人T細胞白血病	271, 524
		整骨療法	118		
スワン・ガンツカテーテル	181, 596	整骨療法士	542	成人T細胞白血病リンパ腫	271, 524
スワン・ネック変形	281	精細管	488		
		精索炎	236	精神的	7
せ		正座不能	298	精神の	36
成育看護学	65	正三角形	39	成人発症型糖尿病	256, 522
精液銀行	242	制酸薬	210		
精液検査	235	正視	131	精神病	37
正円窓	459	精子	235	精神病院	52
清音	156	清拭	89	精神分析	16, 316
声音振盪	158	正色素性	5	精神分析専門医	60
性快感消失	229	精子形成能低下	3	精神保健福祉士	58
生化学	13, 63	静止の	38	精神保健福祉法	46
生化学的酸素要求量	528	精子膨化試験	235, 557	精神療法	7
性格	295	脆弱性骨折	282	ぜいぜい	154
生活環境看護学	66	成熟	244	精製ツベルクリン	586
生活状況	74	正常圧水頭症	111, 306, 577	成績	67
生活の質	92, 590			性腺	488
生活保護	49	正常眼圧緑内障	133, 578	性腺機能低下	235
生活様式	74	正常血圧性	15	性腺機能低下症	254
精管	488	正常呼吸	156	性腺刺激ホルモン	234, 554
正看護師	593	星状細胞腫	313		
精管切除術	242	星状神経節ブロック	123, 190, 597	性腺刺激ホルモン放出ホルモン	234
性感染症	237, 600				
性感染症定点	110	正常洞調律	578	性腺刺激ホルモン放出ホルモン作動薬	241
精管動脈	474	正常範囲内	610		
性器クラミジア感染症	110	精上皮腫	224	性染色質	508
性器ヘルペス	237	青色	39	性染色体	508
性器ヘルペスウイルス感染症	110	生殖子	235	精巣	7, 488, 490
		生殖補助医療	242, 523	精巣炎	236
整形外科	53	精神	7, 37, 293	精巣挙筋反射	301
整形外科医	60	精神安定薬	314	精巣固定術	7, 18, 242
整形外科学	65	精神医学	65	精巣腫瘍	223
清潔間欠自己導尿	224, 534	成人陰毛	245	精巣上体	488
		精神科	53	精巣上体炎	236
清潔間欠導尿	224, 534	精神科医	27, 60	精巣上体精子回収法	242, 571
		精神科ソーシャルワーカー	58, 588		
		精神看護	60	精巣痛	228

精巣摘除術	242	整復	87		112
精巣内精子回収法		生物学的偽陽性	527	脊髄造影法	284
	242, 603	生物学的効果比	591	脊髄損傷	288, 596
精巣の	7	生物学的診断	84	脊髄電気刺激法	123, 596
生存率	92	生物学的製剤	117	脊髄癆	308
声帯	466	生物統計学	65	脊柱	278, 492
声帯炎	144	成分栄養	90, 545	脊柱管	455
生体応答調節剤	528	成分輸血	275	脊柱管狭窄症	288
生態学	63	性別	71	脊柱起立筋	500
生体血縁臓器提供者	226	正方形	39	脊柱後彎	281
生体臓器提供者	226	性ホルモン結合グロブリン	597	脊柱指圧療法	289
声帯ポリープ	144			脊柱前彎	281
声帯麻痺	141	生命維持装置	92	脊柱側彎	281
正多角形	39	生命線	446	脊柱部	452
正中神経	505	生命徴候	75, 609	脊柱変形	278
正中切開	88	生命保険	49	脊椎	7, 492
正中線	454	生命倫理	43	脊椎固定術	291
正中傍切開	88	声門	466	脊椎すべり症	8, 16, 288
正中面	448	声門下喉頭炎	144	脊椎痛	7
成長	244	声門浮腫	141	脊椎の	7
成長曲線	330	性欲	228	脊椎分離症	16, 288
成長障害	244	性欲過剰	296	脊椎分離すべり症	288
成長痛	25, 121	生理学	63	赤白血病	270
成長ホルモン		生理機能検査	78	咳払い	155
	249, 344, 552	生理的食塩水	577	赤面恐怖症	296
成長ホルモン分泌下垂体腺腫	252	政令	46	セグ	31
		世界医師会医の国際倫理綱領	44	ゼク	31
成長ホルモン分泌抑制ホルモン	249, 553			セクレチン試験	202
		世界医師会患者の権利に関するリスボン宣言	44	セザリー症候群	327
成長ホルモン放出ホルモン	249, 553			セシウム	435, 538
		世界保健機関	610	舌	464
性的早熟	244	咳	155	舌痛	18
性同一性障害	240	赤外線の	11, 36	舌圧子	77
青銅色	39	赤芽球	14, 266	舌咽神経	505
制吐薬	211	赤芽球バースト形成細胞	527	舌炎	7, 151, 262
生年月日	71, 542			切開	87
青年期	244	赤芽球癆	270, 587	石灰化	161
精嚢	488	石児	238	石灰化歯原性嚢胞	
精嚢炎	236	赤色	39		151, 536
青斑	502	脊髄	504	石灰化尿毒症性細動脈症	223, 539
性病	237, 608	脊髄空洞症	112, 342		
性病科	53	脊髄くも膜下麻酔	87	切開排膿	561
性病科医	60	脊髄小脳変性症	111, 309, 596	舌下錠	86
性病研究所梅毒血清反応	236, 608			舌下神経	505
		脊髄神経	505	舌下腺	464
性ホルモン結合グロブリン	234	脊髄錐体外路	504	舌下の	597
		脊髄錐体路	504	舌癌	151
西部ウマ脳炎	108, 610	脊髄性筋萎縮症	341, 597	舌痙攣	148
政府管掌健康保険	49	脊髄性進行性筋萎縮症		赤血球	17

赤血球円柱	218	舌動脈	472		539
赤血球吸着ウイルス	160	舌乳頭	148, 464	背骨	278
赤血球吸着試験	161	舌乳頭萎縮	262	セメント質	464
赤血球凝集素	554	舌背	464	セリアック病	206
赤血球凝集反応	81, 554	切迫性尿失禁	217	セリウム	435, 532
赤血球凝集抑制反応		切迫流産	238	セリンプロテアーゼイン	
	81, 556	舌肥厚	11, 148	ヒビター	275, 599
赤血球産生	18	接尾辞	2, 17	セルトリ細胞	488
赤血球産生性プロトポル		舌偏倚	148	セルフケア・ユニット	
フィリン症	335, 547	舌扁桃	465		55, 596
赤血球数	263, 591	説明義務	43	セルロプラスミン	200
赤血球増加	265	背中	444	セレギリン塩酸塩	315
赤血球大小不同	263	セファクロル	531	セレン	434, 596
赤血球沈降速度		セファゾリン	532	セロトニン	250, 559
	266, 529, 548	セファトリジン	533	セロトニン受容体作動薬	
赤血球鉄利用率	269, 592	セファドロキシル	532		122
赤血球濃厚液	275	セファレキシン	532	セロトニン・ドーパミン	
赤血球容積分布幅		セファロチン	532	拮抗薬	316, 596
	263, 592	セフィキシム	533	セロトニン・ノルアドレ	
石鹸浣腸	90, 599	セフェピム	533	ナリン再取り込み阻害	
接合縫合	88	セフォジジム	532	薬	314, 598
舌骨	492	セフォゾプラン	539	腺	36
切歯	464	セフォタキシム	539	線維芽細胞増殖因子	550
摂氏	438, 529	セフォチアム	538	線維芽細胞増殖因子受容	
接辞	2	セフォチアムヘキセチル		体3	550
舌灼熱感	147, 261		538	線維筋異形成症	184, 550
接種	26	セフォペラゾン	537	線維筋腫	239
接種可能の	36	セフカペンピボキシル		線維筋痛症	286, 550
摂取量と排泄量	562		533	線維腫	14, 83
切除	10, 88	セフジトレンピボキシル		線維症	14, 83
舌小帯	464		532	線維腺腫	240
舌小帯短縮	332	セフジニル	533	線維組織	512
切除鏡	226	セフスロジン	533	線維柱帯切開術	137
絶食	577	セフタジジム	531	線維柱帯切除術	137
摂食・嚥下障害看護	61	セフチゾキシム	539	船員保険	49
接触出血(性交時)	229	セフチブテン	532	前腋窩線	454, 516
摂食障害	312	セフテラムピボキシル		前外側の	13
接触蕁麻疹	324		533	前下小脳動脈	472, 520
接触皮膚炎	324, 531	セフトリアキソン	538	腺下垂体	490
舌正中溝	464	セフピラミド	537	前下腿部	453
舌切除術	152	セフピロム	537	腺癌	12, 83
舌尖	464	セフブペラゾン	531	前癌の	12
絶対安静	89	セフポドキシムプロキセ		潜函病	25
切断	88	チル	536	洗眼薬	136
切断四肢重症度スコア		セフミノクス	535	閃輝暗点	126
	282, 571	セフメタゾール	535	漸強性雑音	175
切断術	292	セフメノキシム	535	前胸の	12
舌痛	147, 261	セフロキサジン	539	前胸部圧迫感	172
接頭辞	2, 10	セフロキシムアキセチル		前胸部痛	120

前鋸筋	498	前上膵十二指腸動脈		選択的セロトニン再取り	
占拠性病変	598		474, 524	込み阻害薬	314, 600
前駆期	91	洗浄赤血球	276	選択的腹腔動脈造影法	
前駆症状	12	線条体	503		203, 596
ゼングスターケン・ブレークモア管	212, 595	線条体黒質変性症	112, 308, 598	選択の迷走神経切離術	214, 600
前脛骨筋	500	浅掌動脈弓	472	先端巨大症	
前脛骨静脈	478	線状皮膚萎縮	245		12, 18, 116, 252
前脛骨動脈	476	前上葉区	468	前置胎盤	238
尖圭コンジローマ	25, 110, 237	前上腕部	452	センチネルリンパ節生検	236
前頚三角部	450	染色質	508	センチメートル	438, 535
前掲書中に	579	染色体	13, 508	センチモルガン	510, 535
前頚部	450	染色体地図	510	線虫	199
浅頚リンパ節	478	染色体分析	267	前肘部	452
全血	275, 610	全身	75	前兆	34, 294
全血液量	602	全身性エリテマトーデス	110, 114, 327, 597	仙腸関節	495
全血球計算	263, 531	全身性炎症反応症候群	107, 597	仙腸骨炎	286
鮮血便	195			浅腸骨回旋動脈	476
潜血陽性便	261	全身病	106	仙椎	492, 595
線源皮膚間距離	599	全身浮腫	217	仙椎化	284
前後	522	全身放射線照射	276, 602	仙痛	35, 121
穿孔	198	全身麻酔	87	穿通	198
閃光視	126	全身麻酔後回復室	55, 580	前庭	459
穿孔術	88	仙髄	504	前庭階	459
前交通動脈	471	全生存期間	92, 580	前庭球	489
前交連	502	前脊髄動脈	472	前庭神経	460, 505
仙骨	494	前前腕部	452	前庭神経炎	144
仙骨神経叢	506	全層角膜移植術	138, 585	先天性エプーリス	332
仙骨部	452	漸増抵抗運動	290, 587	先天性横隔膜ヘルニア	338, 532
仙骨麻酔	87	尖足	280	先天性魚鱗癬様紅皮症	116
仙骨リンパ節	479	喘息	154		
潜在性	91	喘息性気管支炎	163	先天性筋ジストロフィー	308, 535
潜在的問題	96	喘息性呼吸	157		
穿刺	17	浅側頭静脈	476	先天性股関節脱白	287, 340, 532, 566
戦死	74	浅側頭動脈	472, 600		
禅式長寿法	118	浅側頭動脈・中大脳動脈吻合術	316, 600	先天性疾患	74, 106
前膝部	453			先天性食道閉鎖	338
漸弱性雑音	175	喘息発作	154	先天性心疾患	183, 338, 533
腺腫	83	腺組織	512	先天性赤芽球性ポルフィリン症	335, 532
前縦隔	468	浅大腿動脈	474, 596		
前十字靱帯	496, 517	前大腿部	452	先天性赤血球生成不全性貧血	269, 532
前収縮期雑音	175	前大脳動脈	471, 517		
全収縮期雑音	175	洗濯室	55	先天性多発性関節拘縮症	341, 521
前縦靱帯骨化症	112, 287, 578	選択視法	334, 585		
		選択的アルドステロンブロッカー	188, 595	先天性胆道閉鎖症	338, 531
腺腫様	12				
腺腫様甲状腺腫	252	選択的エストロゲン受容体修飾薬	241, 289, 596		
浅掌静脈弓	476				

先天性内反足	340	前方椎体間固定術		早期卵巣不全	239, 586
先天性肺囊胞性腺腫様奇形	165, 531		291, 520	早期臨床体験	67
		全末梢血管抵抗	182, 604	装具	289
先天性風疹症候群		喘鳴	154, 157	総頸動脈	471, 531
	109, 338, 538	せん妄	297	象牙質	464
先天性副腎過形成		専門医	57, 59	造血	18
	254, 336, 530	専門医制度	67	造血幹細胞移植	276, 558
先天性溶血性貧血	269	専門看護師	58, 60, 536	造血器系	75, 261
前頭筋	498	専門職間教育	67	造血臓器	261
穿頭孔	317	専門用語	2	造血薬	274
尖頭合指症	341	腺様囊胞癌	83, 517	総合大学	62
前頭骨	492	前立腺	7, 37, 488	総合内科	53
尖頭症	332	前立腺液	217	爪甲白斑	321
前頭側頭型認知症		前立腺炎	7, 223	総合病院	52
	311, 551	前立腺癌	223	造骨性病変	269
尖頭多合指症	341, 518	前立腺結石	223	相互転座	510, 592
尖塔徴候	334	前立腺酸性ホスファターゼ		相互扶助	49
前頭洞	460		219, 581	総コレステロール	
前頭洞炎	144	前立腺腫大硬結	217		250, 602
前頭部	450	前立腺上皮内腫瘍		爪根	462
蠕動不穏	197		223, 584	走査型電子顕微鏡	79, 596
前頭面	448	前立腺痛	216	嘈囃	28
前頭葉	502	前立腺特異抗原	219, 587	走査レーザー検眼鏡	
前頭葉機能検査	303, 548	前立腺の	7		131, 597
セントロメア	510	前立腺肥大症	223	早産	230
前囊下白内障	134, 524	前立腺マッサージ	217	早産児	230
センノシド	211	全リンパ節照射	276, 604	喪失	35
全肺気量	162, 603	前腕	444	爪周囲炎	325
全肺静脈還流異常		前腕切断術	292, 526	早熟	244
	183, 601			双手触診	77
前肺底区	468	そ		双手内診	231
前白血病	271	像	38	爪床	462
前半規管	460	総入れ歯	148	層状角膜移植術	137
全般性不安障害	312, 552	躁うつ病	312	巣状糸球体硬化症	222
全般てんかん	297	造影 X 線撮影法	79	創傷離開	88
浅腓骨神経	506	造影剤増強	532	増殖	83
前部虚血性視神経症		〜増加	71	増殖硝子体網膜症	
	134, 520	爪下血腫	321		135, 590
潜伏精巣	236	総肝管	484	増殖糖尿病網膜症	
浅腹壁動脈	476	総肝動脈	472, 533		135, 583
全部床義歯	152	早期	91	爪切除術	329
前壁心筋梗塞	185	早期胃癌	205, 545	臓側胸膜	468
前壁中隔心筋梗塞	185	臓器移植法	46	爪体	462
前壁中隔の	13	臓器許容量	580	増大	71
前房	456, 517	早期抗原	544	双胎間輸血症候群	
前方	448	早期診断	84		232, 605
前房隅角	456	早期体験	67	相対的瞳孔求心路障害	
前房出血	129	早期破水	238, 587		129, 591
前房蓄膿	129	双極性障害	312	総胆管	484, 531

総胆管空腸吻合術	215	足根骨	494	組織病理学	63
総胆管十二指腸吻合	3	足根三角骨	494	組織プラスミノーゲン活	
総胆管十二指腸吻合術		足根舟状骨	494	性化因子	189, 315, 604
	215	足根中足関節	495	組織ポリペプチド抗原	
総胆管嚢腫	209	即時型過敏反応	322		604
総胆汁酸	200, 601	足趾節骨	494	咀嚼	195
総タンパク	604	束状帯	490	咀嚼筋	498
総腸骨静脈	478	促進心室固有調律		蘇生拒否	542
総腸骨動脈	474, 534		174, 520	疎性結合組織	512
総鉄結合能	268, 603	足底	37, 446, 453	粗大	35
搔爬	88	足底筋	500	卒業証書	67
蒼白	261	足底静脈弓	478	卒業論文	67
蒼白色	39	足底動脈弓	476	卒後医学教育	67
爪白癬	325	足底反射	301	卒後医学教育認定協議会	
爪剝離症	8, 321	側頭筋	498		67, 517
搔破試験	323	側頭骨	492	速効型インスリン	258
爪板	462	側頭動脈炎		卒後臨床研修	67
爪半月	462		111, 114, 187, 601	袖状胃切除術	260
総腓骨神経	506	側頭部	450	ゾニサミド	315, 316, 611
総ビリルビン	199	側頭葉	502	その項を見よ	22, 590
僧帽筋	498	属の	36	その他	21, 548
僧帽弁	470	側脳室	502	そばかす	318
僧帽弁逸脱症	184, 575	足背	446, 453	祖父	73
僧帽弁逆流	574	足背静脈弓	478	ソープ	31
僧帽弁狭窄	184, 574	足背動脈	476	ソフトコンタクトレンズ	
僧帽弁交連切開術	191	足背動脈拍動	177		136
僧帽弁性P波	179	続発緑内障	134	祖母	73
僧帽弁前尖弁後退速度		側腹部	452	ソマトメジン	249
	181, 541	側腹部痛	120, 216	ソマトメジンC	249
僧帽弁置換術	191, 575	足部痛風	5, 286	粗面小胞体	508, 592
僧帽弁閉鎖不全	184, 572	足部白癬	28, 325	ソモジー現象	247
相補性決定領域	532	側壁心筋梗塞	185	空色	39
相補DNA	510, 532	速脈	173	ソラフェニブトシル酸塩	
双面副子	290	属名	36		224
搔痒	27, 37	足浴	89	ソラレン長波長紫外線療	
搔痒感	319	粟粒陰影	161	法	329, 589
総リンパ球数	265, 603	鼠径	26, 444	ゾリンジャー・エリソン	
爪裂症	321	鼠径三角	452	症候群	255, 611
早漏	228	鼠径靭帯	496	損害補償	49
造瘻術	214	鼠径肉芽腫	237	尊厳死	93
添え木	279	鼠径ヘルニア	210, 338	ゾンデ	31, 89
属	36	鼠径リンパ節	479		
側臥位	76	鼠径リンパ肉芽腫	237	た	
足関節	495	組織	512		
足関節上腕血圧比		組織液	512	対	609
	173, 516	組織学	63	ダイアモンド・ブラック	
側胸部	450	組織学的検査	78	ファン貧血	335
俗語	2	組織診断	93	体位	76
足根	38	組織発生	17	胎位	232, 233
				体位性起立性頻拍症候群	

項目	ページ
	174, 586
体位性失神	172
体位性排液法	90, 169
第1横位第1分類(胎位)	233, 568
第1横位第2分類(胎位)	233, 568
第1骨盤位第1分類(胎位)	233, 568
第1骨盤位第2分類(胎位)	233, 568
第1斜位	591
第1心音	595
第1頭位第1分類(胎位)	233, 568
第1頭位第2分類(胎位)	233, 567
第1度熱傷	320
体位変換	90
退院	73
退院時指示	93
退院時指導	93
退院時診断	93
退院時投薬	93
退院時病状	93
退院時要約	93
大陰唇	489
大うつ病性障害	312
体液	512
大円筋	498
大横径	232, 528
体温	75, 529, 604
体温計	77
体温調節	16
胎芽	231
体外限外濾過法	225, 545
体外式膜型人工肺	343, 545
体外受精	242, 563
体外受精胚移植	242, 563
体外循環	192, 544
体外衝撃波砕石術	225, 548
体外心マッサージ	190, 545
体外放射線照射療法	117, 544
体格	76
大学院	62
大学院大学	62
大学入学許可	67
大学病院	52
大顆粒リンパ球	265, 567
体幹	444
体幹ギプス	289
体幹屈曲	333
体幹白癬	325
体幹肥満	245
大臼歯	464
大球性貧血	263
大胸筋	498
大凝集アルブミン	569
太極拳	118
体腔	455
体型	5, 16
台形	39
退形成	10, 34, 83
体血管抵抗	600
大血管転位症	183
対光反射	129
対向流免疫電気泳動法	81, 534
第5病	339
大細胞肺癌	166
第3心音	595
第3大臼歯	464
第3度熱傷	320
第三脳室	502
胎児	231
胎児機能評価	235, 528
胎児機能不全	232, 577
胎児循環遺残	336, 583
胎児心音	232
胎児振動音刺激試験	235
胎児心拍陣痛図	235, 538
胎児心拍数	232, 550
胎児性アルコール症候群	338, 549
胎児赤芽球症	335, 544
胎児切迫仮死	232
胎児胎盤系	231, 551
体質性高ビリルビン血症	208
体質性疾患	74
代謝性アシドーシス	219
代謝性疾患	106
対珠	458
体重	75, 105, 529, 610
体重減少	105
体重増加	105
対称性関節腫脹	280
帯状痛	121
帯状ヘルペス免疫グロブリン	611
帯状疱疹	26, 324
帯状疱疹後神経痛	121, 584
対症療法	118
退職	74
退職者医療制度	49
退職年金	49
対診	84
代診	43
対診医	57
大腎杯	486
大膵動脈	474
体性感覚の	16
体性感覚誘発電位	304, 596
胎生爪皮	462
体性痛	120
耐性伝達因子	594
苔舌	148
苔癬化	320
大泉門	332
大泉門閉鎖	332
対側片麻痺	299
大腿筋膜	501
大腿脛骨角	279, 551
大腿骨	7, 494
大腿骨円靱帯	496
大腿骨頚部骨折	282
大腿骨長	232, 550
大腿骨頭すべり症	287, 596
大腿三角	452
大腿四頭筋	500
大腿静脈	478
大腿神経	506
大腿深動脈	476
大腿切断術	292, 520
大腿直筋	500
大腿痛	7
大腿動脈	474, 548
大腿動脈拍動	176
大腿二頭筋	500
大腿の	7

大腿部膝屈筋腱	501	第2頭位第1分類(胎位)		ダウン症候群	336
大腿ヘルニア	210		233, 593	唾液	147, 512
大腸	482	第2頭位第2分類(胎位)		唾液腺	464
大腸菌	219		233, 593	唾液腺炎	151
大腸憩室症	207	第2度熱傷	320	唾液腺シンチグラフィー	
大腸内視鏡検査	203	耐熱性アルカリホスファ			150
大腸内視鏡的ポリープ切		ターゼ	234, 558	唾液腺造影法	150
除術	212	滞納	49	唾液腺電図	150
大腸ポリープ	206	胎嚢	231, 554	唾液分泌	147
大殿筋	500	大脳	7, 35, 502	唾液分泌減少	148
大転子	494	大脳回	502	楕円形	40
胎動	232	大脳基底核	503	楕円体	40
耐糖能異常	561	大脳脚	504	多角形	39
大頭症	332	大脳溝	502	多価不飽和脂肪酸	589
耐糖能異常	247	大脳動脈輪	471	ダーカム病	245
大動脈	471	大脳の	7	高安動脈炎	111, 187
大動脈炎症候群	114	大脳半球	502	高安病	114, 187
大動脈解離	187	大脳皮質	503	ダカルバジン	543
大動脈冠動脈バイパス		大脳皮質基底核変性症		多汗症	245, 321
	191, 517		116	多関門集積スキャン	575
大動脈弓	471	胎盤	27, 232	タキ	31
大動脈弓症候群	516	胎盤機能不全症候群		濁音	156
大動脈雑音	198		237, 583	濁音移動	197
大動脈縮窄症	183	胎盤早期剥離	238	脱落歯	149
大動脈症候群	111	胎盤部トロホブラスト腫		ダグラス窩	231
大動脈第2音	175	瘍	240, 588	ダグラス窩穿刺術	236
大動脈内バルーン・パン		体表面積	529	タクロリムス水和物	
ピング	192, 559	体表面線	454		288, 328
大動脈弁	470	大伏在静脈	478	多形核好中球	264, 585
大動脈弁逆流	523	胎便吸引症候群	335, 570	多形紅斑	326
大動脈弁狭窄	184, 524	大便失禁	331	多形滲出性紅斑	326, 545
大動脈弁置換術	191, 525	大発作てんかん	297	多系統萎縮症	310, 574
大動脈弁閉鎖不全		大網	482	多形皮膚萎縮	15
	183, 520	大腰筋	500	多血質の	6
大動脈隆起	180	第4心音	595	多血症	11
大動脈輪拡張	183, 516	第4度熱傷	320	多血小板血漿	587
体内総水分量	602	第四脳室	502	多結節の	11
第2横位第1分類(胎位)		対立遺伝子	510	多元酵素免疫測定法	
	233, 594	代理人によるミュンヒハ			81, 546
第2横位第2分類(胎位)		ウゼン症候群	343, 574	多元受容体標的化抗精神	
	233, 594	大菱形筋	500	薬	316, 570
第二言語としての英語		大菱形骨	492	多源性心房頻拍	174, 570
	67, 548	大量ビタミン療法	119	たこ	318
第2骨盤位第1分類(胎		体力指数	583	蛇行	40
位)	233, 594	大彎	480	多幸症	10
第2骨盤位第2分類(胎		多飲	244	多孔性	37
位)	233, 594	ダイン	438, 544	蛇行性	38
第2斜位	565	ダウノルビシン	542	多項目抗原同時検査	
第2心音	595	ダウノルビシン塩酸塩			

	323, 570	多発神経炎	11	単一筋線維筋電図	
ダコスタ症候群	188	多発性筋炎	111, 285, 585		283, 596
多剤耐性	571	多発性筋炎・皮膚筋炎		単一鎖形体の多型	599
多剤耐性結核	165, 571		114	単一探触子ドプラ超音波	
多剤耐性緑膿菌	571	多発性硬化症		診断法	305
多指症	332		111, 308, 574	単一ネフロン糸球体濾過	
多肢選択式試問	67, 570	多発性骨髄腫	273, 572	量	219, 598
多焦点レンズ	135	多発性内分泌腫瘍	571	短胃動脈	474
多食	244	多発性内分泌腫瘍1型		担架	90
打診	77		255	段階的運動負荷試験	180
打診音	156	多発性内分泌腫瘍2型		段階的の患者管理	43
唾石	148		255	単芽球	17
唾石症	151	多発性内分泌腺腫症		短下肢ギプス包帯	289
唾石摘除術	152		255, 571	短下肢装具	290, 519, 597
多関門集積スキャン	181	多発性嚢胞腎	115	単科大学	62
多染性	264	多発性嚢胞腎疾患		胆管炎	209
多臓器不全	107, 573		222, 585	胆管癌	209
多臓器不全症候群		多発ニューロパチー	303	胆管細胞癌	209, 531
	107, 573	ダプソン	541	単眼視	132
多巣性運動ニューロパチ		打撲傷	261	胆管造影法	203
ー	112, 309, 572	ダームスタチウム		ダンカン病	271
タゾバクタム・ピペラシ			436, 543	短期大学	62
リン	601	タムスロシン塩酸塩	224	単球	15, 265
多胎妊娠	229	ため息	154	単極性	15
直ちに	24, 600	多毛	245, 319	単極性うつ病	312
ただれ	318	多毛症	321	タングステン	435, 609
立ちくらみ	293	タモキシフェン	601	単光子放出コンピュータ	
打聴診	580	タモキシフェンクエン酸		断層撮影法	80, 599
脱臼	278	塩	241	炭酸塩	218
脱水	10, 105	ダーモスコピー	322	炭酸脱水酵素阻害薬	
脱水熱	105	タラボルフィンナトリウ			136
脱退一時金	49	ム	170	短時間作用型吸入β_2刺	
脱毛	245, 319	タランピシリン	601	激薬	169, 595
脱毛症	25, 245	タリウム	436, 603	短時間増強感覚指数	
脱力	104	タリウム心筋血流スキャ			142, 597
縦	448	ン	181	単刺試験	323
たとえば	21, 545	タリウムトレッドミル試		短指症	13
ターナー症候群	240	験	181	胆汁	512
ダナゾール	241	ダリエー徴候	320	胆汁うっ滞	13, 19
ダナパロイドナトリウム		ダリエー病	324	胆汁の	35
	275	樽状胸	156	短縦列反復	510, 600
ダニ	38	ダルテパリンナトリウム		断酒会	316, 516
ダニ媒介脳炎	108		275	単純X線撮影法	79
多尿	19, 217, 244	ダルトン	438, 539	単純型先天表皮水疱症	
他人恐怖症	296	ダルベポエチンアルファ			339, 544
多嚢胞性卵巣症候群			274	単純写真	284
	238, 582	多列検出器型コンピュー		単純配列長多型	510, 599
多倍数体	37, 510	タ断層撮影法	79, 571	単純ヘルペス	26, 324
多発関節痛	2	痰	155	単純ヘルペスウイルス	

			322, 559		恥垢	231
単純ヘルペス脳炎		タンパク尿	218		恥骨	494
	307, 558	タンパク分解酵素阻害薬			恥骨後腔	488
巣状糸球体硬化症	550		211		恥骨上	12
炭水化物	533	タンパク漏出性腸症	206		恥骨上切石術	226
胆膵バイパス術	260	短波長紫外線	607		恥骨上痛	216
男性化	240, 244	短腓骨筋	500		恥骨部	452
男性型多毛症	245, 255	ダンピング症候群	206		智歯	147, 464
男性恐怖症	296	単房性	12		致死性家族性不眠症	112
男性性器	488	タンポン	241		致死量	566
男性生殖器系	488	端末表示装置	126, 608		地図状舌	148
弾性組織	512	単麻痺	299		チタン	434, 603
男性様	12	弾力線維性仮性黄色腫			父親	73
胆石	13		328, 590		父方	73
胆石症	209				地中海貧血	269
胆石仙痛	195	ち			腟	489
胆石溶解薬	211	チアゾリジンジオン	606		腟炎	238
炭疽	108	チアゾリジンジオン誘導			腟円蓋	231
炭素	434, 529	体	258		腟鏡	37, 78
淡蒼球	503	チアノーゼ	158		腟鏡検査	236
断層撮影法	79, 161	チアマゾール	258, 572		腟鏡診	231
断続言語	302	チアミンジスルフィド			チック	38, 300
断続性呼吸	157		602		腟痙	229
断続性ラ音	157	チアンフェニコール	604		腟口	232, 489
タンタル	435, 601	地域医療	43		腟式子宮全摘術	243, 606
断端	88	地域医療学	65		腟出血	28, 229
胆道	484	地域医療支援病院	52		腟前庭	489
短頭症	13	地域看護	60		窒素	434, 575
丹毒	326	地域看護学	66		窒息	154
ダントロレンナトリウム		地域保健法	46		窒息する	155
水和物	316	地域立脚型学習	67		腟トリコモナス	235
タンニン酸アルブミン		遅延型過敏反応	323, 543		腟分泌物	228
	211	遅延型皮膚過敏症			知的障害	343
胆嚢	484, 552		323, 540		知的障害者福祉法	46
胆嚢炎	209	チェーン・ストークス呼			千鳥足	294
胆嚢管	484	吸	157		知能検査	303
胆嚢癌	209	チオテパ	603		知能指数	303, 562
胆嚢切除後症候群	209	知覚性神経終末	462		遅発性ウイルス感染症	
胆嚢腺筋腫症	209	知覚異常	301			600
胆嚢造影法	203	知覚過敏	301		遅発性虚血性神経脱落症	
胆嚢摘出術	215	知覚減退	301		候	306, 541
胆嚢動脈	472, 529	知覚消失	294, 301		遅発性内リンパ水腫	113
胆嚢ポリープ	209	恥丘	489		遅反応性アナフィラキシ	
タンパク異化率	582	ちくちくする	121		ー物質	159, 599
タンパク結合ヨウ素	581	チクロピジン塩酸塩			乳房	444
タンパク質・エネルギー			190, 315		痴呆	295
栄養失調症	256	治験コーディネーター			地方病	106
タンパク質分解酵素	17		58, 537		地方病性	35
タンパク同化ステロイド		治験薬	85, 562		緻密骨	494

日本語索引 667

緻密性結合組織	512	中手指節関節	495, 570	腸液	513
遅脈	173	抽出核抗原	546	腸炎	205
チミン	511, 600	中心	448	腸炎ビブリオ	202
チーム看護	89	中心窩	130, 458	超音波検査法	12, 80, 607
チモール混濁試験	605	中心視	132	超音波生体顕微鏡	
チャイルド分類	199	中心静脈圧	182, 539		131, 606
着床前遺伝子診断	85	中心性漿液性脈絡網膜症		超音波内視鏡検査	
着床前診断	85		134, 538		204, 548
チャーグ・ストラウス症		中心性肥満	245	聴覚	139
候群	165	中心・側頭部棘波をもつ		聴覚過敏	139
着床前遺伝子診断	584	良性小児てんかん		聴覚検査	13, 141
チャージ(連合)	533		341, 526	聴覚性鎮痛	13
チャドウィック徴候	231	虫垂	482	聴覚反射	141
チャドック反射	301	虫垂炎	205	聴覚誘発電位	142, 519
チャネル病	106	虫垂切除術	214	長下肢ギプス包帯	289
治癒	91	中枢神経系	502, 536	長下肢装具	290, 564, 567
注意義務	43	中枢性交感神経抑制薬		腸管	480
注意欠陥障害	343, 518		188	腸鉗子	89
注意欠陥多動障害		中枢性摂食異常症	115	腸管出血性大腸菌	
	313, 343, 518	中枢性肺胞低換気症候群			202, 546
中咽頭癌	145		167, 530	腸管出血性大腸菌感染症	
中央滅菌材料部門	538	中性脂肪	250		107
中央材料室	55, 538	中足骨	494	腸管組織侵入性大腸菌	
中央社会保険医療協議会		中足趾節関節	495, 575		202, 546
	49	中大脳動脈	471, 570	腸管の	8
中央滅菌材料部門	55	注腸検査	203	腸管病原性大腸菌	
肘窩	452	中直腸動脈	474		202, 547
中間型インスリン	258	中殿筋	500	腸管付着性大腸菌	
昼間過眠	156, 545	肘頭	452		202, 544
中間冠状症候群	185	中毒性巨大結腸	206	腸間膜	482
中間楔状骨	494	中毒性表皮壊死症		腸間膜リンパ節	479
中間広筋	500		326, 602	腸管連リンパ組織	552
肘関節	495	肘内障	340	聴器	458
肘関節全置換術	292	中年の危機	229	腸偽閉塞	206
中間尿	217	中脳	504	腸球菌	14, 219
中間尿細管	486	中脳水道	502	腸クロム親和性	14
中間物挿入関節形成術		中脳被蓋	504	蝶形紅斑	319
	292	中波長紫外線	329, 607	蝶形骨	492
中結腸動脈	474, 570	中鼻甲介	460	蝶形骨洞	460
中国伝統医学	119	中皮腫	11	蝶形骨洞炎	144
中止	540	中鼻道	460	長結腸症	13
中耳	458	肘部管症候群	285	徴候	120
中耳炎	139	中葉症候群	166	潮紅	319
注射	26	肘リンパ節	478	調合乳	343
注射器	86	中和試験	81, 578	超高比重リポタンパク	
注射硬化療法	212	チューター制	67		608
注射針	86	治癒的治療	118	長後毛様体動脈	472, 568
中縦隔	468	治癒量	531	腸骨	36, 494
中手骨	494	腸	8, 480	腸骨下腹神経	506

用語	ページ
腸骨鼠径神経	506
腸骨大腿靱帯	496
腸骨の	36
腸骨稜	452
腸骨リンパ節	479
腸雑音	198, 529
超自我	38
長時間作用型吸入 β_2 刺激薬	169, 565
腸重積	338
聴診	77
聴診器	77
聴神経	505
聴神経炎	144
聴神経鞘腫	144
聴性脳幹反応	142, 517, 525
調節呼吸	169, 535
調節反射	129
腸腺	483
長端末反復	511, 568
腸チフス	107
超低カロリー食	90, 609
超低出生体重	546
超低出生体重児	331
超低比重リポタンパク	609
超伝導量子干渉素子	599
長頭症	13
腸毒素産生性大腸菌	202, 548
腸内細菌科	202
腸内細菌叢	202
長内転筋	500
長波長紫外線	607
長腓骨筋	500
貼付剤	86
腸閉塞	206
腸壁ヘルニア	210
長方形	39
腸溶(錠)	544
腸腰筋	500
腸腰靱帯	496
聴力	139
聴力図	17, 141
腸瘻造設術	215
腸肋筋	500
直視下生検	78
直視下レーザー前立腺切除術	226, 609
直接クームス試験	267, 540
直接蛍光抗体法	81, 541
直接血液灌流	225, 541
直接抗グロブリン試験	267, 540
直接鼠径ヘルニア	210
直接ビリルビン	199
直線加速器	567
直腸	482
直腸温	75
直腸癌	207
直腸鏡検査	204
直腸肛門科	53
直腸肛門科医	60
直腸子宮窩	489
直腸指診	77, 543
直腸脱・内痔核手術	215, 586
直腸腟診	231
直腸病学	65
直腸瘤	17, 239
直方体	40
直流	540
直角三角形	39
治療の計画	96
治療的診断	85
治療的流産	242
治療的レーザー角膜切除術	137, 589
治療薬濃度測定	86, 602
治療利得係数	603
チロシン尿	333
鎮咳薬	167
沈下歯	149
陳旧性	91
陳旧性心筋梗塞	185, 579
鎮痙薬	210
鎮静薬	314
鎮痛	17, 122
鎮痛薬	25, 122

つ

用語	ページ
ツァンク試験	324
椎間軟骨	496
椎間板	496
椎間板切除術	291
椎間板造影法	284
椎間板ヘルニア	26, 287, 557
椎弓形成術	291
椎弓切除術	291
椎骨	8
椎骨動脈	472, 607
椎骨動脈造影法	305, 607
椎骨の	8
椎骨脳底動脈循環不全	306, 608
対耳輪	458
追伸	587
対麻痺	11, 18, 299
～痛	71
痛覚閾値	121
痛覚過敏	17, 301
痛覚消失	17, 301
痛覚鈍麻	301
通常型間質性肺炎	164, 606
通常の小児期疾患	606
通所介護施設	55
通年性	37
痛風	257
痛風結晶	284, 574
痛風結節	140, 246
痛風性関節炎	286
痛風発作	244
杖	279
ツェンカー憩室	204
使い捨てコンタクトレンズ	136
使い捨て手袋	77
摑まり立ち	330
疲れ目	126
疲れる	104
つぎ足歩行	298
突き指	279
付けまつげ	127
つち骨	36, 459
土踏まず	446
槌指	285
ツッカー	31
つつが虫病	108
ツベルクリン試験	158
つまずく	294
爪	8, 446, 462
爪の	8
ツモール	31

ツリウム	435, 603	
吊り下げギプス包帯	289	
吊り包帯	289	
つわり	229	

て

手	8, 444
手足口病	110, 339, 556
手洗い	87
ディアベ	31
低アルドステロン症	254
定位手術的照射	317, 599
定位放射線照射	600
定位放射線治療	117, 599
帝王切開	243, 538
帝王切開後経腟分娩	243, 608
低カリウム血症	251
低カルシウム血症	251
低カロリー食	90
低換気症候群	166
低緊張性十二指腸造影	203, 555
低形成	83
低血糖	246
低血糖昏睡	256
低血糖症	17
泥膏	328
低吸収域	566
テイコプラニン	602
テイ・サックス病	257, 605
低残渣食	90
低酸素血症	159
低酸素症	11, 159
低酸素性虚血性脳症	334, 556
低酸素性肺血管収縮	558
低色素血	263
ディジタル差分血管造影法	79, 543
低脂肪食	90
低出生体重児	331
テイ症候群	337
泥状便	196
ディジョージ症候群	336
低視力	125
低侵襲心臓外科手術	191, 572

低身長	245, 331
低身長症	245
低心拍出量症候群	185, 568
ディスポ	31
低タンパク血症	219
低タンパク食	224
低張尿	219
ティーツェ症候群	156
ディック試験	323, 334
ディッセ腔	484
低電位	179
低ナトリウム血症	219, 251
ティネル徴候	303
低拍出性心不全	186
低比重リポタンパク	566
低比重リポタンパクコレステロール	250
低分子量ヘパリン	567
低マグネシウム血症	251
低用量ピル	241
定量吸入器	169, 571
定量的CT	283, 590
低リン酸血症	251
ティンパノメトリー	142
デオキシリボ核酸	511, 542
テガフール	551, 603
テガフール・ウラシル	606
滴	554
適応障害	312
適宜	21, 518
出来事	36
デキサメタゾン	541
デキサメタゾン抑制試験	249, 543
摘出	88
デキストロメトルファン臭化水素酸塩	167
笛声音	158
適性検査	67
適正臨床試験実施基準	552
出来高払い方式	49
摘便	90
適法食品(ユダヤ教)	91
テクネチウム	435, 602

手首	444
デシタビン	274, 539
デシベル	540
デシリットル	438, 542
デスγカルボキシプロトロンビン	201, 540
テストステロン	234
デスメ膜	456
デスモプレシン酢酸塩	259, 540
テスラ	439, 600
テタニー	246
データベース	95, 96
鉄	434, 549
鉄芽球	267
鉄芽球性貧血	269
鉄欠乏性貧血	269, 561
鉄剤	274
出っ歯	147
デトーニ・ファンコーニ症候群	337
テトラサイクリン	602
テトラヒドロカンナビノール	603
テニス肘	279
手の平	444
テノホビルジソプロキシルフマル酸	275, 602
テノン嚢	458
デビック病	308
デヒドロエピアンドロステロン	541
テビペネムピボキシル	602
テーピング法	289
デフェロキサミン	274, 541
デブリードマン	88
テーベー	31
デメチルクロルテトラサイクリン	542
デュークス分類	199
デュシェンヌ型筋ジストロフィー	308
デュタステリド	224
デュピュイトラン拘縮	281
デュビン・ジョンソン症候群	208

日本語索引 *671*

デュラフォア潰瘍	205	テンシロン試験	305	頭蓋輪骨盤牽引	291
デューリング病	324	伝染性紅斑	110, 339	動眼神経	505
デュロジェ徴候	177	伝染性単核球症		動悸	172, 244, 261
テリスロマイシン	602		26, 271, 561	同期式間欠的強制換気	
テルソン症候群	130	伝染性膿痂疹	324		170, 597
テルビウム	435, 601	伝染病	106	洞機能不全症候群	600
テルビナフィン塩酸塩		デンタルフロス	147	頭頚部外科	53
	329	点滴静注腎盂造影法		頭頚部再建	146
テール便	196		220, 542	頭頚部腫瘍	145
デルマ	31	点滴静注胆管造影法		頭血腫	13
テルル	435, 602		203, 541	凍結手術	329
デーレ封入体	264	点滴注入	86	洞結節機能回復時間	
テロメア	511	電導収縮解離	176, 583		181, 598
テロメラーゼ	511	点頭てんかん	332	洞結節リエントリー頻拍	
転移	11, 83, 604	デンバー式発達スクリー			174, 598
転位	12	ニング検査	334, 541	凍結融解赤血球	276
転移RNA	511, 605	デンバーシャント	213	糖源生成	14
伝音性難聴	142	点鼻液	145	糖原病	257
電荷結合素子	531	殿部	452	糖原病Ⅰ型	257
てんかん	293	癜風	325	糖原病Ⅱ型	257
てんかん患者	294	添付文書	86, 586	糖原病Ⅲ型	257
転換性障害	312	天疱瘡	116	糖原病Ⅳ型	257
てんかん発作	26, 293	電話番号	71	糖原病Ⅴ型	257
点眼薬	127			瞳孔	456
転帰	93			統合医学用語システム	
電気化学発光免疫測定法		と			3, 606
	81, 545	トランスポゾン	511	瞳孔間距離	129, 562
電気眼振検査法	132, 547	トイレ許可	528	登校拒否	343
電気キモグラフィー	546	銅	434, 539	瞳孔径	129
電気凝固	14	頭位	232, 233	統合失調症	312
電気痙攣療法	316, 548	頭囲	76, 232	瞳孔反射	129
電気歯髄診断器	150	同位元素	11	瞳孔不同	129
電気ショック療法		同化	17	橈骨	492
	316, 548	頭蓋	8, 442	橈骨尺骨の	16
電気水圧式砕石術	546	頭蓋咽頭腫	313	橈骨手根骨の	16
電気生理学的検査		頭蓋X線撮影	251	橈骨静脈	476
	180, 547	頭蓋冠	442	橈骨神経	505
デング熱	108	頭蓋顔面合併切除術	146	橈骨動脈	472
転座	511	頭蓋腔	455	橈骨動脈脈拍	176
点字	125	頭蓋計測	13	同語反復	300
電子カルテ	43, 546	頭蓋牽引	291	陶材インレー	152
電子顕微鏡	79, 546	頭蓋骨	492	倒錯型心室頻拍	179
転子部	452	頭蓋内	36	糖鎖抗原125	529
電子保健医療記録	546	頭蓋内圧	304, 560	糖鎖抗原19-9	201, 529
転写	511	頭蓋内圧亢進	304, 560	陶歯冠	152
点状出血	261	頭蓋内外バイパス		頭字語	56
点状表層角膜炎	133, 599		317, 545	同時視	132, 598
テンションフリー腟メッ		頭蓋内血腫	307, 560	同質性	36
シュ	243, 606	頭蓋内動脈瘤	307	等尺性運動	290
		頭蓋の	8		

同種骨髄移植	276	疼痛の性質	121		159, 595	
凍傷	25, 320	同定	560	動脈血炭酸ガス分圧		
同上	542, 560	動的コンピュータ断層撮			159, 580	
豆状骨	492	影法	79	動脈血中ケトン体比		
動静脈奇形	183, 525	動的副子	290		200, 520	
動静脈交差部	130	等電位線	178	動脈硬化	13, 18, 34	
動静脈の	13, 525	頭殿長	232, 537	動脈硬化症	25	
動静脈吻合	525	糖尿	218, 244	動脈硬化性心血管疾患		
橙色	39	導尿	90, 224		184, 524	
洞徐脈	174	糖尿病	255, 542	動脈硬化性心疾患		
同性愛	231	糖尿病看護	61		184, 524	
透析アミロイドーシス		糖尿病食	91, 258	動脈性	8	
	224	糖尿病性ケトアシドーシ		動脈瘤	187	
透析液	225	ス	256, 542	動脈瘤性骨嚢胞	288, 516	
透析看護	61	糖尿病性昏睡	256	透明中隔	502	
透析関節症	224	糖尿病性腎症	222, 256	投薬	85	
透析器	225	糖尿病性ニューロパチー		糖輸送体	553	
透析困難症候群	224		256	動揺視	126	
透析脳症	224	糖尿病性微小血管症	256	動揺歩行	298	
同前	542	糖尿病網膜症		投与径路	85	
銅線動脈	130		135, 256, 543	投与量制限毒性	542	
凍瘡	27, 320	糖尿病療養指導士	58	同僚検討	43	
痘瘡	107	動肺コンプライアンス		登録看護師	57, 593	
倒像眼底検査	131		532	兎眼	127	
頭側	448	頭髪	442	ドキシサイクリン	543	
橈側	448	逃避	36	ドキシフルリジン	541	
橈側手根屈筋	498	頭皮	442	ドキソルビシン	518, 544	
橈側手根伸筋	498	橙皮様皮膚	231	特異体質	14	
等速性運動	290	洞頻脈	174	特異動の作用	105, 596	
同側半盲	132	頭部	75	読字困難	302	
橈側皮静脈	476	東部ウマ脳炎	108	読書用眼鏡	126	
頭側へ	448	頭部X線規格撮影法	150	毒素性ショック症候群		
同側片麻痺	299	洞不整脈	174		326, 605	
胴体	444	洞不全症候群	183	毒素性ショック症候群毒		
糖タンパク質	14	動物恐怖症	297	素	322, 605	
頭頂	442	動物行動学	65	毒素性ショック様症候群		
頭頂骨	492	頭部の	5		326, 605	
等張性運動	290	頭部白癬	325	特定機能病院	52	
等張の	11	盗癖	18	特定死因死亡比	93, 585	
頭頂部	450	同胞	73	特定疾患	111	
頭頂葉	502	洞房結節	470	特定病原体不在(動物)		
洞調律	173	洞房伝導時間	181, 595		599	
当直医	57	洞房の	595	禿頭	319	
同著者	560	胴回り	196	特発性	14	
疼痛	120	動脈	8, 471, 516	特発性間質性肺炎		
疼痛回避歩行	279	動脈管開存症	183, 582		113, 164, 561	
疼痛管理	122	動脈血ガス	158, 516	特発性器質化肺炎		
疼痛緩和	122	動脈血酸素分圧	159, 581		164, 536	
疼痛許容レベル	121	動脈血酸素飽和度		特発性血小板減少性紫斑		

病	115, 273, 563	
特発性血栓症	115	
特発性高アルドステロン症	253, 561	
特発性細菌性腹膜炎	210, 595	
特発性心筋症	187, 560	
特発性新生児肝炎	335	
特発性ステロイド性骨壊死症	113	
特発性大腿骨頭壊死症	113, 286	
特発性肺線維症	164, 562	
特発性肥大型大動脈弁下狭窄症	187, 561	
特発性門脈圧亢進症	113, 208, 562	
特発性両側性感音性難聴	113	
特別養護老人ホーム	55	
棘	40	
時計方向回転	178, 539	
吐血	195	
ドケルバン病	285	
床ずれ	318	
徒手筋力テスト	281, 573	
徒手整復	289	
土食症	261	
トシリズマブ	289	
トスフロキサシン	603	
ドセタキセル	542, 606	
トーチ症候群	338, 604	
特記すべき疾患なし	575	
突然死	93	
突然変異遺伝子	511	
トッド麻痺	297	
突背	281	
突発痛	121	
届出義務	44	
届出疾患	106	
と共に	529	
ドーナツ	40	
ドナート・ランドシュタイナー試験	268	
ドナーリンパ球輸注	276	
ドネペジル塩酸塩	315	
ドーパミン	250, 539	
ドーパミン塩酸塩	189	
ドーパミン作動薬		

	259, 315	
とびひ	318, 331	
トピラマート	316	
塗布剤	328	
吐物	195	
ドブニウム	436, 540	
ドプラー心エコー図法	181	
ドプラ超音波法	80	
トブラマイシン	604	
ドベーキー分類	182	
トーマス試験	281	
ドミュセー徴候	177	
トモ	32	
どもる	294	
ドライアイ	133	
トライツ靱帯	482	
トラウベ半月部	157	
トラコーマ	133	
トラコーマクラミジア	235	
トラコーマ封入体結膜炎	133, 605	
トラスツズマブ	241	
トラフェルミン	329	
トランスクリプトーム	511	
トランスフェリン	268, 603	
トランスフェリン受容体	268	
トリアージ	44	
トリアージタッグ	44	
トリアゾラム	314	
トリインフルエンザ	108	
トリインフルエンザウイルス	160	
トリウム	436, 603	
トリ型結核菌複合体	160, 569	
トリカルボン酸(回路)	602	
トリグリセリド	250, 603	
トリクロルメチアジド	188	
トリーチャーコリンズ症候群	341	
鳥肌が立つ	318	
ドリペネム	543	

鳥目	126	
トリメトプリム	604	
努力呼気曲線	162	
努力性肺活量	551	
努力肺活量	162, 549	
トリヨードサイロニン	247, 600	
トリヨードサイロニンレジン摂取率	248	
トール	439, 604	
トルエンジイソシアネート	602	
トルコ鞍	251	
トルサードドポアンツ	179, 602	
ドルーゼン	130	
トルソー症候群	177	
トルソー徴候	246	
ドレイン	89	
ドレスラー症候群	186	
トレチノイン	525	
トレッドミル試験	180	
トレミフェン	604	
トレンデレンブルク試験	333	
トレンデレンブルク体位	77	
ドロキシドーパ	315	
トロサ・ハント症候群	307	
トローチ	86	
トロピカミド	136	
トロンビン・アンチトロンビンIII複合体	266, 601	
トロンビン時間	265, 605	
トロンボエラストグラム	602	
トロンボキサン	606	
トロンボテスト	265, 605	
トロンボモジュリン	266, 275, 604	
鈍角三角形	39	
呑気症	197	
ドンペリドン	211	

な

語	ページ
内因子	268
内因性	10
内因性交感神経刺激作用	563
内陰部動脈	474
内科	54
内科医	60
内科学	65
内眼角	456
内眼角贅皮	127
内胸動脈	472, 561, 563
内頸静脈	476
内頸動脈	471, 559
内頸動脈海綿静脈洞瘻	307, 531
内向性の人	296
内耳	459
内耳炎	144
内視鏡医	60
内視鏡下手術	212
内視鏡下生検	78
内視鏡検査	78
内視鏡的(静脈瘤)硬化療法	546
内視鏡の拡張器	213
内視鏡的逆行性胆道膵管造影法	203, 547
内視鏡的逆行性胆道ドレナージ	213, 547
内視鏡的経鼻胆道ドレナージ	213, 546
内視鏡的止血	212
内視鏡的静脈瘤結紮術	212, 548
内視鏡的静脈瘤硬化療法	212
内視鏡的胆道ドレナージ	544
内視鏡的乳頭括約筋切開術	212, 548
内視鏡的乳頭切開術	212, 547
内視鏡的粘膜下層剝離術	212, 548
内視鏡的粘膜切除術	212, 546
内視鏡的ポリープ切除術	212
内視鏡部	54
内耳神経	460
内斜位	128, 547
内斜視	35, 128, 548
内診	231
ナイスタチン	578
内旋	279
内臓	38
内臓脂肪	245
内臓知覚	302
内臓痛	120
内側	448
内側楔状骨	494
内側広筋	500
内側縦束	504, 572
内側上腕皮神経	505
内側前腕皮神経	505
内側足底動脈	476
内側中葉区	468
内側直筋	458
内側肺底区	468
内中膜複合体厚	305, 562
内腸骨静脈	478
内腸骨動脈	474, 561
ナイチンゲール誓詞	44
内転	34, 279
内軟骨腫症	288
内胚葉	10
内反膝	26, 279
内反足	280, 603
内反肘	280
内部寄生動物	10
内腹斜筋	500
内分泌科	54
内分泌科医	60
内分泌学	65
内分泌系	75
内方	448
内包	503
内膜肥厚	305
中指	444
梨	40
梨子地眼底	130
なしに	22, 595
ナジフロキサシン	576
ナースステーション	55
ナースプラクティショナー	58, 577
ナチュラルキラー(細胞)	577
ナテグリニド	258
ナート	32
など	548
ナトリウム	434, 575
ナトリウムチャネル遮断薬	189
ナトリウム排泄分画	220, 549
7価肺炎球菌結合型ワクチン	344
ナノグラム	439, 576
ナノメーター	577
ナファモスタットメシル酸塩	275
ナフトピジル	224
ナブメトン	122
ナプロキセン	122
ナボット囊胞	231
なまず	318
鉛	436, 581
涙	126
ナラトリプタン塩酸塩	122
ナリジクス酸	575
ナルコレプシー	312
軟X線	329
軟膏	328, 606
軟口蓋	464
軟膏剤	86, 579
軟骨	8, 495
軟骨異栄養症	336
軟骨壊死	13
軟骨芽腫	13
骨軟化症	15
軟骨性	8
軟骨組織	512
軟骨肉腫	8, 288
軟骨無形成症	3
難産	230
軟食	90
軟性下疳	237
軟性白斑	130
難治性視神経症	113
難治性ネフローゼ症候群	115
難治性の	121
難聴	139

日本語索引

難病	106, 111
南米出血熱	107
軟便	196
軟膜	14, 504
軟脈	173

に

ニオブ	435, 576
にきび	318
握りこぶし	446
肉眼的血尿	218
肉芽	83
肉芽腫	83
肉腫	16, 83
肉親	73
肉離れ	278
ニコチンアミドアデニンジヌクレオチド	575
ニコチン酸	259
ニコチン貼付剤	169
ニコモール	259
ニコルスキー徴候	321
二酸化炭素ナルコーシス	159
二酸化物	10
二次感染	106
二次救命処置	518, 521
二次性高血圧	184
二次性徴	245
二枝ブロック	179
二重エネルギー X 線吸収法	283, 541
二重焦点眼鏡	135
二重造影法	203
二重瞼	126
二重脈	173
二重免疫拡散法	81, 541
二重らせん	511
二重濾過血漿分離交換法	225, 541
二相性陽性気道内圧	170, 527
二段脈	10, 173
日常語	2, 25
日常生活関連動作	92, 522
日常生活動作	92, 518
ニッケル	434, 576
日光角化症	324
ニッシェ	32, 203
日射性口唇炎	34
日射病	105
ニッスル小体	504
ニッセン噴門形成術	214
二等筋反射	300
二等辺三角形	39
ニトログリセリン	189, 578
ニトロプルシド試験	333
ニトロプルシドナトリウム	189, 598
二倍体	511
ニパウイルス感染症	108
鈍い	121
ニフェカラント塩酸塩	189
ニフェジピン	188
二分脊椎	342
二峰性の	10
二峰性脈	173
日本医学教育学会	67
日本医師会	44, 564
日本医師会医の倫理綱領	46
日本医療機能評価機構	44, 564
日本看護協会	44, 564
日本紅斑熱	108
二本鎖 DNA	511, 543
日本式昏睡尺度	297, 564
日本生命倫理学会	44
日本脳炎	108
日本脳炎ウイルス	564
日本脳炎ワクチン	344
日本版デンバー式発達スクリーニング検査	334, 564
日本病院薬剤師会	44, 564
日本薬剤師会	44, 564
日本薬局方	85, 564
ニーマン・ピック病	257
ニムスチン	518
入院	72, 73
入院経過抄録	93
入院時診断	93
入院前	72, 588
乳癌	240
乳がん看護	61
乳剤性軟膏	328

乳酸デヒドロゲナーゼ	178, 283, 566
乳歯	147
乳児	330
乳児湿疹	339
乳児性骨皮質過形成	340
乳児突然死症候群	339, 597
乳汁漏出	246
乳腺炎	240
乳腺症	240
乳頭	40, 444
乳頭管	486
乳頭陥凹	130
乳頭筋	470
乳頭出血	130
乳頭線	454
乳頭層	462
乳様突起切除術	145
乳頭浮腫	130
乳び胸	478
乳び尿	218
乳び腹水	262
乳房	8, 444
乳房 X 線撮影法	8, 236
乳房温存手術	243
乳房下部	450
乳房形成術	243
乳房再建術	243
乳房自己検診	231, 529
乳房切除術	8, 243
乳房痛	17
乳房パジェット病	240
乳房部	450
乳幼児突発性危急事態	331, 521
乳様突起炎	144
乳輪	450
ニュートン	439, 576
ニューモシスチス・イロベチ	160
ニューモシスチス肺炎	165, 582
ニューヨーク心臓協会分類	178, 578
ニュルンベルク綱領	45
ニューロキニン 1 受容体拮抗薬	211
ニューロレプト鎮痛	123

用語	ページ
ニューロレプト麻酔	87, 577
ニューロン	504
尿	513
尿意	216
尿意切迫	216
尿管	38, 486
尿管炎	223
尿管腎盂移行部	486, 606
尿管切除術	226
尿管膀胱移行部	486, 607
尿器	90
尿細管	486
尿細管間質性腎炎	222, 603
尿細管最大輸送量	220
尿細管性アシドーシス	222, 594
尿細胞診	219
尿酸	606
尿酸結晶	284
尿酸結石	218
尿酸尿	218
尿試験紙	218
尿失禁	216
尿臭	148
尿勢低下	216
尿線	216
尿線細少	216
尿線途絶	216
尿素呼気試験	201, 606
尿中バニリルマンデル酸	333
尿中ホモバニリン酸	333
尿沈渣	218
尿滴下	216
尿道	38, 488
尿道炎	223
尿道海綿体	488
尿道カテーテル法	224
尿道下裂	223
尿道鏡検査	221
尿道形成術	226
尿道ステント留置	224
尿道痛	216
尿道分泌物	217
尿毒症	223
尿毒症性アシドーシス	219
尿毒症性口臭	217
尿の	38
尿培養	219
尿比重測定	219
尿閉	34, 216
尿崩症	253, 541
尿流計	220
尿流測定	220
尿流動態検査法	220, 606
尿流量	220
尿量	216
尿路	486
尿路感染症	223, 607
尿路結石症	16, 223
尿路性器の	16
尿路性器領域	452
二量体	10
二類感染症	107
ニーレ	32
人形の目徴候	298
人間ドック	72
妊娠	229
妊娠悪阻	26, 237
妊娠関連血漿タンパクA	234, 581
妊娠高血圧	238
妊娠高血圧症候群	238, 584
妊娠線	231
妊娠中絶	229
妊娠中毒	238
妊娠糖尿病	256, 552
妊娠反応	235
認知行動療法	316, 531
認知症	295
認知症看護	61
認知症高齢者グループホーム	55
認知症の行動・心理症状	528
人中	460
認定看護師	58, 60, 535
認定専門医	68
妊婦	229

ぬ

用語	ページ
ヌクレオシド系逆転写酵素阻害薬	275, 577
ヌクレオソーム	511
ヌクレオチド	511
ヌーナン症候群	240

ね

用語	ページ
寝汗	105
ネオジム	435, 576
ネオジム・ヤグレーザー	576
ネオン	434, 576
寝返り	330
ネグリ小体	305
ネクる	32
ネーゲレ法則	230
猫恐怖症	297
猫背	278
寝言	104
ネコ鳴き症候群	336
ネザートン症候群	325
ネダプラチン	532
ネチルマイシン	578
熱射病	105
熱傷	320
熱ショックタンパク質	558
熱性痙攣	331
熱帯医学	65
熱帯性	38
熱疲労	105
熱量計	18
ネプツニウム	436, 577
ネブライザー	169
ネフローゼ症候群	221
ネフロン	486
ネーベン	32
ネラトンカテーテル	224
ネルソン症候群	253
粘液	37
粘液水腫	251
粘液水腫性昏睡	251
粘液性	37
粘液嚢胞	148
年金	49
年金受給者	49
捻挫	37, 278
年代順	72
粘着性	38
粘土色便	196
捻髪音	158
粘膜	480, 569

日本語索引

語	ページ
粘膜下下鼻甲介切除術	146
粘膜下層	480, 597
粘膜関連リンパ組織	569
粘膜筋板	480, 572
粘膜皮膚眼症候群	326, 570
粘膜保護薬	210
粘膜レリーフ造影法	203
年齢	71

の

語	ページ
ノイトロ	32
ノイラミニダーゼ	575
ノイラミニダーゼ阻害薬	167
脳	8
脳アミロイド血管症	307, 529
脳炎	8, 14, 26, 307
脳回	35
脳外傷	307
膿痂疹	320
脳幹	504
脳灌流圧	304, 537
膿気心膜症	3
脳弓	502
膿胸	167
脳外科	54
脳外科医	60
脳血管疾患	539
脳血管障害	25, 306, 539
脳血管性認知症	311
脳血管造影法	305
脳血管抵抗	304, 539
脳血管の	13
脳血流量	304, 531
濃厚赤血球	537
脳梗塞	306, 534
脳硬膜動脈血管癒合術	317, 545
脳酸素代謝率	304, 535
脳死	93, 297
脳磁図法	304, 571
脳室	502
脳室鏡検査法	305
脳室周囲器官	502
脳室周囲低吸収域	305, 590
脳室周囲白質軟化症	342, 590
脳室心房短絡	317
脳室穿刺	317
脳室造影法	16, 305
脳室ドレナージ	317
脳室内圧測定	16
脳室内出血	307, 563
脳室腹腔シャント	317, 609
脳室腹腔短絡形成術	317
脳出血	306
脳腫瘍	313, 342, 529
脳神経	505, 535
脳神経外科	54
脳神経外科医	60
脳神経外科学	65
脳振盪	306
脳振盪後症候群	306
脳性ナトリウム利尿ペプチド	178, 528
脳性ナトリウム利尿ペプチド前駆体N端フラグメント	178, 578
脳性麻痺	306, 342, 536
脳脊髄液	304, 513, 538
脳脊髄液減少症	306
脳脊髄の	7, 13
脳卒中	294
脳卒中後うつ状態	312, 587
脳卒中障害評価法	298, 597
脳卒中リハビリテーション看護	61
脳損傷	306
脳底動脈	471, 525
脳動静脈奇形	342
脳動脈瘤	307
脳内出血	306, 560
脳軟化	14, 17
膿尿	218
脳膿瘍	307
脳波	3, 304, 545
脳波記録法	304
脳浮腫	306
嚢胞	83
膿疱	320
膿疱性乾癬	116
嚢胞性線維症	165, 532
嚢胞腺癌	239
嚢胞腺腫	13
嚢胞様黄斑浮腫	130, 535
膿盆	90
脳由来神経栄養因子	526
膿瘍	83
脳瘤	8, 17
脳梁	502
ノギテカン	576
のど	442
のど仏	442
ノーベリウム	436, 577
乗物恐怖症	297
ノルアド	32
ノルアドレナリン	250
ノルアドレナリン作動性・特異的セロトニン作動性抗うつ薬	314, 576
ノルエピネフリン	576
ノルエピネフリン・ドーパミン再取り込み阻害薬	576
ノルフロキサシン	576
ノロウイルス	202
ノンストレステスト	235, 578
ノンレム睡眠	304, 577

は

語	ページ
歯	8, 147, 330, 442, 464
バー（療法）	526
肺	8, 466
肺アスペルギルス症	165
肺アスペルギローム	165
肺移植	171
肺うっ血	176
排液	88
パイエル板	483
肺炎	8, 163
肺炎桿菌	160
肺炎球菌	17, 160
肺炎球菌ワクチン	168
肺炎クラミジア	160
肺炎マイコプラズマ	160
バイオフィードバック	119, 527
背臥位	76

肺活量	162, 608	バイタル	32, 75		116, 166
肺活量計	18, 162	背痛	120	肺胞嚢	466
肺活量測定	162	肺底部	466	ハイムリック法	168
肺癌	166, 566	肺動静脈瘻	183, 581	ハイモア洞	460
肺換気受容体	162	肺動脈	471, 580	肺門陰影	161
肺カンジダ症	165	肺動脈圧	181, 581	肺門部	466
肺気腫	165	肺動脈楔入圧		肺紋理	161
肺機能検査	162, 584		181, 582, 590	肺門リンパ節	478
廃棄物	38	肺動脈第2音	175	肺葉気管支	466
肺吸虫	199	肺動脈弁	470	肺葉切除術	171
肺胸膜嚢胞	161	肺動脈弁狭窄	184, 587	培養と感受性試験	538
配偶子	235	肺動脈弁閉鎖不全		肺容量減少術	171, 569
配偶者	73		184, 587	バイラー病	208
配偶者間人工授精		梅毒	27, 109, 237	排卵痛	228
	242, 520	梅毒血清検査	236, 600	排卵誘発法	241, 242
配偶子卵管内移植		梅毒トレポネーマ	235	肺リンパ脈管筋腫症	
	242, 553	梅毒トレポネーマ運動制			116, 166
肺クリプトコックス症		御試験	236, 604	ハインツ小体	264
	165	梅毒トレポネーマ蛍光抗		パイント	439, 588
肺結核	165	体吸収試験	236, 551	ハウエル・ジョリー小体	
肺血管造影法	161	梅毒トレポネーマ赤血球			264
肺血管抵抗	182, 590	凝集試験	236, 604	ハウスキーピング遺伝子	
敗血症	27, 107	排尿	216		511
肺高血圧症	166, 584	排尿筋・括約筋協調不全		バウヒン弁	482
肺好酸球浸潤	164, 584		223, 543	バウフ	32
肺梗塞	166	排尿困難	216	破壊性脊椎関節症	
肺サーファクタント	343	排尿時灼熱感	216		224, 543
肺静脈	476	排尿時膀胱尿道造影法		バカンピシリン	526
肺水腫	166, 176		221, 608	吐き気	195
胚性幹細胞	548	排尿遅延	216	歯ぎしり	147
肺性心	7, 186, 536	排尿痛	216	バーキットリンパ腫	272
肺清掃	169	肺の	8	パーキンソン病	
肺性肥厚性骨関節症		排膿管	89		27, 112, 308, 582
	158, 558	這い這い	330	吐く	28
肺性P波	179	背腹方向の	14	白衣高血圧	173
排泄	10	排便	196	歯茎	147, 442
肺尖	466	排便痛	196	博士号	584
肺腺癌	166	肺胞	466	白色	39
肺尖区	468	肺胞気-動脈血ガス分圧		白色帯下	18, 27, 228
肺尖後区	468	較差	159	白線	501
肺全摘除術	15, 171	肺胞気-動脈血酸素分圧		白癬	38, 325
肺尖帽	161	較差	159, 516	白癬症	28
肺臓学	65	肺胞気-動脈血窒素分圧		薄層クロマトグラフィー	
背側	448	較差	159, 516		81, 603
背側膵動脈	474	肺胞気-動脈血二酸化炭		白内障	134
肺塞栓血栓症	166, 589	素分圧較差	159, 516	白内障嚢外摘出術	
肺塞栓症	166, 583	肺胞呼吸音	157		137, 545
肺塞栓除去術	171	肺胞タンパク症	165, 581	白内障嚢内摘出術	
背側の	14	肺胞低換気症候群			137, 560

日本語索引

白斑	319	ハーツー	32	発達緑内障	134
白板症	14, 148	発育	244, 330	パッチテスト	323
白皮症	326	発育性股関節形成異常		ハッチンソン三徴	237
白毛	321		340, 540	ハッチンソン歯	149
剥離	88	発育遅延	244	発痛点注射	123
バークリウム	436, 527	発育不全	331, 551	バッド・キアリ症候群	
剥離骨折	282	発育良好な	76, 610		113, 208
剥離細胞診	78	八角形	40	発熱	105
剥離性間質性肺炎		麦角誘導体	122	発病	72
	164, 542	発汗	105, 244	発病年齢	72
パクリタキセル	589	発癌	15, 17	発病率	36
麦粒腫	26, 133	発癌物質	13	抜毛	35
歯車様呼吸	157	発汗療法	10	バト	32
激しい	121	パッキオニ小体	504	波動	197
ハーゲマン因子	556	白金	436, 588	ハードコンタクトレンズ	
跛行	298	白血球	14, 610		136
跛行する	294	白血球アルカリホスファ		鳩胸	27, 156
破壺共鳴	156	ターゼ	265, 565	バトル徴候	141
破骨細胞活性化因子	578	白血球円柱	218	鼻	8, 442, 460
破砕赤血球	264	白血球関連抗原	268, 566	鼻かぜ	155
鋏	88	白血球減少	265	鼻声	140
はさみ脚歩行	298	白血球除去療法	212	バナジウム	434, 607
バザン病	325	白血球数	263	鼻茸	141
はしか	330	白血球増加	18, 265	鼻血	261
把持鉗子	89	白血球走化性ケモカイン		鼻づまり	140
バシトラシン	526		601	鼻の	8
橋本病	251	白血球尿	218	鼻水	139
バージャー病	114, 187	白血球破砕皮膚血管炎		バーナー・モリソン症候	
播種	83		111	群	255
播種性血管内凝固		白血球分画	263	歯並び	147
	274, 541	白血病	17, 270	パニック障害	312
播種性表在性光線性汗孔		白血病性細網内皮症		パニペネム・ベタミプロ	
角化症	327, 543		271, 568	ン	581
バー小体	508	発語緩慢	302	パネート細胞	483
破傷風	27, 109	発語困難	294	ばね指	285
破傷風免疫グロブリン		発語障害	18, 35	歯の	8
	603	ハッサル小体	490	母親	73
破水	232	抜歯	147, 152	母方	73
パスカル	439, 580	ハッシウム	436, 558	ハバース管系	494
パズフロキサシン	590	発症	72	羽ばたき振戦	197
派生語	2	抜髄	152	ハバードタンク	290
バセドウ病	251	発生学	63	パパニコロー・スミア試	
バーセル指数	92, 527	発声訓練	145	験	235, 581
バゾプレシン	259	発生順	72	馬尾	506
肌色	39	発声障害	35, 140	馬尾腫瘍	288
バーター症候群	254	バッセン・コーンツヴァ		バビンスキー反射	301
破綻出血	239	イク症候群	256	ハプトグロビン	266, 558
パチニ小体	462	発達指数	331, 543		
ばち指	158	発達性言語障害	343		

ハフニウム	435, 556	バルプロ酸	316, 609	ロフィー	311, 594
歯ブラシ	147	ハルン	32	反射性尿失禁	217
ハプロタイプ	511	バルーン拡張式血管内ステント	191, 526	斑状歯	149
ハマン徴候	158			斑状出血	261
ハマン・リッチ症候群	164	バルーン血管形成術	190	板状無気肺	161
		バルーン心房中隔裂開	191, 526	半身不随	294
ハミルトンうつ病評価尺度	303, 555	バルーン閉塞下逆行性経静脈的塞栓術	213, 528	ハンスフィールド単位	79, 559
				伴性遺伝	74
ハム試験	268	バルーン弁形成術	192	伴性リンパ増殖症候群	271, 610
腹	8, 444	バレー徴候	246		
パラアミノサリチル酸	581	破裂	198	ハンセン病	328
		バレット食道	205	絆創膏	328
パラアミノサリチル酸カルシウム	581	バレー・リエウ症候群	285	半側麻痺	11, 18
				反対咬合	149
パラアミノ馬尿酸	581	パロキセチン塩酸塩水和物	314	反対側性	10
パラアミノ馬尿酸クリアランス	220			ハンタウイルス肺症候群	108
		半陰陽	240, 254		
ばら色粃糠疹	325	半円形	40	ハンター症候群	337
パラインフルエンザウイルス	160	反回神経麻痺	144	ハンター舌炎	151, 262
		汎下垂体機能低下	11, 252	パンチ症候群	270
パラジウム	435, 582	半規管	460	パンチ生検	78
バラシクロビル塩酸塩	329, 607	半奇静脈	476	反跳痛	197
		半球体	40	ハンチントン病	112, 310, 555
ハーラー症候群	337	反響言語	300		
パラチフス	107	半月型	12	ハンチントン舞踏病	310
バラニー検査	143	汎血球減少	11, 265	反時計方向回転	178, 531
バラニー指示試験	143	半月体形成性糸球体腎炎	221	ハンド・シュラー・クリスチャン病	342
パラフィン浴	289				
パラメーター	37	半腱様筋	500	ハント症候群	299
バリウム	435, 525	反抗挑戦性障害	313, 526	パンヌス	128, 280
バリウム注腸造影	203, 526	半固形便	196	反応性関節炎	286
		パンコースト症候群	158	晩発性小脳皮質萎縮症	310, 566
針恐怖症	297	バンコマイシン	608		
鍼師	58	バンコマイシン耐性黄色ブドウ球菌	609	晩発性皮膚ポルフィリン症	328, 582
バリズム	300				
ハリソン溝	156	バンコマイシン耐性黄色ブドウ球菌感染症	109	汎発性流行病	106
針電極	283			汎発流行性	35
パリノー症候群	301	バンコマイシン耐性腸球菌	609	反復運動過多損傷	285, 594
パリビズマブ	344				
鍼療法	119	バンコマイシン耐性腸球菌感染症	109	反復拮抗運動不能	300
バリント症候群	301			反復せよ	592
バルサルバ法	190	瘢痕	83	半分	599
パルスオキシメトリー	158	瘢痕拘縮	281	ハンマー	77
		半昏睡	12	ハンマー状足趾	280
ハルステッド手術	243	反射	300	半盲	132
ハルトマン手術	214	反社会的人格障害	313, 524	汎網膜光凝固術	136, 587
バルトリン腺	489				
バルトリン腺炎	238	反射性交感神経性ジスト			
バルビツレート	314				

日本語索引　　**681**

ひ

語	ページ
ピアペネム	527
非アルコール性脂肪性肝炎	208, 576
非アルコール性脂肪性肝疾患	207, 575
ヒアルロン酸	200
ヒアルロン酸ナトリウム	289
緋色	39
鼻咽腔検査	143
鼻咽頭癌	145
非 ST 上昇型心筋梗塞	185, 578
非エステル結合型脂肪酸	576
ピエール・ロバン症候群	332
ピエロ	32
鼻炎	8
ピオグリタゾン塩酸塩	258
ビオー呼吸	157
皮下	12, 596
被害妄想	293
皮下気腫	156
被殻	503
比較ゲノムハイブリダイゼーション	82, 533
皮下結節	280
皮下骨折	282
皮下脂肪	245
皮下脂肪組織	462
皮下組織	462
皮下注射	86
非活動性問題	96
鼻カニューレ	168
光凝固術	582
光刺激	304
光力学療法	583
ビカルタミド	224
非観血的整復	289
非器質性雑音	175
ひきずり歩行	298
引き出し徴候	280
ひきつけ	331
脾機能亢進症	270
鼻鏡	77
火恐怖症	297
ビグアナイド薬	258
鼻腔	460
ピクウィック症候群	156
脾屈曲部	482
非経口栄養	91, 585
非経口的	37
鼻形成術	18, 146
非結核性抗酸菌	160, 578
非結核性抗酸菌症	165
鼻孔	460
鼻甲介	460
鼻甲介切除術	146
粃糠疹	320
肥厚性幽門狭窄	338
ピコグラム	439, 584
ピコスルファートナトリウム	211
腓骨	494
尾骨	494
鼻骨	492
腓骨静脈	478
尾骨神経叢	506
腓骨動脈	476
腓骨の	37
非コレラビブリオ	202, 576
鼻根	460
膝	36, 446
非細菌性血栓性心内膜炎	186, 576
非再呼吸式マスク	168
微細脳機能障害	343, 570
肘	444
皮質骨	494
皮質脊髄の	13
皮質脳波	304, 544
ピシバニール	579
脾腫	8, 18, 198, 262
比重	598
鼻汁	16, 18
鼻出血	26, 140
鼻出血焼灼	146
尾状核	503
微小管	508
微小管形成中心	508, 574
微小管結合タンパク質	569
微小血管症性溶血性貧血	270, 572
非小細胞肺癌	166, 577
微少残存病変	271, 574
微小循環	11
微小物恐怖症	297
微小変化型ネフローゼ症候群	222, 570
微小変化群	222, 570
脾静脈	478, 600
尾状葉	484
非侵襲的陽圧換気	170, 577
非浸潤性小葉癌	240, 566
非浸潤性乳管癌	240, 540
脾髄	485
ヒス束	470
ヒス束心電図	180, 555
ヒステリー	17, 296
ヒステリー性	36
非ステロイド系抗炎症薬	122, 288, 577
ヒストン	511
ビスホスホネート	289, 528
ビスマス	436, 527
鼻声	16, 18
非正視	131
微生物	27
微生物学	63
非接触眼圧計	131, 576
鼻尖	460
鼻洗浄	145
鼻前庭	460
ヒ素	434, 524
鼻疽	108
脾臓	8, 36, 485
脾臓の	37
腓側	448
尾側	448
尾側へ	448
額	442
肥大	19, 83
肥大型心筋症	115, 187, 555
肥大型非閉塞性心筋症	187, 557
肥大型閉塞性心筋症	187, 557
肥大吸虫	199

非対称	10	ヒト絨毛性ゴナドトロピン	234, 555	泌尿器科	54
非代償性肝硬変	208	ヒト上皮増殖因子受容体2型	234, 556	泌尿器科医	60
非対称性緊張性頚反射	333, 524	ヒト心臓由来脂肪酸結合タンパク	178, 556	泌尿器科学	65
ひだ集中	203	ヒト成長ホルモン	556	泌尿器系	486
ビタミンK欠乏時産生タンパク	584	ヒト組織適合白血球抗原	557	泌尿生殖器系	75
ビタミンD	289	ヒト胎盤性乳腺刺激ホルモン	234, 558	泌尿生殖器の	554
ビタミンD依存性くる病	337, 608	ヒトチロトロピンアルファ	248	避妊	230
ビタミンD受容機構異常症	115	ヒトTARC定量	323	避妊具	241
ビタミンB$_6$	274	ヒトT細胞白血病	559	避妊薬	241
ビタミンB$_{12}$	268, 274	ヒトTリンパ球向性ウイルス1型	267, 559	非ヌクレオシド系逆転写酵素阻害薬	275, 577
ビダラビン	329, 523	ヒトTリンパ球向性ウイルス2型	267, 559	ビネー式知能検査	334
左回旋枝	471, 566	ヒト白血球抗原	557	脾の	8
左下腹部	452, 567	ヒトパピローマウイルス	235, 558	ビノレルビン	609
左下肋部	450	ヒトパピローマウイルスワクチン	242	鼻背	460
左利き	294	ヒトパルボウイルスB19	334	非配偶者間人工授精	242, 520
左結腸曲	482	ビトー斑	128	疲憊する	37
左上腹部	452, 568	ヒト閉経期ゴナドトロピン	234, 557	非びらん性胃食道逆流症	204, 576
左前下行枝	471, 565	ヒト免疫グロブリン	344	皮膚	8, 75, 318, 462
左側臥位	77	ヒト免疫不全ウイルス	557	鼻部	460
左鼠径部	452	ヒドララジン塩酸塩	189	皮膚移植片	329
左の	565	一人歩き	330	皮膚エリテマトーデス	327, 534
鼻柱	460	ヒドロキシカルバミド	559	皮膚炎	8, 324
鼻中隔	460	ヒドロキシプロリン	283, 559	皮膚科	54
鼻中隔矯正術	146	ヒドロキシメチルグルタリル補酵素A	557	皮膚科医	60
鼻中隔穿孔	141	ヒドロキシメチルグルタリル補酵素A還元酵素阻害薬	259	皮膚介達牽引	291
鼻中隔彎曲	141			皮膚科学	13, 17, 65
非中毒性甲状腺腫	251	ヒドロキシメチルビレーン合成酵素	557	皮膚関連リンパ組織	595
尾椎	492			皮膚筋炎	111, 327, 542
ピック病	308	皮内注射	86	腓腹筋	500
必須アミノ酸	544	皮内テスト	323	腓腹筋痙攣	25
必要時	23, 24, 587, 598	鼻軟骨	495	腓腹部	453
非定型的腺腫様過形成	166, 516	泌尿器	486	皮膚生検	324
ビデオ下胸腔鏡手術	170, 608			皮膚知覚帯	301
脾摘後重症感染症	274, 579			皮膚貼布剤	189
脾摘出術	215, 276			皮膚T細胞性リンパ腫	272, 538
鼻道	460			皮膚電位図	324, 545
脾動脈	474, 595			皮膚電気反射	304, 554
非特異性間質性肺炎	164, 578			皮膚電気反応聴力検査	141, 547
ヒト血清アルブミン	558			皮膚軟化剤	328
ヒトゲノム計画	556			皮膚粘膜リンパ節症候群	340, 570, 572
人差指	444			皮膚の	8
				皮膚・排泄ケア	61

項目	ページ
皮膚描記症	13, 35, 319
ピブメシリナム	585
被扶養者	49
皮膚良性リンパ節症	327, 565
飛蚊症	126
鼻閉	140
非閉塞性腸管虚血症	206, 577
ピペミド酸	586
ピペラシリン	584
ピベリデン	315
非弁膜症性心房細動	174, 578
被包筋膜	500
非抱合型ビリルビン	199
被包性	10
被包性腹膜硬化症	224, 547
ヒポキサンチングアニンホスホリボシルトランスフェラーゼ	556
ヒポクラテス顔貌	76
ヒポクラテスの誓い	45
被保険者	49
非ホジキンリンパ腫	272, 576
飛沫感染	105
ピマリシン	585
肥満	12, 105, 244
肥満学	260
肥満細胞白血病	271
肥満指数	245, 528
びまん性	35
びまん性軸索損傷	307
びまん性大細胞B細胞リンパ腫	272, 542
びまん性肺胞傷害	166, 540
びまん性汎細気管支炎	113, 164, 328
びまん性閉塞性肺症候群	543
びまん性レヴィー小体病	542
肥満低換気症候群	115, 156
非免疫性胎児水腫	335, 577
百日咳	27, 110, 330
百万分率	587
日焼け	318
日焼け止め指数	318, 599
ピュストー術式	215
ヒューストン弁	482
ヒューナー試験	235
秒	439, 595
病院	52
病院医	57
病院情報システム	44, 556
病因診断	84
病院内職掌	59
病院部門	53
病院薬剤師	58
病因論	35
評価	96, 598
病臥	72
病気	72
美容外科	54
美容外科医	60
美容外科学	65
表現型	511
病原性	15
表在痛	120
表在反射	301
病死	74
美容歯科学	152
標識フルオロデオキシグルコース	80
表示せよ	597
被用者保険	49
標準化死亡比	44, 93, 598
標準誤差	596
標準失語症検査	304, 597
標準偏差	596
標準模擬患者	68, 598
表情筋	498
氷食症	261
ひょう疽	326
病巣	35
病巣感染	106
病態修飾性抗リウマチ薬	288, 542
病態生理学	15
病的	35
病的の骨折	282
標的細胞	264
病的反射	301
病棟	55
病棟看護師	59
表皮	462
表皮水疱症	116, 327, 544
表皮剥脱	320
表皮肥厚	320
表面電極	283
表面麻酔	87
病理医	60
病理学	17, 63, 65
病理学的検査	78
病理診断	84
病理部	54
氷冷	289, 593
病歴	559
病歴室	55
病歴と身体的検査	558
病歴の	36
鼻翼	460
日和見感染	106
ピラジナミド	168, 590
ヒラメ筋	500
ピラルビシン	603
びらん	320
ひりひりする	121
鼻瘤	141
微粒子計数免疫凝集測定法	82, 582
粟粒腫	319
微量アルブミン尿	218
ビリルビン尿	218
鼻涙管	456
鼻涙管狭窄症	133
ヒル・サックス病変	284
ピルフェニドン	168
昼間過眠	104
ビルロートⅠ法	214, 525
ビルロートⅡ法	214, 525
披裂軟骨	495
疲労	104
鼻漏	139
疲労骨折	282
広場恐怖症	297
ピロミド酸	580
ピロリン酸カルシウム	284, 537
ヒルシュスプルング病	338
ヒル徴候	173

ビンクリスチン	608	フィルグラスチム	274	ゼン病	313
ビンクリスチン硫酸塩		風疹	27, 109, 325, 330	～不快感	71
	274	風土病	106	不可逆性	91
貧血	25, 261	封入体	559	不可算名詞	329
頻呼吸	16, 154	封入体筋炎	285, 559	不活化	11
瀕死	76	フェイススケール	122	不活化ポリオウイルスワ	
品質管理	590	フェニトイン	315, 584	クチン	562
ビンスワンガー病	311	フェニトイン歯肉増殖症		不感症	229
ピンセット	89		149	不完全脚ブロック	
ビンデシン	608	フェニルケトン尿	333		179, 559
頻尿	216	フェニルケトン尿症	585	～不規則	71
頻発月経	228	フェノバルビタール		吹き抜け骨折	528
ビンブラスチン	609		315, 581	腹圧下尿漏出圧	220, 521
頻脈	16, 172, 245	フェノール	212	腹圧性排尿	216
		フェノールスルホンフタ		腹囲	76, 196, 232, 517
ふ		レイン試験	220, 588	副院長	59
ファウラー体位	77	フェリチン	268	腹会陰式	12
ファーター乳頭	482	フェルティー症候群		腹会陰式直腸切除術	214
ファブリ病	113, 336		111, 286	腹横筋	500
ファムシクロビル		フェルミウム	436, 550	腹臥位	76
	329, 549	フェンタニル	122	副学長	62
ファラド	438, 548	フェンタニルクエン酸塩		副学部長	62
ファル	32		122	腹腔	455
ファレン試験	282	フォヴィーユ症候群	299	腹腔鏡	14, 18
ファロー四徴症	183, 604	不応性貧血	115, 270, 591	腹腔鏡下胃緊縛術	
ファロペネム	551	フォーカスチャーティン			214, 260, 567
不安	295	グ	89	腹腔鏡下生検	204
ファンコーニ貧血	336	フォガティー・カテーテ		腹腔鏡下胆嚢摘出術	
不安障害	312	ル	191		213, 566
不安定狭心症	185	フォークト・小柳・原田		腹腔鏡検査	204
不安定糖尿病	256	症候群	134	腹腔鏡補助下結腸切除術	
不安定な	36	ぶどう膜炎	134		214, 565
ファンネンスチール切開		フォスターケネディー症		腹腔鏡補助下手術	565
	88	候群	130	腹腔鏡補助下腟式子宮摘	
部位	37, 450	フォーダイス斑	149	出術	243, 566
部位診断	85	フォーリーカテーテル		腹腔・静脈短絡術	
フィッシャー症候群			225		213, 589
	112, 310	フォルクマン拘縮	281	腹腔神経叢ブロック	123
フィッシュバーグ濃縮試		フォレスター分類	182	腹腔穿刺	12, 204
験	220	フォレスティエ病	287	腹腔動脈	472, 529
フィッツヒュー・カーテ		フォンウィルブランド因		腹腔内	562
ィス症候群	232	子	266, 609	腹腔内注射	86
フィート	438, 551	フォンウィルブランド病		腹腔妊娠	237
フィブラート	259		273, 609	腹腔の	8
フィブリノゲン	266	フォンギールケ病	257	副交感神経	506
フィブリン分解産物		フォンタン手術	191	複合筋活動電位	304, 535
	266, 549	フォンヒッペル・リンダ		複合樹脂インレー	152
フィラデルフィア染色体		ウ病	313, 608	副甲状腺	490
	267, 584	フォンレックリングハウ		副甲状腺機能亢進症	252

日本語索引　　685

副甲状腺機能低下症	252	
副甲状腺摘出術	259	
副甲状腺ホルモン	248, 589	
副甲状腺ホルモン関連タンパク質	248, 589	
複合性局所疼痛症候群	121, 302, 538	
伏在神経	506	
副雑音	157	
複雑骨折	281	
複雑部分発作	297, 537	
副子	279	
複視	125	
副耳	332	
腹式呼吸	154	
腹式子宮全摘術	243, 601	
福祉大学	62	
副腎	490	
副腎アンドロゲン	250	
副腎機能不全	254	
副腎偶発腫	255	
副腎クリーゼ	254	
副神経	505	
副腎酵素欠損症	115	
副腎髄質	490	
副腎性器症候群	240, 254, 519	
副腎性高血圧	184	
副腎脊髄末梢神経障害	12	
副腎低形成	115	
副腎摘除術	259	
副腎の	10	
副腎白質ジストロフィー	521	
副腎皮質	490	
副腎皮質機能亢進症	253	
副腎皮質機能低下症	254	
副腎皮質刺激ホルモン	13, 248, 518	
副腎皮質の	12	
腹水	196, 197, 217, 512	
副膵管	484	
複製	511	
腹側	448	
腹側外側の	16	
腹側の	16	
腹直筋	498	
腹痛	120, 195	

副半奇静脈	476	
副鼻腔	460	
副鼻腔炎	27, 144	
副鼻腔気管支症候群	163, 596	
腹部	25	
腹部腱膜	501	
腹部コンパートメント症候群	199, 518	
腹部大動脈	472	
腹部大動脈瘤	187, 516	
腹部単純撮影	202	
腹部超音波検査	202	
腹部痛	120	
腹部の	8	
腹部浮球感	198	
腹部膨満	196	
腹部膨隆	197	
腹壁破裂	339	
腹壁反射	301	
腹壁ヘルニア	210	
腹膜	483	
腹膜炎	210	
腹膜偽粘液腫	210	
腹膜後腔	12	
腹膜透析	225, 582	
腹膜の	37	
腹鳴	196, 198	
服薬遵守	86	
服薬不履行	86	
服用	594	
ふくらはぎ	446	
ふけ	318	
父系	73	
不顕性感染	106	
腐骨	284	
腐骨形成	284	
ブコローム	259	
プシ	32	
フシジン酸	548	
不治の病	107	
ブシャール結節	280	
浮腫	83, 173	
ブシラミン	288	
婦人科医	60	
婦人科学	14, 65	
不随意運動	294	
ブスルファン	529	
不正咬合	36, 149, 245	

腐性ブドウ球菌	219	
不整脈	172, 174	
不整脈原性右室異形成	187, 523	
不全骨折	281	
不全麻痺	298	
付属器腫瘍	239	
双子	229	
ブタ由来インフルエンザウイルスA型	160, 598	
ブラリドキシム	581	
普通食	90	
二日酔い	195	
物質依存	312	
フッ素	152, 434, 548	
物理療法学	65	
不定愁訴	104	
不定愁訴症候群	104	
不定症状	104	
ブデソニド	169, 529	
舞踏アテトーシス	300	
ブドウ球菌	17	
ブドウ球菌性熱傷様皮膚症候群	600	
ブドウ糖液	544	
ブドウ糖負荷試験	247, 554	
舞踏病	299	
舞踏病性歩行不能	300	
不等辺三角形	39	
不等辺四辺形	39	
ぶどう膜	456	
太腿	446	
太りすぎの	105	
不妊	229	
不妊症看護	61	
～不能	71	
プパール靱帯	496	
ブプレノルフィン塩酸塩	123	
部分入れ歯	148	
部分寛解	92, 587	
部分再呼吸マスク	168	
部分床義歯	152	
部分の椎弓切除術	291	
部分的肺静脈還流異常	183, 581	
部分的脾動脈塞栓術	213, 588	

部分トロンボプラスチン時間	265, 589	
不変	91	
不飽和鉄結合能	268, 606	
不眠(症)	104	
不明熱	105, 551	
浮遊物	126	
フライ試験	323	
フライ症候群	151	
プライマー	511	
プライマリーナーシング	89	
プライマリヘルスケア	584	
ブラウン-セカール症候群	299	
ブラウント病	287	
プラークコントロールレコード	150	
フラジオマイシン	551	
プラスミド	511	
プラスミノーゲン	266	
プラスミノーゲンアクチベーターインヒビター1	266, 581	
プラスミン	266	
プラスミン・αプラスミンインヒビター複合体	266, 587	
プラセオジム	435, 587	
プラセボ	85	
プラゾシン塩酸塩	188	
プラダー・ウィリ症候群	338, 590	
ブラッシュフィールド斑	128	
ブラディ	32	
プラバスタチンナトリウム	259	
フラビンアデニンヌクレオチド	548	
ブラマー病	251	
ブラマー・ヴィンソン症候群	262	
ブラロック・トーシグ手術	191	
フランシウム	436, 551	
ブランルカスト水和物	167	
フリクテン	128
振子様眼振	129
プリズム曲光度	582
プリック・プリック試験	323
フリードライヒ運動失調症	310
プリミドン	316, 587
フリーラジカルスカベンジャー	315
ブリンクマン指数	156, 527
プリングル病	116, 326
プリンツメタル型狭心症	185
ふるえ	294
フルオレセインイソチオシアネート	550
フルオロウラシル	551
ブルガダ症候群	174
プルキンエ線維	470
ブルークロス	50
フルコナゾール	550
フルシトシン	549
ブルーシールド	50
ブルジンスキー徴候	298
プルス	32
ブルセラ症	108
フルダラビン	550
フルチカゾンプロピオン酸エステル	145, 169, 551
ブルート	32
プルトニウム	436, 589
ブルトン病	335
フルニエ壊疽	237
ブルヌヴィーユ病	326
ブルーム症候群	336
プルリフロキサシン	589
フルンケル	26
ブルンネル腺	483
ブルンベルグ徴候	197
ブレオマイシン	527
プレグナンジオール	234
プレセニリン	588
プレセニリン遺伝子	511
プレチスモグラフィー	162
プレート	32
プレドニゾロン	588
ブレー反射	333
フレーリッヒ症候群	253
フレロキサシン	550
フレンツェル眼鏡	132
ブレンナー腫瘍	239
フロイント完全アジュバント	549
フロイント不完全アジュバント	550
プロカインアミド塩酸塩	189
ブローカ失語症	302
ブローカ中枢	503
プロカルシトニン	248, 582
プロカルバジン	582
プロクロルペラジン	211
プロゲステロン	234, 241
プロコラーゲンⅢペプチド	200, 586
フローサイトメトリー	549
フローシート	96
プロスタグランジン	189, 241, 584
プロスタグランジンアナログ	210
プロスタグランジンE	584
プロスタグランジンF	584
フロセミド	188
プロテアーゼ阻害薬	275
プロテインC	266, 582
プロテインS	266, 587
プロテオーム	511
プロトアクチニウム	436, 580
プロードベント徴候	176
プロトロンビン時間	265, 588
プロトンポンプ阻害薬	210, 587
プロピルチオウラシル	258, 589
プロブコール	259
プロプラノロール塩酸塩	188

日本語索引　687

プロベネシド	259	
フローボリューム曲線	162	
フロマン徴候	303	
プロメチウム	435, 585	
フロモキセフ	550	
ブロモクリプチン	259	
ブロモクリプチンメシル酸塩	241, 315	
プロラクチン	234, 249, 587	
プロラクチン分泌異常症	113	
プロラクチン放出因子	234	
プロラクチン放出ホルモン	249, 587	
プロラクチン抑制ホルモン	249, 584	
ブロンコ	32	
分	438, 572	
分化	84	
噴火口	40	
分化抗原群	531	
吻合	88	
吻合器	89	
吻合の	34	
吻合部潰瘍	205	
粉砕骨折	282	
分散分析	522	
分子遺伝学	63	
分枝鎖アミノ酸	200, 211, 526	
分枝鎖アミノ酸・チロシンモル比	200	
分枝鎖ケト酸	526	
分枝鎖ケト酸尿	333	
分子生物学	63	
分子病	106	
分子標的療法	117	
噴出性出血	261	
文章完成法検査	304, 596	
分子量	575	
分析	10	
分節核好中球	264	
分泌過多	12	
糞便	196	
分娩	230	
分娩鉗子	89	
分娩施設	52	
分娩室	55	
分娩前の	10	
糞便中ヘリコバクター・ピロリ抗原	202	
分娩予定日	230, 545	
噴霧剤	328	
噴門	480	
噴門筋切開術	214	
分葉	40	
分離した	35	
分類不能型免疫不全症	273, 539	
分裂赤血球症	264	

ヘ

柄	37	
平滑筋	498	
平滑筋抗体	597	
平滑筋腫	18	
ベイカー嚢胞	280	
平均一日の過ごし方	96	
平均赤血球ヘモグロビン濃度	263, 570	
平均赤血球ヘモグロビン量	263, 570	
平均赤血球容積	263, 570	
平均動脈圧	75, 569	
平均尿流率	220	
平均余命	92	
閉経期	15, 27, 229	
閉経後出血	229, 585	
平衡機能検査	143	
平衡砂	460	
平行四辺形	39	
平衡障害	139	
平衡斑	460	
平行六面体	40	
米国医師会	521	
米国医師会倫理綱領	45	
米国医師免許試験	68, 607	
米国看護協会	522	
米国軍病理研究所	519	
米国国立衛生研究所	577	
米国国立癌研究所	576	
米国疾病対策センター	532	
米国食品医薬品局	549	
米国心臓協会	519	
米国対癌協会	518	
米国病院協会患者の権利章典	45	
米国保健社会福祉省	541	
米国保健福祉省	50	
米国麻薬取締局	541	
米国薬局方	85, 607	
米国リウマチ協会	523	
米国臨床腫瘍学会	524	
閉鎖	88	
閉鎖型質問	68	
閉鎖骨折	282	
閉鎖式病院	52	
閉鎖神経	506	
閉鎖動脈	474	
閉所恐怖症	18, 297	
閉塞	198	
閉塞性血栓血管炎	187, 601	
閉塞性睡眠時無呼吸症候群	167, 580	
閉塞性動脈硬化症	187, 524	
閉塞性肺疾患	163	
平坦な	197	
平面視野計	132	
ペイロニー病	237	
ペインクリニック	54	
ペインブリッジ反射	177	
ベカナマイシン	520	
ペガプタニブナトリウム	136	
ヘガール徴候	231	
壁細胞	480	
壁側胸膜	468	
へき地診療	44	
ペグインターフェロン	211, 583	
ベクトル心電図	180, 608	
ベクレル	438, 528	
ベクロメタゾンプロピオン酸エステル	169, 526	
ベザフィブラート	259	
ベスタチン	529	
ペスト	107	
ベスニエ痒疹	324	
臍	37, 444	
ベーチェット病	111, 114, 150	

ペチジン塩酸塩	122	ヘモグロビン症	269	変形性膝関節症	286
ベツォルト三徴	142	ヘモグロビン尿	218	変形性脊椎症	288
ベッカー型筋ジストロフィー	309	ヘモクロマトーシス	209, 257	変更遺伝子	511
別居	74	ベーラー角	280	偏光顕微鏡検査	284
ベックウィズ・ウィーデマン症候群	339	ヘラー手術	214	便失禁	196
ベック三主徴	176	ペラミビル	168	偏食	261
ベッケン	32	ヘリウム	434, 555	ベンジルペニシリン	582
ペッサリー	241	ヘリオトロープ疹	319	ベンジルペニシリンベンザチン	540
ヘッセルバッハ三角	452	ヘリカルコンピュータ断層撮影法	79	ベンスジョーンズタンパク質	263, 527
ペディキュア	15	ヘリコバクター・ピロリ	201, 558	片頭痛	120
ベドナーアフタ	332	ヘリコバクター・ピロリ除菌療法	211	ベンズブロマロン	259
ペニシリン	581	ベリー症候群	308	変性	84
ペニシリン耐性肺炎球菌	160, 587	ベリリウム	434, 526	変性関節疾患	542
ペニシリン耐性肺炎球菌感染症	110	ペル・エプスタイン熱	262	変性疾患	106
ベネズエラウマ脳炎	108, 608	ペルオキシソーム病	112	便潜血	199, 550
ベネディクト症候群	299	ヘルクスハイマー反応	233	ベンゼンヘキサクロリド	527
ヘノッホ・シェーンライン紫斑病	340, 558	ペルゲル・フエット核異常	264	ベンゾイルチロシルパラアミノ安息香酸	529
ヘバーデン結節	280	ペルゴリドメシル酸塩	315	片側胸部	36
ヘパプラスチンテスト	265, 558	ベルジェ病	221	片側頭痛	11, 120
ヘパリン	189	ヘルシンキ宣言	45	片側バリズム	300
ヘパリン起因性血小板減少症	273, 556	ベルタン柱	486	ベンゾジアゼピン	314
ヘパリン添加血	275	ヘルツ	32, 438, 559	変態	11
蛇恐怖症	297	ベルテポルフィン	136	ペンタゾシン	123
ベビーベッド	330	ヘルテル眼球突出計	131	胼胝	28, 34, 320
ペプシノーゲンⅠ	200, 584	ベルナール・スーリエ症候群	273	胼胝性	34
ペプシノーゲンⅡ	200, 584	ヘルニア	26	鞭虫	199
ペプロマイシン	583	ヘルニア縫合術	18, 215	ベンチュリマスク	168
ヘマト	32	ヘルパンギーナ	110, 339	便通	196, 527
ヘマトキシリンエオジン染色	555	ヘールフォルト症候群	165	扁桃	465
ヘマトクリット	263, 555	ベル麻痺	299	扁桃アデノイド手術	146, 601
ヘマトポルフィリン誘導体	136	ベロ毒素	609	扁桃炎	144
ペメトレキセドナトリウム水和物	168	ベロ毒素産生性大腸菌	334, 609	扁桃窩	465
ヘモ	32	便	196	扁桃周囲炎	144
ヘモグロビン	263, 555	変異	511	扁桃周囲膿瘍	144, 588
ヘモグロビンA1c	247, 555	便器	90	扁桃腫大	141
		変形性関節症	285, 539	扁桃腺	140
		変形性股関節症	285	扁桃摘出術	146
		変形性骨関節症	578	ペントスタチン	540
				ヘンドラウイルス感染症	108
				便秘	196
				扁平円柱上皮境界	480, 596
				扁平上皮癌	84, 166, 596

日本語索引 689

扁平上皮内病変	239, 597
扁平足	5, 280
扁平苔癬	325
片麻痺	299
片麻痺歩行	298
ヘンリー	438, 554
偏菱形	39
ヘンレループ	486

ほ

保育器	343
保育士	58
ポイツ・ジェガース症候群	207
法医学	63
包括医療	44
包括的機能評価スケール	92, 552
傍胸骨線	454
包茎	231, 237
方形葉	484
剖検	78
方向	448
縫合	88
膀胱	8, 486
膀胱炎	223
膀胱拡張	217
抱合型ビリルビン	199
膀胱下閉塞	223, 528
膀胱鏡	8, 18
膀胱鏡検査	13, 221
縫工筋	500
膀胱三角	486
膀胱腫瘍	223, 529
方向性冠動脈粥腫切除術	191, 540
膀胱洗浄	225
膀胱摘除術	226
膀胱内圧測定	220
膀胱尿管逆流	223, 609
膀胱の	8, 38
膀胱瘤	239
芳香療法	118
放散痛	121
傍糸球体装置	486, 564
傍糸球体の	14
房室回帰頻拍	174, 525
房室間の	525
房室結節	470, 525
房室結節リエントリー頻拍	174, 525
房室束	470
房室の	525
房室ブロック	179
房室弁	470
放射型コンピュータ断層撮影	545
放射酵素測定法	82, 592
放射状角膜切開術	137, 138, 603
放射性アレルゲン吸着試験	323, 591
放射性医薬品	79
放射線核種	79
放射性クロム標識赤血球半減期	269
放射性同位元素	80, 593
放射性免疫吸着試験	82, 323, 593
放射性ヨウ素	258, 591
放射性ヨウ素摂取試験	248, 591
放射性ヨウ素標識ヒト血清アルブミン	593
放射線医学	65
放射線科	54
放射線科医	60
放射線直腸炎	206
放射線治療	117, 594
放射線透過性	16, 161
放射線肺炎	164
放射線皮膚炎	324
放射線不透過性	161
放射能	16
放射免疫測定法	82, 593
傍腫瘍性小脳変性症	309, 582
傍腫瘍性神経症候群	309, 586
傍腫瘍性多発ニューロパチー	309
胞状奇胎	238
帽状腱膜	501
膨疹	320
紡錘	40
法制	46
乏精子症	235
傍脊椎線	454
ホウ素	434, 525
蜂巣	40
蜂巣炎	325
蜂巣状肺	161
包帯交換	90
傍大動脈	11
膨大部	34
乏尿	15, 217
包皮	488
放屁	26, 197
膨満痛	195
訪問看護	44, 61
法律	46
膨隆した	197
ボエルハーヴェ症候群	205
ボーエン病	327
頬	442
頬の	34
頬骨	442
補完代替療法	118, 530
ポークウィードマイトジェン	590
北米看護診断協会	68, 575
ほくろ	318
黒子	319
母系	73
保健医療システム	44
保健医療施設	52
保健医療大学	62
保健衛生大学	62
保険会社	49
保険給付	49
保険金受給者	49
保険契約者	49
保健師	58, 584
保健師助産師看護師法	46
保健師	52
保険証	48
保険証券番号	71
保険証書	49
保健所法	46
保険料	49
歩行	34, 77
歩行器	90, 290
歩行困難	294
歩行の	34
保護眼鏡	135
星	40

母指	444	勃起	228	ウム	211
母趾	446	勃起不全	237, 545	ボリコナゾール	609
母指球	446	ボックダレックヘルニア		ポリソムノグラフィー	162, 588
ホジキン病	272, 555		338		
ホジキンリンパ腫		発作	36	ホリナートカルシウム	
	272, 557	発作後錯乱	297		568
母子保健センター	52	発作性寒冷血色素尿症		ポリビニルピロリドン	
母子保健法	46		270, 582		590
補充現象	142	発作性心房頻拍	174, 581	ポリープ	40
補充療法	117	発作性夜間血色素尿症		ポリープ状	37
補助人工心臓	607		270, 586	ポリープ状脈絡膜血管症	
補助人工心臓システム		発作性夜間呼吸困難			135, 582
	192, 607		172, 585	ポリペク	32
補助の	34	発疹	318	ポリミキシンB	585
ホスアンプレナビルカル		発疹チフス	108	ポリメラーゼ連鎖反応	
シウム	275, 551	発端者	73		82, 582
歩数計	15	ポット骨折	282	ボルグ指数	156
ホスピス	55	ポット病	287	ホルター心電計	180
ホスファチジルグリセロ		ボツリヌス症	108	ボルテゾミブ	274
ール	234, 584	火照り	229	ボルト	439, 607
ホスファチジルコリン		ポートフォリオ	68	ホルネル症候群	158
	581	母乳栄養	343	ホールパイク法	141
ホスファチジルセリン		哺乳瓶	343	ポール・バンネル試験	
	587	骨	37, 492		267
ホスフェストロール	541	歩幅	294	ポルフィマーナトリウム	
ホスフルコナゾール	550	母斑	25, 27, 319		170
ホスホグルコムターゼ		母斑症	326	ポルフィリン症	257
	584	ポビドン	590	ポルフォビリノーゲン	
ホスホジエステラーゼ		ポビドンヨード	152, 590		250, 581
	583	ホフマン徴候	301	ボールマン分類	199
ホスホジエステラーゼ阻		ホーマンズ徴候	177	ホルミウム	435, 557
害薬	189, 583	ボーマン嚢	486	ホルミウムレーザー前立	
ホスホマイシン	551	ホームズ現象	300	腺核出術	226, 557
ホスホリボシルピロリン		ホメオ遺伝子	511	ホルミウムレーザー前立	
酸	587	ホメオパシー	14, 119	腺蒸散術	226, 557
母性看護	60	ホモシスチン尿	333	ホルモン補充療法	
母性看護学	66	ホモバニル酸	559		241, 558
ボー線	321	ポリアクリルアミド・ゲ		ホルモン療法	117
保存血	275	ル電気泳動法	82, 582	ポロニウム	436, 586
保存的療法	117	ボーリウム	436, 527	本態性血小板血症	
補体	35, 529	ポリエチレングリコール			271, 548
補体価	533		583	本態性高血圧	184
補体結合抗体	532	ポリエチレンテレフタレ		ポンド	438, 566
補体結合反応	82, 532, 533	ート	192, 583	奔馬調律	175
補体受容体	537	ポリ塩化ビニル	589	ポンペ病	257
補体調節タンパク質	531	ポリ塩素化ビフェニル		翻訳	511
母体保護法	46		582		
ボタン穴変形	281	ポリオワクチン	344	**ま**	
補聴器	145	ポリカルボフィルカルシ		毎朝	23, 579

マイクロアレイ	511	麻酔科医	60	マルファン症候群	337
マイクログラム	439, 572	麻酔科学	65	マールブルグ熱	107
マイクロサテライト不安定性	511, 574	マスター２階段試験	180	マロリー体	204
		股擦れ	319	マロリー・ワイス症候群	204
マイコプラズマ肺炎	110	待合室	55		
毎時	23, 590	マッカードル病	257	マンガン	434, 573
マイスネル神経叢	483	末期	91	満期自然分娩	230
マイトジェン活性化プロテインキナーゼ	569	末期医療	118	満月顔貌	245
		末期腎不全	222, 548	慢性	91
マイトネリウム	436, 574	マッキューン・オールブライト症候群	252	慢性胃炎	205
マイトマイシンＣ	572			慢性炎症性脱髄性多発神経炎	112
毎日	23, 590	睫毛	127, 456		
毎晩	23, 579	マッサージ	289	慢性炎症性脱髄性多発ニューロパチー	309, 534
毎分回転数	439, 594	マッサージ療法	119		
埋没歯	149	末梢	448	慢性活動性肝炎	207, 530
マイボーム腺	456	末梢血幹細胞移植	276, 581	慢性肝炎	207
マイル	438, 572			慢性間質性腎炎	222, 534
マイルズ手術	214	末梢血管疾患	187, 589	慢性気管支炎	165
前髪	442	末梢血リンパ球	265, 581	慢性機能性腹痛	196, 533
前歯	147, 442	末梢神経系	505, 586	慢性血栓塞栓性肺高血圧症	166, 538
マーカスガン瞳孔	129	末梢神経ブロック	123		
巻尺	78	末梢動脈疾患	187, 580	慢性好酸球性肺炎	164, 532
マキューイン徴候	333	末梢浮腫	177, 217		
膜侵襲複合体	569	末端デオキシヌクレオチド転移酵素	267, 602	慢性甲状腺炎	251
膜性腎症	221, 573			慢性好中球性白血病	271, 536
膜性増殖性糸球体腎炎	221, 573	マットレス縫合	88		
		松葉杖	279	慢性呼吸不全	166
マグネシア乳	573	マトリックスメタロプロテイナーゼ３	283, 573	慢性骨髄性白血病	271, 535
マグネシウム	434, 571				
マクバーニー切開	88	マネージドケア	48	慢性骨髄増殖性疾患	270, 535
マクバーニー徴候	197	まばたき	127		
膜迷路	459	麻痺	294, 298	慢性骨髄単球性白血病	271, 535
マクロファージ	265	麻痺性疼痛	294		
マクロファージ活性化因子	569	マーフィー徴候	197	慢性糸球体腎炎	221, 533
		まぶしい	127	慢性疾患看護	60
マクロファージ走化因子	570	まぶた（瞼）	126, 442	慢性疾患に伴う貧血	269, 517
		麻薬	27, 122		
マクロファージ遊走阻止試験	572	麻薬及び向神経薬取締法	47	慢性進行性外眼筋麻痺	135, 536
		眉	456		
マーゲン	32	眉毛	442	慢性腎臓病	222, 534
マーシャル・マーケティ・クランツ手術	226	マラリア	36, 108	慢性腎不全	222, 537
		マリオット盲点	132	慢性膵炎	114, 209
麻疹	109, 325, 330	マリー・シュトリュンペル病	287	慢性石灰化膵炎	210
麻疹・風疹混合ワクチン	344			慢性単純性苔癬	325
		マルク	32	慢性肉芽腫病	533
麻疹・流行性耳下腺炎・風疹混合ワクチン	573	マルチスライスコンピュータ断層撮影法	79, 574	慢性肺血栓塞栓症	116
				慢性非化膿性破壊性胆管炎	208, 536
麻酔	87	マルピギー小体	486		
麻酔科	54			慢性疲労症候群	104, 533

慢性閉塞性肺疾患	164, 536
慢性リンパ性白血病	271, 535
マントー反応	158
マンニトール	315
マンニトール・アデニン・リン酸(液)	569
マンマ	32

み

ミエリン塩基性タンパク	305, 570
ミエロ	32, 33
ミエロペルオキシダーゼ	268, 573
ミオクローヌス	300
ミオグロビン	178, 283
ミオシン軽鎖	178
未解決問題	96
味覚	147
味覚異常	147
味覚器	464
味覚減退	147
味覚試験	150
見掛けの年齢	76
三日月形	40
ミカファンギン	570
右下腹部	452, 593
右(左)下腹部痛	120
右下肋部	450
右利き	294
右利きの	13
右結腸曲	482
右上腹部	452, 594
右(左)上腹部痛	120
右前斜位	591
右側臥位	76
右鼠径部	452
右の	590
ミクリッツ症候群	151
ミグリトール	258
ミクロノマイシン	570
眉間	442
ミコナゾール	329, 570
ミコフェノール酸モフェチル	572
未婚	74
未熟児	331

未熟児慢性呼吸不全	336, 537
未熟児網膜症	135, 593
水	523
みずいぼ	330
水制限試験	250
ミーズ線	321
水チャネル	523
水治療法	119, 289
水ぶくれ	318
水ぼうそう	330
水虫	318
未成熟	244
みぞおち	444
ミソプロストール	210
三日ばしか	330
三日目毎	23, 541
みつくち	147
三つ子	229
密封小線源治療	117
密封貼布試験	323
密封包帯法	328, 579
密閉剤	152
ミデカマイシン	571
ミトキサントロン	572
ミトコンドリア	508
ミトコンドリア DNA	511, 574
ミトコンドリア脳筋症	311
ミトコンドリア脳筋症・乳酸アシドーシス・脳卒中様発作	571
ミトコンドリア病	113
水俣病	309
ミニサテライト	511
ミネソタ多面的性格検査	303, 573
ミノサイクリン	572
ミノドロン酸水和物	289
未分化	12, 84
未萌出歯	149
耳	9, 442, 458
みみず脹れ	318
耳たぶ	442
耳だれ	139
耳の	9, 34
ミーム	511
脈	172, 173

脈圧	75
脈拍	75, 173, 604
脈拍欠損	173
脈拍数	75, 587
脈波伝播速度	178
脈絡叢	504
脈絡膜	35, 458
脈絡膜黒色腫	135
脈絡膜新生血管	130, 536
脈絡膜剝離	134, 531
ミュア・トレ症候群	207
ミュンヒハウゼン症候群	313
見よ	607
ミラー・アボット管	212
ミラール・ギュブレ症候群	299
ミリグラム	438, 571
ミリグラム当量	438, 571
ミリッツィ症候群	198
ミリメートル	438, 572
ミリモスチム	274
ミルタザピン	314
ミルナシプラン塩酸塩	314
ミルロイ病	177
ミロン試験	333
民間療法	118
眼前	23, 558

む

無意識の	12
無医地区	44
無塩食	90
無害性雑音	175
無害の	36
無顆粒球症	265
無汗症	321
無関心の	295
無気肺	165
無嗅覚	140
無菌室	526
無菌性	25, 34
無菌性髄膜炎	110
無菌操作	87
むくみ	173, 216
無形成	34, 84
無月経	228
無鉤条虫	199

向こう脛	446	ムンテラ	33	メディケア・メディケイドセンター	50, 535
無鉤鑷子	89			メディケイド	50
無呼吸	154	**め**		メトトレキセート	288, 575
無呼吸指数	162, 520	眼	9, 75, 442, 456	メトホルミン塩酸塩	258
無呼吸低換気指数	163, 520	迷走神経	505	メートル	438, 569
ムコ多糖症	337, 573	迷走神経刺激法	316, 609	メドロキシプロゲステロン	573
ムコ多糖類	573	迷入	10	メドロキシプロゲステロン酢酸エステル	241
無再発生存期間	92, 592	迷路	459	メニエール病	113, 144
無酸素閾値	524	迷路摘出術	145	メネトリエ病	205
無酸素症	10	眼鏡	126	眼の	9
無資格診療	44	メキシレチン塩酸塩	189	メビウス徴候	246
虫下し	211	メーグス症候群	233	メピチオスタン	573
無刺激食	90	目薬	127	メープルシロップ尿	333
虫刺され	318	メサドン塩酸塩	123	メープルシロップ尿症	336, 574
無歯の	149	メサラジン	211		
虫歯	147	メサンギウム	486	めまい	28, 139, 172, 261, 293
矛盾語法	47	メージ症候群	311	目やに	126
無症候期間	92	メシル酸イマチニブ	274	メラス症候群	311
無症候性キャリア	517	メス	88	メラトニン	249
無症候性心筋虚血	185, 598	メズサの頭	5, 197	メラニン減少症	319
無褥ギプス包帯	289	メタ	33	メラニン細胞	15
無水晶体眼	129	メタボリック症候群	256	メラニン細胞刺激ホルモン	574
息子	73	メタヨードベンジルグアニジン	572	メルケル細胞	462
娘	73	メチシリン感受性黄色ブドウ球菌	574	メルセブルグ三徴候	246
夢精	27, 228			メルファラン	568
無精子症	235	メチシリン耐性黄色ブドウ球菌	574	メロキシカム	122
無増悪生存期間	92, 584			メロペネム	571
むち打ち症	279	メチシリン耐性黄色ブドウ球菌感染症	110	面	448
むち打ち損傷関連障害	285, 610	メチシリン耐性表皮ブドウ球菌	574	免疫科	54
無痛性	9	メチマゾール	258	免疫学	63
無痛性甲状腺炎	251	メチラポン試験	250	免疫学的検査	78
無頭体	331	メチルドパ	189	免疫グロブリン	561
無尿	217	メチルフェニデート塩酸塩	314	免疫グロブリンE	323, 561
胸	444			免疫専門医	60
無熱の	105	メチルメチオニンスルホニウムクロライド	573	免疫電気泳動法	82, 561
胸の	5	メチレンジオキシメタンフェタミン	571	免疫粘着赤血球凝集反応	82, 559
胸やけ	27, 195			免疫放射定量測定	563
無脳体	331	メチレンジフェニルジイソシアナート	571	免疫反応性インスリン	247, 563
無病生存期間	92, 541	メッケル憩室	206	免疫反応性グルカゴン	247, 563
ムピロシン	575	メッセンジャーRNA	511, 574		
無ベータリポタンパク血症	256, 516	メディエーター抑制薬	167		
夢遊症	104	メディケア	50		
夢遊症者	104				
無抑制収縮	223, 606				
無力	104				

免疫反応性 C ペプチド	網膜上膜 130, 547	モロー反射 333
247, 537	網膜静脈分枝閉塞症	問題解決 95
免疫比濁法 82, 603	134, 528	問題基盤型学習 68, 581
免疫表現型判定 268	網膜新生血管 130	問題志向型医療情報システム 95
免疫複合体 559	網膜正常対応 132, 577	問題志向型看護記録 95
免疫放射定量測定 82	網膜中心静脈閉塞症	問題志向型システム
免疫抑制性酸性タンパク	134, 538	68, 95, 586
559	網膜中心動脈 472, 537	問題志向型診療録
免疫抑制薬 274	網膜中心動脈圧 132, 530	68, 95, 586
免疫抑制療法 117	網膜中心動脈閉塞症	問題・知見カプラー 95
綿花様白斑 130, 539	134, 537	問題番号 96
免責額 49	網膜電図 132, 547	問題リスト 95, 96
メンデルソン症候群 163	網膜動脈圧 132, 591	モンテジア骨折 282
メンデレビウム 436, 570	網膜動脈分枝閉塞症	モンドール病 177
面皰 25, 320	134, 528	文部科学省 68
	網膜内細小血管異常	門脈 478, 589
も	130, 563	門脈下大静脈吻合術
	網膜剥離 135, 592	215, 582
毛幹 462	網膜復位術 137	
盲係蹄症候群 206	毛様体 458	**や**
蒙古斑 331	模擬患者 68, 598	
毛根 462	モキシフロキサシン 571	夜間遺精 27
毛細管脆弱 266	模擬装置 68	夜間恐怖症 297
毛細血管拡張症 17	黙想法 119	夜間呼吸困難 154
網状赤血球 264	モスキート鉗子 89	夜間多尿 37, 217
網状層 462	モートン病 285	夜間痛 195
網状帯 490	モノアミンオキシダーゼ	夜間病院 52
毛舌 148	569	夜間頻尿 37, 217
網赤血球 263	モノアミンオキシダーゼ	夜間勃起 235, 577
網赤血球増加 265	阻害薬 315, 569	ヤギ声 157
毛瘡 37, 325	モノクローナル抗体 569	野牛の肩瘤 246
妄想 293	物差し 78	夜驚症 331
毛巣嚢胞 326	ものもらい 127	薬学部 62
盲腸 482	モノヨードチロシン	薬剤師 58
盲腸の 35	248, 572	薬剤師法 46
盲点 132	物忘れ 295	薬剤性過敏症症候群
毛嚢 462	もみあげ 442	327, 541
毛嚢炎 325	桃色 39	薬剤耐性緑膿菌感染症
網嚢孔 482	もやもや病 111, 307	110
毛根様細胞白血病	モラクセラ・カタラーリス 160	薬剤部 55
271, 555	モリソン窩 483	薬剤誘発リンパ球刺激試験 323, 542
毛包性角化症 324	モリブデン 435, 573	薬剤溶出性ステント
網膜 458	モル 438, 573	191, 541
網膜異常対応 128, 523	モルガニー孔 466	薬事法 46
網膜炎 134	モルガニーヘルニア 338	薬疹 324
網膜芽細胞腫 135, 342	モルヒネ塩酸塩 122	薬草療法 119
網膜色素変性症	モルヒネ硫酸塩水和物	薬物送達システム 541
113, 135, 593	122	薬物動態学・薬力学 585
網膜出血 130		
網膜症 18		

薬物療法	117	誘発筋電図	283	用手の	8
薬理学	63	誘発耳音響放射	334, 547	用手補助腹腔鏡手術	
やけど	318	幽門	480		213, 554
焼けるような	121	幽門狭窄	205	養生法	292
痩せた	36, 105	幽門形成術	214	痒疹	319
野戦病院	53	幽門洞	480	腰神経叢	505
矢田部・ギルフォード性		幽門リンパ節	478	腰髄	504
格検査	303, 611	遊離サイロキシン		羊水鏡検査	236
薬科大学	62		247, 551	羊水指数	235, 519
薬局	55	遊離サイロキシン指数		羊水穿刺	236
薬局長	59		247, 551	陽性反応適中度	587
ヤード	439, 611	遊離脂肪酸	550, 576	腰仙椎装具	290, 568
野兎病	108	遊離トリヨードサイロニ		ヨウ素	435, 559
夜尿症	26, 34, 217	ン	248, 551	ヨウ素標識ヒト血清アル	
薮医者	45	有料老人ホーム	55	ブミン	561
夜盲症	126	ユウロビウム	435, 548	腰帯	494
ヤング症候群	235	ユーグロブリン溶解時間		腰椎	492, 565
			266	腰椎化	284
ゆ		輸血	275	腰椎牽引	291
ユーイング肉腫	288	輸血関連急性肺傷害		腰椎穿刺	568
誘因	72		166, 604	腰椎麻酔	87
憂うつ	295	輸血関連循環過負荷	601	腰痛	120, 216, 278, 566
有害事象	44	輸血後肝炎	207, 589	腰痛体操	290
有害事象共通用語基準		輸血副作用	274	陽電子放出断層撮影法	
	538	油脂性軟膏	328		80, 583
有害薬物反応	44, 518	輸入脚症候群	206	幼年期	36
有郭乳頭	464	指	9	腰部	452
有棘赤血球	264	指関節部	446	腰部脊柱管狭窄症	
有棘赤血球増加	264	指先	444		288, 568
有棘赤血球を伴う舞踏病		指しゃぶり	330	羊膜	232
	116, 310	指の	9	要約	70
有棘層	462	指鼻試験	300	腰リンパ節	478
有鉤骨	492	夢	104	溶連菌感染後急性糸球体	
有鉤条虫	199	揺りかご	330	腎炎	221, 587
有鉤鑷子	89			養老保険	49
有効量	545	**よ**		ヨガ	119
有歯の	149	陽陰圧換気	170, 586	翼状頸	332
有水晶体眼内レンズ	137	ヨウ化カリウム	258	翼状片	127
疣贅	176, 320	ヨウ化カリウム溶液	599	抑制性シナプス後電位	
優性遺伝子	511	溶血	17, 262		562
融像	133	溶血性尿毒症症候群		抑制帯	90
遊走腎	223		273, 559	よく注意せよ	576
有痛脂肪症	245	溶血性貧血	115	横	448
誘導結合プラズママス		溶骨性病変	269	予後	85
スペクトロメトリー		養護老人ホーム	55	よこね	228
	82, 560	葉酸	268, 274	横腹	444
有頭骨	492	幼児	330	よたよた歩く	294
誘導分娩	241	幼児型多発性囊胞腎	339	よだれ	147
尤度比	568	陽子線治療	117	よちよち歩く	330

予備吸気量	162, 563	ラテックス凝集反応		卵巣嚢胞	238
予備呼気量	547		82, 565	ランソン判定基準	204
予備的診断	84	ラテン語	21	ランダム化比較試験	592
予防医学	65	ラドン	436, 593	ランタン	435, 565
予防看護学	66	ラニビズマブ	136	ランドルト環	131
予防接種	36, 343	ラニムスチン	570	ランバート・イートン筋	
予防接種法	47	ラパ	33	無力症候群	158, 566
予防の治療	118	ラパコレ	33	ランベール縫合	88
予防法	12	ラボ	33	卵胞刺激ホルモン	
よろめく	294	ラマーズ法	230		234, 249, 551
四類感染症	107	ラミブジン	211	卵胞膜	35
		ラモセトロン塩酸塩	211		
ら		ラモトリギン	316	**り**	
来院	72	ラロキシフェン塩酸塩		リウマチ	278
来院時死亡	542		289	リウマチ性心疾患	
来院時心肺停止	536	卵円孔開存	183, 584		184, 592
ライエル症候群	326	卵円窓	459	リウマチ性多発筋痛症	
ライ症候群	339	卵管	9, 488		286, 585
ライソゾーム病	112	卵管炎	27, 238	リウマチ熱	110, 340, 592
ライター症候群	286	卵管鏡検査	236	リウマチ病医	60
ライディッヒ細胞	490	卵管結紮術	242	リウマチ病科	54
ライノウイルス	160	卵管采	488	リウマチ病学	65
ライフェンスタイン症候		卵管造影法	9	リウマトイド因子	
群	240	卵管疎通性検査	236		283, 592
ライム病	108	卵管通気性検査	236	リウマトイド結節	281
雷鳴恐怖症	297	卵管妊娠	9, 237	利害関係	44
ライル島	502	卵管卵巣摘出術	243	理学士	68, 528
ラインケ浮腫	141	卵管留水症	238	理学修士	68, 574
ラウン・ギャノン・レバ		卵管留膿症	238	理学療法	118, 588
イン症候群	178, 567	卵形	40	理学療法士	58, 588
ラ音	157	卵形嚢	460	理学療法部	55
裸眼視力	131	ランゲルハンス細胞組織		リガーゼ連鎖反応	82, 566
落屑	320	球症	114, 342, 566	リガ・フェーデ病	332
ラクナ梗塞	306	ランゲルハンス島	490	罹患	72
ラザホージウム	436, 592	卵細胞質内精子注入法		裏急後重	196
ラジアン	439, 591		242, 560	リクター症候群	271
ラジウム	436, 591	乱視	125	リコール	33
ラジオアイソトープレノ		卵子	235	離婚	74
グラム	221	乱視矯正角膜切開術		梨状陥凹	466
ラジオ波焼灼療法			137, 520	リスフラン関節	495
	214, 592	卵巣	9, 488, 490	リスペリドン	316
ラセーグ徴候	281	卵巣炎	238	リセルグ酸ジエチルアミ	
螺旋	40	卵巣過剰刺激症候群		ド	568
裸体恐怖症	297		239, 579	リソソーム	508
ラタモキセフ	567	卵巣癌	239	離脱症候群	196, 303
ラッサ熱	107	卵巣子宮内膜症	239	離断	88
ラッド症候群	338	卵巣上体	488	離断性骨軟骨炎	286, 578
ラテックスアレルギー		卵巣摘出術	9	利胆薬	211
	324	卵巣の	9	リチウム	434, 567

立位	76	
リッサウイルス感染症		
	108	
立体覚	302	
立体覚認知障害	302	
立体視	132	
律動性眼振	129	
リットル	438, 565	
立方骨	494	
立方センチメートル		
	438, 531	
立方体	40	
立毛	6	
立毛筋	462	
リーデル甲状腺腫	252	
リドカイン	123, 189	
リード・ステルンベルグ		
細胞	269	
リトナビル	594	
リドル症候群	254	
リトル病	306	
離乳	343	
離乳食	343	
利尿	35	
利尿薬	35, 188, 224	
リネゾリド	569	
リハ	33	
リパーゼ	17, 202	
リハビリ	33	
リハビリテーション医学		
	65	
リバビリン	211	
離被架	90	
リヒターヘルニア	210	
リー病	307	
リファブチン	591	
リファンピシン	168, 592	
リフトバレー熱	108	
リプマン・サックス心内		
膜炎	186	
リボ核酸	511, 593	
リボ核タンパク質		
	511, 593	
リボスタマイシン	594	
リポソーマルドキソルビ		
シン	566	
リボソーム	508	
リボソーム RNA		
	511, 594	

リポ多糖	568	
リポタンパク質	14, 250	
リポタンパク質リパーゼ		
	250, 568	
リポトロピン	568	
リュイ体	503	
流感	155	
流行性角結膜炎		
	110, 133, 546	
流行性耳下腺炎		
	26, 110, 151, 330	
流行性耳下腺炎ワクチン		
	344	
流行病	106	
流産	229	
硫酸亜鉛混濁試験	611	
硫酸アルミニウムカリウ		
ム・タンニン酸		
	212, 521	
硫酸キニジン	189	
硫酸ストレプトマイシン		
	168	
硫酸モルヒネ	574	
粒子凝集反応	82, 580	
留置カテーテル	90, 225	
流動食	90	
流動物	194	
流涙	126	
流涙症	133	
両価性	10	
両側肺門リンパ節腫大		
	527	
両眼	23, 580	
両眼視	132, 529	
両脚ブロック	179, 526	
菱形	39	
菱形窩	502	
両肩峰の	10	
両耳	22, 525	
両耳音の大きさバランス		
検査	142, 516	
両耳側半盲	132	
良心	35	
両心室補助装置	192, 529	
良性	84	
良性前立腺肥大	528	
良性単クローン性免疫グ		
ロブリン症	272, 527	
良性頭蓋内圧亢進症		

	306, 527	
良性発作性頭位性めまい		
	144, 528	
両側性	10	
両側肺門リンパ節腫大		
	161	
両手利き	10	
両鼻側半盲	132	
量不足	590	
両麻痺	299	
療養所	52	
療養費	49	
緑色	39	
緑色蛍光タンパク質	552	
緑内障	133	
緑膿菌	219	
旅行医学	65	
リルゾール	315	
履歴書	68, 539	
理論的根拠	37	
リン	434, 580	
淋菌	235	
淋菌感染症	110	
淋菌性眼炎	26	
淋菌性関節炎	286	
リンコマイシン	566	
リン酸塩	218	
リン酸コデイン	167	
臨時追加投与	123	
臨床医	57	
臨床医学	63	
臨床学習	68, 529	
臨床看護学	66	
臨床技能	68, 538	
臨床教授	62	
臨床検査	78	
臨床検査技師	58, 574	
臨床現場即時検査	78, 586	
臨床工学技士	59	
臨床診断	84	
臨床心理士	59	
輪状臍	210	
臨床知識	68, 534	
臨床的認知症尺度		
	303, 532	
輪状軟骨	495	
臨床病理医	60	
臨床病理学	65	
臨床病理検討会	68, 536	

臨床病理部	54	ルテニウム	435, 594	レジオネラ症	108
臨床免疫学	65	ルードウィッヒアンギーナ	151	レジオネラ・ニューモフィーラ	160
鱗屑	320	ルートプレーニング	152	レシチン	581
リンネ試験	142	ルドロフ徴候	282	レシチン・コレステロール・アシルトランスフェラーゼ	566
リンパ	512	ルビジウム	434, 591		
リンパ管	478	ループス抗凝固因子	322, 565		
リンパ球	264			レーシック	33
リンパ球減少	265	ループス腎炎	221	レジデント	59
リンパ球混合培養	572	ループ利尿薬	188	レジンスポンジ摂取率	594
リンパ球混合培養反応	572	ルーメン	438, 567		
リンパ球刺激試験	323, 568	ルリーシュ症候群	177	レスピ	33
		ルー・ワイ吻合	214	レセ	33
リンパ球性間質性肺炎	164, 567	ルンゲ	33	レセプト	33
		ルンバール	33	レチウス腔	488
リンパ球性脈絡髄膜炎ウイルス	566	ルンペル・レーデ現象	262	レチノール結合タンパク質	591
リンパ球様	18			レッグ・カルベ・ペルテス病	286, 566
リンパ系	478	**れ**			
リンパ腫 WHO 分類	263	霊安室	55	レックリングハウゼン病	116
リンパ節	478, 567, 604	冷罨法	289		
リンパ節腫	262	冷凍療法	329	裂肛	207
リンパ節腫大	262	レイノー現象	321	裂孔ヘルニア	204
リンパ節摘除術	276	レイノルズ五徴	196	レッシュ・ナイハン症候群	337
リンパ浮腫	177	レヴィ小体	305		
リンパ脈管筋腫症	565	レヴィ小体型認知症	312, 542	裂傷	320
淋病	26, 237			劣性遺伝子	512
リンホカイン活性化キラー細胞	565	レヴィン管	211	劣等感	296
		レオパード症候群	325, 566	レット症候群	313
倫理委員会	44			レットレル・ジーベ病	342
倫理綱領	44	レオポルド操作	232		
		レーザー	565	裂毛症	326, 605
る		レーザー角膜内切削形成術	137, 565	裂離	281
涙液層破壊時間	129, 529			裂離歯	149
類軋音	158	レーザー凝固	329	レナンピシリン	565
類宦官	231	レーザー隅角形成術	137, 567	レニウム	435, 592
類語反復	371			レニン・アンギオテンシン系	591
涙腺	456	レーザー屈折矯正角膜切除術	137, 587		
るいそう	105, 244			レノグラム	16
類洞	484	レーザー血管形成術	190	レノックス・ガストー症候群	332
類肉腫	16, 18	レーザー紅彩切開術	137, 567		
涙囊	456			レーバー遺伝性視神経症	135
涙囊炎	133	レーザー線維柱帯形成術	137, 568		
涙囊鼻腔狭窄症	133			レプ	592
涙囊鼻腔吻合術	136, 540	レーザー・トレラー徴候	321	レフグレン症候群	161
類鼻疽	108			レフスム病	311
ルーカス徴候	332	レーザー光凝固術	136	レプトスピラ症	109
ルクス	438, 569	レーザー免疫測定法	82, 567	レプリーゼ	330
ルテチウム	435, 568			レフルノミド	288

レプレッサー遺伝子	512	労作性呼吸困難	154	肋骨横隔膜角鈍化	161
レフレル症候群	164	老視	125	肋骨下	12
レフレル心内膜炎	186	老視者	125	肋骨弓	450
レーベル	33	老人医療費	49	肋骨脊柱角	452, 539
レーベンベルク徴候	177	老人介護支援センター	55	肋骨脊柱角圧痛	217
レボチロキシンナトリウム	258	老人環	128, 245	肋骨の	9
レボドーパ製剤	315	老人看護	60	ロート斑	130
レボフロキサシン	569	老人性難聴	143	ロピナビル	568
レボホリナートカルシウム	567	老人短期入所施設	55	ロピニロール塩酸塩	315
レム	592	老人病院	53	ロブシング徴候	197
レム睡眠	304, 592	老人福祉センター	55	ロペラミド塩酸塩	211
レム睡眠時行動障害	302, 591	老人福祉法	47	濾胞性リンパ腫	272, 550
レルミット徴候	298	老人保健法	47	濾胞腺腫	252
連結形	2, 12	老衰	74, 244	ロマノ・ワード症候群	183
連結母音	2	労働安全衛生法	47	ロメフロキサシン	567
連合弁膜症	184, 539	労働者災害補償保険	49	ローランド溝	502
連合野	503	漏斗胸	156	ロールシャッハテスト	304
連鎖球菌感染後急性糸球体腎炎	340, 523	老年	244	ロルフィング	119
連鎖球菌性咽頭炎	27	老年医学	65	ローレル指数	331
連鎖球菌発熱外毒素	322, 599	老年科	54	ローレンシウム	436, 568
レンズ核	503	老年看護学	66	ローレンス・ムーン・ビードル症候群	253
連銭形成	264	老年痴呆	295	ロンベルグ試験	300
連続携行式腹膜透析	225, 530	老年病専門医	60		
連続サイクル式腹膜透析	225, 531	蝋様円柱	218	わ	
連続性雑音	175	老齢・遺族・障害者年金および健康保険	50, 578	ワイセ	33
連続性ラ音	158	老齢基礎年金	49	ワイル病	208
連続多項目分析装置	597	濾過分画	220, 550	ワイル・フェリックス反応	322
連続縫合	88	ロキシスロマイシン	595	若木骨折	282
レントゲニウム	436, 592	ロキタマイシン	593	わきが腋臭	321
レントゲン	439, 590	ロキタンスキー・アショッフ洞	484, 591	腋毛	444
		肋頚動脈	472	わきの下	444
ろ		肋軟骨	496	ワクシニア免疫グロブリン	608
ロイコ	33	ロジウム	435, 592	ワクチン関連麻痺性ポリオ	607
ロイコトリエン	159, 568	濾出	84	鷲手	298
ロイコトリエン拮抗薬	167	ローション	23, 568	ワセリン	328
ロイシンアミノペプチダーゼ	200, 565	ローション剤	86, 328	ワッセルマン反応	610
ロイマ	33	六角形	39	ワット	439, 610
聾	139	肋間筋	498	ワトソン・シュウォーツ試験	250
労災	49	肋間腔	175, 560	ワルダイエル輪	465
労作性狭心症	185, 544	肋間神経	505	ワルデンシュトレーム・マクログロブリン血症	273
		肋間神経痛	121		
		肋間動脈	472		
		肋間の	11		
		ロッキー山紅斑熱	109, 593		
		肋骨	9, 492		
		肋骨縁	450		

ワールデンブルグ症候群 337	ワーレンベルグ症候群 306	腕橈骨筋 5, 498
ワルトン管 464	彎曲カテーテル 90	腕橈骨筋反射 300
ワルファリンカリウム 189	腕神経叢 505	腕頭静脈 476
	腕神経叢障害 311, 528	腕頭動脈 472
割れるような 121	腕神経叢ブロック 123	

英語索引

1-deamino-8-D-arginine vasopressin	259, 540
1,5-anhydroglucitol	247
3 dimensional computed tomography	79
5-bromouridine-2′-deoxyrebose	529
5′-deoxy-5-fluorouridine	541
5′-doxifluridine	429
5-fluorocytosine	549
5-fluorodeoxyuridine	551
5-fluorouracil	430
5-hydroxyindoleacetic acid	250
5-hydroxytryptamine	559
5-year survival rate	92
6-mercaptopurine	431
11-deoxycorticosterone	249
17-hydroxycorticosteroid	249
17-ketosteroid	249
^{18}F-fluorodeoxyglucose	80
24-hour urine specimen	218

A

a-	10, 71
a feeling of ~	71
a feeling of inferiority	296
a fit of convulsions	331
a posteriori	21
a priori	21
a sensation of ~	71
ab-	10
abdomen	8, 25, 444
abdominal	8
abdominal aorta	472
abdominal aortic aneurysm	187
abdominal aponeurosis	501
abdominal ballottement	198
abdominal cavity	455
abdominal circumference	76, 232
abdominal compartment syndrome	199
abdominal distention	196, 332
abdominal girth	76, 196
abdominal hernia	210
abdominal leak point pressure	220
abdominal pain	120, 195
abdominal paracentesis	204
abdominal pregnancy	237
abdominal reflex	301
abdominal respiration	154
abdominal ultrasonography	202
abdomino-	12
abdominocentesis	12
abdominocyesis	237
abdominoperineal	12
abdominoperineal resection of rectum	214
abducens nerve	505
abduction	9, 34, 279
aberration	10
abetalipoproteinemia	256
ablactation	343
abnormal	10
abnormal secretion of ADH	114
abnormal secretion of gonadotropin	113
abnormal secretion of prolactin	113
abnormally frequent menstruation	228
ABO blood group	267
abortion	229
above-elbow amputation	292
above-knee amputation	292
abrasion	88, 320
abruptio placentae	238
abscess	83
absence epilepsy	297
absorption	34
absorption ointment	328
academic degree	66
academic standing	67
acalculia	302
acanthocyte	264
acanthocytosis	264
acanthosis	320
acanthosis nigricans	327
acarbose	258
acathisia	298
accelerated idioventricular rhythm	174
acceptable daily intake	518

accessory ear	332	acrodynia	12, 18
accessory hemiazygos vein	476	acromegaly	12, 18, 116, 252
accessory nerve	505	acromioclavicular joint	495
accessory pancreatic duct	484	acromion	492
accident	73	acronym	56
accident insurance	49	acrophobia	18, 296
accommodation reflex	129	act	46
accompany	72	actin	34
accountability	43	actinic	34
Accreditation Council for Graduate		actinic cheilitis	34
Medical Education	67	actinic keratitis	133
acephalus	331	actinic keratosis	324
acetaminophen	122	actinium	436
acetazolamide	136, 188	actinomycin D	429
acetic	34	actinotherapy	343
acetohexamide	258	activated coagulation time	265
acetone odor	148	activated partial thromboplastin	
acetylcholine	517	time	265
acetylcholine esterase	517	activated protein C	266
acetylcysteine	167	active exercise	290
acetylsalicylic acid	122, 288	active problem	96
achalasia	205	activities of daily living	92
ache	120	activities parallel to daily living	92
-ache	71	acupressure	118
achondroplasia	3	acupuncture	119
acid dyspepsia	195	acupuncturist	58
acid phosphatase	219	acute	91
acid stomach	26, 195	acute abdomen	210
acid-fast bacillus	519	acute anterior poliomyelitis	25
aclarubicin	429	acute arterial occlusive disease	187
acne	245, 318	acute bacterial endocarditis	186
acne rosacea	141	acute basophilic leukemia	271
acne vulgaris	25, 324	acute cerebellar ataxia	339
acoustic maculae	460	acute coronary syndrome	184
acoustic nerve	505	acute disseminated encephalomyeli-	
acoustic neurinoma	144	tis	307
acoustic neuritis	144	acute encephalitis	109
acoustic reflex	141	acute eosinophilic leukemia	271
acoustic shadow	523	acute eosinophilic pneumonia	164
acquired cystic disease of kidney		acute epiglottitis	340
	222	acute fatty liver in pregnancy	207
acquired hemolytic anemia	270	acute gastric mucosal lesion	205
acquired immunodeficiency syn-		acute gastritis	205
drome	109, 237, 270	acute glomerulonephritis	221
acral enlargement	245	acute hemorrhagic colitis	206
acro-	12	acute hemorrhagic conjunctivitis	
acrocephalopolysyndactyly	341		110, 133
acrocephalosyndactyly	341	acute hemorrhagic pancreatitis	209
acrocephaly	332, 341	acute hepatitis	207

acute infectious endocarditis	186	adduction	34, 279
acute inflammatory demyelinating polyneuropathy	309	adductor longus muscle	500
		adefovir pivoxil	211
acute intermittent porphyria	257	adenine	509
acute interstitial nephritis	222	adenine arabinoside	329
acute interstitial pneumonia	164	adeno-	12
acute kidney injury	222	adeno-associated virus	516
acute laryngotracheobronchitis	340	adenocarcinoma	12
acute lung injury	166	adenocarcinoma of lung	166
acute lymphocytic leukemia	270	adenohypophysis	490
acute megakaryocytic leukemia	270	adenoid cystic carcinoma	83
acute monocytic leukemia	270	adenoidectomy	146
acute myelogenous leukemia	270	adenoma	83
acute myelomonocytic leukemia	270	adenomatous	12
acute myocardial infarction	185	adenomatous goiter	252
acute necrotizing pancreatitis	210	adenosine deaminase	518
acute necrotizing ulcerative gingivitis	151	adenosine diphosphate	518
		adenosine monophosphate	521
acute nonlymphocytic leukemia	270	adenosine triphosphate	524
acute obstructive suppurative cholangitis	209	*Adenovirus*	160
		adherence	86
acute otitis media	143	adhesive bandage	328
acute pancreatitis	209	adiadochokinesis	300
acute phase reactant	523	adiaphoresis	321
acute physiology and chronic health evaluation	92	adipo-	12
		adiponectin	250
acute poliomyelitis	107	adipose	12
acute posterior multifocal placoid pigment epitheliopathy	135	adipose tissue	512
		adiposis	245
acute poststreptococcal glomerulonephritis	340	adiposis dolorosa	245
		adiposity	12, 245
acute promyelocytic leukemia	270	adjustment disorder	312
acute renal failure	222	admitting diagnosis	93
acute respiratory distress syndrome	166	adnerval	10
		adnexa uteri	489
acute respiratory failure	166	adnexal tumor	239
acute retinal necrosis	135	adolescence	244
acute thyroiditis	251	adrenal	10
acute triangle	39	adrenal androgen	250
acute tubular necrosis	222	adrenal cortex	490
acyclovir	329	adrenal crisis	254
ad	22	adrenal enzyme deficiency	115
ad-	10	adrenal gland	490
ad hoc	21	adrenal hypertension	184
ad libitum	21	adrenal incidentaloma	255
adalimumab	289	adrenal insufficiency	254
Adam's apple	442	adrenal medulla	490
adapalene	329	adrenalectomy	259
adde	22	adrenaline	189, 250

Term	Page
adreno-	12
adrenocortical	12
adrenocortical hyperfunction	253, 254
adrenocortical insufficiency	254
adrenocorticotropic hormone	248
adrenogenital syndrome	240, 254
adrenomyeloneuropathy	12
adsorption	34
adult nursing	66
adult pubic hair	245
adult Still disease	114
adult T-cell leukemia	271
adult T-cell leukemia/lymphoma	271
adult-onset diabetes mellitus	256
advanced glycation end product	247
advanced stage	91
adventitious sounds	157
adverse drug reaction	44
adverse event	44
aerophagia	18, 197
aerophagy	197
aerophobia	296
aerosol	86, 169
aerospace medicine	64
afebrile	105
afferent	34
afferent loop syndrome	206
afferent neuron	504
affiliated hospital	52
affix	2
afterbirth	27
aftercataract	134
after-hours practice	43
against medical advice	521
age	71
age of onset	72
agenda	390
age-related macular degeneration	113, 135
aggravation	91
aging society	43
agnosia	302
agonizing	121
agoraphobia	297
agranulocytosis	265
agraphia	302
AHA Patients' Bill of Rights	45
AIDS-related complex	523
ailurophobia	297
air bronchogram	161
air conduction	142
air douche	145
airborne infection	105
air-fluid level	203
airway obstruction	156
airway reversibility test	162
akathisia	298
ala nasi	460
alanine aminotransferase	199
albinism	326
albumin tannate	211
albumin-globulin ratio	200
albuminuria	19
alcohol dependence	296
alcoholic liver disease	207
Alcoholics Anonymous	316
alcoholism	17, 296
aldehyde dehydrogenase	521
aldolase	283
aldosterone	249
aldosterone to renin activity ratio	249
aldosterone-producing adenoma	253
alendronate sodium hydrate	289
alert	76
-algesia	17
-algia	17, 71
alimentary canal	480
alkaline phosphatase	199
alkalosis	34
allele	510
allelic gene	510
allergen	17
allergic bronchopulmonary aspergillosis	165
allergic conjunctivitis	133
allergic granulomatous angiitis	111, 114
allergic rhinitis	25, 144
allergist	59
allergology	63
allied health personnel	59
allodynia	120
allogenic bone marrow transplantation	276
allopathy	119
allopurinol	259
alopecia	25, 245

alopecia areata	326
α-adrenergic antagonist	188
α-adrenergic blocking agent	188
α-adrenoreceptor antagonist	188
α-fetoprotein	201
α-glucosidase inhibitor	258
α-hemolytic streptococcal pharyngitis	109
alteplase	189, 315
alternate binaural loudness balance test	142
alternating cover test	128
alternating hemiplegia	299
alternating hemiplegia in infants	342
alternating pulse	173
alternative dispute resolution	43
altitudinal hemianopia	132
aluminium	434
aluminum potassium sulfate-tannic acid	212
alveolar abscess	151
alveolar hypoventilation syndrome	116, 166
alveolar pyorrhea	151
alveolar sac	466
alveolar-arterial carbon dioxide difference	159
alveolar-arterial gas tension difference	159
alveolar-arterial nitrogen difference	159
alveolar-arterial oxygen difference	159
Alzheimer disease assessment scale	303
AMA Code of Ethics	45
amalgam restoration	152
amantadine hydrochloride	168, 315
amaurosis	125
amaurosis fugax	134
amaxophobia	297
ambi-	10
ambidexterity	10
ambivalence	10
amblyopia	125
Ambu bag	190
ambulance	34
ambulate	407
ambulation	34
ambulatory	34
ambulatory blood pressure monitoring	75
amebic dysentery	109
amelioration	91
ameloblastoma	148
amenorrhea	228
America's Health Insurance Plans	50
American Medical Association	45
americium	436
ametropia	125, 131
amikacin	422
amine precursor uptake and decarboxylation	523
aminoaciduria	218
aminoglycoside	519
aminophylline	167
amiodarone hydrochloride	189
amlodipine besilate	188
ammonia	200
amnesia	295
amniocentesis	236
amnion	232
amnioscopy	236
amniotic fluid index	235
amoxicillin	422
amoxicillin/clavulanic acid	422
ampere	438
amphetamine	27
amphophilic	269
amphoric resonance	156
amphotericin B	422
ampicillin	422
ampicillin/cloxacillin	422
ampicillin/sulbactam	422
ampule	22, 34
ampulla	22, 34
amputation	88, 292
amrubicin	429
amyl nitrite	189
amylase	2, 202
amylase creatinine clearance ratio	202
amylase isozyme	202
amyloid precursor protein	305
amyloidosis	114, 257
amyloid β-protein	305
amyotrophic lateral sclerosis	112, 308

an-	10, 71	anginal attack	172
ana	22	angio-	12
ana-	10	angiocardiography	182
anabolic steroid	274	angiography	6, 12, 17, 79
anabolism	17	angioimmunoblastic lymphadenopathy with dysproteinemia	272
anal	448		
anal atresia	338	angioneurotic	12
anal bleeding	195	angioplasty	18
anal canal	482	angiotensin	250
anal fissure	207	angiotensin II type I receptor blocker	188
anal fistula	207		
anal region	452	angiotensin-converting enzyme inhibitor	188
anal sphincter	482		
anal sphincter tone	198	angle of anterior chamber	456
analgesia	17, 122, 301	angle-recession glaucoma	134
analgesic	25, 122	angular cheilitis	150, 262
analysis	10	angular cheilosis	153
analysis of covariance	522	angular stomatitis	150
analysis of variance	522	anhedonia	229
anaplasia	10, 34, 83	anhidrosis	321
anasarca	217	anion exchange resin	259
anastomosis	88	anion gap	159, 219
anastomotic	34	*Anisakis*	199
anastrozole	429	anisocoria	129
anatomic	34	anisocytosis	263
anatomical diagnosis	84	anisophoria	128
anatomical position	448	ankle	446
anatomy	63	ankle clonus	301
Ancylostoma	199	ankle jerk	300
andro-	12	ankle joint	495
androgen	12	ankle swelling	173
androgen deprivation therapy	224	ankle-brachial index	173
androgen-insensitivity syndrome	240	ankle-foot orthosis	290
android	12	ankylosing spinal hyperostosis	287
androphobia	296	ankylosing spondylitis	287
anemia	25, 261	ankylosis	34
anemia of chronic disease	269	annuity	49
anemic	261	annular cartilage	495
anencephalus	331	annular pancreas	210
anesthesia	87, 294, 301	annuloaortic ectasia	183
anesthesia dolorosa	294	annulus	40
anesthesiologist	60	anodyne	122
anesthesiology	65	anomalous retinal correspondence	128
aneurysm	187		
aneurysmal bone cyst	288	anomaly	83
angeion	6	anorectic	194
angina at rest	185	anorexia	194
angina of effort	185	anorexia nervosa	312
angina pectoris	185	anosmia	140

anoxia	10	anthrax	108
antacid	210	anti-	10
antalgic gait	279	anti-acetylcholine receptor antibody	303
ante-	10		
ante cibum	22	anti-agalactosyl IgG antibody	283
ante meridiem	22	antianxiety agent	314
antegrade	10	antiarrhythmic	189
antemortem diagnosis	84	antibacterial agent	117
antepartum	10	antibacterial substance	117
anterior	448	antibiotic	10
anterior antebrachial region	452	antibiotic therapy	117
anterior axillary line	454	antibiotic-associated colitis	206
anterior basal segment (S^8)	468	antibiotic-associated diarrhea	196
anterior brachial region	452	antibiotics	117
anterior cerebral artery	471	antibody	10, 34
anterior cervical region	450	antibody deficiency syndrome	519
anterior cervical triangle	450	antibody-dependent cellular cytotoxicity	518
anterior chamber	456		
anterior commissure	502	anti-cardiolipin antibody	322
anterior communicating artery	471	anticentromere antibody	322
anterior cruciate ligament	496	anticholinergic	210
anterior crural region	453	anticholinergic agent	315
anterior cubital region	452	anticoagulant	189
anterior femoral region	452	anticoagulant therapy	189
anterior fontanelle (fontanel)	332	anticonvulsant	314
anterior inferior cerebellar artery	472	anticonvulsive	314
		anti-cyclic citrullinated peptide antibody	283
anterior interbody fusion	291		
anterior ischemic optic neuropathy	134	antidepressant	314
		antidepressive drug	314
anterior knee region	453	antidiarrheals	211
anterior mediastinum	468	antidiuretic hormone	249
anterior myocardial infarction	185	anti-DNA antibody	321
anterior segment (S^3)	468	anti-double stranded DNA antibody	322
anterior semicircular canal	460		
anterior spinal artery	472	anti-EBV-early antigen antibody	267
anterior subcapsular cataract	134	anti-EBV-nuclear antigen antibody	267
anterior superior pancreaticoduodenal artery	474		
		anti-EBV-viral capsid antigen antibody	267
anterior tibial artery	476		
anterior tibial vein	478	antiemetic	211
antero-	13	antiepileptic drug	315
anterolateral	13	anti-extractable nuclear antigen antibody	322
anteroseptal	13		
anteroseptal myocardial infarction	185	antifungal agent	117
		anti-GAD antibody	247
anthelix	458	antigen	17
anthelmintic	211	antigen-antibody reaction	516
anthracycline	274	antigen-binding fragment	548

antigen-presenting cell	522	antisocial personality disorder	313
antiglobulin test	267	antispasmodic	210
anti-glomerular basement membrane nephritis	221	antistreptokinase	524
		antistreptolysin O	283
anti-glutamic acid decarboxylase antibody	247	antithrombin III	266, 275
		antithymocyte globulin	276
anti-HAV antibody	200	antithyroglobulin antibody	248
anti-HBc antibody	200	antithyroid agent	258
anti-HBe antibody	200	anti-thyroid peroxidase antibody	248
anti-HBs antibody	200	antitopoisomerase I antibody	322
anti-HCV antibody	201	antitragus	458
anti-Helicobacter pylori antibody	201	antitubercular agent	117
antihelix	458	antituberculous agent	117
anti-herpes simplex virus antibody	322	antitussive	167
		anti-varicella-zoster virus antibody	322
antihistamine	145		
anti-human T-lymphotropic virus 1 antibody	268	antiviral agent	117, 314
		anuresis	34
antihypertensive	188, 224	anuria	217
anti-influenza virus antibody	160	anus	482
anti-Jo-1 antibody	283	anvil	459
anti-Ku antibody	283	anxiety	295
antilymphocyte globulin	276	anxiety disorder	312
anti-measles virus antibody	334	aorta	471
antimicrosomal antibody	248	aortic arch	471
antimitochondrial antibody	201	aortic arch syndrome	516
antimony	435	aortic bruit	198
anti-mumps virus antibody	334	aortic dissection	187
antimuscarinic agent	224	aortic knob	180
antineutrophil cytoplasmic antibody	219	aortic regurgitation	183
		aortic second sound	175
antineutrophil cytoplasmic myeloperoxidase antibody	219	aortic stenosis	184
		aortic valve	470
antinuclear antibody	283, 321	aortic valve insufficiency	183
antinuclear factor	522	aortic valve replacement	191
antiphospholipid antibody	322	aortic valve stenosis	184
antiphospholipid antibody syndrome	111, 114	aortitis syndrome	111, 114
		aortocoronary bypass	191
antiplatelet agent	189	ape hand	298
antipsychotic agent	314	apertura pelvis inferior	232
antipyresis	117	apertura pelvis superior	232
antipyretic	117	apex beat	175
anti-rubella virus antibody	334	apex cardiogram	180
anti-Sjögren syndrome-A/Ro antibody	149	apex nasi	460
		apex of the lung	466
anti-Sjögren syndrome-B/La antibody	150	apex of tongue	464
		aphagia	34
anti-Sm antibody	322	aphakia	129
anti-smooth muscle antibody	524	aphakic eye	129

aphasia	18, 34, 302	areolar tissue	512
apheresis	315	argentaffinoma	255
aphonia	18, 140, 302	arginine vasopressin	249
aphtha	147	argon	434
aphthous stomatitis	150	aripiprazole	316
apical cap	161	arm	444
apical segment (S^1)	468	armpit	444
apicoectomy	152	aromatherapy	118
apicoposterior segment (S^{1+2})	468	arrector muscles of hairs	462
aplasia	34, 84	arrector pili muscle	462
aplastic anemia	115, 269	arrhythmia	172, 174
apnea	154	arrythmogenic right ventricular dysplasia	187
apnea index	162		
apnea-hypopnea index	163	arsenic	434
apocrine gland	462	artēria	8
apolipoprotein	250	arterial	8
aponeurosis	501	arterial blood gas	158
apoplexy	294	arterial carbon dioxide tension	159
apoptosis	82	arterial keton body ratio	200
apparent age	76	arterial oxygen saturation	159
apparent life-threatening event	331	arterial oxygen tension	159
appendectomy	214	arterio-	13
appendicitis	205	arteriole	8
appendix	482	arteriosclerosis	13, 18, 25, 34
appetite	194	arteriosclerosis obliterans	187
applanation tonometer	131	arteriosclerotic cardiovascular disease	184
apposition suture	88		
apprehensive	295	arteriosclerotic heart disease	184
appropriate-for-dates infant	331	arteriovenous	13
appropriate-for-gestational-age infant	331	arteriovenous anastomosis	525
		arteriovenous crossing	130
apraxia	300	arteriovenous malformation	183
aptitude test	67	artery	471
aqua	22	artery of ductus deferens	474
aquaporin	523	arthralgia	17, 120, 278
aqueous humor	512	arthralgia in children	25
arachnephobia	296	arthresthesia	302
arachnodactylia	17	arthritis	5, 17, 278
arachnodactyly	9	arthro-	13
arachnoid	504	arthrocentesis	284
arachnophobia	296	arthrodesis	291
arbekacin	422	arthrography	284
arch	446	arthrogryposis	281
arcuate ligament of diaphragm	496	arthrogryposis multiplex congenita	341
arcus senilis	128, 245		
area of cardiac dullness	175	arthrometer	283
area postrema	502	arthron	5
area under the curve	525	arthroplasty	13, 291
areola mammae	450	arthroscope	5

Term	Page
arthroscopy	13, 284
articular cartilage	496
artificial abortion	229
artificial arm	279
artificial blood vessel	192
artificial dialysis	225
artificial eye	126
artificial heart	192
artificial heart-lung	192
artificial insemination	242
artificial insemination by donor	242
artificial insemination by husband	242
artificial joint	292
artificial kidney	225
artificial leg	279
artificial limb	279
artificial limb fitter	58
artificial liver support	212
artificial lung	171
artificial pancreas	259
artificial respiration	169
artificial tears	136
artificial tooth	148
arytenoid cartilage	495
asbestos exposure	156
asbestosis	165
Ascaris	199
ascending aorta	471
ascending colon	482
ascending pharyngeal artery	472
ascending reticular activating system	523
ascites	196, 197, 217
ascitic	197
ascitic fluid	512
-ase	17
aseptic	25, 34
aseptic meningitis	110
aspartate aminotransferase	199
asphyxia	154
asphyxia neonatorum	334
aspiration biopsy	78
aspiration biopsy cytology	78
aspiration cytology	78
aspiration pneumonia	163
aspirin	190
aspoxicillin	422
assessment	96
assignment	67
assistant professor	62
assisted reproductive technology	242
assisted ventilation	169
associate dean	62
associate professor	62
association area	503
astatine	436
astereognosis	302
asterixis	197
asthenia	104
asthenic	104
asthenopia	126
asthma	154
asthmatic breathing	157
asthmatic bronchitis	163
astigmatic keratectomy	137
astigmatism	125
astrocytoma	313
astromicin	422
asymmetrical tonic neck reflex	333
asymmetry	10
asymptomatic infection	106
ataractic	314
ataxia	299
ataxic	299
ataxic gait	298
atazanavir sulfate	525
atelectasis	165
atherosclerosis	18, 34
athetosis	299
athlete's foot	28, 318
atlantoaxial dislocation	287
atlantoaxial joint	495
atlantoaxial sublaxation	287
atlantooccipital joint	495
atomic mass unit	439
atopic dermatitis	324
atrial extrasystole	174
atrial fibrillation	174
atrial flutter	174
atrial myxoma	188
atrial natriuretic peptide	178
atrial premature complex (contraction)	174
atrial septal defect	183
atrioventricular block	179
atrioventricular bundle	470

atrioventricular nodal reentrant tachycardia	174
atrioventricular nodal reentry tachycardia	174
atrioventricular node	470
atrioventricular reciprocating tachycardia	174
atrioventricular valve	470
atrium	470
atrophic rhinitis	144
atrophoderma striatum	245
atrophy	19, 82
atrophy of lingual papillae	262
attempted suicide	296
attending physician	57
attention deficit disorder	343
attention obligation	43
attention-deficit hyperactivity disorder	313, 343
atto-	20
attrition	149
atypia	82
atypical adenomatous hyperplasia	166
atypical epithelium	205
atypical fibroxanthoma	327
atypical lymphocyte	265
audio-	13
audioanalgesia	13
audiogram	17, 141
audiometer	141
audiometry	13, 141
audit	95
auditory brainstem response	142
auditory evoked potential	142
auditory hallucination	293
auditory organ	458
auditory ossicles	459
auditory sense	139
auditory tube	458
aura	34, 294
aural	9, 34
aures unitas	22
auricle	458
auricular cartilage	495
auricular concha	458
auricular deformity	140
auricular lobule	458
auricular tubercle	140
auris	9
auris dextra	22
auris sinistra	22
auris utreque	23
auscultation	77
autism	296
autistic	296
autistic disorder	313, 343
auto-	10
autogenic training	316
autoimmune disease	106
autoimmune hemolytic anemia	270
autoimmune hepatitis	113, 207
autoimmune pancreatitis	210
autoimmunity	10
autologous bone marrow transplantation	276
autologous mixed lymphocyte reaction	521
autologous stem cell transplantation	276
autologous transfusion	275
autolysis	83
automated external defibrillator	190
automated perimeter	132
automated peritoneal dialysis	225
automatic atrial tachycardia	174
automatic implantable cardioverter-defibrillator	190
autonomic nervous system	506
autonomously functioning thyroid nodule	251
autonomy	10
autophobia	296
autophonia	139
autophony	139
autopsy	78
autoradiography	523
autosomal dominant inheritance	73
autosomal dominant polycystic kidney disease	222
autosomal recessive inheritance	74
autosomal recessive polycystic kidney disease	222
autosome	508
autotransfusion	275
auxiliary	34
average urinary flow rate	220
avian influenza	108

avian influenza virus	160
aviation medicine	64
avulsed tooth	149
avulsion	281
avulsion fracture	282
awareness	293
axillary	34
axillary artery	472
axillary fossa	450
axillary hairs	444
axillary lymph node dissection	243
axillary nerve	505
axillary nodes	478
axillary region	450
axillary temperature	75
axillary vein	476
axis deviation	178
axon	504
Ayurveda	118
azidothymidine	275
azithromycin	422
azoospermia	235
azotemia	219
aztreonam	422
azulene sulfonate sodium	152
azure	39
azygos	193
azygos fissure	193
azygos lobe	193
azygos vein	476

B

B virus disease	108
babies' sore eyes	26
baby	330
baby produced by artificial insemination	25
baby teeth	147
bacampicillin	422
Bachelor of Science	68
bachelor's degree	66
bacillary dysentery	107
bacilluria	218
bacitracin	422
back	444
back of hand	444, 452
back of the head	442
back pain	120
back teeth	147
back tooth	442
backache	120
backbone	278
back-formation	407
backside	444
bacterial cast	218
bacterial infection	106
bacterial meningitis	110
bacterial vaginosis	238
bacteriological examination	78
bacteriology	63
bacteriophobia	296
bacteriuria	218
bad blood	27
bad breath	26, 147
balanced diet	90, 194
balanitis	237
bald	319
bald head	319
bald-headedness	319
baldness	25, 245, 319
ball of the thumb	446
ballism	300
ballismus	300
ballistocardiogram	181
balloon angioplasty	190
balloon atrial septostomy	191
balloon valvuloplasty	192
balloon-expandable intravascular stent	191
balloon-occluded retrograde transvenous obliteration	213
ballottement of the patella	280
balneotherapy	118
band neutrophil	264
band-like pain	172
banked blood	275
bar(o)-	260
barbers' itch	27
barbiturate	314
bariatric surgery	260
bariatrics	260
barium	435
barium enema	203
barrel chest	156
barrenness	229
bartholinitis	238
basal acid output	201
basal blood pressure	75

basal body temperature	231
basal cell carcinoma	327
basal diet	90
basal energy expenditure	526
basal ganglia	503
basal layer	462
basal metabolic rate	246
basal supported oral therapy	258
base excess	159
base of the lung	466
base pair	510
base sequence	510
basic calcium phosphate	284
basic fetoprotein	201
basic fibroblast growth factor	527
basic life support	527
basic medicine	63
basic nursing	65
basilar artery	471
basilic vein	476
basophil	264
basophilic stippling	264
bassinet	330
bathyanesthesia	302
bathyesthesia	302
BCG vaccine	344
beard	442
bearing-down pains	121
beclomethasone dipropionate	169
becquerel	438
bed bath	89
bed rest	89
bedpan	90
bedridden	72
bedside learning	68
bedsore	25, 318
bed-wetting	26, 331
beef tapeworm	199
before admission	72
behavioral and psychological symptoms of dementia	295
behavioral observation audiometry	334
behavioral science	63
bekanamycin	422
belching	26, 195
belief	74
belly	25, 444
belonephobia	297
below-elbow amputation	292
below-knee amputation	292
bends	25
beneficiary	49
benefits	48
benign epilepsy of childhood with centrotemporal spikes	341
benign intracranial hypertension	306
benign migratory glossitis	148
benign monoclonal gammopathy	272
benign paroxysmal positional vertigo	144
benign prostatic hypertrophy	223
benignancy	84
benzbromarone	259
benzodiazepine	314
benzylpenicillin	427
benzylpenicillin benzathine	424
berkelium	436
berry aneurysm	307
beryllium	434
β-adrenergic blocking agent	188
β-blocker	188
β-hemolytic streptococcus	334
β_2-microglobulin	219
bevacizumab	433
bezafibrate	259
bezoar	209
bi-	10
biapenem	422
bicalutamide	224
bicarbonate concentration	158
biceps brachii muscle	498
biceps femoris muscle	500
biceps reflex	300
bicuspid tooth	464
bicycle ergometer	180
bifascicular block	179
bifocal glasses	126, 135
bifocals	126
bifurcation of the trachea	466
big toe	446
bigeminal pulse	173
bigeminy	10, 173
biguanide	258
bilateral	10
bilateral bundle branch block	179
bilateral hilar lymphadenopathy	161
bile	512

bile duct cancer	209
biliary colic	195
biliary tract	484
biliopancreatic diversion	260
bilirubin encephalopathy	335
bilirubinuria	218
bimanual palpation	77
bimanual pelvic examination	231
binasal hemianopia	132
binocular vision	132
bio-	13
biochemical oxygen demand	528
biochemistry	13, 63
bioethics	43
biofeedback	119
biological diagnosis	84
biological drug	117
biological false positive	527
biological product	117
biophysical profile score	235
biopsy	13, 138
biostatistics	65
biparietal diameter	232
biperiden	315
biphasic positive airway pressure	170
bipolar disorder	312
birth canal	232
birth certificate	74
birth control	230, 241
birth place	74
birthing assistant	58
birthing center	52
birthing room	55
birthmark	25, 318, 319
bis-	10
bis in die	23
bisacromial	10
bisferious	10
bisferious pulse	173
bismuth	436
bisphosphonate	289
bitemporal hemianopia	132
bite-wing radiography	150
biventricular assist device	192
black	39
black hairy tongue	148
black substance	504
black tongue	148
black-and-blue	25
black-and-blue mark	261
blackhead	25
blackish	39
blackout	28
bladder	486
bladder irrigation	225
bladder outlet obstruction	223
bladder tumor	223
bland diet	90
-blast	17
bleb	161, 320
bleeder's disease	26
bleeding	83, 261
bleeding time	265
bleomycin	429
blepharedema	217
blepharitis	133
blepharochalasis	127
blepharophimosis	127
blepharoptosis	2, 18, 127
blepharospasm	127
blind loop syndrome	206
blind spot	132
blinding	127
blindness	125
blink	127
blister	28, 318, 320
bloating	196
blockage	198
blood	512
blood bank	275
blood cell counter	263
blood chemistry test	78
blood clot	262
blood coagulation	262
blood component transfusion	275
blood donation	262
blood dyscrasias	261
blood group	267
blood group incompatibility	267
blood platelet count	263
blood pressure	172, 173
blood pressure cuff	77
blood pressure manometer	77
blood purification	225
blood relative	73
blood sedimentation	266
blood test	78

blood transfusion	275	bone transplantation	292
blood type	267	bone-specific alkaline phosphatase	283
blood urea nitrogen	219		
blood volume	529	bony birth canal	232
blood-brain barrier	526	bony labyrinth	459
blood-forming organs	261	bony tissue	512
bloodletting	276	borborygmus	196, 198
blood-poisoning	27	borderline hypertension	184
bloody	261	borderline personality disorder	313
bloody stool	196	born	34
bloody sputum	155	borne	34
blot hemorrhage	261	boron	434
blue	39	bortezomib	274, 433
Blue Cross	50	bottle-feeding	343
Blue Shield	50	Botulinum A toxin	315
blues	25	botulism	108
bluish	39	boutonnière deformity	281
blunting of the costophrenic angle	161	bovine spongiform encephalopathy	307
blurring	125	bowel	480
B-mode ultrasonography	80	bowel movement	196
board certified oncology pharmacy specialist	58	bowel sounds	198
		bowleg	26, 279
board certified pharmacist in oncology pharmacy	58	brachial	5
		brachial artery	472
body cast	289	brachial muscle	498
body cavity	455	brachial plexopathy	285
body fluid	512	brachial plexus	505
body mass index	245	brachial plexus block	123
body of the pancreas	484	brachial plexus neuropathy	311
body weight	75	brachial vein	476
bohrium	436	brachiocephalic artery	472
boil	26, 318	brachiocephalic vein	476
bolus	34	brachiōn	5
bone	492	brachioradial muscle	498
bone biopsy	251, 284	brachioradialis	5
bone conduction	142	brachioradialis reflex	300
bone densitometry	283	brachium	5
bone elongation	291	brachy-	13
bone grafting	292	brachycephaly	13
bone marrow aspirate	266	brachydactyly	13
bone marrow biopsy	266	brachytherapy	117
bone marrow puncture	266	brady-	13
bone marrow suppression	266	bradycardia	13, 172
bone marrow transplantation	276	bradycardia-tachycardia syndrome	174
bone mineral density	527		
bone pain	120	bradykinesia	299
bone remodeling	282	bradylalia	302
bone scintigraphy	284	bradypnea	13

brady-tachy syndrome	174	broad ligament of uterus	488
braille	125	bromine	434
brain abscess	307	bromocriptine	259
brain death	93, 297	bromocriptine mesilate	315
brain edema	306	bromocriptine mesylate	241
brain fever	26	bronchial	5, 34
brain injury	306	bronchial arterial embolization	170
brain natriuretic peptide	178	bronchial arterial infusion	170
brain stem	504	bronchial arteriography	161
brain surgeon	60	bronchial artery	472
brain tumor	313, 342	bronchial asthma	163
brain-derived neurotrophic factor	526	bronchial hyperreactivity test	162
brainstem auditory evoked potential	142	bronchial sounds	157
		bronchiectasis	17, 164
branch retinal artery occlusion	134	bronchiole	466
branch retinal vein occlusion	134	bronchiolitis obliterans with organizing pneumonia	164
branched-chain amino acid	200, 211		
branched-chain amino acid-tyrosine molar ratio	200	bronchioloalveolar cell carcinoma	166
		bronchitis	17, 25, 163
branched-chain ketoacid	526	broncho-	13
branched-chain ketoaciduria	333	bronchoalveolar lavage	163
branchial	34	bronchoalveolar lavage fluid	163
brand name	86	bronchodilator	13, 167
brash	195	bronchogenic carcinoma	166
BRCA1 gene	508	bronchography	5, 161
BRCA2 gene	508	bronchophony	157
breach of confidence	43	bronchopneumonia	13
breach of confidentiality	43	bronchopulmonary dysplasia	336
breakthrough bleeding	239	bronchopulmonary hygiene	169
breakthrough dose	123	bronchopulmonary lavage	169
breakthrough pain	121	bronchopulmonary segments	468
breast	444	bronchos	5
breast cancer	240	bronchoscopy	163
breast cancer nursing	61	bronchovesicular sounds	157
breast reconstruction	243	bronchus	5, 466
breast self-examination	231	brontophobia	297
breast-conserving surgery	243	bronze	39
breast-feeding	343	bronzy	39
breath sounds	157	brother	73
breathing	154	brow presentation	232
breathing exercise	169	brown	39
breathing movements	156	brownish	39
breech delivery	230	brucellosis	108
breech presentation	232	bruise	25, 261, 318
bridge prosthodontics	152	bruit	198
British Medical Association	527	bruit de diable	176
brittle diabetes	256	bruxism	147
broad base	40	bubo	228
		buccal	34

buccal region	450	calcium	434
bucillamine	288	calcium antagonist	188
buck teeth	147	calcium channel blocker	188
bucolome	259	calcium folinate	430
budesonide	169	calcium oxalate calculus	218
buffalo hump	246	calcium paraaminosalicylate	427, 581
bug	27, 28	calcium pyrophosphate dihydrate	284
bulbar conjunctiva	456	calf	446
bulbocavernosus reflex	231	calf cramps	25
bulbus oculi	456	caliber	34
bulbus vestibuli	489	calices renales	486
bulimia nervosa	312	californium	436
bulla	320	calipers	34
bullous	34	callous	34
bullous pemphigoid	327	callus	34, 318, 320
bundle branch block	526	caloric test	143
buprenorphine hydrochloride	123	calorie	438
burn	318, 320	calvaria	442
burning	121	calx	34, 453
burning tongue	261	calyx	34
burping	26	*Campylobacter jejuni*	202
burr cell	264	cancellous	34
burr hole	317	cancellous bone	494
bursitis	285	cancer	34, 83
business office	54	cancer center	52
busulfan	429	cancer chemotherapy nursing	61
butterfly rash	319	cancer insurance	48
buttocks	444	cancer nursing	60
buttonhole deformity	281	cancer pain management nursing	61
		cancerophobia	296
C		cancerous	34
cabergoline	315	cancrphobia	296
cabinet order	46	candela	438
cachectic	76	candesartan cilexetil	188
cachexia	76	*Candida albicans*	235
cadaveric kidney	226	cane	279
cadmium	435	canine	464
caesium	435	canine tooth	464
café-au-lait spot	153, 298	cannabis	124
cafeteria	54	cannonball pulse	173
caffeine	27	canthus	456
caisson disease	25	capillary fragility	266
calcaneal region	453	capitate bone	492
calcaneus	494	capricious	295
calcific uremic arteriolopathy	223	capsula	23
calcification	161	capsula interna	503
calcifying odontogenic cyst	151	capsule	86
calciphylaxis	223	capsule endoscopy	204
calcitonin	248, 289		

captopril	188
caput	5
caput medusae	5, 197
caput succedaneum	332
carbamazepine	315
carbohydrate antigen 19-9	201
carbohydrate antigen 125	529
carbon	434
carbon dioxide narcosis	159
carbonate	218
carbonic anhydrase inhibitor	136
carboplatin	429
carboxyhemoglobin	267
carcino-	13
carcinoembryonic antigen	201
carcinogen	13
carcinogenesis	17
carcinoid syndrome	255
carcinoma	18, 83
carcinoma of the tongue	151
carcinomatosis	13
cardia	480
cardiac	480
cardiac arrest	172, 176
cardiac catheterization	182
cardiac enlargement	175
cardiac event recorder	180
cardiac failure	185
cardiac index	181
cardiac insufficiency	185
cardiac murmur	173, 175
cardiac muscle	470
cardiac output	181
cardiac pacemaker	190
cardiac pacing	190
cardiac rehabilitation	190
cardiac resynchronization therapy	190
cardiac sounds	175
cardiac stimulant	189
cardiac surgeon	60
cardiac surgery	64
cardiac symptoms	172
cardiac troponin I	178
cardiac troponin T	178
cardio-	13
cardio-ankle vascular index	180
cardiogenic shock	176
cardiologist	59
cardiology	7, 64
cardiomegaly	175
cardiomyopathy	186
cardiomyotomy	214
cardiopulmonary	13
cardiopulmonary arrest	176
cardiopulmonary arrest on arrival	536
cardiopulmonary bypass	192
cardiopulmonary resuscitation	190
cardio-renal-anemia syndrome	222
cardiothoracic ratio	180
cardiotocography	235
cardiotonic	189
cardiovascular	13
cardiovascular disease	184
cardiovascular system	75
cardioversion	190
cardioverter	190
care house	55
care manager	57
carmofur	430
carmustine	526
carorimeter	18
carotid angiography	305
carotid artery stenting	316
carotid bruit	176
carotid cavernous fistula	307
carotid endarterectomy	316
carotid pulse wave	180
carotid sinus syndrome	184
carpal bone	492
carpal tunnel syndrome	285
carpometacarpal joint	495
carteolol hydrochloride	136
cartilage	495
cartilaginous tissue	512
cartilago	8
carumonam	424
case conference	392
case presentation	392, 405
case report	392
case study	392
cashier	54
cast	279
casting	289
casualty	35
casuistry	35
cata-	10

catabolism	10	cefotiam	424
cataplexy	10	cefotiam hexetil	424
cataract	134	cefozopran	424
catchment area	43	cefpiramide	424
cat-cry syndrome	336	cefpirome	424
catechol O-methyltransferase	536	cefpodoxime proxetil	424
catecholamine	189, 250	cefroxadine	424
cathartic	211	cefsulodin	423
catheter ablation	191	ceftazidime	422
catheter coudé	90	cefteram pivoxil	423
catheterization	90	ceftibuten	423
catheterized urine	218	ceftizoxime	424
catilaginous	8	ceftriaxone	424
cauda equina	506	cefuroxime axetil	424
cauda equina tumor	288	-cele	17
caudad	448	celiac	8
caudal	448	celiac artery	472
caudate lobe	484	celiac disease	206
caudate nucleus	503	celiac plexus block	123
cauliflower	40	cell	508
causal therapy	117	cell marker	267
causalgia	121	cell membrane	508
cauterization	87	cellulitis	325
cauterization of nosebleeds	146	cementum	464
caveolae	508	center for maternal and child health	52
cavernous breath sounds	157		
cavernous sinus	476	Centers for Medicare and Medicaid Services	50
cavitation	161		
Cavitron Ultrasonic Surgical Aspirator	539	-centesis	17
		centi-	20
cavity	161	centimeter	438
cecal	35	centimorgan	510
cecum	482	central	448
cefaclor	422	central alveolar hypoventilation syndrome	167
cefadroxil	423		
cefatrizine	423	central arterial pressure of retina	132
cefazolin	423		
cefbuperazone	422	central eating disorder	115
cefcapene pivoxil	423	central fovea	130, 458
cefdinir	423	central nervous system	502
cefditoren pivoxil	423	central obesity	245
cefepime	423	central pontine myelinolysis	309
cefixime	423	central retinal artery	472
cefmenoxime	423	central retinal artery occlusion	134
cefmetazole	423	central retinal vein occlusion	134
cefminox	423	central serous chorioretinopathy	134
cefodizime	423	Central Social Insurance Medical Council	49
cefoperazone	424		
cefotaxime	424	central sterile supply department	55

central supply room	55	cerebrospinal fluid	304, 513
central sympatholytic	188	cerebrospinal fluid hypovolemia	306
central venous pressure	182	cerebrospinal fluid pressure	304
central vision	132	cerebrospinal fluid protein	305
centromere	510	cerebrovascular	13
centrosome	508	cerebrovascular disease	539
cephalad	448	cerebrum	7, 35, 502
cephalalgia	120	cerium	435
cephalexin	423	certified care worker	57
cephalic	5	certified diabetes educator	58
cephalic presentation	232, 233	certified mental health and welfare worker	58
cephalic vein	476		
cephalo-	13	certified nurse	58, 60
cephalohematoma	13	certified nurse specialist	58, 60
cephalometric radiography	150	certified respiratory therapist	58
cephalometry	13	certified social worker	58
cephalopelvic disproportion	232	certified specialist	68
cephalothin	423	ceruloplasmin	200
cerebellar	7	cerumen	25, 139
cerebellar gait	298	cervical carcinoma	239
cerebellar peduncle	504	cervical cord	504
cerebellopontine	7	cervical erosion	239
cerebellum	7, 35, 504	cervical intraepithelial neoplasia	239
cerebral	7	cervical laceration	239
cerebral amyloid angiopathy	307	cervical mucus	235
cerebral aneurysm	307	cervical orthosis	290
cerebral angiography	305	cervical plexus	505
cerebral aqueduct	502	cervical polyp	239
cerebral arterial circle	471	cervical region	450
cerebral arteriovenous malformation	342	cervical spondylotic myelopathy	287
		cervical spondylotic radiculopathy	287
cerebral blood flow	304		
cerebral concussion	306	cervical traction	291
cerebral cortex	503	cervical vertebra	492
cerebral crus	504	cervicitis	238
cerebral edema	306	cervicobrachial syndrome	285
cerebral hemisphere	502	cervix uteri	489
cerebral hemorrhage	306	cesarean section	243
cerebral infarction	306	cetuximab	433
cerebral metabolic rate of oxygen	304	chafing	319
		chalazion	133
cerebral palsy	306, 342	chancre	34, 231
cerebral perfusion pressure	304	chancroid	237
cerebral tumor	313	change of life	27, 229
cerebral vascular accident	25, 306	channel disease	106
cerebral vascular resistance	304	channelopathy	106
cerebral ventricle	502	chaotic atrial tachycardia	174
cerebro-	13	chaps	318
cerebrospinal	7, 13	character	295

character of a pain	121
charge nurse	59
charge-coupled device	531
charley horse	25
checkup	72
cheek	442
cheekbone	442
cheilitis	6, 150
cheilognathopalatoschisis	338
cheilognathouranoschisis	150
cheiloplasty	152
cheilos	6
cheiloschisis	150
cheir	8
chelation therapy	118
chemical peeling	328
chemiluminescent enzyme immunoassay	80
chemiluminescent immunoassay	80
chemo-	13
chemoreceptor trigger zone	539
chemosis	127
chemotaxis	13
chemotherapy	13, 118
chenodeoxycholic acid	211
chest	444
chest colds	25
chest leads	178
chest pain	120, 155, 172
chest physiotherapy	169
chest roentgenogram	161, 180
chest x-ray	161, 180
chewing	195
chicken breast	27, 156
chickenpox	28, 330
chief cell	480
chief complaint	70, 95
Chief Concern	70
chilblain	27, 318, 320, 331
child	73
child abuse	343
child care	330
child care person	58
child health nursing	60
child molestation	343
child rearing	330
Child Welfare Act	46
childbed	230
childbed fever	27
childbirth	230
childhood illnesses	73
children's hospital	52
chill	105
chin	442
Chinese herbal medicine	118
chiropractic	118, 289
Chlamydia trachomatis	235
chlamydial inclusion bodies	235
chlamydial pneumonia	110
chlamydial urethritis	237
Chlamydophila pneumoniae	160
chloasma	319
chloramphenicol	423
chlorine	434
chlorpheniramine maleate	145
choked disk	130
cholagogue	211
cholangiocarcinoma	209
cholangiocellular carcinoma	209
cholangiography	203
cholangitis	209
chole-	13
cholecystectomy	215
cholecystitis	209
cholecystography	203
choledochal cyst	209
choledochoduodenostomy	3, 215
choledochojejunodenostomy	215
cholelithiasis	13, 209
cholera	107
choleretic	211
cholestasis	13, 19
cholesteatoma	143
cholic	35
choline acetyltransferase	530
cholinesterase	200
chondro-	13
chondroblastoma	13
chondrodermatitis noduralis helicis	140
chondrodystrophy	336
chondronecrosis	13
chondros	8
chondrosarcoma	8, 288
chord	35
chordae tendineae	470
chorditis	144
chorditis vocalis	144

chorditis vocalis inferior	144	cholangitis	208
chorea	299	chronic obstructive pulmonary disease	164
chorea with acanthocytes	116, 310	chronic pancreatitis	114
choreic	299	chronic pancreatitis	209
choreic abasia	300	chronic progressive external ophthalmoplegia	135
choreoathetosis	300		
chorioamnionitis	238	chronic pulmonary insufficiency of prematurity	336
choriocarcinoma	239		
chorion	232	chronic pulmonary thromboembolism	116
chorionic villi sampling	235		
choroid	35, 458	chronic renal failure	222
choroid plexus	504	chronic respiratory failure	166
choroidal detachment	134	chronic thromboembolic pulmonary hypertension	166
choroidal melanoma	135		
choroidal neovascularization	130	chronic thyroiditis	251
Christian Science	118	chylomicron	250
chromatin	508	chylous ascites	262
chromium	434	chyluria	218
chromo-	13	cibophobia	296
chromophobe	13	cicatricial contracture	281
chromosome	13, 508	cicatrix	83
chromosome analysis	267	ciclacillin	422
chromosome map	510	cilia	127, 456
chronic	91	ciliary body	458
chronic active hepatitis	207	cillosis	127
chronic bronchitis	165	cilostazol	315
chronic calcific pancreatitis	210	cimetidine	210
chronic calcifying pancreatitis	210	cineangiocardiography	182
chronic care nursing	60	cingulum membri inferioris	494
chronic eosinophilic pneumonia	164	cingulum membri superioris	492
chronic fatigue syndrome	104	cinoxacin	423
chronic functional abdominal pain	196	ciprofloxacin	424
		circa	21
chronic gastritis	205	circadian rhythm sleep disorder	312
chronic glomerulonephritis	221	circle	40
chronic granulomatous disease	533	circulating immune complex	322
chronic hepatitis	207	circulation	173
chronic inflammatory demyelinating polyneuropathy	112, 309	circum-	10
		circumcision	242
chronic interstitial nephritis	222	circumference	10
chronic kidney disease	222	circumscribed	10
chronic lymphocytic leukemia	271	circumventricular organs	502
chronic myelocytic leukemia	271	cirrhosis	35
chronic myelomonocytic leukemia	271	cirrhosis of the liver	208
		cisplatin	429, 532
chronic myeloproliferative disorders	270	cisterna chyli	478
		citrated blood	275
chronic neutrophilic leukemia	271	city hospital	52
chronic nonsuppurative destructive			

Term	Page
c-kit gene	508
cladribine	429
clamp	88
clap	26
clarithromycin	422
claustrophobia	18, 297
clavicle	25
clavicula	6, 492
clavicular	6
clavus	25, 318
clawhand	298
clean catch urine	218
clean intermittent catheterization	224
clean intermittent self-catheterization	224
clean-voided urine	218
cleft lip	150, 332
cleft palate	150, 332
cleidotomy	6
clerk	59
click	175
climacteric	229
clindamycin	423
clinic	52
clinic return date	93
clinical clerkship	67
clinical dementia rating	303
clinical diagnosis	84
clinical early exposure	67
clinical engineering technologist	59
clinical immunology	65
clinical informatics	64
clinical knowledge	68
clinical medicine	63
clinical nursing	66
clinical pathologist	60
clinical pathology	65
clinical pathway	89
clinical practice guideline	43
clinical professor	62
clinical psychologist	59
clinical research coordinator	58
clinical skills	68
clinical teacher	57
clinical test	78
clinical thermometer	77
clinical trainee	59
clinical-pathological conference	68
clinician	57, 59
clitoris	489
clockwise rotation	178
clomiphene citrate	241
clonazepam	316
cloning	510
Clonorchis sinensis	199
clonus	300
clopidogrel sulfate	315
closed chest cardiac massage	190
closed fracture	282
closed hospital	52
closed patch test	323
closed question	68
closed reduction	289
closure	88
closure of the anterior fontanelle	332
clot retraction	265
cloudy urine	216
clover	40
clozapine	316
clubbed finger	158
clubbing of digits	158
clubfoot	280
cluster headache	120
cluster of differentiation	531
coagulase-negative staphylococci	536
coagulating ability	262
coagulation factor	265
coagulation time	265
coagulum	262
coaptation splint	290
coaptation suture	88
coarctation of the aorta	183
coarse	35
coarse crackles	157
coated tongue	148
cobalt	434
cocaine	25
cocaine hydrochloride	122
coccidioidomycosis	108
-coccus	17
coccygeal plexus	506
coccygeal vertebra	492
coccyx	494
cochlea	459
cochlear duct	459
cochlear implant	146

cochlear microphonic potential	142	colostomy	19, 215
cochlear microphonics	142	colostrum	343
cochlear nerve	460, 505	colpitis	238
code of ethics	44	colposcopy	236
codeine phosphate	122, 167	columnae renales	486
codon	510	columnella nasi	460
coeur en sabot	180	coma	76, 297
coffee-ground materials	195	comatose	76
cognitive behavioral therapy	316	combination inhaled corticosteroid and long-acting inhaled $\beta 2$-agonist	169
cogwheel breathing	157		
coil embolization	317		
coin lesion	161	combined valvular disease	184
coition	228	combining form	2, 12
coitus	228	combining vowel	2
colchicine	259	comedical	61
cold	155	comedo	25, 320
cold agglutinin disease	270	comminuted fracture	282
cold compress	289	commode	90
cold hemagglutinin	268	common achievement tests	66
cold sore	26, 150	common acute lymphoblastic leukemia antigen	268
colectomy	214		
colestyramine	259	common bile duct	484
colic	35, 121	common carotid artery	471
colicky pain	121	common cold	155
colistin	423	common cold syndrome	163
collagen disease	106, 110	common hepatic artery	472
collapsing pulse	173	common hepatic duct	484
collarbone	25	common iliac artery	474
collecting duct	486	common iliac vein	478
college	62	common peroneal nerve	506
college of nursing	62	common variable immunodeficiency	273
college of nutrition	62		
colloid	35	communicable disease	106
colloid osmotic pressure	536	community health care	43
collyrium	136	Community Health Law	46
coloboma	131	community health nursing	60, 66
colon	6, 482	community medicine	43, 65
colonic	6	community-acquired infection	105
colonic cancer	207	community-acquired pneumonia	163
colonic diverticulosis	207	community-based learning	67
colonic polyp	206	comorbidity	106
colonoscope	6	compact bone	494
colonoscopic polypectomy	212	comparative genomic hybridization	82
colonoscopy	203		
colony-forming unit	533	competitive protein binding analysis	81
colony-stimulating factor	538		
color	39	complement	35
color vision	125	complement control protein	531
color vision test	131	complement fixation	82

complement receptor	537	condyloma acuminatum	25, 110, 237
complementarity-determining region	532	cone	40
		cone biopsy	78
complementary and alternative medicine	118	confabulation	302
		conference room	54
complementary DNA	510	confero	21
complement-fixing antibody	532	confidentiality	43
complete bed rest	89	confinement	230
complete blood cell count	263	conflict of interest	44
complete blood count	263	confluence of sinuses	476
complete denture	152	confused	297
complete fracture	281	confusion	297
complete left bundle branch block	179	congelation	25, 320
		congenital adrenal hyperplasia	254, 336
complete physical examination	72	congenital biliary atresia	338
complete remission	92	congenital clubfoot	340
complete right bundle branch block	179	congenital cystic adenomatoid malformation of lung	165
complex partial seizure	297	congenital diaphragmatic hernia	338
complex regional pain syndrome	121, 302	congenital disease	74, 106
compliance	86	congenital dislocation of the hip	287, 340
complications	93		
composite resin inlay	152	congenital dyserythropoietic anemia	269
compound fracture	281	congenital epulis	332
compound muscle action potential	304	congenital erythopoietic porphyria	335
comprehensive geriatric assessment	533	congenital esophageal atresia	338
comprehensive medical care	44	congenital heart disease	183, 338
comprehensive physical examination	72	congenital hemolytic anemia	269
		congenital hypothyroidism	336
compress	289	congenital ichthyosiform erythroderma	116
compression	289		
compression fracture	282	congenital muscular dystrophy	308
computed tomography	79	congenital rubella syndrome	109, 338
computer-based testing	67	congenital vascular nevus	25
computerized axial tomography	79	congestion	82
COMT inhibitor	315	congestive cardiomyopathy	187
con-	10	congestive heart failure	185
concave	197	conical cornea	128
concentrated red blood cells	275	conjoined	10
concentration	10	conjugated bilirubin	199
conception	229	conjunctiva	456
concha nasalis	460	conjunctival edema	127
condition at discharge	93	conjunctival injection	127
condom	230	conjunctival pallor	262
conductive deafness	142	conjunctival suffusion	262
conductive hearing loss	142	conjunctivitis	25

conjunctivochalasis	133
connecting peptide	247
connective tissue	512
consanguineous marriage	74
consanguinity	73
conscience	35
conscious	35, 76
consciousness	293
consensual light reflex	129
conservative therapy	117
consolidation	161
constipation	196, 215
constitutional disease	74
constitutional hyperbilirubinemia	208
constricting pain	172
constriction	173
constrictive pericarditis	186
consultant	57
consultation	84
consumption	28
contact bleeding	229
contact dermatitis	324
contact lens	126
contact urticaria	324
contagious disease	106
continued fever	105
continuing medical education	66
continuous ambulatory peritoneal dialysis	225
continuous arteriovenous hemofiltration	225
continuous cyclic peritoneal dialysis	225
continuous fever	105
continuous glucose monitoring	258
continuous hemodiafiltration	225
continuous hemofiltration	533
continuous hepatic arterial infusion	213
continuous murmur	175
continuous passive motion	290
continuous positive airway pressure	170
continuous positive pressure breathing	170
continuous positive pressure ventilation	170
continuous sounds	158
continuous subcutaneous insulin infusion	258
continuous suture	88
continuous traction	291
continuous venovenous hemofiltration	225
contra-	10
contraception	230, 241
contraceptive	241
contraceptive agent	241
contraceptive device	241
contracted kidney	223
contraction of visual field	132
contraction stress test	235
contracture	278
contraindication	10
contralateral	10
contralateral hemiplegia	299
contrast enhancement	532
contrast material	79
contrast medium	79
contrast radiography	79
controlled mechanical ventilation	169
contusion	25
convalescence	92
convergence of the folds	203
convergent strabismus	128
conversion disorder	312
convolution	35
convulsion	25, 35, 293
convulsive	293
convulsive status epilepticus	331
co-payment	48
co-payment rate	48
copernicium	436
copper	434
copper-wire artery	130
coprolalia	300
coprophobia	296
cor	7
cor pulmonale	7, 186
coracoacromial ligament	496
coracoclavicular ligament	496
cord	35
cord blood stem cell transplantation	276
core curriculum	67
corium	462
corn	25, 318
cornea	456

corneal abrasion	128	cosmetic dentistry	152
corneal erosion	128	cosmetic surgeon	60
corneal foreign body	128	cosmetic surgery	65
corneal leukoma	128	costa	9, 492
corneal opacity	128	costal	9
corneal reflex	301	costal arch	450
corneal sensitivity	128	costal cartilage	496
corneal transplantation	137	costal margin	450
corneal ulcer	128	costal respiration	154
Cornell Medical Index	303	costalgia	120
corniculate cartilage	495	costocervical trunk	472
corona dentis	464	costovertebral angle	452
coronal plane	448	costovertebral angle tenderness	217
coronary	27	cotton-wool patches	130
coronary angiography	182	cotton-wool spots	130
coronary arteriosclerosis	184	cough	155
coronary artery	471	cough medicine	167
coronary artery bypass graft	191	coughing	155
coronary artery bypass grafting	191	coulomb	438
coronary artery disease	184	counseling	316
coronary care unit	54	counterclockwise rotation	178
coronary heart disease	184	counterimmunoelectrophoresis	81
coronary sinus	476	counting fingers	127
coronary T wave	179	course	35, 91
Coronavirus	160	cover test	128
corpulent	105	cover-uncover test	128
corpus	5	coxal bone	494
corpus callosum	502	coxalgic gait	279
corpus cavernosum penis	488	coxarthrosis	285
corpus luteum	5	C-peptide	247
corpus luteum cyst	238	C-peptide immunoreactivity	247
corpus spongiosum penis	488	cracked-pot resonance	156
corpus striatum	503	cracks	318
corpus unguis	462	cradle	90, 330
corpus uteri	488	cramp	278, 293
corrected vision	126	cramps	25, 121
corrective exercise	290	cranial	8, 448
cortical bone	494	cranial bone	492
cortico-	13	cranial cavity	455
corticobasal degeneration	116	cranial nerves	505
corticospinal	13	craniofacial resection	146
corticotropin	13, 248	craniopharyngioma	313
corticotropin-like intermediate lobe peptide	248	craniotomy	8, 317
corticotropin-releasing hormone	248	cranium	8, 442
corticotropin-releasing hormone test	249	crater	40
		craving for ice	261
cortisol	249	crawl	330
coryza	155	C-reactive protein	537
		cream	86

creatine kinase	178, 283	crystalline lens	456
creatine kinase isoenzyme BB	534	crystallizable fragment	549
creatine kinase isoenzyme MB	178	crystalluria	218
creatine kinase isoenzyme MM	534	CT angiography	79
creatine phosphokinase	178	cube	40
creatinine clearance	219	cubic centimeter	438
credential society	66	cubital fossa	452
credentialism	66	cubital nodes	478
credibility	71	cubital tunnel syndrome	285
cremasteric reflex	301	cubitus valgus	280
crenated erythrocyte	264	cubitus varus	280
crenocyte	264	cuboid bone	494
creola body	159	culdocentesis	236
crescendo murmur	175	culdoscopy	236
crescent	40	cum	21
crescentic glomerulonephritis	221	cuneiform cartilage	495
CREST syndrome	111, 328	cup-disk ratio	130
cretinism	251, 336	cupping of the disk	130
cri du chat syndrome	336	curative dose	531
crib	330	curative treatment	118
crib death	339	cure	91
cribriform tissue	512	curettage	88
cricoid cartilage	495	curium	436
Crimean-Congo hemorrhagic fever	107	curriculum vitae	68
		cut	318
critical care nursing	60, 65	cutaneous	8
critical condition	76	cutaneous leukocytoclastic vasculitis	111
critical flicker frequency	131		
crocodile tongue	148	cutaneous lupus erythematosus	327
cross match	267	cutaneous lymphoid hyperplasia	327
cross-eye	27	cutaneous T-cell lymphoma	272, 327
cross-eyed	125	cutis	8, 318, 462
croup syndrome	340	cyanosis	158
crown	148	cyanotic	158
crown restoration	152	cyclic adenosine monophosphate	530
crown-rump length	232	cyclic citrulinated peptide	531
crural hernia	210	cyclic guanosine monophosphate	178
crus	446	cyclooxygenase-2 inhibitor	122
crush syndrome	222	cyclophosphamide	429
crust	318, 320	cycloserine	168, 424
crutch	279	cyclosporin A	276
cryosurgery	329	cylinder	40
cryotherapy	329	cylindruria	218
cryptogenic organizing pneumonitis	164	cynophobia	296
		cyst	83
cryptorchidism	236	cystadenocarcinoma	239
cryptorchism	236	cystadenoma	13
cryptosporidiosis	109	cystatin C	219
crystal-induced arthritis	286	cystectomy	226

cystic artery	472
cystic duct	484
cystic fibrosis	165
cystic fibrosis of pancreas	114, 210
cystine calculus	218
cystitis	223
cysto-	13
cystocele	239
cystoid macular edema	130
cystometry	220
cystoscope	8, 18
cystoscopic urography	220
cystoscopy	13, 221
cytapheresis	212, 276
cytarabine	429
cytarabine ocfosfate	431
-cyte	17
cytidine diphosphate	532
cytidine monophosphate	535
cyto-	13
cytochemistry	268
cytogenetics	63
cytokeratin 19 fragment	539
cytologic diagnosis	84
cytological examination	78
cytology	35, 78
cytomegalovirus	535
cytopathic effect	536
cytoplasm	13, 508
cytosine	510
cytotoxic	13
cytotoxic T-lymphocyte	538

D

D dimer	159, 266
dacarbazine	429
dacryocystitis	133
dacryocystorhinostenosis	133
dacryocystorhinostomy	136
daktylos	9
dalteparin sodium	275
dalton	438
danaparoid sodium	275
danazol	241
dandruff	318
dantrolene sodium hydrate	316
dapsone	541
darbepoetin alfa	274
dark glasses	126

dark-field microscopy	236
darmstadtium	436
darting	121
dasatinib	433
data	390
data base	95
date of birth	71
daughter	73
daunorubicin	429
daunorubicin hydrochloride	274
dawn phenomenon	246
day services center for the elderly	55
dazzling	127
de-	10
de facto	21
de novo	21
dead on arrival	542
deafferentation pain	121
deafness	139
dean of the school of medicine	62
death	74
death certificate	84
death with dignity	93
debility	104
debridement	88
deca-	20
decayed tooth	147
deceased	35
decerebrate rigidity	298
decerebration	10
deci-	20
deciduous tooth	149
deciliter	438
decimal reduction time	539
decitabine	274
Declaration of Helsinki	45
decline in ～	71
decompensated liver cirrhosis	208
decompression	87
decongestant	145
decrease in ～	71
decreased breath sounds	157
decreased position sense	262
decrescendo murmur	175
decubitus	318, 324
decubitus ulcer	25
deductible	49
deep artery of thigh	476

deep brain stimulation	316	delusion	293
deep cervical nodes	478	dementia	295
deep circumflex iliac artery	474	dementia nursing	61
deep fascia of thigh	501	demethylchlor-tetracycline	424
deep neck abscess	144	demography	35
deep pain	120	demonophobia	296
deep palmar arterial arch	472	demophobia	296
deep palmar venous arch	476	dendrite	40, 504
deep peroneal nerve	506	dengue	108
deep sensation	302	dengue fever	108
deep tendon reflex	300	dens	8
deep vein thrombosis	177	dense connective tissue	512
defecation	196	dental	8
deferoxamine	274	Dental Act	46
defibrillator	190	dental alveolus	465
deficiency disease	106	dental calculus	147
defined contribution pension	48	dental caries	147, 149
defined data base	96	dental cavity	149
definite diagnosis	84	dental cement	464
deformity	278	dental college	62
defuse	35	dental crown	464
degeneration	84	dental cusp	465
degenerative arthritis	285	dental enamel	464
degenerative disease	106	dental floss	147
degenerative joint disease	542	dental fluorosis	149
degree Celsius	438	dental formula	149
degree Fahrenheit	438	dental hygiene	147
dehydrated	105	dental hygienist	58
dehydration	10, 105	dental prosthesis	148
dehydration fever	105	dental pulp	464
dehydroepiandrosterone	541	dental root	464
déjà vue	293	dental technician	58
delayed cutaneous hypersensitivity	323	dental university	62
		dentin	464
delayed endolymhatic hydrops	113	dentinum	464
delayed growth	244	dentist	57, 59
delayed ischemic neurological deficit	306	dentistry	64
		dentition	149
delayed sleep phase syndrome	104	dentulous	149
delayed-type hypersensitivity reaction	323	denture	148
		Denver Developmental Screening Test	334
delirious	297		
delirium	297	Denver shunt	213
delirium tremens	25, 308	deoxycorticosterone acetate	542
delivery	230	deoxyribonucleic acid	511
delivery room	55	department head	59
deltoid ligament	496	D. of Allergy	53
deltoid muscle	498	D. of Anesthesiology	54
deltoid region	452	D. of Brain Surgery	54

D. of Cardiac Surgery	53
D. of Cardiology	53
D. of Cardiovascular Surgery	53
D. of Clinical Pathology	54
D. of Cosmetic Surgery	54
D. of Dentistry	53
D. of Dermatology	54
D. of Endocrinology	54
D. of Endoscopy	54
D. of Gastroenterology	53
D. of General Internal Medicine	53
D. of General Surgery	53
D. of Geriatrics	54
D. of Head and Neck Surgery	53
Department of Health	50
Department of Health and Human Services	50
D. of Hematology	53
D. of Hepatology	53
D. of Immunology	54
D. of Infectious Disease	53
D. of Internal Medicine	54
D. of Medicine	54
D. of Nephrology	53
D. of Neurological Surgery	54
D. of Neurology	53
D. of Neurosurgery	54
D. of Nuclear Medicine	53
department of nursing	54
D. of Obstetrics and Gynecology	53
D. of Oncology	53
D. of Ophthalmology	53
D. of Oral Surgery	53
D. of Orthodontics	53
D. of Orthopedic Surgery	53
D. of Orthopedics	53
D. of Oto(rhino)laryngology	53
D. of Pathology	54
D. of Pediatric Surgery	53
D. of Pediatrics	53
D. of physical therapy	55
D. of Plastic Surgery	53
D. of Proctology	53
D. of Psychiatry	53
D. of Psychosomatic Medicine	53
D. of Pulmonary Disease	53
D. of Radiology	54
D. of Respiratory Medicine	53
D. of Rheumatology	54
D. of Surgery	53
D. of Thoracic Surgery	53
D. of Transplant Surgery	53
D. of Urology	54
D. of Vascular Surgery	53
D. of Venereology	53
dependent	49
dependent edema	177
depilation	35, 245
depletion	35
depressed fracture	282
depression	25
depressive	295
depth electroencephalogram	304
deputizing service	43
derivative	2
derm(at)o-	13
derma	8
-derma	17
dermatitis	8, 324
dermatitis medicamentosa	324
dermatographism	319
dermatologist	60
dermatology	13, 17, 65
dermatome	301
dermatomyositis	111, 114, 327
dermis	318, 462
dermographism	319
dermography	13, 35, 319
dermoscopy	322
descending aorta	472
descending colon	482
descending genicular artery	476
descending part of the duodenum	482
desiccated thyroid gland	258
desmopressin acetate	259
desquamation	320
desquamative interstitial pneumonia	164
destructive spondyloarthropathy	224
des-γ-carboxy prothrombin	201
deterioration	91
detrusor-sphincter dyssynergia	223
detur	23
deuterium	539
development	244, 330
development nursing	65
developmental dysplasia of the hip	

	340	diaphragmatic hernia	25, 204
developmental glaucoma	134	diaphragmatic myocardial infarction	185
developmental language disorder	343	diaphragmatic respiration	154
developmental quotient	331	diaphysis	494
dexamethasone suppression test	249	diarrhea	196, 215
dextro-	13	diascopy	319
dextrocardia	13, 183	diastema	149
dextromanual	13	diastolic blood pressure	75
dextromethorphan hydrobromide hydrate	167	diastolic descent rate	181
di-	10	diastolic heart failure	186
dia-	10	diastolic murmur	175
diabetes insipidus	253	diathermy	10
diabetes mellitus	255	diazepam	314
diabetes nursing	61	diazoxide	258
diabetic coma	256	dibekacin	424
diabetic diet	91, 258	dichlorodiphenyltrichloroethane	541
diabetic ketoacidosis	256	diclofenac sodium	122
diabetic microangiopathy	256	dicrotic pulse	173
diabetic nephropathy	222, 256	didanosine	275
diabetic neuropathy	256	dideoxycytidine	275
diabetic retinopathy	135, 256	dideoxyinosine	275
diagnose	407	diebus alternis	23
diagnosis	70, 84, 401	diebus tertiis	23
diagnosis by exclusion	85	diencephalon	503
diagnosis ex juvantibus	85	diet	90, 194
diagnosis procedure combination	49	diet instructions	93
diagnosis-related group	49	diet therapy	117
Diagnostic and Statistical Manual of Mental Disorders	303	dietary habits	74
		dietary therapy	117
diagnostic criteria	84	dietetics	64
diagnostic error	85	diethylenetriamine pentaacetic acid	543
diagnostic imaging	64		
diagnostic impression	84	diethylstilbestrol	541
diagnostic parsimony	19	diethyltryptamine	541
diagnostic peritoneal lavage	204	dietician	57
diagnostic plan	96	diet-induced thermogenesis	105
diagnostician	57	dietitian	57
dialysate	225	differential blood count	263
dialysis amyloidosis	224	differential diagnosis	85
dialysis arthropathy	224	differentiation	84
dialysis encephalopathy	224	difficulty in ~	71
dialysis nursing	61	diffuse	35
dialyze	407	diffuse alveolar damage	166
dialyzer	225	diffuse axonal injury	307
diaper rash	318, 330	diffuse idiopathic skeletal hyperostosis	287
diaphoresis	10, 105		
diaphoretic	105	diffuse large B cell lymphoma	272
diaphragm	241, 444, 455, 466	diffuse Lewy body disease	542

diffuse panbronchiolitis	113, 164	director	59
diffusing capacity of the lung for carbon monoxide	162	director of nursing	59
		direct-vision biopsy	78
digestion	194	dirt-eating	261
digestive organ	480	dis-	10
digestive tract	480	disability of ~	71
digital	9	disability pension	49
digital rectal examination	77	disability-adjusted life year	539
digital subtraction angiography	79	disarticulation	10
digitalis	189	disaster medical assistance team	43
digitalization	189	disaster medical center	52
digitus	9	disc hemorrhage	130
dihydrotestosterone	234	discharge	73
dihydroxyphenylalanine	543	discharge diagnosis	93
diiodotyrosine	248	discharge instructions	93
dilatation and curettage	242	discharge medication	93
dilated cardiomyopathy	115, 187	discharge orders	93
dilation	87	discharge summary	93
dimer	10	discoid lupus erythematosus	327
dimercaptosuccinic acid	542	discomfort in ~	71
dimethyl sulfoxide	542	discontinuous sounds	157
dimple	442	discreet	35
dining room	54	discrete	35
dinitrochlorobenzene	542	discus nervi optici	130
dinitrochlorobenzene test	323	disdialysis syndrome	224
dinitrophenylhydrazine test	333	disease	72
diopter	539	diseased	35
diosopyrobezoar	209	disease-free interval	92
dioxide	10	disease-free survival	92
dipeptidyl peptidase	543	disease-modifying antirheumatic drug	288
diphenhydramine hydrochloride	145		
diphtheria	107	diseases of blood	261
diphtheria-tetanus-pertussis vaccine	343	diseases of medical practice	106
		disequilibrium	139
diplegia	299	disinfection	10
diploid	511	diskectomy	291
diploma	67	diskography	284
diplopia	125	dislocation	278
dipstick	218	disodium cromoglycate	167, 543
direct antiglobulin test	267	disorder	72
direct bilirubin	199	disoriented	76
direct Coombs test	267	disposable contact lens	136
direct current	540	disposable gloves	77
direct fluorescent antibody technique	81	dissecting aneurysm	187
		dissection	87
direct hemoperfusion	225	disseminated intravascular coagulation	274
direct inguinal hernia	210		
directional coronary atherectomy	191	disseminated spinal canal stenosis	112

disseminated superficial actinic porokeratosis	327
dissemination	83
dissertation	66
dissociative disorder	312
distal	448
distal interphalangeal joint	495
distal pancreatectomy	215
distal tubule	486
distant metastasis	82
distended	197
distended bladder	217
distention of the abdomen	197
distoclusion	149
distraction	297
distraught	297
distress	71
ditto	21
diuresis	35
diuretic	188, 224
diuretic agent	224
diuretics	35
divergent strabismus	128
diverticulitis	205
divorce	74
dizziness	28, 139, 172, 293
docetaxel	429, 431
doctor	57
Doctor of Medicine	66
Doctor of Philosophy	66
doctor on call	57
doctor's office	54
doctorless area	44
dolicho-	13
dolichocephaly	13
dolichocolon	13
doll's eye sign	298
dominant gene	511
domperidone	211
donepezil hydrochloride	315
donor lymphocyte infusion	276
dopamine	250
dopamine agonist	259, 315
dopamine hydrochloride	189
dope	27
doripenem	424
dorsal	14, 448
dorsal decubitus	76
dorsal pancreatic artery	474
dorsal venous arch	478
dorsalis pedis artery	476
dorsalis pedis pulse	177
dorso-	14
dorsosacral position	77
dorsoventral	14
dorsum manus	452
dorsum of foot	453
dorsum of hand	452
dorsum of the nose	460
dorsum of tongue	464
dorsum pedis	453
dose-limiting toxicity	542
dotage	295
double eyelid	126
double helix	511
double immunodiffusion	81
double noun	485
double renal pelvis	223
double vision	125
double-contrast radiography	203
double-filtration plasmapheresis	225
double-stranded DNA	511
doubt	85
douche	289
doughnut	40
doxorubicin	429, 430
doxycycline	424
doxyfluridine	541
doze	104
drain	89
drainage	88
drawer sign	280
dream	104
dressing changes	90
dribbling	216
drinking	74
drip infusion	86
drip infusion cholangiography	203
drip infusion pyelography	220
drivel	147
drool	147
drop foot	280
drop hand	298
drop-foot gait	298
droplet infection	105
drowsiness	297
droxidopa	315
drug eruption	324

英語索引　735

drug therapy	117	dysmenorrhea	10, 25, 228
drug-eluting stent	191	dysosmia	140
drug-induced hypersensitivity syndrome	327	dyspareunia	229
		dyspepsia	10, 26, 194
drug-induced lymphocyte stimulation test	323	dysphagia	35, 195
		dysphagia nursing	61
drug-resistant pseudomonas infection	110	dysphasia	18, 35
		dysphonia	35, 140
drusen	130	dysphoria	35
dry cough	155	dyspnea	18, 154, 172
dry eye	133	dyspnea at rest	154
dual-energy x-ray absorptiometry	283	dyspnea on exertion	154
		dysprosium	435
dubnium	436	dysthymic disorder	312
duct of Steno	464	dystocia	230
ductal carcinoma in situ	240	dysuria	216
due date	230		
dull	121, 156	**E**	
dullness	156		
dumbbell	40	ear	442, 458
dumping syndrome	206	ear discharge	139
duodenal bulb	482	ear speculum	77
duodenal diverticulum	205	earache	120, 139
duodenal juice	512	eardrum	139, 458
duodenal papilla	482	earlobe	442, 458
duodenal ulcer	205	early antigen	544
duodenitis	205	early diagnosis	84
duodenoscopy	203	early diastolic murmur	175
duodenum	482	early exposure	67
duplex Doppler ultrasonography	305	early gastric cancer	205
duplicated renal pelvis	223	early stage	91
dura mater	504	early systolic murmur	175
dural sinuses	476	early-morning hyperglycemia	246
dutasteride	224	earwax	25, 139
dwarfism	245	Eastern equine encephalitis	108
dynamic computed tomography	79	easy bruisability	261
dynamic lung compliance	532	eating disorder	312
dynamic splint	290	ebastine	145
dynamometer	283	Ebola hemorrhagic fever	107
dyne	438	ecchymosis	261
-dynia	17, 71	eccrine gland	462
dys-	10, 71	echinococcosis	108
dysarthria	302	*Echinococcus*	199
dyscalculia	302	echinocyte	264
dyschromatopsia	125	echocardiogram	181
dysfunctional uterine bleeding	239	echocardiography	181
dysgeusia	147	echolalia	300
dyslexia	302	eclampsia	238
dyslipidemia	256	ecology	63
		-ectasis	17

Term	Page
ecto-	10
ectoderm	10
-ectomy	17
ectopic	10
ectopic ACTH syndrome	253
ectopic atrial tachycardia	174
ectopic pregnancy	237
ectropion	127
ectropium	127
eczema	319
edaravone	315
edema	83, 173, 216
edentate	148
edentulous	148, 149
edrophonium chloride test	305
education	74
Educational Commission for Foreign Medical Graduates	66
educational objective	66
educational plan	96
efavirenz	275
effective dose	545
efferent	34
efferent neuron	504
effort angina	185
egophony	157
eicosapentaenoic acid	547
einsteinium	436
ejaculation	228
ejaculatory duct	488
ejection fraction	182
ejection murmur	175
ejection sound	175
elastase 1	202
elastic tissue	512
elbow	444
elbow joint	495
elbowed catheter	90
electric pulp tester	150
electric response audiometry	141
electric shock therapy	316
electro-	14
electrocardiogram	17, 178
electrocardiography	17, 178
electrochemiluminescent immunoassay	81
electrocoagulation	14
electrocochleography	142
electroconvulsive therapy	316
electrocorticogram	304
electrodermal audiometry	141
electrodermogram	324
electroencephalogram	3, 304
electroencephalography	304
electrokymography	546
electromyogram	14, 283
electron microscope	79
electronic health record	546
electronic medical record	43
electronystagmography	132
electro-oculogram	132
electro-olfactogram	143
electrophysiologic study	180
electroretinogram	132
electrosalivogram	150
electroshock therapy	316
elemental diet	90
elevation	289
elicit	35
elimination diet	90
elixir	86
ellipse	40
ellipsoid	40
elusion	36
emaciated	105
emaciation	105, 244
embedded tooth	149
embryo	231
embryology	63
embryonic stem cell	547
emergency and critical care center	52
emergency contraceptive	241
emergency department	54
emergency hospital	52
emergency medical technician	58
emergency medicine	64
emergency nursing	60
emergency room	54
emerging infectious disease	106
emesis	195
emesis basin	90
EMG syndrome	339
-emia	17
emission computed tomography	545
emmetropia	131
emollient	328
emotional instability	295

emotional lability	295	endoscopic examination	78
empiric therapy	118	endoscopic hemostasis	212
employees' health insurance	49	endoscopic injection sclerotherapy for varices	212
employees' pension insurance	48		
employer's name	71	endoscopic mucosal resection	212
emporiatrics	65	endoscopic nasobiliary drainage	213
empty sella syndrome	313	endoscopic operation	212
empty-nest syndrome	229	endoscopic papillotomy	212
emtricitabine	275	endoscopic polypectomy	212
emulsion ointment	328	endoscopic retrograde biliary drainage	213
en-	10		
encapsulated	10	endoscopic retrograde cholangio-pancreatography	203
encapsulating peritoneal sclerosis	224		
encephalitis	8, 14, 26, 307	endoscopic sphincterotomy	212
encephalo-	14	endoscopic submucosal dissection	212
encephalocele	8, 17		
encephaloduroarteriosynangiosis	317	endoscopic surgical procedure	212
encephalomalacia	14, 17	endoscopic ultrasonography	204
encephalon	8	endoscopic variceal ligation	212
enchondromatosis	288	endoscopist	60
encopresis	331	endoscopy	78
end-diastolic pressure	182	Endoscopy Unit	54
end-diastolic volume	182	endosteum	494
endemic	35, 106	endotracheal intubation	168
endemic disease	106	endotracheal tube	168
endo-	10	endovaginal ultrasonography	236
endobronchial ultrasonography	163	endovascular treatment	192
endocardial cushion defect	183	endowment insurance	49
endocarditis	186	end-stage renal disease	222
endocardium	470	end-systolic pressure	182
endocochlear potential	142	end-systolic volume	182
endocrine organ	490	enema	90
endocrine system	75	enema syringe	90
endocrine therapy	117	English as a foreign language	66
endocrinologist	60	English as a second language	67
endocrinology	65	English for medical purposes	2
endoderm	10	enkephalos	7, 8
endodontics	152	enlarged lymph nodes	262
endogenous	10	enlargement of ~	71
endometrial biopsy	236	enocitabine	429
endometrial carcinoma	239	enophthalmos	128
endometriosis	239	enoxacin	425
endometritis	238	entacapone	315
endomyocardial fibrosis	187	entecavir hydrate	211
endoplasmic reticulum	508	enteral nutrition	91, 212
endoscopic biliary drainage	544	enteric cytopathogenic human orphan virus	545
endoscopic biopsy	78		
endoscopic dilator	213	enteric-coated tablet	544
		enteritis	205

entero-	14	ephelis	319
enteroadherent *Escherichia coli*	202	epi-	10
Enterobacteriaceae	202	epicanthal folds	127
Enterobius vermicularis	199	epicanthus	127
enterochromaffin	14	epicardium	470
enterococcus	14	epicranial aponeurosis	501
Enterococcus	219	epidemic	106
enterocolitis	8	epidemic disease	106
enterohemorrhagic *Escherichia coli*	202	epidemic keratoconjunctivitis	110, 133
enterohemorrhagic Escherichia coli infection	107	epidemic parotitis	26, 110, 151, 330
enteroinvasive *Escherichia coli*	202	epidemiology	63
enteron	8	epidermal burn	320
enteropathogenic *Escherichia coli*	202	epidermal growth factor	546
enteroscopy	203	epidermal growth factor receptor	546
enterostomy	215	epidermis	462
enterotoxigenic *Escherichia coli*	202	epidermolysis bullosa	116, 327
ento-	10	epidermolysis bullosa simplex	339
entomophobia	296	epididymis	488
entotic	10	epididymitis	236
entozoon	10	epidural	10
entrapment neuropathy	282, 285	epidural anesthesia	87
entropion	127	epidural block	123
entropium	127	epidural blood patch	316
enucleation	87, 137	epidural hematoma	307
enureis	34	epidural hemorrhage	307
enuresis	26, 217, 331	epiduroscopy	123
enviomycin	425	epigastralgia	120
environmental health	63	epigastric pain	120
environmental health nursing	66	epigastric pain syndrome	195
Environmental Law	46	epigastric region	450
environmental medicine	64	epigastrium	444, 450
environmental pollution	43	epigenetics	510
enzyme	10	epiglottic cartilage	495
enzyme immunoassay	81	epiglottis	466
enzyme multiplied immunoassay technique	81	epiglottitis	144
enzyme-linked immunosorbent assay	81	epilation	245
eosinophil	264	epilepsy	293
eosinophilia	18, 265	epileptic	293, 294
eosinophilia-myalgia syndrome	286	epileptic seizure	26, 293
eosinophilic cationic proteins	159	epiloia	326
eosinophilic fasciitis	114, 285	epiluminescence microscopy	322
eosinophiluria	218	epimacular membrane	130
epalrestat	258	epinephrine	189, 250
ephelides	26	epiphora	126, 133
		epiphysial ischemic necrosis	286
		epiphysis	494
		epiploic foramen	482

epiretinal membrane	130	erythrocyte	17
epirubicin	430	erythrocyte count	263
episcleritis	133	erythrocyte sedimentation rate	266
episiotomy	243	erythrocytosis	265
epistaxis	26, 140, 261	erythroderma	14, 17, 319
epithalamus	503	erythrodermia	319
epithelial cast	218	erythroleukemia	270
epithelial membrane antigen	546	erythromycin	425
epithelial pearls	332	erythrophobia	296
epithelial tissue	512	erythropoiesis	18
epithelium	10	erythropoietic protoporphyria	335
epitrochlear nodes	478	erythropoietin	268
eplerenone	188	*Escherichia coli*	219
epoetin alfa	274	esophageal	7
epoetin beta	274	esophageal artery	472
eponychium	462	esophageal cancer	205
eponym	38	esophageal diverticulum	204
epoophoron	488	esophageal intraluminal pressure	201
epulis	149	esophageal manometry	202
equilateral triangle	39	esophageal speech	145
equilibrium test	143	esophageal varix	204
equinia	108	esophagectomy	214
equivocal symptom	104	esophagitis	7
erbium	435	esophagogastric junction	480
erect position	76	esophagogastroduodenoscopy	203
erectile dysfunction	237	esophagus	26, 480
erection	228	esophoria	128
erector spinae muscles	500	esotropia	35, 128
ergot derivatives	122	essential hypertension	184
ergotamine tartrate	122	essential thrombocythemia	271
erlotinib	168, 433	established diagnosis	84
erosion	318, 320	estetrol	234
erotomania	18	esthetic dentistry	152
eructation	26, 195	estimated blood loss	544
eruption	318	estimated delivery date	230
erysipelas	326	estimated glomerular filtration rate	
erythema	319		219
erythema exudativum multiforme		estradiol	234, 241
	326	estramustine	430
erythema induratum	325	estriol	234
erythema infectiosum	339	estrogen	234
erythema multiforme	326	estrogen receptor	234
erythema multiforme exudativum		estrogen replacement therapy	241
	326	estrone	234
erythema nodosum	326	et alii	21
erythrasma	325	et cetera	21
erythro	14	et sequens	21
erythroblast	14, 266	etanercept	288
erythroblastosis fetalis	335	ethambutol	425

ethambutol hydrochloride	168		190
ethanol	548	excision	10, 88
ethics committee	44	excision of the breast	243
ethionamide	168, 425	excitable	295
ethmoid sinusitis	144	excitatory postsynaptic potential	547
ethmoidal sinus	460	excoriation	320
ethmoiditis	144	excrement	196
ethology	65	excretion	10
ethosuximide	316	exempli gratia	21
ethyl icosapentate	259	exercise	67
ethylene oxide gas	547	exercise stress test	180
ethylenediaminetetraacetic acid	545	exercise test	180
ethylenediaminetetraacetic acid infusion test	250	exercise therapy	117
		exercise-induced asthma	163
etiologic diagnosis	84	exertional dyspnea	154
etiology	35	exfoliative cytology	78
etoposide	430, 432	exhaustion	104
etymology	2, 35	exo-	11
etymon	2	exocrine	11
eu-	10, 94	exomphalos	339
euglobulin lysis time	266	exomphalos-macroglossia-gigantism syndrome	546
eunuchism	231		
eunuchoid	231	exon	510
euphoria	10	exophoria	128
europium	435	exophthalmic ophthalmoplegia	135
eustachian salpingitis	143	exophthalmos	26, 128, 246
eustachian tube	459	exoskeleton	6
euthanasia	26, 93, 94	exotropia	11, 35, 128
euthyroid	10	expandable metallic stent	213
evaluation of medical practice	42	expectant mother	229
eversion of the eyelids	127	expectant treatment	118
evidence-based medicine	67	expected date of confinement	230
evidence-based nursing	67	expected date of delivery	230
evoked electromyogram	283	expectorant	167
evoked otoacoustic emission	334	expectoration	155
ex-	10	expensive care	48
exa-	20	experimental medicine	63
examination room	54	expiration	154
examining room	54	expiratory reserve volume	162
exanthem	318	expired carbon dioxide tension	162
exanthema	318	expired carbon monoxide concentration	162
exanthema subitum	110, 339		
excavatio rectouterina	231	expired nitric oxide concentration	162
excessive ~	71		
excessive daytime sleepiness	104, 156	expired-air analysis	162
excessive flow	228	exploration	87
excessive menstrual bleeding	228	exploratory laparotomy	214
exchange transfusion	343	exposure of the palpebral conjunctiva	127
excimer laser coronary angioplasty			

extended family	73
extension	279
extension contracture	281
extensor	448, 498
extensor carpi radialis	498
extensor carpi ulnaris	498
extensor digitorum	498
extensor retinaculum	498
extensor tendon	501
external	448
external auditory canal	458
external cardiac massage	190
external carotid artery	471
external ear	458
external genitals	444
external iliac artery	474
external iliac vein	478
external jugular vein	476
external oblique muscle of abdomen	500
external otitis	143
external pudendal artery	476
external rotation	279
external strabismus	128
external urethral orifice	488, 489
external-beam radiation therapy	117
extirpation	88
extra-	11
extracapsular cataract extraction	137
extracellular	11
extracellular fluid	512
extracorporeal circulation	192
extracorporeal membrane oxygenation	343
extracorporeal shock wave lithotripsy	225
extracorporeal ultrafiltration method	225
extracranial-intracranial bypass	317
extractable nuclear antigen	546
extrahepatic portal obstruction	113, 208
extraocular movement	129
extraocular muscles	458
extrapyramidal syndrome	299
extrauterine pregnancy	237
extravasation	11
extravascular fluid	512
extravascular lung water	162
extremely low birth weight infant	331
extremitas inferior	447
extremitas sternalis claviculae	447
extremitas superior	447
extremitas superior testis	447
extremity	447
extrovert	296
exudate	26
exudation	83
exudative retinitis	134
exude	319
eye	442, 456
eye bank	138
eye chart	131
eye drops	127
eye mucus	126
eyeball	442, 456
eyebrow	442, 456
eyeground	458
eyelash	127, 456
eyelid	126, 442, 456
eyepatch	136
eyesight	125
eyesight test	131
eyesight test chart	131
eyestrain	126
eyewash	136
ezetimibe	259

F

face	442
face presentation	232
face scale	122
facial	5, 35
facial artery	472
facial nerve	505
facial pain	120
facial paralysis	294
facial plethora	262
facial vein	476
facies	5
faculty development	66
faculty of medicine	62
failure to thrive	331
fainting	293
faith	74
falciform ligament of liver	484
fallopian pregnancy	237

fallopian tube	488
false joint	282
false pains	121
falter	294
famciclovir	329
familial	35
familial adenomatous polyposis	207
familial amyloid polyneuropathy	309
familial combined hyperlipidemia	256
familial disease	106
familial polyposis coli	207
familial sudden death syndrome	113
familiar	35
family	73
family doctor	57
family health nursing	60
family history	70, 95, 397
family medicine	64
family nursing	65
family physician	57
family problems	96
family tree	73
farad	438
farcy	108
faropenem	425
farsighted glasses	126
far-sightedness	125
fascia	500
fascia investiens	500
fascia lata	501
fascial	35
fascicular zone	490
Fasciolopsis	199
fasting blood sugar	246
fat	105
fat embolism syndrome	549
fatal familial insomnia	112
father	73
father-in-law	73
fatigability	104
fatigable	104
fatigue	104
fatigue fracture	282
fatness	105
fatty cast	218
fatty liver	207
fatty tissue	512
faucial tonsil	465
favus	318

febrile convulsions	331
febrile seizure	331
fecal Helicobacter pylori antigen	202
fecal incontinence	196, 331
fecal occult blood	199
feces	196
fee for medical services	49
feebleness	104
feeding	89
fee-for-service plans	49
feeling	295
feet	438
felon	326
female genital organ	488
female genitalia	488
female reproductive system	488
feminism	244
feminization	244
feminizing syndrome	240
femoral	7
femoral artery	474
femoral hernia	210
femoral neck fracture	282
femoral nerve	506
femoral pulse	176
femoral triangle	452
femoral vein	478
femorotibial angle	279
femto-	20
femur	7, 494
femur length	232
fenestra cochleae	459
fenestra vestibuli	459
fenestration	87, 291
fentanyl	122
fentanyl citrate	122
fermium	436
ferritin	268
fester	319
festering	318
festinating gait	298
festination	298
fetal alcohol syndrome	338
fetal distress	232
fetal heart rate	232
fetal heart tone	232
fetal movement	232
fetal presentation	232, 233
fetoplacental unit	231

fetor hepaticus	197	fissure fracture	282
fetus	231	fissure in ano	207
fever	105	fissured tongue	148
fever of unknown origin	105	fist	446
fever sore	26	fits	25, 26
feverless	105	fixation	87
fibrates	259	fixed bridge	152
fibric acid derivatives	259	fixed partial denture	152
fibrin degradation product	266	flaccid paralysis	298
fibrinogen	266	flank	444
fibro-	14	flank pain	120, 216
fibroadenoma	240	flap operation	152
fibroblast growth factor	550	flapping tremor	197
fibroblast growth factor receptor 3	550	flashlight	77
		flat	197
fibrodysplasia ossificans progressiva	116, 341	flat plate	203
		flatfoot	280
fibroid	239	flatulence	26, 196
fibroidectomy	243	flatus	26, 197
fibroma	14, 83	flaval ligaments	496
fibromuscular dysplasia	184	flavin adenine dinucleotide	548
fibromyalgia	286	fleeting blindness	125
fibromyoma	239	fleroxacin	425
fibrosis	14, 83	flesh-colored	39
fibrous tissue	512	flexion	279
fibula	494	flexion contracture	281
fibular	448	flexion deformity	279
field hospital	53	flexor	448, 498
field of vision	132	flexor carpi radialis	498
fifth disease	339	flexor carpi ulnaris	498
filgrastim	274	flexor retinaculum	498
filiform papilla	464	flexor surface of hand	452
filling	87	floaters	126
filling defect	203	floating kidney	223
filtration fraction	220	floating patella	280
fimbriae tubae	488	flomoxef	425
final diagnosis	84	floor	55
fine crackles	158	floor nurse	59
fine needle aspiration	78	flow cytometry	549
fine-needle biopsy	78	flow sheet	96
finger cot	77	flow-volume curve	162
fingerbreadth	549	flu	26, 155
finger-nose test	300	fluconazole	425
fingerprint	444	fluctuation	197
fingers	444	flucytosine	425
fingertip	444	fludarabine	430
finger-to-nose test	300	fluid ounce	438
first cranial nerve	505	fluid wave	197
first-degree burn	320	fluorescein angiography	132

fluorescence in situ hybridization	81	foreign body	127
fluorescence microscope	79	foreign-body sensation	126
fluorescence polarization immunoassay	81	forelock	442
		forensic medicine	63
fluorescent antibody	548	foreskin	488
fluorescent antibody technique	81	forgetfulness	295
fluorescent antinuclear antibody	549	form pus	319
fluorescent enzyme immunoassay	81	formula	343
fluorescent immunoassay	81	fornix	480, 502
fluorescent treponemal antibody absorption test	236	fornix of vagina	231
		fornix vaginae	231
fluoride	152	fosamprenavir calcium	275
fluorine	434	fosfestrol	429, 541
flushing	319	fosfluconazole	425
fluticasone propionate	145, 169	fosfomycin	425
flying flies	126	fossa	35
focal epilepsy	297	fossae	35
focal glomerulosclerosis	222	foul breath	147
focal infection	106	fourchette	489
focal nodular hyperplasia	550	fourth ventricle	502
foci	35	fourth-degree burn	320
focus	35	fovea	35
focus charting	89	fovea centralis	130, 458
focused ultrasound surgery	551	foveated chest	156
foetoe ex ore	148	foveola gastricae	480
folic acid	268, 274	fraction of inspired oxygen	162
folk remedies	118	fractional excretion of sodium	220
follicle-stimulating hormone	234, 249	fracture	278
follicular adenoma	252	Fracture Risk Assessment Tool	278
follicular keratosis	324	fradiomycin	425
follicular lymphoma	272	fragmented red blood cell	264
folliculitis	325	francium	436
fonticulus major	332	freckles	26, 318
fonticulus minor	332	free radical scavenger	315
food	194	free thyroxine	247
food poisoning	196	free thyroxine index	247
Food Sanitation Act	46	free triiodothyronine	248
food stamp program	50	French-American-British classification	262
food substitution table	258		
foot	438, 446	frenulum labiorum pudendi	489
foot bath	89	fresh frozen plasma	276
foot clonus	301	Freund complete adjuvant	549
forced expiratory volume	162	frigidity	229
forced expiratory volume in one second	162	frigotherapy	329
		front teeth	147
forceps	88	front tooth	442
forceps delivery	230	frontal assessment battery	303
forearm	444	frontal bone	492
forehead	442	frontal lobe	502

frontal muscle	498
frontal plane	448
frontal region	450
frontal sinus	460
frontal sinusitis	144
frontotemporal dementia	311
frostbite	25, 318, 320
frozen shoulder	278
frozen-thawed red blood cells	276
full denture	152
full pulse	173
full-term spontaneous delivery	230
full-thickness burn	320
fulminant hemolytic streptococcus infection	109
fulminant hepatitis	113, 207
fulminant type 1 diabetes mellitus	255
functional brace	289
functional disease	106
functional dyspepsia	204
functional electrical stimulation	291
functional independence measure	92
functional murmur	175
functional neck dissection	146
functional neuromuscular stimulation	316
functional orthosis	289
functional residual capacity	162
functional uterine bleeding	239
fundus oculi	458
fundus uteri	488
funduscopy	131
fungal lung disease	165
fungous	36
fungus	36
funiculitis	236
funnel chest	156
funny bone	497
furosemide	188
furred tongue	148
furrowed tongue	148
furuncle	26, 318
fusidic acid	425
fusion	133

G

gabapentin	316
gadolinium	79, 435
gag reflex	141
gait	77
galactorrhea	246
galactosemia	333
galea aponeurotica	501
galeophobia	297
gallbladder	484
gallbladder adenomyomatosis	209
gallbladder cancer	209
gallbladder polyp	209
gallium	434
gallon	438
gallop rhythm	175
galvanic skin reflex	304
gamete	235
gamete intrafallopian transfer	242
Gamma Knife	317
γ-aminobutyric acid	552
γ-glutamyltransferase	199
γ-hydroxybutyric acid	552
gamophobia	296
ganglion	285, 504
ganglion geniculi nervi facialis	505
gangrenous stomatitis	151
Gardnerella vaginalis	235
garenoxacin	425
gargle	86, 147, 152, 344
gargling	147
gargoylism	344
gas	26
gas chromatography	80
gas chromatography-mass spectrometry	80
gas pains	195
gaseous distention	196
gash	318
gas-liquid chromatography	80
gas-oxygen-ether anesthesia	87
gas-oxygen-fluothane anesthesia	87
gas-oxygen-isoflurane anesthesia	87
gasp	154
gasserian ganglion	505
gassiness	196
gas-solid chromatography	80
gastēr	5

gastrectomy	17, 214	gemsitabine hydrochloride	168
gastric	5	gemtuzumab ozogamicin	433
gastric adenoma	205	-gen	17
gastric analysis	201	gender identity disorder	240
gastric angle	480	gene	508
gastric antral vascular ectasia	205	gene amplification	509
gastric antrum	480	gene arrangement	509
gastric biopsy	204	gene conversion	509
gastric body	480	gene deletion	509
gastric bypass	260	gene expression	509
gastric cancer	205	gene fusion	509
gastric fundus	480	gene locus	509
gastric gland	480	gene map	509
gastric hyperacidity	26	gene pool	509
gastric inhibitory polypeptide	247	gene therapy	117
gastric irrigation	211	genealogical tree	73
gastric juice	512	geneion	5
gastric lavage	211	general anesthesia	87
gastric pits	480	general hospital	52
gastric polyp	205	general instructional objective	66
gastric submucosal tumor	205	general manager	59
gastric ulcer	205	General Medical Council	553
gastritis	14	general practitioner	57
gastro-	14	general surgeon	59
gastrocnemius muscle	500	generalist	57
gastroduodenal artery	474	generalized anxiety disorder	312
gastroenterologist	59	generalized epilepsy	297
gastroenterology	64	generic	36
gastroesophageal reflux disease	204	generic drug	85
gastrogavage	212	generic name	86
gastrointestinal endocopy	203	-genesis	17
gastrointestinal stromal tumor	205	genetic	36
gastrointestinal symptoms	194	genetic code	509
gastrointestinal system	75	genetic engineering	63
gastrointestinal tract	26, 480	genetically modified organism	553
gastrojejunostomy	14, 214	genetics	63
gastrolith	5, 209	genicular	7
gastropexy	18	geniculate ganglion	505
gastroptosis	18, 205	geniohyoid	5
gastroschisis	339	genital chlamydial infection	110
gastroscopy	203	genital herpes	237
gateway drug	124	genital herpes simplex	237
gatifloxacin	425	genital herpesvirus infection	110
gauss	438	genital ulcer	231
gauze	89	genitofemoral nerve	506
gavage	212	genitourinary system	75
gefitinib	168, 433	genome	510
gelatinous tissue	512	genomic imprinting	510
gemcitabine	430	genomics	510

genophobia	296	Glasgow Coma Scale	297
genotype	509	Glasgow Outcome Scale	92
gentamicin	425	glasses	126
genu	7, 36	glaucoma	133
genu valgum	26, 280	glenoid cavity	495
genu varum	26, 279	glenoid fossa of scapula	495
genupectoral position	77	glial fibrillary acidic protein	305
genus	36	glibenclamide	258
geographic tongue	148	glimepiride	258
geophagia	261	glioblastoma	313
geriatric hospital	53	glioma	313
geriatric nursing	66	Global Assessment of Functioning	
geriatrician	60	scale	92
geriatrics	65	globus pallidus	503
German measles	27, 109, 330	glomerular basement membrane	486
germanium	434	glomerular filtration rate	219
germ-free	25	glomerular zone	490
gerontological nursing	60	glomerulonephritis	26
gerontology	65	glomerulus	486
gerontoxon	128	gloomy	295
gestational diabetes mellitus	256	glōssa	7
gestational hypertension	238	glossalgia	147, 261
gestational sac	231	glossectomy	152
get goosebumps	318	glossitis	7, 151, 262
get gooseflesh	318	glossodynia	18, 147, 261
giant cell arteritis	187	glossopharyngeal nerve	505
giant cell tumor	288	glossophytia	148
giant lymph node hyperplasia	272	glossopyrosis	147, 261
giant papillary conjunctivitis	133	glossospasm	148
giant platelet syndrome	273	glottis	466
giardiasis	109	glottis edema	141
gibbosity	281	glucagon-like peptide	247
gibbus	281	glucocorticoid receptor anomaly	115
giddiness	139	glucocorticoid-remediable aldoster-	
giga-	20	onism	254
gigantism	245	glucose tolerance test	247
gingiva	7, 147, 464	glucose transporter	553
gingival	7	glucosuria	218
gingival hemorrhage	149	glutamic acid decarboxylase	552
gingival hypertophy	262	glutamic-oxaloacetic transaminase	
gingivitis	7, 151		553
girdle pain	121	glutamic-pyruvic transaminase	553
glabella	442	glutathione disulfide	554
gland	36	gluteal region	452
glandular fever	26	gluteus maximus muscle	500
glandular tissue	512	gluteus medius muscle	500
glans	36	gluteus minimus muscle	500
glans penis	488	glycated hemoglobin	247
glaring	127	glycemic index	244, 247

Term	Page
glycerin enema	90
glyco-	14
glycoalbumin	247
glycogen storage disease	257
glycogen storage disease type I	257
glycogen storage disease type II	257
glycogen storage disease type III	257
glycogen storage disease type IV	257
glycogen storage disease type V	257
glycogenesis	14
glycogenosis	257
glycoprotein	14
glycosuria	218, 244
glycosylated hemoglobin	247
gnawing	121
gobbledygook	4
goiter	246
gold	436
gold salts	288
gonad	488
gonadotropic hormone	234
gonadotropin-releasing hormone	234
gonadotropin-releasing hormone agonist	241
gonalgia	278
gonarthrosis	286
gonatocele	7
goniometer	283
gonioscopy	131
goniosynechiolysis	137
gonitis	286
gonococcal arthritis	286
gonococcal infection	110
gonococcus	235
gonorrhea	26, 237
gonorrheal arthritis	286
gonorrheal ophthalmia	26
gony	7
good clinical practice	552
goserelin acetate	224
gout	257
gouty arthritis	286
gouty attack	244
government hospital	52
government-managed health insurance	49
grade	67
graded exercise test	180
graduate school	62
graduation thesis	67
graft	9
graft-versus-host disease	274
grain	438
gram	438
-gram	17
gram-negative bacillus	202
gram-positive cocci	553
grand mal epilepsy	297
grandfather	73
grandmother	73
granisetron hydrochloride	211
granular cast	218
granular cell tumor	552
granular layer	462
granulation	83
granule	83, 86
granulocyte	17, 264
granulocyte colony-stimulating factor	552
granulocyte transfusion	276
granulocyte-macrophage colony-stimulating factor	276
granulocytopenia	265
granuloma	83
granuloma inguinale	237
-graphy	17
grasping forceps	89
gravida	229
gray	39, 438
gray hair	319
grayish	39
graze	318
great pancreatic artery	474
great saphenous vein	478
great toe	446
greater curvature	480
greater omentum	482
greater trochanter	494
green	39
green fluorescent protein	552
greenish	39
greenstick fracture	282
gridiron incision	88
grip	278
grip dynamometer	283
griping	121
grippe	155
griseofulvin	329, 425

groin	26, 444
gross hematuria	218
ground glass appearance	161
group checkup	72
group home for the elderly with dementia	55
group practice	43
growing pains	25, 121
growling	196
growth	244, 330
growth curve	330
growth disorder	244
growth hormone	249
growth hormone-inhibiting hormone	249
growth hormone-releasing hormone	249
growth hormone-secreting pituitary adenoma	252
growth retardation	244
guanine	510
guanosine diphosphate	552
guanosine monophosphate	553
guanosine triphosphate	554
guarding	198
guided bone regeneration	153
guided tissue regeneration	152
gullet	26
gum	126, 147, 442
gum bleeding	261
gum hypertrophy	262
gunshot wound	554
gurgling	196
gurney	90
gustation	147
gustation test	150
gustatory hypesthesia	147
gustatory organ	464
gut-associated lymphoid tissue	552
guts	26
gutta	23
guttae	23
gymnophobia	297
gyncology	14
gyneco-	14
gynecologist	60
gynecology	65
gynecomastia	14, 197, 246
gynephobia	296
gyrus of cerebrum	502

H

H$_1$-receptor antagonist	145
H$_2$ blocker	210
H$_2$-receptor antagonist	210
habits	74
habitual abortion	238
hacking cough	155
Haemophilus influenzae	159
Haemophilus influenzae type b vaccine	344
hafnium	435
haima	6
hair	462
hair (of the head)	442
hair folliculus	462
hair root	462
hair shaft	462
hairiness	245
hairless	319
hairy	319
hairy tongue	148
hairy-cell leukemia	271
half-life for radiochromium-labeled red blood cells	269
halitosis	26, 148
hallucination	293
hallux	446
hallux valgus	280
halo vision	126
halo-pelvic traction	291
hamartoma	83
hamartophobia	296
hamate bone	492
hammer	77, 459
hammer toe	280
hamstring tendon	501
hand	444
hand lens	78
hand movement	127
hand-assisted laparoscopic surgery	213
hand-foot-and-mouth disease	110, 339
hanging arm cast	289
hangover	195
hantavirus pulmonary syndrome	108
haploid	509
haplotype	511

haptoglobin	266
hard contact lens	136
hard exudate	130
hard palate	464
hard pulse	173
hardening of the arteries	25
hare's eye	127
harelip	147
hassium	436
haustra coli	482
haustra of colon	482
haversian system	494
hay fever	25, 27, 140, 144
head	442
head and neck reconstruction	146
head and neck tumor	145
head circumference	76, 232
head cold	155
head doctor	27
head line	446
head mirror	77
head nurse	59
head of the pancreas	484
head pharmacist	59
head presentation	232
head technologist	59
headache	120, 244
healing	91
health	104
Health and Medical Service Law for the Elderly	47
health care cost	42
health care cost control program	42
health care coverage	48
health care facility for the elderly	55
health care system	44
Health Center Act	46
health certificate	67
health examination	72
health expenditure	49
health food	194
health insurance	48, 71
health insurance certificate	48
Health Insurance Portability and Accountability Act	50
health insurance reimbursement	48
health insurance society	48
health maintenance organization	50

Health Policy Bureau	43
Health Promotion Law	46
health university	62
health-care facilities	52
health-care team	95
healthy	104
hearing	139
hearing acuity	139
hearing aid	145
hearing test	141
heart	470
heart attack	27, 172
heart catheterization	182
heart failure	172, 185
heart failure with normal left ventricular ejection fraction	186
heart line	446
heart murmur	173, 175
heart rate	75
heart sound	175
heart transplantation	192
heart trouble	172
heartbeat	172
heartburn	27, 195
heart-lung machine	192
heart-type fatty acid-binding protein	178
heat exhaustion	105
heat rash	27, 318, 330
heat shock protein	558
heat stroke	105
heat-stable alkaline phosphatase	234
heaving	195
heavy chain disease	273
heavy ion therapy	117
hecto-	20
heel	446
heel-knee test	300
heel-to-knee test	300
height	76
helical computed tomography	79
Helicobacter pylori	201
Helicobacter pylori eradication therapy	211
heliotrope eruption	319
helium	434
helix	40, 458
HELLP syndrome	238
hemadsorption test	161

hemadsorption virus	160
hemagglutination	81
hemagglutination inhibition	81
hemagglutinin	554
hemangioma	83, 326
hemarthrosis	280
hematemesis	195
hematinics	274
hematochezia	195
hematocrit	263
hematologic test	78
hematologist	59
hematology	2, 64
hematoma	261
hematometra	239
hematopoiesis	18
hematopoietic organs	261
hematopoietic stem cell transplantation	276
hematopoietic system	75, 261
hematoporphyrin derivative	136
hematoxylin and eosin stain	555
hematuria	216
hemi-	11
hemianopia	132
hemianopsia	132
hemiazygos vein	476
hemiballism	300
hemicrania	11, 120
hemimandibulectomy	3
hemiplegia	11, 18, 294, 299
hemiplegic	299
hemiplegic gait	298
hemisphere	40
hemithorax	36
hemo-	14
hemochromatosis	209, 257
hemodiafiltration	225
hemodialysis	6, 225
hemodialysis-associated amyloidosis	224
hemofiltration	225
hemoglobin	263
hemoglobin A1c	247
hemoglobinopathy	269
hemoglobinuria	218
hemolysis	17, 262
hemolytic anemia	115
hemolytic disease of the newborn	335
hemolytic uremic syndrome	273
hemophagocytic lymphohistiocytosis	272
hemophagocytic syndrome	272
hemophilia	14, 26, 274
hemophilic arthritis	286
hemoptysis	155
hemorrhage	83, 261
hemorrhagic fever with renal syndrome	108
hemorrhagic shock and encephalopathy syndrome	339
hemorrhoid	207
hemorrhoidectomy	215
hemorrhoids	26
hemostasis	19, 36, 87, 262
hemostat	89
hemostatic forceps	89
hemothorax	14, 36, 167
Hendra virus infection	108
henry	438
hepaplastin test	265
hēpar	5
heparin	189
heparin-induced thrombocytopenia	273
heparinized blood	275
hepatectomy	215
hepatic	5
hepatic abscess	208
hepatic blood flow	201
hepatic encephalopathy	208
hepatic failure	208
hepatic fetor	148
hepatic flexure	482
hepatic lobule	484
hepatic portal	484
hepatic vein	478
hepatitis	2, 26
hepatitis A	107
hepatitis A (B, C, D, E)	207
hepatitis A (B, C, D, E, G) virus	200
hepatitis B core antigen	200
hepatitis B envelope antigen	200
hepatitis B immune globulin	555
hepatitis B surface antigen	200
hepatitis B virus DNA quantification	201

hepatitis C virus RNA detection by amplification with RT-PCR	201
hepatitis C virus serotype	201
hepatitis E	107
hepatitis virus marker	200
hepatitis-associated antigen	200
hepato-	14
hepatocellular	14
hepatocellular carcinoma	208
hepatocyte growth factor	200
hepatojugular reflux	175
hepatolenticular degeneration	209
hepatologist	59
hepatology	64
hepatoma	208
hepatomegaly	5, 14, 198, 262
hepatorenal syndrome	222
hepatosplenomegaly	3
heptavalent pneumococcal conjugate vaccine	344
herbal medicine	119
herbalism	119
hereditary angioedema	324
hereditary angioneurotic edema	324
hereditary coproporphyria	257
hereditary disease	73, 106
hereditary elliptocytosis	269
hereditary erythroblastic multinuclearity associated with positive acidified serum	269
hereditary hemorrhagic telangiectasia	274
hereditary motor and sensory neuropathy	309
hereditary nonpolyposis colorectal cancer	207
hereditary nonspherocytic hemolytic anemia	269
hereditary progressive arthro-ophthalmopathy	341
hereditary sensory and autonomic neuropathy	309
hereditary spherocytosis	269
hermaphrodism	240, 254
hermaphroditism	240, 254
hernia	26
herniated intervertebral disk	287
herniated nucleus pulposus	287
herniation of the intervertebral disc	26
herniorrhaphy	18, 215
herpangina	110, 339
herpes labialis	150
herpes simplex	26, 324
herpes simplex encephalitis	307
herpes simplex virus	322
herpes zoster	26, 324
hertz	438
hetero-	14
heteroantibody	14
heterochromia iridis	128
heterologous insemination	242
heteronym	38
heteronymous hemianopia	132
heterophile	14
heterophoria	128
heterotopia	36, 82
heterotopic pancreas	210
heterotropia	36, 125
hexagon	39
hiatal hernia	204
hiatus hernia	204
hiccup	27, 155
high blood sugar	26
high calorie diet	90
high fiber diet	90
high medical expenses	48
high protein diet	90
high right atrial electrogram	180
high tibial osteotomy	292
high-altitude cerebral edema	306
high-altitude pulmonary edema	166
high-cost medical care	48
high-density lipoprotein	555
high-density-lipoprotein cholesterol	250
high-frequency oscillation	170
high-frequency ventilation	556
high-intensity focused ultrasound	226
highly active antiretroviral therapy	275
highly-advanced medical technology	48
high-output heart failure	186
high-performance liquid chromatography	81
high-power field	558

Term	Page
high-resolution computed tomography	79
hilar nodes	478
hilar shadow	161
hilum of the lung	466
hip	444
hip joint	495
hip osteoarthritis	285
hippocampus	502
hippocratic face	76
Hippocratic Oath	45
hirci	444
hircismus	321
hirsute	319
hirsutism	245, 255
histogenesis	17
histological diagnosis	93
histological examination	78
histology	63
histone	511
histopathology	63
historical	36
history of present illness	70
histrionic personality disorder	313
hives	28, 318
hoarse voice	140
hoarseness	140, 244
hobbies	74
hobble	294
hollow foot	280
holmium	435
holmium laser ablation of the prostate	226
holmium laser enucleation of the prostate	226
holosystolic murmur	175
home address	71
home blood pressure	75
home care	43
home enteral nutrition	91
home for the elderly with a moderate fee	55
home health care	43
home oxygen therapy	169
home parenteral nutrition	91
home remedies	118
home-based medical care	43
homeo-	14
homeopathy	14, 119
homeostasis	14, 36
homeostasis model assessment of insulin resistance	247
homeotic gene	511
home-visit nursing care	44
homework	67
homocystinuria	333
homogeneous	36
homogenous	36
homologous insemination	242
homonym	38
homonymous hemianopia	132
homophone	38
homosexuality	231
honeycomb	40
honeycomb lung	161
honeycomb ringworm	318
hookworm	199
hora	23
hora somni	23
hordeolum	26, 133
horizontal	448
horizontal fissure	466
horizontal infection	106
horizontal plane	448
hormonal therapy	117
hormone replacement therapy	241
hormone therapy	117
horny layer	462
horrors	25
hospice	55
hospital	52
hospital information system	44
hospital pharmacist	58
hospital staff	59
hospital-acquired pneumonia	163
hospitalist	57
hospitalization	72
hot flashes	229
hot pack	289
house physician	57
housekeeping gene	511
HOX genes	508
HTLV-1-associated myelopathy	116, 309
human chorionic gonadotropin	234
human epidermal growth factor receptor type 2	234
human genome project	556

human growth hormone	556	hygienics	63
human histocompatibility leukocyte antigen	557	hyoid bone	492
		hypalgesia	301
human immunodeficiency virus	556	hypalgia	301
human leukocyte antigen	667	hyper-	11, 71
human menopausal gonadotropin	234	hyperacidity	195
		hyperacusis	139
human normal immunoglobulin	344	hyperadrenocorticism	253
Human papillomavirus	235	hyperalgesia	17, 301
human papillomavirus vaccine	242	hyperalgia	301
human parvovirus B19	334	hyperbaric medicine	64
human placental lactogen	234	hypercalcemia	251
human serum albumin	558	hypercapnia	159
human T-lymphotropic virus 1	267	hypercholesterolemia	256
human T-lymphotropic virus 2	267	hyperchromia	263
humerus	492	hypercoagulability	266
humming-top murmur	176	hypercorticalism	253
humoral hypercalcemia of malignancy	251	hyperemesis gravidarum	26, 237
		hyperemia	83
humpback	278	hypereosinophilic syndrome	271
hunger	194	hyperesthesia	301
hunger pain	195	hyperextension	279
hyaline cast	218	hyperglycemia	26, 246
hyaline membrane disease	334	hyperglycemic hyperosmolar nonketotic coma	256
hyaluronate sodium	289		
hyaluronic acid	200	hyperhidrosis	245, 321
hydatid mole	238	hyperkalemia	219, 251
hydatidiform mole	238	hyperlipidemia	3, 256
hydralazine hydrochloride	189	hyperlipoproteinemia	256
hydrarthrosis	280	hypermagnesemia	251
hydro-	14	hypermenorrhea	228
hydrocele testis	237	hypermetrope	125
hydrocephalus	14, 306, 332	hypermetropia	125
hydrocephaly	332	hypernatremia	251
hydrogen	14, 434	hypernephroma	223
hydrogen ion concentration	158	hyperope	125
hydrogen ion exponent	584	hyperopia	125
hydronephrosis	223	hyperosmolar nonketotic coma	256
hydrophilic contact lens	136	hyperparathyroidism	252
hydrophilic ointment	328	hyperphagia	194
hydrophobia	108	hyperphosphatemia	251
hydrophobic contact lens	136	hyperpituitarism	252
hydrosalpinx	238	hyperplasia	18, 82
hydrotherapy	119, 289	hyperprolactinemia	253
hydrothorax	167	hypersensitivity pneumonia	163
hydroxycarba-mide	430	hypersexuality	296
hydroxymethylglutaryl-Coenzyme A reductase inhibitor	259	hypersomatotropism	253
		hypersomnia	312
hydroxyproline	283	hypersplenism	270

hypertension	11, 184, 217	hypophyseal dwarf	253
hypertensive heart disease	184	hypophysectomy	259
hypertensive retinopathy	135	hypophysial fossa	461
hyperthermia	11	hypophysis	490
hyperthyroidism	2, 251	hypopituitarism	116, 252
hypertrichosis	245, 321	hypoplasia	83
hypertriglyceridemia	256	hypoplastic left heart syndrome	338
hypertrophic cardiomyopathy	115, 187	hypoproteinemia	219
hypertrophic nonobstructive cardiomyopathy	187	hypoptyalism	148
		hypopyon	129
hypertrophic obstructive cardiomyopathy	187	hyposmia	140
		hypospadia	223
hypertrophic pulmonary osteoarthropathy	158	hypospermatogenesis	3
		hyposthenuria	219
hypertrophic pyloric stenosis	338	hypothalamic-pituitary-adrenal axis	558
hypertrophy	19, 83		
hyperuricemia	250	hypothalamus	490, 503
hyperventilation syndrome	166	hypothyroidism	11, 251
hyperviscosity syndrome	559	hypotonic duodenography	203
hypesthesia	301	hypoventilation syndrome	166
hyphema	129	hypoxemia	159
hypnotherapy	118	hypoxia	11, 159
hypnotic	117, 314	hypoxic-ischemic encephalopathy	334
hypo-	11	hystera	6
hypoadrenocorticism	115, 254	hysterectomy	17
hypoaldosteronism	254	hysteria	17, 296
hypoalgesia	301	hysterical	36
hypocalcemia	251	hystero-	14
hypochondriac	36	hysteropexy	6, 14, 243
hypochondrium	36	hysterosalpingectomy	243
hypochromia	263	hysterosalpingography	3, 236
hypocoagulability	266	hysteroscope	14
hypodermis	462	hysteroscopic insemination into tube	242
hypogastrium	452		
hypoglossal nerve	505	hysteroscopic selective hydrotubation	242
hypoglycemia	17, 246		
hypoglycemic coma	256	hysteroscopy	236
hypogonadism	235, 254		
hypokalemia	251	**I**	
hypomagnesemia	251	-ia	17
hypomelanosis	319	iatro-	14
hypomenorrhea	228	iatrogenic	14
hyponatremia	219, 251	iatrogenic disease	106
hypo-osmotic swelling test	235	ibidem	21
hypoparathyroidism	252	ibritumomab tiuxetan	433
hypopharyngeal cancer	145	ibuprofen	122
hypophosphatemia	251	ice	289
hypophyseal adenoma	313	ice pack	289
		ichthyophobia	296

ichthyosis	320	ileocolic artery	474
ichthyosis vulgaris	325	ileum	36, 482
ICM Code of Ethics for Midwives	44	ileus	206
		iliac	36
ICN Code of Ethics for Nurses	44	iliac crest	452
icosapentaenoic acid	562	iliac nodes	479
icteric	197	ilial	36
icterometer	333	iliocostal muscle	500
icterus	26, 36, 196, 197	iliofemoral ligament	496
ictus	36	iliohypogastric nerve	506
id est	21	ilioinguinal nerve	506
idarubicin	430	iliolumbar ligament	496
idem	21	iliopsoas muscle	500
identification	71	ilium	36, 494
identifying information	70	illacrimation	133
idio-	14	illicit	35
idiopathic	14	illness	72
idiopathic bilateral sensorineural hearing loss	113	illusion	36
		imaging diagnosis	84
idiopathic cardiomyopathy	187	imatinib mesilate	274, 433
idiopathic hyperaldosteronism	253	imidafenacin	224
idiopathic hypertrophic subaortic stenosis	187	imipenem/cilastatin	425
		imipramine hydrochloride	314
idiopathic interstitial pneumonia	113, 164	immature	244
		immediate hypersensitivity reaction	322
idiopathic necrosis of the femoral head	113		
		immune adherence hemagglutination	82
idiopathic neonatal hepatitis	335		
idiopathic osteonecrosis due to corticosteroid	113	immune complex	559
		immunization	343
idiopathic osteonecrosis of the femoral head	286	Immunization Law	47
		immunoelectrophoresis	82
idiopathic portal hypertension	113, 208	immunoglobulin E	323
		immunological test	78
idiopathic pulmonary fibrosis	164	immunologist	60
idiopathic thrombocytopenic purpura	115, 273	immunology	63
		immunophenotyping	268
idiopathic thrombosis	115	immunoradiometric assay	82
idiosyncrasy	14	immunoreactive glucagon	247
ifosfamide	430	immunoreactive insulin	247
IgA nephropathy	115, 221	immunosuppressant	274
IgM class antibody to hepatitis A virus	201	immunosuppressive acidic protein	559
		immunosuppressive therapy	117
IgM class antibody to hepatitis B core antigen	201	impacted cerumen	140
		impacted fracture	282
ileac	36	impaction	140
ileal	36	impaired fasting glucose	247
ileal artery	474	impaired glucose tolerance	247
ileocecal valve	482		

impaired hearing	139
impaired vision	125
imperforate anus	338
impetigo	318, 320, 331
impetigo contagiosa	324
impingement syndrome	284
implant denture	152
implantable cardioverter-defibrillator	190
implantable insulin pump	258
implantable pacemaker	190
implanted pacemaker	190
impotence	228
improvement	91
in-	11
in chronological order	72
in situ	21
in toto	21
in utero	21
in vitro	21
in vitro fertilization	242
in vitro fertilization and embryo transfer	242
in vivo	22
inability of ~	71
inactivated poliovirus vaccine	562
inactivation	11
inactive problem	96
inborn genetic disease	106
incarcerated hernia	198
incarceration	9
incentive spirometry	169
inch	438
incidence	36
incidents	36
incision	87
incision and drainage	560
incisive tooth	464
incisor	464
inclusion body	559
inclusion body myositis	285
incomplete bundle branch block	179
incomplete fracture	281
incontinence	11
incontinent	196
incoordination	300
increase in ~	71
incretin	247
incubator	343
incurable disease	107
incus	459
indemnity	49
index case	73
index finger	444
indifferent	295
indigestion	26, 194
indirect antiglobulin test	267
indirect bilirubin	199
indirect Coombs test	267
indirect fluorescent antibody technique	80
indirect hemagglutination	80
indirect inguinal hernia	210
indirect ophthalmoscopy	131
indium	435
indocyanine green test	200
indolent	9
indomethacin	122
induced abortion	229
induced delivery	241
induced pluripotent stem cell	562
inducing cause	72
inductively coupled plasma mass spectrometry	82
Industrial Safety and Health Act	47
indwelling catheter	90, 225
infancy	36
infant	330
infant respiratory distress syndrome	339
infantile autism	343
infantile cortical hyperostosis	340
infantile eczema	339
infantile paralysis	294, 331
infantile polycystic kidney	339
infantile spasm	332
infarction	83
infection	105
infection control	61
infection control nurse	560
infection control nursing	60
infection control team	560
infection of the tubes	27
infectious arthritis	286
infectious disease	106, 107
infectious endocarditis	186
infectious endophthalmitis	133
infectious enterocolitis	206

infectious erythema	110, 339	infrequent menstruation	228
infectious gastroenteritis	110	ingrowing toenail	281
infectious mononucleosis	26, 271	ingrown nail	281
infective endocarditis	186	ingrown toenail	281
inferior	448	inguen	26
inferior epigastric artery	474	inguinal hernia	210, 338
inferior extensor retinaculum	500	inguinal ligament	496
inferior lingular segment (S^5)	468	inguinal nodes	479
inferior mesenteric artery	474	inguinal triangle	452
inferior mesenteric vein	478	inhalation anesthesia	87
inferior myocardial infarction	185	inhalation therapy	169
inferior nasal meatus	460	inhalator	169
inferior oblique muscle	458	inhaled corticosteroids	169
inferior pancreaticoduodenal artery	474	inhaler	169
inferior rectus muscle	458	inherited disease	73
inferior sagittal sinus	476	inhibitor of intesitinal cholesterol transporter	259
inferior turbinate	460	inhibitory postsynaptic potential	562
inferior vena cava	478	in-home care	43
inferior vesical artery	474	initial plan	95
inferiority complex	296	initial stage	91
infertility	229	initial symptom	72
infertility nursing	61	initialism	56
infiltrate	161	initiation	36
infiltration	83	injection	26
infiltration anesthesia	87	injection of trigger points	123
inflammation	82	injection sclerotherapy	212
inflammation of a testis	236	injure	407
inflammation of the glans penis	237	injury	73
inflammation of the spermatic cord	236	injury severity score	76
inflammatory bowel disease	206	inlay restoration	152
inflammatory cells	82	innocent murmur	175
inflection	2	innocuous	36
infliximab	211, 289	inoculable	36
influenza	26, 109, 155	inoculation	26, 343
Influenza A virus	160	inorganic murmur	175
Influenza B virus	160	inquiry-based learning	67
influenza vaccine	344	insect bite	318
influenza virus antigen	160	insomnia	104
information source	71	insomniac	104
informed consent	95	inspection	77
infra-	11	inspiration	154
inframammary region	450	inspiratory capacity	162
infraorbital	11	inspiratory reserve volume	162
infraorbital region	450	instep	446
infrared	11, 36	institution	36
infrascapular region	452	institutional review board	43
infraclavicular region	450	instrumental activities of daily living	92

insufficiency fracture	282	interferon-gamma release assay	160
insulin antibody	247	interleukin	561
insulin glargin	258	intermaxillary fixation	290
insulin glulicine	258	intermediate coronary syndrome	185
insulin resistance	247	intermediate cuneiform bone	494
insulin sensitivity test	250	intermediate tubule	486
insulin tolerance test	250	intermediate-acting insulin	258
insulin-dependent DM	255	intermenstrual	11
insulinlike growth factor-I	249	intermenstrual bleeding	229
insulinlike growth factors	249	intermenstrual pain	228
insulinoma	255	intermenstrual spotting	229
insurance benefits	49	intermittent claudication	173
insurance company	49	intermittent fever	105
insurance ID number	71	intermittent hydronephrosis	339
insurance policy	49	intermittent mandatory ventilation	170
insurance premium	49	intermittent peritoneal dialysis	225
insured	49	intermittent positive pressure breathing	170
insured person	49	internal	448
intake and output	562	internal capsule	503
integument	75, 318, 462	internal carotid artery	471
integumentum commune	462	internal derangement of the elbow joint	340
intelligence quotient	303	internal derangement of the knee joint	286
intelligence test	303	internal ear	459
intense	121	internal iliac artery	474
intensity-modulated radiation therapy	117	internal iliac vein	478
intensive care	61	internal jugular vein	476
intensive care unit	54	internal medicine	65
inter-	11	internal oblique muscle of abdomen	500
interarticular cartilage	496	internal pacemaker	190
interatrial septum	470	internal pudendal artery	474
intercostal	11	internal rotation	279
intercostal artery	472	internal strabismus	128
intercostal muscle	498	internal thoracic artery	472
intercostal nerve	505	International Cancer Genome Consortium	560
intercostal neuralgia	121	International Classification for Nursing Practice	4
intercostal space	175	International Classification of Diseases	85
interdental brush	147	International Classification of Functioning, Disability, and Health	92
interdental space	149	International Confederation of Midwives	44
interdisciplinary	66	International Council of Nurses	44
interferon	211		
interferon alfa	430		
interferon alfa-2b	430		
interferon beta	430		
interferon gamma-1a	430		
interferon gamma-n1	430		
interferon regulatory factor	509		
interferon sensitivity determining region	201		

international normalized ratio	562	intracapsular cataract extraction	137
International Pharmacopeia	85	intracardiac injection	86
International Prognostic Index	263	intracellular	11
international prostate symptom score	217	intracellular adhesion molecule	560
		intracellular fluid	512
International Red Cross	562	intracerebral hemorrhage	306
International Scientific Vocabulary	4	intracoronary thrombolysis	190
International Statistical Classification of Diseases and Related Health Problems, Tenth Revision	3	intracranial	36
		intracranial aneurysm	307
		intracranial hematoma	307
		intracranial hypertension	304
International Unit	563	intracranial pressure	304
internist	60	intractable	121
interposition	87	intractable disease	106, 111
interposition arthroplasty	292	intractable nephrotic syndrome	115
interprofessional education	67	intractable optic neuropathy	113
interpupillary distance	129	intracytoplasmic sperm injection	242
interrupted breathing	157	intradermal injection	86
interrupted suture	88	intradermal test	323
interruption of pregnancy	229	intraductal papillary mucinous neoplasm	562
interscapular region	452		
intersexuality	254	intraductal ultrasonography	204
interspinal ligament	496	intrahepatic bile duct	484
interstitial cell-stimulating hormone	249	intrahepatic cholelithiasis	114, 209
		intrahepatic cholestasis	208
interstitial fluid	512	intramedullary nailing	291
interstitial lung disease	164	intramuscular injection	86
interstitial pneumonia	164	intraocular lens	137
intertrigo	320	intraocular pressure	129
intertrigo labialis	153	intraoperative radiotherapy	117
interventional radiology	117	intraperitoneal injection	86
interventricular septum	470	intraperitoneal pregnancy	237
intervertebral cartilage	496	intraretinal microvascular abnormality	130
intervertebral disk	496		
intestinal	8	intrathecal	563
intestinal clamps	89	intrathecal baclofen	315
intestinal flora	202	intrathecal injection	86
intestinal gland	483	intrauterine adhesion	239
intestinal juice	513	intrauterine contraceptive device	241
intestinal obstruction	206		
intestinal pseudo-obstruction	206	intrauterine device	241
intestinal tract	480	intrauterine fetal death	232
intestine	480	intrauterine growth retardation	232
intestinum	8	intravascular ultrasonography	182
intimal thickening	305	intravenous	11
intima-media thickness	305	intravenous anesthesia	87
intra-	11	intravenous hyperalimentation	91, 212
intra-aortic balloon pumping	192		
intra-articular injection	86	intravenous injection	86

intravenous pyelography	220
intraventricular hemorrhage	307
intrinsic factor	268
intrinsic sympathomimetic activity	563
introduction	392
introitus	232
intron	510
introvert	296
intussusception	338
Inulead	220
inulin clearance	220
inverted T wave	179
investigational new drug	85
investing layer	500
involuntary motion	294
involuntary movement	294
iodine	435
ipsilateral hemiplegia	299
irbesartan	188
iridium	436
iridocyclitis	134
iridology	118
irinotecan	429
iris	456
iritis	134
iron	434
iron preparations	274
iron-deficiency anemia	269
irregular ~	71
irregular menstruation	228
irregular pulse	172
irregularity in ~	71
irreversibility	91
irreversible	91
irritable	295
irritable bowel syndrome	206
ischemia	83
ischemic colitis	206
ischemic contracture	281
ischemic heart disease	184
ischemic optic neuropathy	134
ischiatic neuralgia	121
ischiofemoral ligament	496
ischium	494
ischuria	216
isepamicin	425
islet cell adenoma	255
islet cell antibody	247
islet cell surface antibody	247
islet cell tumor	210
islet transplantation	259
-ism	17
iso-	11
isoelectric line	178
isokinetic exercise	290
isolation hospital	52
isometric exercise	290
isoniazid	168, 425
isoniazid sodium methanesulfonate	425
isonicotinic acid hydrazide	168
isosceles triangle	39
isosorbide dinitrate	189
isosorbide mononitrate	189
isotonic	11
isotonic exercise	290
isotope	11
isthmus uteri	488
itch	27
itching	27, 319
-itis	17
itraconazole	329, 426
ixabepilone	433

J

jacksonian epilepsy	297
Japan Association for Bioethics	44
Japan Coma Scale	297
Japan Council for Quality Health Care	44
Japan Medical Association	44
Japan Pharmaceutical Association	44
Japan Society for Medical Education	67
Japanese B encephalitis vaccine	344
Japanese edition of Denver Developmental Screening Test	334
Japanese encephalitis	108
Japanese encephalitis virus	564
Japanese Nursing Association	44
Japanese Pharmacopoeia	85
Japanese Society of Hospital Pharmacists	44
Japanese spotted fever	108
jargon	2
jaundice	26, 196, 197, 262
jaw	442

jecur	5
jejunal artery	474
jejunum	482
jerk nystagmus	129
JMA Code of Medical Ethics	45
job	74
jockstrap itch	27, 318
joint	495
Joint Commission International	43
Joint Commission on Accreditation of Healthcare Organizations	42
joint loose body	280
joint mobility	280
joint mouse	280
joint pain	120, 278
joint replacement	291
joint sense	302
joint space narrowing	284
joint swelling	278
josamycin	426
joule	438
judo therapist	58
jugular pulse wave	180
jugular venous distention	174
jumper's knee	279
junctura	5
junior college	62
juvenile emphysema	114
juvenile rheumatoid arthritis	340
juvenile-onset diabetes mellitus	255
juxta-	14
juxta-articular	14
juxtaglomerular	14
juxtaglomerular apparatus	486

K

kanamycin	426
kardia	7
karyo-	14
karyolysis	14
karyorrhexis	18
karyotype	508
karyotyping	14
kelvin	438
kephalē	5
keratic precipitates	128
keratinization	320
keratitis	14, 36
kerato-	14
keratoconjunctivitis sicca	133
keratoconus	128
keratodermia	321
keratodermia tylodes palmaris progressiva	324
keratoplasty	137
keratosis	14, 36, 320
kernicterus	335
ketoacidosis	247
ketoconazole	329, 426
ketone body	247
ketonuria	218
ketotifen fumarate	145
key hospital for AIDS treatment	52
kidney	486
kidney calculus	223
kidney calices	486
kidney stone	223
kidney transplantation	226
kidney trouble	216
kilo-	20
kilobase	510
kilogram	438
kilometer	438
kin	73
kinesitherapy	117
Klebsiella pneumoniae	160
kleis	6
kleptomania	18
knee	446
knee clonus	301
knee jerk	300
knee joint	495
knee osteoarthritis	286
knee-ankle-foot orthosis	290
kneecap	27
knee-chest position	77
kneippism	118
knēmē	6
knocked-out tooth	149
knock-knees	26, 280
knuckles	446
koilia	8
koilonychia	262, 321
kolon	6
kranion	8
K-ras gene	508
krestin	431
krypton	434

Kyasanur forest disease	108
kyphosis	281
kystis	8

L

labia majora	489
labia minora	489
labial	6, 36
labile	36, 295
labile hypertension	184
labium	6, 464
labium majus pudendi	489
labium minus pudendi	489
labor	230
labor pains	121, 230
laboratory	54
laboratory and imaging findings	400
laboratory animal science	63
laboratory diagnosis	84
laboratory findings	70, 95
Labour and Welfare	43
labyrinth	459
labyrinthectomy	145
labyrinthitis	144
laceration	320
lack of ~	71
lacrimal gland	456
lacrimal sac	456
lacrimation	126
lactate dehydrogenase	178, 283
lactic acid dehydrogenase	178
lacunar infarction	306
lagophthalmos	127
lamellar keratoplasty	137
lamina muscularis mucosae	480
laminagraphy	161
laminectomy	291
laminography	79, 161
laminoplasty	291
laminotomy	291
lamivudine	211
lamotrigine	316
lancinating	121
lanthanum	435
laparo-	14
laparoscope	18
laparoscopic biopsy	204
laparoscopic cholecystectomy	213
laparoscopic gastric banding	214, 260
laparoscopically assisted vaginal hysterectomy	243
laparoscopic-assisted colectomy	214
laparoscopy	14, 204
laparotomy	14, 19, 214
lapatinib	433
large bowel	482
large cell lung carcinoma	166
large granular lymphocyte	265
large intestine	482
large-for-dates infant	331
large-for-gestational-age infant	331
laryngeal	6
laryngeal cancer	145
laryngeal cartilage	495
laryngectomy	146
laryngismus	144
laryngitis	28, 144
laryngoplasty	146
laryngoscopy	6, 143
laryngospasm	144
laryngostroboscope	143
laryngotomy	146
larynx	6, 466
laser	565
laser angioplasty	190
laser coagulation	329
laser gonioplasty	137
laser immunoassay	82
laser iridotomy	137
laser photocoagulation	136
laser trabeculoplasty	137
laser-assisted in-situ keratomileusis	137
L-asparaginase	430, 565
Lassa fever	107
lassitude	104
last menstrual period	228
latamoxef	426
late cortical cerebellar atrophy	310
latent	91
latent infection	106
late-onset hypogonadism	237
lateral	448
lateral abdominal region	452
lateral basal segment (S^9)	468
lateral canthus	456
lateral cuneiform bone	494
lateral decubitus	76

lateral myocardial infarction	185
lateral pectoral region	450
lateral plantar artery	476
lateral rectus muscle	458
lateral segment (S^4)	468
lateral semicircular canal	460
lateral ventricle	502
latex agglutination	82
latex allergy	324
latissimus dorsi muscle	500
laundry	55
Law concerning Autopsy and Preservation of Corpse	46
Law for the Prevention of Infectious Diseases and the Medical Care of People Suffering from Infectious Diseases	46
Law for the Welfare of the People with Intellectual Disability	46
Law for the Welfare of the People with Physical Disabilities	46
Law on Mental Health and Welfare for People with Mental Disorders	46
lawrencium	436
laxative	27, 211
lay terms	25
lazy eye	125
L-dopa	315
LE cell	321
lead	436
leaky heart	28
lean	36, 105
lean body mass	245
learning disability	302
Leber hereditary optic neuropathy	135
lecithin	581
lecture	67
lecturer	62
leflunomide	288
left anterior descending branch	471
left anterior fascicular block	179
left anterior hemiblock	179
left anterior oblique position	565
left atrial enlargement	179
left atrium	470
left bundle branch block	179
left circumflex branch	471
left colic artery	474
left coronary artery	471
left flexure of colon	482
left gastric artery	474
left gastric vein	478
left gastroepiploic artery	474
left hepatic artery	474
left hypochondriac region	450
left inguinal region	452
left lobe	484
left lower lobe	466, 468
left lower quadrant	452
left lung	466
left main trunk	471
left posterior fascicular block	179
left posterior hemiblock	179
left sternal border	175
left upper lobe	466, 468
left upper quadrant	452
left ventricle	470
left ventricular assist device	192
left ventricular ejection fraction	182
left ventricular end-diastolic pressure	182
left ventricular end-diastolic volume	182
left ventricular end-systolic pressure	182
left ventricular end-systolic volume	182
left ventricular failure	185
left ventricular hypertrophy	175
left ventriculography	182
left-handedness	294
left-sided heart failure	185
leg	446
legal medicine	63
Leggett's tree	420
Legionella pneumophila	160
legionellosis	108
legionnaires disease	108, 165
legislation	46
leiomyoma	18
leiomyoma of the uterus	239
lema	127
lenampicillin	426
length of the hospital stay	93
lens	456
lens opacity	129

lenticular opacity	129	lichen simplex chronicus	325
lentiform nucleus	503	lichenification	320
lentigo	319	lid lag	127
LEOPARD syndrome	325	lid retraction	127
lepto-	14	lidocaine	123, 189
leptocephalia	14	lien	8, 36
leptomeninx	14	lienal	8, 37
leptospirosis	109	life expectancy	92
lesser curvature	480	life insurance	49
lesser occipital nerve	505	life line	446
lesser omentum	482	life prolongation	92
lesser trochanter	494	life style	74
let-down reflex	232	life support system	92
lethal dose	566	ligament	496
lethargy	297	ligamentum falciforme hepatis	484
leucine aminopeptidase	200	ligamentum latum uteri	488
leucocytosis	18	ligamentum teres hepatis	484
leukemia	17, 270	ligase chain reaction	82
leukemic reticuloendotheliosis	271	ligation	87
leuko-	14	light microscope	78
leukocytapheresis	212	light perception	127
leukocyte	14	light reflex	129, 458
leukocyte alkaline phosphatase	265	light-headedness	172, 261, 293
leukocyte cast	218	likelihood ratio	568
leukocyte common antigen	268	limb lead	178
leukocyte count	263	limp	294, 298
leukocytosis	265	limping	298
leukocyturia	218	lincomycin	426
leukoderma	319	linea alba	501
leukonychia	321	linear accelerator	567
leukopenia	265	linear atrophy	245
leukoplakia	14, 148	lines of the hand	446
leukorrhea	18, 27, 228	linezolid	426, 569
leukotriene	159	lingua	7, 464
leukotriene antagonist	167	lingual	7
levator muscle of scapula	500	lingual artery	472
level of consciousness	297	lingual cancer	151
levo-	14	lingual frenulum	464
levocardia	14	lingual frenum	464
levodopa	315	lingual papilla	464
levofloxacin	426	lingual papillae	148
levofolinate calcium	430	lingual tonsil	465
levothyroxine sodium	258	liniment	328
levoversion	14	lip	442, 464
libido	228	lipase	17, 202
licensed practical nurse	57	lipid	250
lichen planus	325	lipidosis	256
lichen sclerosus et atrophicus	114, 325	lipo-	14
		lipoma	14, 83

lipoprotein	14, 250	long QT syndrome	113, 183
lipoprotein lipase	250	long terminal repeats	511
lipotropic hormone	568	long-acting inhaled β_2-agonist	169
liquefied natural gas	567	long-acting insulin	258
liquefied petroleum gas	568	long-acting thyroid stimulator	248
liquid diet	90	longissimus muscle	500
liquid food	194	longitudinal	448
liquid medicine	86	long-term care insurance	48
liquid nitrogen	329	long-term care insurance facility	55
liquor	23	loop diuretic	188
liter	438	loop of Henle	486
lithiasis	15	loose bowels	196
lithium	434	loose connective tissue	512
litho-	15	loose tooth	149
lithopedion	238	loperamide hydrochloride	211
lithotomy position	77	lordosis	281
lithotripsy	15, 19	loss of ~	71
little finger	444	loss of hair	319
liver	484	loss of vibratory sensation	262
liver abscess	208	lotio	23
liver biopsy	204	lotion	86, 328
liver breath	197	loupe	78
liver cirrhosis	208	louse	318
liver dullness	198	low back exercise	290
liver flap	197	low back pain	120, 216, 278
liver fluke	199	low backache	278
liver function test	199	low birth weight infant	331
liver transplantation	215	low blood count	25
living conditions	74	low calorie diet	90
living donor	226	low fat diet	90
living related donor	226	low output syndrome	185
lobar bronchus	466	low protein diet	224
lobular carcinoma in situ	240	low residue diet	90
lobulation	40	low salt diet	90
local anesthesia	87	low vision	125
local anesthetic	123	low voltage	179
localized gingival enlargement	149	low-density lipoprotein	566
lockjaw	27, 148	low-density-lipoprotein cholesterol	250
locomotor syndrome	278	low-dose oral contraceptive	241
locomotor system	278	lower digestive tract	480
locum tenens	43	lower esophageal sphincter	480
locus ceruleus	502	lower esophageal sphincter pressure	201
locus control region	509	lower extremity	446
-logy	17	lower eyelid	456
loins	444	lower jaw	442
lomefloxacin	426	lower leg	446
long leg brace	290	lower limb	446
long leg cast	289		
long posterior ciliary artery	472		

lower lip	442
lower urinary tract	486
lower urinary tract symptoms	216
low-molecular-weight heparin	567
low-output heart failure	186
low-power field	568
lozenge	86
lubricant	78
lumbago	120, 278
lumbar anesthesia	87
lumbar cord	504
lumbar nodes	478
lumbar pain	120
lumbar plexus	505
lumbar puncture	568
lumbar region	452
lumbar spinal canal stenosis	288
lumbar traction	291
lumbar vertebra	492
lumbarization	284
lumbosacral orthosis	290
lumen	438
lumpectomy	243
lump-sum withdrawal payment	49
lunate bone	492
lung cancer	166
lung fluke	199
lung markings	161
lung transplantation	171
lung volume reduction surgery	171
lunula	462
lunule	462
lupus anticoagulant	322
lupus erythematosus	566
lupus miliaris disseminatus faciei	328
lupus nephritis	221
luteinized unruptured follicle syndrome	239
luteinizing hormone	234, 249
luteinizing hormone-releasing hormone	249
luteinizing hormone-releasing hormone agonist	224
luteinizing hormone-releasing hormone test	234
lutetium	435
lux	438
luxatio coxae congenita	287
lying position	76
lying-in hospital	52
Lyme disease	108
lymph	512
lymph node	478
lymph node excision	276
lymph vessel	478
lymphadenectomy	276
lymphadenopathy	262
lymphadenosis benigna cutis	327
lymphatic system	478
lymphatic vessel	478
lymphedema	177
lymphocyte	264
lymphocyte stimulation test	323
lymphocytic choriomeningitis virus	566
lymphocytic interstitial pneumonia	164
lymphocytopenia	265
lymphogranuloma venereum	237
lymphoid	18
lymphokine-activated killer cell	565
lymphopenia	265
-lysis	17
lysosomal storage diseases	112
lysosome	508
Lyssavirus infection	108

M

macro-	11
macroaggregated albumin	569
macrobiotics	118
macrocephalus	332
macrocephaly	332
macrocheiria	8
macrocytic anemia	263
macroglossia	11, 148, 245
macromolecule	11
macrophage	265
macrophage chemotactic factor	570
macrophage migration inhibition test	572
macrophage-activating factor	569
macroscopic hematuria	218
macula	130, 458
macula lutea	130, 458
macula retinae	458
macular edema	130

Term	Page
macular hole	130
magnesium	434
magnetic resonance angiography	79
magnetic resonance cholangiopancreatography	203
magnetic resonance imaging	79
magnetic resonance spectroscopy	574
magnetoencephalography	304
magnifying glass	78
main en griffe	298
main pancreatic duct	484
maintenance therapy	118
major aortopulmonary collateral artery	183
major calyx	486
major depression	312
major depressive disorder	312
mal-	11
malabsorption syndrome	206
-malacia	17
malaise	104
malaria	36, 108
male genital organ	488
male genitalia	488
male reproductive system	488
malformation	11, 83
malignancy	82
malignant disease	106
malignant fibrous histiocytoma	571
malignant hyperthermia	105
malignant lymphoma	272
malignant melanoma	327
malignant neoplasm	106
malignant rheumatoid arthritis	114
malignant syndrome	314
malignant tumor	106
malleolus	36
mallet finger	285
malleus	36, 108, 459
malnutrition	11, 244
malocclusion	36, 149, 245
malpighian corpuscle	486
malpractice	42
Malpractice Council	42
malpractice insurance	48
malpractice litigation	42
malpractice suit	42
Malta fever	108
mamillary line	454
mamma	8
mammaplasty	243
mammary region	450
mammectomy	243
mammillary line	454
mammography	8, 236
managed care	48
mandible	492
mandibula	492
mandibular nerve	505
mandibular protrusion	149
mandibular region	450
mandibular retrusion	149
mandibulofacial dysostosis	341
manganese	434
mangled extremity severity score	282
-mania	18
manic-depressive psychosis	312
manifest anxiety scale	303
manipulation	289
manipulative reduction	289
mannitol	315
mannitol-adenine-phosphate solution	569
manometer	304
manual	8
manual muscle test	281
manubrium of sternum	492
manubrium sterni	492
manus	8
manuscriptum	22
maple syrup urine	333
maple syrup urine disease	336
Marburg fever	107
marijuana	124
marital status	74
married	74
masculinization	240, 244
masked hypertension	173
mass screening	72
massage	289
massage therapy	119
masseter muscle	498
masseur	57
mast cell leukemia	271
mastectomy	8, 243
Master of Science	68

master's degree	67
mastication	195
masticatory muscle	498
mastitis	240
mastodynia	17
mastoidectomy	145
mastoiditis	144
mastopathy	240
mastos	8
masturbation	228
maternal	73
Maternal and Child Health Law	46
Maternal Protection Law	46
maternal-child nursing	66
maternity home	52
maternity hospital	52
maternity leave	230
maternity nurse	58
maternity ward	54
matriculation	67
matrilineal	73
matrix metalloproteinase-3	283
matrix unguis	462
mattress suture	88
maturation	244
maturity	244
maturity-onset diabetes of youth	255
maxilla	492
maxillary artery	472
maxillary nerve	505
maxillary protrusion	149
maxillary region	450
maxillary retrusion	149
maxillary sinus	460
maxillary sinus cancer	144
maxillary sinusitis	144
maximal acid output	201
maximal blood pressure	75
maximal expiratory flow-volume curve	162
maximal mid-expiratory flow rate	162
maximal voluntary ventilation	575
maximum androgen blockade	224
maximum capacity of tubular transport	220
maximum permissible dose	573
maximum tolerated dose	574
maximum urinary flow rate	220
meal	90, 194
mean arterial pressure	75
mean corpuscular hemoglobin	263
mean corpuscular hemoglobin concentration	263
mean corpuscular volume	263
measles	109, 325, 330
measles-mumps-rubella vaccine	573
measles-rubella vaccine	344
measurement prefixes	20
mechanical ventilation	169
mechanical ventilator	169
mechanocardiogram	180
meconium aspiration syndrome	335
medevac	51
medial	448
medial antebrachial cutaneous nerve	505
medial basal segment (S^7)	468
medial brachial cutaneous nerve	505
medial canthus	456
medial cuneiform bone	494
medial longitudinal fasciculus	504
medial plantar artery	476
medial rectus muscle	458
medial segment (S^5)	468
median incision	88
median line	454
median nerve	505
median plane	448
median sagittal plane	448
median sulcus of tongue	464
mediastinal emphysema	167
mediastinal nodes	478
mediastinal tumor	167
mediastinitis	167
mediastinoscopy	163
mediastinum	468
mediator inhibitor	167
Medicaid	50, 51
medical accident	42
medical administration	42
medical argot	2
medical assistance	42
medical audit	42
medical bioengineering	63
medical care	42
medical care facility for the elderly	55

medical care in remote site (in less populated area)	44
medical care plan	42
medical care standard	42
medical care system for retirees	49
medical center	52
medical certificate	43
medical climatology	64
medical college	62
medical corporation	43
medical dispute	42
medical economics	63
medical education	63
medical electronics	571
medical engineering	571
medical English	2
medical ethics	43, 64
Medical Ethics Council	42
medical examiner	57
medical expenditure for the elderly	49
medical expenses	49
medical expenses deduction	48
medical facilities	52
medical faculty	62
medical fee points	49
medical genetics	63
medical informatics	63
medical information	42
medical information disclosure	43
medical inspection	42
medical insurance system	48
medical insurance system for people aged 75 and older	48
medical interview	66
medical jargon	2
medical juridical person	43
medical law	46
medical lawsuit	42
medical licensure	66
Medical Literature Analysis and Retrieval System	571
medical malpractice	42
medical mycology	63
medical physicist	57
medical practice	42
Medical Practitioners Law	46
medical problems	96
medical professional liability insurance	42
medical professionals	57
medical record administrator	58
medical record library	55
medical representative	57
medical school	62
Medical Service Law	46
medical social worker	57
medical sociology	63
medical staff	59
Medical Subject Headings	3
medical system	42
medical technologist	58
medical technology assessment	42
medical terminology	2
medical terms	2
medical treatment insurance	48
medical trial	42
medical university	62
medical waste	42
medical zoology	63
medicalese	2
medically underserved area	44
medically unexplained symptom	104, 575
Medicare	50
medication	85
Medicinae Doctor	66
medicinal treatment	117
meditation	119
medroxyprogesterone	431
medroxyprogesterone acetate	241
medulla oblongata	504
medulla spinalis	504
medullary carcinoma	252
medullary cavity	494
mega-	11, 20
megacolon	11
megakaryoblast	267
megakaryocyte	11, 266
megaloblastic anemia	269
-megaly	18
megavitamin therapy	119
meibomian gland	456
meiosis	37
meitnerium	436
melancholic	295
melanism	319
melano-	15

melanocyte	15	mental retardation	303, 343
melanocyte-stimulating hormone	574	mentoplasty	5
melanoglossia	148	mentum	5, 442
melanoma	15	mepitiostane	431
melanosis	319	meralgia	7
MELAS syndrome	311	mercury	436
melatonin	249	mercy killing	26, 94
melena	195	meropenem	426
melioidosis	108	mēros	7
meloxicam	122	mesalazine	211
melphalan	430	mesangium	486
membrane attack complex	569	mesencephalon	504
membrane rupture	232	mesenchyma	512
membranoproliferative glomerulo-nephritis	221	mesenchymal stem cell	574
		mesenchymal tissue	512
membranous labyrinth	459	mesenteric nodes	479
membranous nephropathy	221	mesentery	482
membrum inferius	447	mesioclusion	36, 149
membrum superius	447	meso-	11
meme	511	mesocolon	11, 483
memorize	295	mesothelioma	11
memory	295	messenger RNA	511
memory loss	295	meta-	11
menarche	228	metabolic acidosis	219
mendelevium	436	metabolic disease	106
meninges	504	metabolic syndrome	256
meningioma	313	metacarpal bone	494
meningitis	307	metacarpophalangeal joint	495
meningo-	15	metachromatic leukodystrophy	307
meningomeningocele	342	metamorphosis	11
meningococcal meningitis	109	metaphyseal-diaphyseal angle	280
meningococcus	15	metaphysis	494
meningorrhagia	15	metaplasia	18, 83
meniscectomy	291	metastasis	11, 83
meniscus	496	metatarsal bone	494
meno-	15	metatarsophalangeal joint	495
menopausal disorder	229	meteorism	196, 197
menopause	15, 27, 229	meter	438
menorrhagia	228	-meter	18
menorrhalgia	121, 228	metered-dose inhaler	169
menoschesis	15	metformin hydrochloride	258
mens	7	methadone hydrochloride	123
menses	228	methicillin-resistant staphylococcus aureus infection	110
menstrual pain	121, 228		
menstrual periods	228	methimazole	258
menstruation	27, 228	methotrexate	288, 431
mental	7, 36	methyldopa	189
mental hospital	52	methylphenidate hydrochloride	314
mental region	450	metrorrhagia	229

metrorrhexis	18	middle turbinate	460
metyrapone test	250	midecamycin	426
mexiletine hydrochloride	189	midlife crisis	229
micafungin	426	midline	454
miconazole	329, 426	midline incision	88
micro-	11, 20	midriff	444
microalbuminuria	218	midscapular line	454
microaneurysm	130	midspinal line	454
microangiopathic hemolytic anemia	270	midsternal line	454
		midstream urine	217
microarray	511	midsystolic murmur	175
microbe	27	midwife	58
microbiology	63	midwifery	65
microcephalus	332	miglitol	258
microcephaly	332	migraine	120
microcirculation	11	mile	438
microcytic anemia	263	miliaria	36, 320
micrognathia	149, 332	miliary shadow	161
micrognathism	149	military antichock trousers	290
microgram	439	milium	319
micromandible	332	milk ejection reflex	232
micronomicin	426	milk of magnesia	573
microphobia	297	milk teeth	147
microsatellite instability	511	milli-	20
microscope	11	milliequivalent	438
microscopic diagnosis	84	milligram	438
microscopic hematuria	218	millimeter	438
microscopic polyangiitis	111	milnacipran hydrochloride	314
microsurgical epididymal sperm aspiration	242	mimetic muscle	498
		mind	293
microtia	332	minimal blood pressure	75
microtubule	508	minimal brain dysfunction	343
microtubule organizing center	508	minimal change disease	222
micturition	216	minimal change nephrotic syndrome	222
micturition desire	216		
midaxillary line	454	minimal erythema dose	324
midbrain	504	minimal identifiable odor	143
midclavicular line	454	minimal lethal dose	572
mid-diastolic murmur	175	minimal residual disease	271
middle cerebral artery	471	minimally invasive cardiac surgery	191
middle colic artery	474		
middle ear	458	Mini-Mental State Examination	303
middle finger	444	minimum audible field	141
middle lobe syndrome	166	minimum audible threshold	142
middle mediastinum	468	minipill	241
middle nasal meatus	460	minisatellite	511
middle of the eyebrows	442	ministroke	294
middle pain	228	Ministry of Education, Culture, Sports, Science and Technology	
middle rectal artery	474		

	68	moisturizer	328
Ministry of Health	43	molar	464
Minnesota Multiphasic Personality Inventory	303	molar tooth	464
		molars	147
minocycline	426	mole	27, 318, 438
minodronic acid hydrate	289	molecular biology	63
minor calyx	486	molecular disease	106
minute	438	molecular genetics	63
miosis	37, 129	molecular weight	575
miotic	37	molecularly targeted therapy	117
miotics	136	molluscum contagiosum	330
mirimostim	274	molybdenum	435
mirtazapine	314	mongolian blue spot	331
miscarriage	229	mongolian spot	331
misce	23	moniliasis	27
misdiagnosis	85	monkeypox	108
misoprostol	210	mono-	15
missed abortion	238	monoamine oxidase	569
missed periods	228	monoamine oxidase inhibitor	315
missing tooth	149	monoblast	17
mitochondria	508	monoclonal gammopathy of uncertain significance	273
mitochondrial disease	113		
mitochondrial DNA	511	monocular vision	132
mitochondrial encephalomyopathy	311	monocyte	15, 265
		monoiodotyrosine	248
mitomycin C	431	monophobia	296
mitotic	37	monoplegia	299
mitoxantrone	430	monopolar	15
mitral commissurotomy	191	monosodium urate monohydrate	284
mitral P wave	179	mons pubis	489
mitral regurgitation	184	mood	76, 295
mitral stenosis	184	mood disorder	312
mitral valve	470	moon face	245
mitral valve insufficiency	184	moon-shaped face	245
mitral valve prolapse	184	*Moraxella catarrhalis*	160
mitral valve replacement	191	morgue	55
mitral valve stenosis	184	moribund	76
mittelschmerz	228	morning sickness	26, 229
mixed connective tissue disease	111, 116, 328	morphine hydrochloride	122
		morphine sulfate	574
mixed lymphocyte culture	572	morphine sulfate hydrate	122
mixed lymphocyte reaction	572	mortality rate	93
mixed passive hemagglutination	81	mortuary	55
mixed venous oxygen tension	182	mosquito clamp	89
M-mode echocardiography	181	mother	73
mnemonic	317	mother-in-law	73
mobilization	87	motion sense	302
modifier gene	511	motive	72
moistening agent	328	motor aphasia	302

motor area	503
motor speech center	503
mottled fundus	131
mottled tooth	149
motus manus	127
moustache	442
mouth	442, 464
mouth breathing	140
mouth-to-mouth breathing	190
mouthwash	147
movement sense	302
moxibustion	118
moxibustionist	58
moxifloxacin	426
moyamoya disease	111, 307
MR sialography	150
MRC dyspnea scale	158
mucocutaneous lymph node syndrome	340
mucocutaneous ocular syndrome	326
mucopolysaccharide	573
mucopolysaccharidosis	337
mucosa	480
mucosa-associated lymphoid tissue	569
mucosal protective agent	210
mucosal relief radiography	203
mucous	37
mucous cyst	148
mucous membrane	480
mucus	37
multi-	11
multiacting receptor targeted antipsychotic	316
multidetector-row computed tomography	79
multidisciplinary therapy	118
multidrug-resistant tuberculosis	165
multifocal atrial tachycardia	174
multifocal lens	135
multifocal motor neuropathy	112, 309
multigravida	229
multi-infarct dementia	311
multinodular	11
multipara	11, 230
multiple antigen simultaneous test	323
multiple endocrine adenomatosis	255
multiple endocrine neoplasia type 1	255
multiple endocrine neoplasia type 2	255
multiple myeloma	273
multiple organ failure	107
multiple pregnancy	229
multiple sclerosis	111, 308, 317
multiple sleep latency test	163, 304
multiple system atrophy	310
multiple-choice question	67
multiple-gated acquisition scan	181
multiple-organ dysfunction syndrome	107
multislice computed tomography	79
mumps	26, 110, 151, 330
mumps vaccine	344
municipal hospital	52
municipal ordinance	46
mupirocin	426
muscae volitantes	126
muscle	498
muscle action potential	304
muscle biopsy	284
muscle pain	120, 278
muscle relaxant	289
muscle strain	278
muscle weakness	261
muscular	5
muscular atrophy	278
muscular contracture	281
muscular defense	198
muscular pain	120
muscular rigidity	198
muscular tissue	512
muscular wasting	278
muscular weakness	278
muscularis mucosae	480
musculoskeletal system	75
musculus	5
music therapist	57
mustache	442
mutant gene	511
mutation	511
mutual aid	49
mutual aid association health insurance	48
myalgia	120, 278
myasthenia gravis	111, 310
mycobacterium avium complex	160

Mycobacterium kansasii	160
Mycobacterium tuberculosis	160
Mycoplasma pneumoniae	160
mycoplasmal pneumonia	110
mycosis fungoides	272, 327
mydriasis	129
mydriatics	136
myelin basic protein	305
myelo-	15
myeloblast	266
myelocyte	266
myelodysplastic syndrome	115, 270
myelofibrosis	15, 115, 271
myelography	284
myeloperoxidase	268
myelopoiesis	15
myeloproliferative disorders	270
myelosuppressive therapy	276
myiodesopsia	126
myo-	15
myocardial contrast echocardiography	181
myocardial infarction	27, 185
myocardial perfusion imaging	181
myocarditis	15, 186
myocardium	470
myoclonus	300
myoclonus epilepsy with ragged red fibers	311
myodesopsia	126
myofibroma	15
myoglobin	178, 283
myoma	5, 83
myonephropathic metabolic syndrome	187
myope	125
myopia	125
myopic	37
myosin light chain	178
myositis	285
myositis ossificans	285
myringitis	143
myringoplasty	145
myringotomy	145
mys	5
mysophobia	296
myxedema	251
myxedema coma	251

N

nabothian cyst	231
nabumetone	122
N-acetylcystein	575
N-acetylglucosaminidase	219
nadifloxacin	426
nadir	91
nafamostat mesilate	275
naftopidil	224
nagging	121
nail	446, 462
nail bed	462
nail body	462
nail excision	329
nail plate	462
nail root	462
nalidixic acid	426
name	71
nano-	20
nanogram	439
nanometer	577
nap	104
nape	444
naproxen	122
naratriptan hydrochloride	122
narcissistic personality disorder	313
narcolepsy	312
narcotic	27, 122
Narcotic and Psychotropic Drugs Control Law	47
naris	460
narrative notes	96
narrowing	198
nasal	8
nasal blockage	140
nasal bone	492
nasal cannula	168
nasal cartilages	495
nasal cavity	460
nasal congestion	140
nasal continuous positive airway pressure	170
nasal discharge	139
nasal douche	145
nasal drop	145
nasal hemorrhage	261
nasal irrigation	145
nasal meatus	460

nasal obstruction	140	needle	86
nasal polyp	141	needle biopsy	78
nasal prongs	168	needle electrode	283
nasal region	450	needle holder	89
nasal septum	460	negative predictive value	577
nasal speculum	77	negative T wave	179
nasal stuffiness	140	*Neisseria gonorrhoeae*	235
nasal tone	140	nematode	199
nasal vestibule	460	neo-	11
nasal voice	140	neodymium	435
nasogastric tube	211	neon	434
nasolacrimal duct	456	neonatal	11
nasolacrimal duct stenosis	133	neonatal alloimmune thrombocytopenia	335
nasopharyngeal cancer	145	neonatal asphyxia	334
nasopharyngoscopy	143	neonatal blennorrhea	336
nasotracheal suctioning	169	neonatal hyperbilirubinemia	335
nasus	8	neonatal intensive care	61, 343
nateglinide	258	neonatal intensive care unit	55, 343
national examination for medical practitioner	66	neonatal jaundice	335
National Health Insurance	48	neonatal necrotizing enterocolitis	336
National Health Service	50	neonatal respiratory distress syndrome	334
National Health Service and Community Care Act	50	neonate	330
national hospital	52	neoplasm	11
National Hospital Organization	52	neovascularization	130
national pension insurance	48	nephrectomy	226
native valve endocarditis	186	nephritis	7
natural death	93	nephro-	15
natural killer cell	577	nephrologist	60
natural thymocytotoxic autoantibody	578	nephrology	64
naturopathy	118	nephron	486
nausea	195	nephropathy	18
nauseous feeling	195	nephropexy	15, 226
navel	37, 444	nephroptosis	223
navicular bone	494	nephros	7
N-benzoyl-L-tyrosyl-paraaminobenzoic acid test	202	nephrosclerosis	223
Nd-YAG laser	576	nephrotic syndrome	221
near-sightedness	125	nephrotoxicity	15
nebulizer	169	neptunium	436
neck	442	nerve action potential	304
neck brace	290	nerve block	123
necrophilia	18	nerve conduction velocity	283, 304
necrophobia	296	nerve excitability test	304
necrosis	82	nerve growth factor	576
necrotizing enteroclitis	576	nerve growth factor receptor	576
nedaplatin	429, 532	nervous	7, 295
		nervous breakdown	27, 295

nervous system	75, 293	nicotinamide adenine dinucleotide	575
nervous tissue	512	nicotine patches	169
nervousness	295	nicotinic acid	259
nervus	7	nifedipine	188
neuralgia	17, 120, 294	nifekalant hydrochloride	189
neurally mediated syncope	184	night hospital	52
neuraminidase	575	night sweat	105
neuraminidase inhibitor	167	night terrors	331
neurilemma	506	night-blindness	126
neurinoma	313	Nightingale Pledge	44
neuro-	15	nightmare	104
neuroblastoma	15, 342	NIH Stroke Scale	298
neurocirculatory asthenia	187	nil disease	222
neurofibril	504, 506	nil per os	23
neurofibromatosis	313	nilotinib	433
neurofibromatosis type 1	116	nimustine	429
neurofibromatosis type 2	116	niobium	435
neurogenic bladder	223	Nipah virus infection	108
neurohypophysis	490	nipple	444
neurokinin-1 receptor antagonist	211	nitric oxide synthase	577
neuroleptanalgesia	123	nitrogen	434
neuroleptanesthesia	87	nitroglycerin	189
neuroleptic	314	nitroprusside test	333
neuroleptic malignant syndrome	314	niveau diagnosis	85
neurologist	60	no change	91
neurology	7, 64	nobelium	436
neuroma	83	noctiphobia	297
neuromuscular unit	283	nocturia	37, 217
neuron	7, 504	nocturnal dyspnea	154
neuron-specific enolase	578	nocturnal emission	27, 228
neuropathic pain	294	nocturnal pain	195
neurosurgeon	60	nocturnal penile tumescence	235
neurosurgery	65	nocturnal pollution	228
neurosyphilis	308	node	40, 83
neurotology	64	nodule	40, 83
neurotropic	15	nogitecan	431
neutralization test	81	noma	151
neutropenia	18, 265	nonalcoholic fatty liver disease	207
neutrophil	264	nonalcoholic steatohepatitis	208
neutrophil alkaline phosphatase	265	nonbacterial thrombotic endocarditis	186
neutrophil chemotactic factor	576	nonchalant	295
nevus	27, 319	noncholera vibrios	202
New York Heart Association classification	178	noncompliance	86
newborn	330	noncontact tonometer	131
newton	439	non-erosive reflux disease	204
niche	203	non-esterified fatty acid	576
nickel	434	nonimmune hydrops fetalis	335
nicomol	259		

Term	Page
non-insulin-dependent DM	255
noninvasive positive pressure ventilation	170
nonnucleoside reverse transcriptase inhibitor	275
nonocclusive mesenteric ischemia	206
nonpayment	49
nonpitting	177
nonpitting edema	246
non-prescription drug	85
nonproductive cough	155
non-rapid eye movement sleep	304
nonreassuring fetal status	232
nonrebreathing mask	168
nonseasonal allergic rhinitis	144
non-small cell lung carcinoma	166
nonspecific interstitial pneumonia	164
nonspecific symptom	104
non-ST-elevation myocardial infarction	185
nonsteroidal antiinflammatory drug	288
nonsteroidal anti-inflammatory drug	122
non-stress test	235
non-toothed forceps	89
nontoxic goiter	251
nontuberculous mycobacteriosis	165
nontuberculous mycobacterium	160
non-valvular atrial fibrillation	174
noradrenaline	250
noradrenergic and specific serotonergic antidepressant	314
norepinephrine	250, 576
norepinephrine-dopamine reuptake inhibitor	576
norfloxacin	426
normal retinal correspondence	132
normal saline	577
normal-pressure hydrocephalus	111, 306
normal-tension glaucoma	133
normo-	15
normochromic	15
normotensive	15
Norovirus	202
North American Nursing Diagnostic Association	68
nose	442, 460
nosebleed	26, 140, 261
nosocomial infection	105
nosocomial pneumonia	163
nosophobia	296
nostril	460
nota bene	22
notifiable disease	106
nourishment	76
N-terminal pro-brain natriuretic peptide	178
nuchal region	452
nuchal rigidity	298
nuclear envelope	508
nuclear factor-activated T cell	576
nuclear family	73
nuclear magnetic resonance	577
nuclear medicine	64
nucleic acid	510
nucleic acid amplification technique	80
nucleic acid base	510
nucleolus	508
nucleoplasm	508
nucleoside reverse transcriptase inhibitor	275
nucleosome	511
nucleotide	511
nucleus	508
nudophobia	297
number sign	97
numbness	294
numerus digitorum	127
Nuremberg Code	45
nurse	57
nurse practitioner	58
nurse's aide	59
nurse's station	55
nursery	54
nursing	65, 89, 343
nursing administration	65
nursing art	89
nursing audit	89
nursing bottle	343
nursing care	89
nursing care plan	89
nursing diagnosis	84
nursing education	65

nursing epidemiology	65	Occam's razor	19
nursing ethics	65	occipital artery	472
nursing home for the elderly	55	occipital bone	492
nursing intervention	89	occipital lobe	502
Nursing Interventions Classification	89	occipital muscle	498
		occipital nodes	478
Nursing Outcomes Classification	89	occipital region	450
nursing procedure	89	occiput	442
nursing process	89	occlusion of the circle of Willis	111
nursing record	89	occlusive dressing technique	328
nursing service	89	occult-blood positive stool	261
nursing skill	89	occupation	71, 74
nursing standard	89	occupational disease	106
nursing university	62	occupational medicine	64
nursing-care facilities	55	occupational physician	57
nutrition	76, 90	occupational therapist	58
nutrition and food services	54	occupational therapy	117
nutrition university	62	ochlophobia	296
nyctalopia	126	octagon	40
nyctophobia	296	octothorp	97
nycturia	37, 217	octreotide acetate	258
nystagmus	129	ocular	9
nystatin	427	ocular albinism	134
		ocular bobbing	298
O		ocular chamber	456
obese	105	ocular fundus	458
obesity	105, 244	ocular hypertension	133
obesity-hypoventilation syndrome	115	ocular myopathy	135
		oculi unitas	23
objective data	96	oculocutaneous albinism	326
objective structured clinical examination	66	oculomotor nerve	505
		oculus	9
oblique fissure	466	oculus dexter	23
obsessive-compulsive disorder	578	oculus sinister	23
obsessive-compulsive neurosis	312	oculus uterque	23
obstetric canal	232	odontalgia	120
obstetrical forceps	89	odontodynia	120
obstetrician	59	odontogenic	8
obstetrician's hand	298	odontogenic cyst	151
obstetrics	64	odontogenic maxillary sinusitis	152
obstetrics and gynecology	64	odontoma	148
obstipation	196	odous	8
obstruction	198	-odynia	18
obstructive lung disease	163	oesophagus	7
obstructive sleep apnea syndrome	167	office blood pressure	75
		ofloxacin	427
obturator artery	474	ohm	439
obturator nerve	506	-oid	18
obtuse triangle	39	ointment	86, 328

oisophagos	7	oozing	261
old	91	opacitas corporis vitrei	129
Old Age, Survivors, Disability, and Health Insurance	50	open fracture	281
		open heart surgery	191
old myocardial infarction	185	open hospital	52
old tuberculin	580	open patch test	323
old-age basic pension	49	open reading frame	510
oleaginous ointment	328	open reduction	291
olecranon	452, 497	open reduction and internal fixation	291
olfaction	140		
olfactometry	143	open-ended question	66
olfactory nerve	505	opening snap	175
olfactory organ	460	operating room	54
oligo-	15	operating room nurse	59
oligodendroglia	15	operation	73, 86, 93
oligomenorrhea	228	operative cholangiography	203
oligospermia	235	operative note	87
oligozoospermia	235	operative treatment	118
oliguria	15, 217	operator	510
olivopontocerebellar atrophy	310	operator gene	510
-oma	18	opere citato	22
omalizumab	167	ophidiophobia	297
omental foramen	482	ophthalmalgia	120, 125
omeprazole	211	ophthalmectomy	137
omni mane	23	ophthalmia	9
omni nocte	23	ophthalmic artery	472
omphalocele	6	ophthalmic nerve	505
omphalos	6	ophthalmo-	15
Omsk hemorrhagic fever	108	ophthalmodynamometry	132
onanism	228	ophthalmodynia	125
on-call doctor	57	ophthalmologist	59
onco-	15	ophthalmology	64
oncogene	510	ophthalmoplegia	15, 135
oncogenesis	15	ophthalmos	9
oncogenic osteomalacia	255	ophthalmoscope	77
oncologist	59	ophthalmoscopy	15, 131
oncology	64	opioid	123
oncovirus	15	opium	122
onom-	38	opium alkaloid hydrochlorides	122
onset	72	opportunistic infection	106
onset of menses	228	oppositional defiant disorder	313
onychectomy	329	opsoclonus	332
onycholysis	8, 321	optic atrophy	130
onychorrhexis	321	optic chiasm	458
onyx	8	optic disc	130
oophorectomy	9	optic disk	130, 458
oophoritis	238	optic nerve	458, 505
oophoron	9	optic neuritis	134
ooze	319	optic neuromyelitis	308

optic papilla	458	organum vasculosum of lamina terminalis	502
optic tract	458	orientation	76
optical coherence tomography	132	oriented	76
optokinetic nystagmus	129	oropharyngeal cancer	145
optometry	131	orphan drug	85
ora serrata	458	ortho-	15
oral	6, 34, 448	orthodontics	64, 152
oral antihyperglycemic drug	258	orthodontist	59
oral appliance	168	orthokeratology	137
oral candidiasis	150	orthopedic surgeon	60
oral case presentation	392	orthopedics	65
oral contraceptive pill	241	orthopedist	60
oral contraceptives	230	orthopnea	15, 18, 154
oral examination	67	orthoptics	136
oral glucose tolerance test	247	orthoptist	58
oral hygiene	147	orthosis	289
oral hypoglycemic agent	258	orthostatic	15
oral region	450	orthostatic dysregulation	341
oral rehydration therapy	117	orthostatic hypotension	184, 262
oral surgeon	59	os	6, 37
oral surgery	64	oscillating nystagmus	129
oral temperature	75	oscillopsia	126
oral-facial-digital syndrome	338	oseltamivir phosphate	168
orange	39	-osis	18
orbicularis oculi muscle	498	osmidrosis	321
orbicularis oris muscle	498	osmium	435
orbit	456	osmole	439
orbita	456, 492	osmotic diuretics	136
orbital evisceration	137	osmotic fragility test	266
orbital floor blow-out fracture	135	osseous	6
orbital margin	127	osseous tissue	512
orbital region	450	ossiculectomy	145
orchialgia	228	ossiculoplasty	145
orchidectomy	242	ossification	6
orchidopexy	242	ossification of anterior longitudinal ligament	112, 287
orchiectomy	242		
orchiodynia	228	ossification of ligamentum flavum	287
orchiopexy	7, 18, 242		
orchis	7	ossification of posterior longitudinal ligament	112, 287
orchitis	236		
order	70	ossification of yellow ligament	112, 287
ordinance of the ministry	46		
organ of touch	462	ostalgia	120
organ tolerance dose	580	osteo-	15
Organ Transplantation Law	46	osteoarthritis	285
organelle	508	osteoarthrosis deformans	285
organic disease	106	osteoblast	17
organic food	194	osteoblastic lesion	269
organic murmur	175		

osteocalcin	283	ovarian cyst		238
osteochondritis dissecans	286	ovarian endometriosis		239
osteochondrosis	286	ovarian hyperstimulation syndrome		
osteoclast activating factor	578			239
osteogenesis imperfecta	288	ovarium	9,	488
osteology	63	ovary	488,	490
osteolytic lesion	269	overactive bladder		223
osteoma	83	overall survival		92
osteomalacia	15, 17, 255, 288	overeating		194
osteomyelitis	15	overflow incontinence		217
osteon	6, 494	over-the-counter drug		85
osteopath	58	overweight		105
osteopathic medicine	65	overwhelming postsplenectomy infection		274
osteopathy	118	ovulation induction	241,	242
osteopenia	284	ovulatory pain		228
osteophyte	284	ovum		235
osteoporosis	255, 288	oxalate		218
osteosarcoma	288	oxaliplatin		430
osteosynthesis	291	oxycodone hydrochloride		122
osteotomy	291	oxygen		434
ostomy	214	oxygen inhalation therapy		168
ostomy and continence nursing	61	oxygen mask		168
otalgia	120, 139	oxygen saturation by pulse oximetry		159
otitis externa	143	oxygen tent		168
otitis media	139	oxygen therapy		168
otitis media with effusion	143	oxygen under high pressure		579
oto(rhino)laryngologist	59	oxymoron		47
otoacoustic emission	142	oxyntic cell		480
otolith	460	oxytetracycline		427
otolithic organ	460	oxytocin	241,	249
otomycosis	144	oxytocin challenge test		235
otorhinolaryngology	3, 64	ozena		144
otorrhea	9, 139			
otosclerosis	144			
otoscope	77	**P**		
otoscopy	141			
oulon	7	P mitrale		179
ounce	439	P pulmonale		179
ous	9	pacchionian body		504
outcome	93	pachy-		11
out-of-hospital cardiac arrest	176	pachydermia		11
out-of-pocket maximum	48	pachyglossia	11,	148
out-of-pocket medical expenses	48	pachymeningitis		307
outpatient department	54	pacinian corpuscle		462
ova of parasites	199	packed red blood cells		275
oval	40	paclitaxel		431
oval window	459	padded cast		289
ovarian	9	pagophagia		261
ovarian cancer	239	pain		120

pain clinic	54		palpebral edema	217
pain control	122		palpitation	172, 244, 261
pain in ~	71		palsy	298
pain in a testis	228		p-aminohippurate clearance	220
pain on inspiration	156		p-aminohippuric acid	581
pain on pressure	197		p-aminosalicylic acid	581
pain relief	122		pan-	11
pain reliever	122		pancreas	7, 484, 490
pain threshold	121		pancreatectomy	259
pain tolerance level	121		pancreatic	7
painful menstruation	228		pancreatic cancer	210
painkiller	25, 122		pancreatic cyst	210
painless thyroiditis	251		pancreatic function diagnostant	202
palatal torus	150		pancreatic function test	202
palate	464		pancreatic juice	512
palatine	464		pancreatic oncofetal antigen	201
palatine tonsil	465		pancreatic pseudocyst	210
palatoplasty	152		pancreatic secretory trypsin inhibitor	202
palatoschisis	332		pancreaticoduodenectomy	215
palatum	464		pancreaticojejunostomy	19, 215
palatum durum	464		pancreatitis	7
palatum molle	464		pancreatolithiasis	210
pale	39		pancytopenia	11, 265
pale palmar creases	262		pandemic	35, 106
palilalia	300		pandemic disease	106
palivizumab	344		panhypopituitarism	11, 252
palladium	435		panic disorder	312
pallesthesia	302		panipenem/betamipron	427
palliative care	61		panitumumab	433
palliative care unit	54		pankreas	7
palliative therapy	118		panniculitis	245
pallid	261		panniculus adiposus	245
pallium	502		pannus	128, 280
pallor	261		panoramic radiography	150
palm	444, 452		panretinal photocoagulation	136
palmar	444		pansystolic murmur	175
palmar erythema	197		pant	154
palmar muscles	498		panting	154
palmar region	452		pantomography	150
palmoplantar pustulosis	327		Pap smear	235
palpable	37		Pap test	235
palpable kidney	217		papilla	40
palpable mass	198		papillary duct	486
palpation	77		papillary layer	462
palpebra	456		papillary muscles	470
palpebra inferior	456		papilledema	130
palpebra superior	456		papule	319
palpebral	37		para	230
palpebral conjunctiva	456			

para-	11	parietal lobe	502
paraaortic	11	parietal pleura	468
paracentesis	17, 204	parietal region	450
paradoxic pulse	173	parity	232
paradoxical incontinence	217	paronychia	325
paraffin bath	289	parotid duct	464
parageusia	147	parotid gland	464
Paragonimus	199	parotid nodes	478
parainfluenza virus	160	parous	37, 232
parallelepiped	40	paroxetine hydrochloride hydrate	314
parallelogram	39		
paralysis	294, 298	paroxysmal atrial tachycardia	174
paralytic	298	paroxysmal cold hemoglobinuria	270
paramedian incision	88	paroxysmal nocturnal dyspnea	172
paramedic	61	paroxysmal nocturnal hemoglobinuria	270
paramedical staff	59		
parameter	37	parrot fever	108
parametric	37	partial anomalous pulmonary venous return	183
paranasal sinus	460		
paraneoplastic cerebellar degeneration	309	partial denture	152
		partial rebreathing mask	168
paraneoplastic neurological syndrome	309	partial remission	92
		partial splenic embolization	213
paraneoplastic polyneuropathy	309	partial thromboplastin time	265
paraplegia	11, 18, 299	partial-thickness burn	320
parasitology	63	particle agglutination	82
parasomnia	104	particle counting immunoassay	82
parasternal line	454	parts per million	587
parasympathetic nerve	506	parturient canal	232
parathormone	248	parturient woman	230
parathyroid gland	490	pascal	439
parathyroid hormone	248	passive cutaneous anaphylaxis	324
parathyroid hormone-related hormone	248	passive exercise	290
		passive hemagglutination	80
parathyroidectomy	259	passive incontinence	217
paratyphoid fever	107	past history	70, 95, 396
paraumbilical vein	478	past medical history	70
paravertebral line	454	paste	328
parenkephalida	7	patch	86
parent	73	patch test	323
parental	37	patella	27, 494
parenteral	37	patellar clonus	301
parenteral nutrition	91	patellar hammer	77
paresis	298	patellar reflex	300
paresthesia	301	patellar region	453
paretic	298	patellar tendon	501
parietal bone	492	patellar tendon bearing	290
parietal cell	480	patellar tendon reflex	300
parietal hernia	210	patellofemoral dysfunction	279

patent ductus arteriosus	183	pediatric surgeon	60
patent foramen ovale	183	pediatric surgery	64
paternal	73	pediatrician	60
patho-	15	pediatrics	64
pathogenic	15	pediatrist	37
pathognomonic	84	pedicle	37
pathognomy	84	pediculosis	325
pathologic fracture	282	pediculus	37
pathologic reflex	301	pedicure	15
pathological diagnosis	84	pedigree	73
pathological examination	78	pedo-	15
pathologist	60	pedodontics	15
pathology	17, 63, 65	pedometer	15
pathophobia	296	pedophilia	15
pathophysiology	15	peduncle	40
-pathy	18	peer review	43
patient	588	pegaptanib sodium	136
Patient Care Partnership	45	peginterferon	211
patient controlled analgesia	123	pellis	6
patient controlled epidural analgesia	123	pelvic	6
patient identification	70	pelvic arteriography	236
patient package insert	86	pelvic cavity	455
patient profile	95, 394	pelvic examination	231
patient-centered medicine	95	pelvic floor	231, 500
patrilineal	73	pelvic girdle	494
patulous eustachian tube	144	pelvic inflammatory disease	238
pavor nocturnus	331	pelvic inlet	232
PAX genes	509	pelvic obliquity	279
pazufloxacin	427	pelvic outlet	232
peak acid output	201	pelvic pain	228
peak expiratory flow	162	pelvic peritonitis	238
peak expiratory flow rate	162	pelvic presentation	232, 233
peak flow meter	162	pelvimetry	6, 234
pear	40	pelvis	6, 494
peau d'orange	231	pemetrexed sodium hydrate	168
peau d'orange fundus	130	pemphigus	116
pectoral nerve	505	pemphigus vulgaris	327
pectoral region	450	pendular nystagmus	129
pectoralgia	120	penetrating keratoplasty	138
pectoralis major muscle	498	penetration	198
pectoralis minor muscle	498	-penia	18
pectoriloquy	157	penicillin-resistant pneumococcal infection	110
pectus carinatum	27, 156	penicillin-resistant *Streptococcus pneumoniae*	160
pectus excavatum	156		
pedagogy	66	penis	488
pediatric emergency nursing	61	penlight	77
pediatric intensive care unit	343	pension	49
pediatric nursing	65	pensioner	49

pentagon	39
pentazocine	123
pentostatin	429
pep pill	27
peplomycin	431
pepsinogen I	200
pepsinogen II	200
peptic ulcer	205
peptic ulcer disease	205
per	22
per-	11
per annum	22
per anum	23
per capita	22
per os	23
per se	22
peramivir	168
percent of one second forced expiratory volume	162
perceptive deafness	142
percussion	77
percussion hammer	77
percussion sound	156
percutaneous	11
percutaneous balloon aortic valvuloplasty	192
percutaneous cardiopulmonay support	192
percutaneous coronary intervention	190
percutaneous endoscopic gastrostomy	213
percutaneous ethanol injection therapy	213
percutaneous microwave coagulation therapy	213
percutaneous nephrolithotomy	225
percutaneous nephrostomy	225
percutaneous nephroureteral lithotomy	225
percutaneous nucleotomy	291
percutaneous transhepatic biliary drainage	213
percutaneous transhepatic cholangiography	203
percutaneous transhepatic cholangioscopy	204
percutaneous transhepatic gallbladder drainage	213
percutaneous transhepatic obliteration of esophageal varices	213
percutaneous transhepatic portography	589
percutaneous transluminal angioplasty	317
percutaneous transluminal coronary angioplasty	190
percutaneous transluminal coronary recanalization	190
percutaneous transluminal renal angioplasty	225
percutaneous transvenous mitral commissurotomy	191
perennial	37
perennial allergic rhinitis	144
perforation	198
perforation of the nasal septum	141
performance status	92
pergolide mesilate	315
peri-	11
periarteritis nodosa	585
pericardial effusion	186
pericardial fluid	512
pericardial friction rub	176
pericardial tamponade	186
pericarditis	186
pericardium	11, 470
pericoronitis	151
perimetry	132
perinatal	230
perinatology	64
perineal	37
perineal pain	216, 228
perineal region	452
perineorrhaphy	18
period	27
period pains	25
periodic acid-Schiff stain	581
periodic paralysis	311
periodontal ligament	465
periodontal membrane	465
periodontal pocket	149
periodontitis	151
periodontosis	152
periods	228
perioperative nursing	61
perioral region	450
periorbital region	450

periosteum	494	pervasive developmental disorder		313
peripheral	448	pes		5
peripheral anterior synechia	129	pes planus		5, 280
peripheral arterial disease	187	pessary		241
peripheral blood lymphocyte	265	peta-		20
peripheral blood stem cell transplantation	276	petechia		261
peripheral edema	177, 217	petechial hemorrhage		261
peripheral iridectomy	137	pethidine hydrochloride		122
peripheral nerve block	123	petit mal epilepsy		297
peripheral nervous system	505	-pexy		18
peripheral vascular disease	187	phacoemulsification and aspiration		136
peripheral vision	132	phacomatosis		326
peritoneal	37	-phagia		18
peritoneal dialysis	225	phagocyte		265
peritoneovenous shunt	213	phagophobia		296
peritoneum	483	phakic intraocular lens		137
peritonitis	210	phakomatosis		326
peritonsillar abscess	144	phalanges of fingers		494
peritonsillitis	144	phalanges of toes		494
periumbilical region	450	phalanx		446
perivascular	11	phantom limb pain		121
periventricular leukomalacia	342	phantom pain		121
periventricular lucency	305	Pharmaceutical Affairs Law		46
perleche	150, 153, 262	Pharmaceutical and Food Safety Bureau		42
permanent teeth	147	pharmaceutical university		62
permanent threshold shift	142	Pharmaceuticals and Medical Devices Agency		42
pernicious anemia	269	pharmacist		58
pernio	27, 320	Pharmacists Law		46
peroneal	37	pharmacobezoar		209
peroneal artery	476	pharmacodynamics		585
peroneal vein	478	pharmacokinetics		585
peroneus brevis muscle	500	pharmacology		63
peroneus longus muscle	500	pharmacotherapy		117
peroral	11	pharmacy		55
peroral endoscopy	78	pharyngalgia		120
peroxisomal disorder	112	pharyngeal injection		141
persistent fetal circulation	336	pharyngeal reflex		141, 301
persistent pulmonary hypertension of the newborn	336	pharyngeal tonsil		465
persistent vegitative state	590	pharyngectomy		146
personal health record	43	pharyngitis		28, 144
personal history	96	pharyngoconjunctival fever		109
personal hygiene	77	pharyngotympanic tube		458
personality	295	pharynx		465
personality disorder	313	phase microscope		79
personalized health care	118	-phasia		18
perspiration	105, 244			
pertussis	27, 110, 330			

phenobarbital	315	physical examination	70
phenol	212	physical findings	95, 398
phenolsulfonphthalein test	220	physical medicine	65
phenotype	511	physical therapist	58
phenylketonuria	333	physical therapy	118
phenytoin	315	physician	57
phenytoin-induced gingival hyperplasia	149	Physicians' Desk Reference	583
		physiological function test	78
pheochromocytoma	254	physiology	63
Philadelphia chromosome	267	physiotherapy	118
-philia	18	physique	76
Philosophiae Doctor	66	phytobezoar	209
philtrum	460	pia mater	504
phimosis	231, 237	pica	261
phlebitis	7, 15	picibanil	431
phlebo-	15	pickwickian syndrome	156
phlebotomy	15, 276	pico-	20
phlegm	155, 479	picogram	439
phlegmatic	479	picture archiving and communication system	580
phleps	7		
phlyctenule	128	piercing	121
phobia	35, 296	pigeon chest	156
-phobia	18	pigmentation	245, 319
phobias	296	pigmented spot	319
phobic	296	pigmented villonodular synovitis	286
-phonia	18	piles	26
phonocardiography	180	pills	230
phosphate	218	pilocarpine hydrochloride	136
phosphatidylglycerol	234	piloerection	6
phosphatidylserine	587	pilonidal cyst	326
phosphodiesterase	583	pilus	6, 462
phosphodiesterase inhibitor	189	pimaricin	427
phosphoglucomutase	584	pimple	25, 318
phosphoribosyl pyrophosphate	587	pineal body	490
phosphorus	434	pineal gland	490
photic stimulation	304	pinguecula	127
photocoagulation	582	pink	39
photodynamic therapy	136, 170	pink eye	25
photopatch test	323	pinkie	444
photophobia	127	pinkish	39
photopsia	126	pinna	458
photopsy	126	pint	439
photorefractive keratectomy	137	pinworm	199
photosensitivity	320	pioglitazone hydrochloride	258
photosensitivity test	323	pipemidic acid	427
phototherapeutic keratectomy	137	piperacillin	427
phototherapy	343	pirarubicin	431
physic	27	pirfenidone	168
physical diagnosis	84	piriform	40

piriform recess	466		588
piromidic acid	427	plasmalemma	508
pisiform bone	492	plasmapheresis	225, 276
pit of the stomach	444	plasmid	511
pitting	177	plasmin	266
pitting edema	177	plasminogen	266
pituitary	490	plasminogen activator inhibitor-1	266
pituitary adenoma	252	plasmin-α plasmin inhibitor complex	266
pituitary dwarfism	253	plaster	86, 328
pituitary fossa	461	plaster cast	279
pituitary gigantism	253	plaster of Paris	279
pituitary gland	490	plastic surgeon	59
pituitary neuroadenolysis	123	plastic surgery	64
pityriasis	320	-plasty	18
pityriasis rosea	325	plate	148
pityriasis versicolor	325	platelet aggregation test	265
pivmecillinam	427	platelet concentrate	276
placebo	85	platelet inhibitor	189, 314
placenta	27, 232	platelet peroxidase	268
placenta previa	238	platelet-activating factor	265
placental abruption	238	platelet-derived growth factor	583
placental dysfunction syndrome	237	platelet-derived growth factor receptor	583
placental site trophoblastic tumor	240	platelet-rich plasma	587
plague	107	platelike atelectasis	161
plain abdominal radiograph	202	platinum	436
plain chest radiography	161	-plegia	18
plain films	284	pleocytosis	305
plain radiography	79	pleonasm	371
plan	70, 96, 403	pleoptics	136
planta	453	plethysmography	162
plantar	446	pleura	9, 468
plantar arterial arch	476	pleural	9, 37
plantar muscle	500	pleural cavity	468
plantar reflex	301	pleural effusion	158, 217
plantar venous arch	478	pleural empyema	167
plaque	147	pleural fluid	512
plaque control record	150	pleural friction rub	158
-plasia	18	pleural lavage	169
plasma	512	pleural malignant mesothelioma	167
plasma aldosterone concentration	249	pleuralgia	120
plasma cell	265	pleurisy	167
plasma exchange	225, 276	pleuritic pain	120, 156
plasma iron turnover rate	269	pleuritis	37, 167
plasma membrane	508	pleurodesis	170
plasma protein fraction	586	pleurodynia	17, 120, 156
plasma renin activity	219	pleurolysis	170
plasma thromboplastin component		pleuropneumonia-like organism	587

Term	Page
plutonium	436
plyometrics	290
-pnea	18
pneumatic antichock garment	290
pneumo-	15
pneumococcal vaccine	168
pneumococcus	17
Pneumococcus	160
pneumoconiosis	165
Pneumocystis jiroveci	160
pneumocystis pneumonia	165
pneumoencephalography	305
pneumomediastinography	161
pneumomediastinum	167
pneumōn	8
pneumonectomy	15
pneumonia	8, 163
pneumothorax	15, 167
pneumoventriculography	305
podagra	5, 286
podiatrist	37
POEMS syndrome	273
-poiesis	18
poikilo-	15
poikilocyte	15
poikilocytosis	264
poikiloderma	15
point of maximal impulse	175
point-of-care testing	78
pokeweed mitogen	590
polarizing microscopy	284
police doctor	57
policy-holder	49
polio	25, 331
polio-	15
polioencephalitis	15
poliomyelitis	15
poliosis	321
poliovirus vaccine	344
pollakiuria	216
pollen allergy	140
pollenosis	27, 144
pollinosis	27, 144
pollution	228
polonium	436
poly-	11
polyacrylamide gel electrophoresis	82
polyarteritis nodosa	111, 114
polyarthralgia	2
polycarbophil calcium	211
polychromasia	264
polycystic kidney	115
polycystic kidney disease	222
polycystic ovary syndrome	238
polycythemia	11
polycythemia vera	271
polydactyly	332
polydipsia	244
polyethylene terephthalate	192
polygon	39
polymenorrhea	228
polymerase chain reaction	82
polymorphonuclear neutrophil	264
polymyalgia rheumatica	286
polymyositis	111, 114, 285
polymyxin B	427
polyneuritis	11
polyneuropathy	303
polyp	40
polyphagia	18, 244
polyploid	37, 510
polypoid	37
polypoidal choroidal vasculopathy	135
polysomnography	162, 304
polytrichia	245
polytrichosis	321
polyunsaturated fatty acid	589
polyuria	19, 217, 244
pompholyx	324
pons	504
pontine	504
popeyes	26
popliteal artery	476
popliteal fossa	453
popliteal nodes	479
popliteal pulse	176
popliteal vein	478
porcelain crown	152
porcelain inlay	152
porfimer sodium	170
pork tapeworm	199
porous	37
porphobilinogen	250
porphyria	257
porphyria cutanea tarda	328
porta hepatis	484

portacaval shunt	215
portal vein	478
portfolio	68
portion	37
portmanteau word	51
position	76
position sense	302
positional change	90
positive end-expiratory pressure	170
positive negative pressure ventilation	170
positron emission tomography	80
post-	12
post cibum	23
post meridiem	23
post mortem	22
post operationem	22
post partum	22
post scriptum	22
postanesthesia care unit	55
postcholecystectomy syndrome	209
postcoital contraceptive	241
postcoital test	235
postconcussion syndrome	306
postconcussional syndrome	306
posterioanterior	15
posterior	448
posterior antebrachial region	452
posterior auricular artery	472
posterior axillary line	454
posterior basal segment (S^{10})	468
posterior brachial region	452
posterior cerebral artery	471
posterior cervical triangle	450
posterior chamber	456
posterior communicating artery	471
posterior cruciate ligament	496
posterior crural region	453
posterior cubital region	452
posterior femoral region	453
posterior fontanelle (fontanel)	332
posterior inferior cerebellar artery	472
posterior knee region	453
posterior lumbar interbody fusion	291
posterior mediastinum	468
posterior myocardial infarction	185
posterior rhinoscopy	143
posterior segment (S^2)	468
posterior semicircular canal	460
posterior subcapsular cataract	134
posterior superior pancreaticoduodenal artery	474
posterior tibial artery	476
posterior tibial pulse	176
posterior tibial vein	478
posterior vitreous detachment	134
postero-	15
posterolateral	15
postgastrectomy syndrome	206
postgraduate clinical training	67
postgraduate medical education	67
postherpetic neuralgia	121
postictal confusion	297
post-marketing surveillance	585
postmenopausal bleeding	229
postmortem	12
postmortem examination	78
postnasal drip	139
postoperative	12
postprandial	586
postprandial distress syndrome	195
postprandial pain	195
poststreptococcal acute glomerulonephritis	221
post-stroke depression	312
post-transfusion hepatitis	207
posttraumatic stress disorder	312
postural change	90
postural drainage	90, 169
postural orthostatic tachycardia syndrome	174
postural syncope	172
posture	76
potassium	434
potassium iodide	258
potential problems	96
potion	37
pound	438
pounding	121
pous	5
povidone	590
povidone-iodine	152
powder	86
pox	27
PPD test	158
practitioner	57

practitioner of acupuncture	58	premenstrual syndrome	228
practitioner of amma-massage-acupressure	57	premium	49
practitioner of moxibustion	58	premolar tooth	464
pranlukast hydrate	167	prenatal	230
praseodymium	435	prenatal diagnosis	85
pravastatin sodium	259	prenatal screening	236
prazosin hydrochloride	188	preoperative diagnosis	84
pre-	12	prepuce	488
preauricular region	450	preputium penis	488
precancerous	12	presbyacusia	143
preceptor	57	presbyacusis	143
precipitate	72	presbyope	125
precocious	244	presbyopia	125
precocious puberty	254, 343	prescribe	37
precordial	12	prescribed drug	85
precordial leads	178	prescription drug	85
precordial oppression	172	presenilin gene	511
precordial pain	120	present illness	70, 95, 395
predeposit autologous transfusion	275	presenting symptom	72
		preservation	87
prediastolic murmur	175	preserved blood	275
preeclampsia	238	president	62
prefectural hospital	52	press through package	86
prefectural ordinance	46	pressing pain	172
preferential looking	334	pressure sores	318
preferred providers organization	50	pressure support ventilation	170
prefix	2, 10	pressure-volume relation	182
pregnancy	229	presumptive diagnosis	84
pregnancy test	235	presystolic murmur	175
pregnancy-associated plasma protein A	234	preterm	230
		preterm delivery	230
pregnancy-induced hypertension	238	preterm infant	230
pregnanediol	234	pretibial pitting edema	217
pregnant woman	229	preventive medicine	65
preimplantation diagnosis	85	preventive nursing	66
preimplantation genetic diagnosis	85	preventive treatment	118
preleukemia	271	previous illnesses	73
preliminary diagnosis	84	priapism	228
premature atrial contraction	174	prick test	323
premature birth	230	pricking	121
premature ejaculation	228	prickle cell layer	462
premature infant	230, 331	prickling	121
premature ovarian failure	239	prickly heat	318, 330
premature rupture of membranes	238	prick-to-prick test	323
		primary aldosteronism	115, 253
premature ventricular contraction	174	primary angle-closure glaucoma	133
		primary atypical pneumonia	163
		primary biliary cirrhosis	113, 208
premenstrual dysphoric disorder	237	primary cardiomyopathy	187

primary ciliary dyskinesia	164	procedure room	54
primary hyperlipidemia	113	prochlorperazine	211
primary immunodeficiency syndrome	114	procollagen-3-peptide	200
		proctologist	60
primary lateral sclerosis	116, 308	proctology	65
primary nursing	89	proctoscopy	204
primary open-angle glaucoma	133	prodromal stage	91
primary physician	57	prodrome	12
primary pulmonary hypertension	116, 166	productive cough	155
		professional mechanical tooth cleaning	152
primary sclerosing cholangitis	114, 208	professor	62
primary suture	88	progesterone	234, 241
primer	511	prognathism	149, 245
primidone	316	prognosis	85
primigravida	229	progress notes	70, 91, 95
primipara	230	progression	91
primitive neuroectodermal tumor	342	progression-free survival	92
		progressive	91
principal	37	progressive bulbar palsy	308
principal diagnosis	84	progressive diaphyseal dysplasia	341
principle	37	progressive external ophthalmoplegia	135
prior to admission	72		
private health insurance	48	progressive multifocal leukoencephalopathy	112, 307
private hospital	52		
private nursing home	55	progressive muscular dystrophy	308
private parts	444	progressive patient care	43
pro-	12	progressive resistance (resistive) exercise	290
pro re nata	23		
proband	73	progressive spinal muscular atrophy	112, 309
probe	89		
probenecid	259	progressive supranuclear palsy	112, 308
problem list	95, 96		
problem number	96	progressive systemic sclerosis	328
problem-based learning	68	projectile bleeding	261
Problem-Knowledge Coupler	95	prolactin	234, 249
Problem-oriented Medical Information System	95	prolactin-inhibiting hormone	249
		prolactin-releasing factor	234
problem-oriented medical record	68, 95	prolactin-releasing hormone	249
		proliferation	83
problem-oriented nursing record	95	proliferative diabetic retinopathy	135
problem-oriented system	68, 95	proliferative vitreoretinopathy	135
problem-solving	95	prolonged expiration	157
probucol	259	prolonged PR interval	178
procainamide hydrochloride	189	prolonged pulse	173
procalcitonin	248	promethium	435
procarbazine	431	prominent eyes	246
procedure for prolapse and hemorrhoids	215	promontory of tympanic cavity	458
		pronation	279

pronator teres muscle	498
prone position	76
proper hepatic artery	472
proper muscle layer	480
prophylactic treatment	118
prophylaxis	12, 118
proportionate mortality rate	93
propositus	73
propranolol hydrochloride	188
proprioception	302
proprioceptive neuromuscular facilitation	290
proprioceptive sensation	302
proptosis	128
propylthiouracil	258
proscribe	37
prosōpon	5
prosopoplegia	5
prostaglandin	189, 241
prostaglandin analog	210
prostata	7
prostate	37, 488
prostatēs	7
prostate-specific antigen	219
prostatic	7
prostatic acid phosphatase	219
prostatic cancer	223
prostatic intraepithelial neoplasia	223
prostatic massage	217
prostatic secretions	217
prostatitis	7, 223
prostatodynia	216
prostatolithiasis	223
prosthesis	279
prosthetic arm	279
prosthetic foot	279
prosthetic valve endocarditis	186
prosthetics	64
prosthetist and orthotist	58
prosthodontics	152
prostrate	37
prostration	104
protactinium	436
protease	17
protease inhibitor	211, 275
protective glasses	135
protein C	266
protein catabolic rate	582
protein induced by vitamin K absence-II	201
protein restricted diet	224
protein S	266
protein-calorie malnutrition	256
protein-energy malnutrition	256
protein-losing enteropathy	206
proteinuria	218
proteome	511
prothrombin time	265
proto-	16
protodiastolic	16
proton beam therapy	117
proton pump inhibitor	210
proto-oncogene	510
protoplasm	16, 508
protruding	197
protruding teeth	147
protrusion of the jaws	245
protuberant	197
provisional diagnosis	84
proximal	448
proximal interphalangeal joint	495
proximal tubule	486
prulifloxacin	427
prurigo	319
pruritus	27, 37, 319
pseudarthrosis	282
pseudo-	12
pseudoarthrosis	282
pseudobulbar palsy	308
pseudogene	510
pseudogout	286
pseudohermaphroditism	240
pseudohypertrophic muscular dystrophy	308
pseudohypoaldosteronism	115, 254
pseudohypoparathyroidism	12, 115, 252
pseudomembrane	12, 141
pseudomembranous colitis	206
Pseudomonas aeruginosa	219
pseudomyxoma peritonei	210
pseudophakia	137
pseudoxanthoma elasticum	328
psittacosis	108
psoas major muscle	500
psoas minor muscle	500
psoralen-ultraviolet A therapy	329
psoriasis vulgaris	327

psoriatic arthritis	286	pulmonary	8
psyche	7, 293	pulmonary alveolar proteinosis	165
psychiatric mental health nursing	60	pulmonary alveolus	466
psychiatric nursing	66	pulmonary angiography	161
psychiatric social worker	58	pulmonary arteriovenous fistula	183
psychiatrist	27, 60	pulmonary artery	471
psychiatry	65	pulmonary artery pressure	181
psychic	293	pulmonary aspergilloma	165
psycho-	16	pulmonary aspergillosis	165
psychoanalysis	16, 316	pulmonary candidiasis	165
psychoanalyst	60	pulmonary capillary wedge pressure	181
psychological problems	96	pulmonary congestion	176
psychoneurosis	27	pulmonary cryptococcosis	165
psychophysiological disorder	312	pulmonary edema	166, 176
psychosis	37	pulmonary embolectomy	171
psychosomatic	16	pulmonary embolism	166
psychosomatic disease	312	pulmonary emphysema	165
psychosomatic medicine	64	pulmonary function test	162
psychostimulant	314	pulmonary hypertension	166
psychotherapy	7	pulmonary infarction	166
pterygium	127	pulmonary infiltration with eosinophilia	164
pterygium colli	332	pulmonary lobectomy	171
-ptosis	18	pulmonary lymphangioleiomyomatosis	116, 166
ptyalolithiasis	151	pulmonary markings	161
puberty	244, 330	pulmonary P wave	179
pubes	444	pulmonary rehabilitation	169
pubic	37	pulmonary stenosis	184
pubic area	444	pulmonary surfactant	343
pubic hairs	444	pulmonary thromboembolism	166
pubic region	452	pulmonary toilet	169
pubis	494	pulmonary tuberculosis	165
public assistance	49	pulmonary valve	470
public health	63	pulmonary valve insufficiency	184
public health administration	43	pulmonary valve stenosis	184
public health center	52	pulmonary vascular resistance	182
public health insurance	48	pulmonary vein	476
public health nurse	58	pulmonary wedge pressure	181
Public Health Nurse, Midwife and Nurse Law	46	pulmonic regurgitation	184
public hospital	52	pulmonic second sound	175
public pension	48	pulmonis	8
pudendal nerve	506	pulmonology	65
pudendal plexus	506	pulp removal	152
puerile breathing	157	pulpa dentis	464
puerperal fever	230	pulpitis	151
puerperal period	230	pulsation	172
puerperal sepsis	27	pulse	75, 172, 173
puerperium	230		
puffiness	216		

pulse deficit	173
pulse oximetry	158
pulse pressure	75
pulse rate	75
pulse wave velocity	178
pulseless electrical activity	176
pulsus alternans	173
pulsus bigeminus	173
pulsus bisferiens	173
pulsus celer	173
pulsus duplex	173
pulsus durus	173
pulsus mollis	173
pulsus paradoxus	173
pulsus plenus	173
pulsus tardus	173
pulsus vacuus	173
pulvis	23
punch biopsy	78
pupil	456
pupil diameter	129
pupilla	456
pupillary constriction	129
pupillary dilatation	129
pupillary reflex	129
pure red cell aplasia	270
pure tone audiometry	142
purgative	211
purified protein derivative	158, 586
purple	39
purplish	39
purpura	261, 319
purse-string suture	88
pustular psoriasis	116
pustule	320
pustulosis palmaris et plantaris	327
putamen	503
pyelonephritis	223
pyloric antrum	480
pyloric nodes	478
pyloric stenosis	205
pyloroplasty	214
pylorus	480
pyogenic arthritis	286
pyogenic spondylitis	287
pyopneumopericardium	3
pyosalpinx	238
pyothorax	167
pyramid	40
pyramidalis muscle	500
pyrazinamide	168, 427
pyrexia	105
pyriform sinus	466
pyrophobia	297
pyrosis	27, 195
pyuria	218

Q

Q fever	108
QRS complex	179
quack	45
quackery	45
quadrate lobe	484
quadriceps femoris muscle	500
quadriceps reflex	300
quadrilateral	39
quadriplegia	299
quality of health care	42
quality of life	92
QuantiFERON-TB test	160
quantitative computed tomography	283
quantum libet	23
quantum satis	23
quantum sufficit	23
quaque	23
quaque die	23
quaque hora	23
quaque quarta hora	23
Quarantine Act	46
quart	439
quater in die	23
quazepam	314
quick pulse	173
quickening	232
quinidine sulfate	189
quinupristin/dalfopristin	427
quod vide	22

R

rabbit fever	108
rabies	108
rachiodynia	7
radial	448
radial artery	472
radial keratotomy	137
radial nerve	505
radial pulse	176

radial vein	476	rainbow vision	126
radian	439	rale	157
radiating pain	121	raloxifene hydrochloride	289
radiation dermatitis	324	ramosetron hydrochloride	211
radiation pneumonitis	164	randomized controlled trial	592
radiation proctitis	206	range of motion	280
radiation therapy	117	range of motion exercise	290
radiation therapy nursing	61	ranibizumab	136
radical	37	ranimustine	430, 570
radical hysterectomy	243	ranula	148
radical mastectomy	243	rape	229
radical neck dissection	146	rapid eye movement sleep	304
radical treatment	118	rapid heartbeat	172
radicle	37	rapid plasma reagin test	236
radicular cyst	151	rapid pulse	172
radio-	16	rapid urease test	201
radioactive iodine	258	rapid-acting insulin	258
radioactive iodine uptake test	248	rapidly progressive glomerulonephritis	115, 221
radioactivity	16	rash	318
radioallergosorbent test	323	rational	37
radiocarpal	16	rationale	37
radiodermatitis	324	raucous	140
radioenzymatic assay	82	re-	12
radiofrequency ablation	214	reactive arthritis	286
radiograph	79	reading glasses	126
radioimmunoassay	82	rebound tenderness	197
radioimmunosorbent test	82, 323	reception desk	54
radioiodinated human serum albumin	593	receptive aphasia	302
radioisotope	80	recessive gene	512
radioisotope renogram	221	recipe	23
radiologic examination	78	reciprocal help	49
radiological technologist	58	reciprocal translocation	510
radiologist	60	recombinant DNA	510
radiology	65	recombinant human erythropoietin	224, 274
radiolucency	16, 161	recombinant immunoblot assay	593
radionuclide	79	recombinant tissue plasminogen activator	315
radionuclide sialography	150	recommended dietary allowance	592
radionuclide study	79	reconstruction	87
radiopacity	161	recovery	91, 92
radiopharmaceutical	79	recovery room	54
radiotherapy	117	recruitment	142
radioulnar	16	rectal cancer	207
radium	436	rectal temperature	75
radius	492	rectangle	39
radix dentis	464	rectangular solid	40
radix nasi	460	rectocele	17, 239
radix unguis	462		
radon	436		

rectouterine pouch	231, 489	registered dietician (dietitian)	58
rectovaginal examination	231	registered nurse	57
rectum	482	regular diet	90
rectus abdominis muscle	498	regular polygon	39
rectus femoris muscle	500	regurgitation	195
recumbent posture	76	rehabilitation medicine	65
recuperation	92	reinfection	12
recurrence	91	relapse	91
recurrent	91	relapse-free survival	92
recurrent laryngeal nerve paralysis	144	relapsing fever	108
		relapsing polychondritis	144
red	39	relation	73
red blood cell cast	218	relative	73
red blood cell count	263	relative afferent pupillary defect	129
red cell distribution width	263	relative biological effectiveness	591
red cell iron utilization	269	relief	91
red herring	146	religion	74
reddish	39	REM sleep behavior disorder	302
reduced glutathione	554	remember	295
reduced nicotinamide adenine dinucleotide	575	remembrance	295
		remittent fever	105
reducible hernia	198	remote-controlled afterloading system	591
reducing diet	91		
reduction in ~	71	ren	7, 486
reel	294	renal	7, 37
re-emerging infectious disease	106	renal angiomyolipoma	223
referral	73	renal arteriography	221
referral letter	418	renal artery	474
referral rate	73	renal artery stenosis	222
referral response	419	renal artery thrombosis	222
referral system	43	renal atrophy	223
referred pain	121	renal biopsy	221
referring physician	71	renal blood flow	220
reflex	300	renal bruit	217
reflex hammer	77	renal calices	486
reflex incontinence	217	renal cell carcinoma	223
reflex sympathetic dystrophy	311	renal colic	216
reflux esophagitis	204	renal columns	486
refractive error	125	renal corpuscle	486
refractometry	131	renal fascia	501
refractory anemia	115, 270	renal function test	219
refractory anemia with excess blasts	270	renal hilus	486
		renal osteodystrophy	223
regeneration	83	renal papilla	486
regenerative medicine	118	renal pelvis	486
regime	292	renal plasma flow	220
regimen	292	renal ptosis	223
region of interest	593	renal scintigraphy	221
regional anatomy	68	renal sinus	486

renal stone	223	respiratory distress syndrome	592
renal transplantation	226	respiratory excursions	156
renal tubular acidosis	222	respiratory medicine	64
renal tubule	486	respiratory muscles training	169
renal vein	478	respiratory quotient	594
renal vein thrombosis	222	respiratory sinus arrhythmia	174
rending	121	respiratory stimulant	167
reno-	16	respiratory symptoms	154
renogram	16	respiratory syncytial virus	334
renovascular	16	respiratory system	75
renovascular hypertension	184, 222	respiratory therapy	167
reoperation	12	respiratory tract	466
repair	87	rest	289
repetatur	24	restless legs syndrome	279
repetitive strain injury	285	restlessness	295
repetitive stress injury	285	restraint	90
replacement	87	restriction enzyme	510
replacement arthroplasty	291	restriction fragment length poly-	
replacement therapy	117	morphism	510
replication	511	restrictive cardiomyopathy	113, 187
reportable disease	106	restrictive lung disease	163
reporting responsibility	44	résumé	68
repressor gene	512	retch	195
reprise	330	retching	195
rescue dose	123	reticular layer	462
research assistant	62	reticular tissue	512
research institute	62	reticular zone	490
research personnel	62	reticulocyte	263, 264
researcher	57	reticulocytosis	265
resection	88	reticuloendothelial system	265
resectoscope	226	reticulum cell	267
resident	59	retina	458
resident physician	59	retinal arterial pressure	132
residual urine	220	retinal detachment	135
residual volume	162	retinal hemorrhage	130
resin sponge uptake	248	retinal neovascularization	130
resistance transfer factor	594	retinal pigmentary degeneration	135
resolved problem	96	retinitis	134
resonance	156	retinitis pigmentosa	113, 135
resonant	156	retinoblastoma	135, 342
Resource Utilization Groups	42	retinol-binding protein	591
respiration	75, 154	retinopathy	18
respiration rate	75	retinopathy of prematurity	135
respirator	169	retinopexy	137
respiratory acidosis	159	retinoscopy	131
respiratory bronchiole	466	retirement	74
respiratory bronchiolitis-associated		retirement pension	49
interstitial lung disease	164	retracted	197
respiratory care	167	retractor	89

retro-	12	rhinitis	8
retroauricular nodes	478	rhino-	16
retroauricular region	450	rhinophonia	18
retrocochlear hearing loss	143	rhinophony	16
retroflexion	12	rhinophyma	141
retrognathism	149	rhinoplasty	18, 146
retrograde ejaculation	228	rhinorrhea	16, 18, 139
retrograde pyelography	220	*Rhinovirus*	160
retrograde urethrography	221	rhis	8
retrograde urography	220	rhodium	435
retrolental fibroplasia	134	rhomboid	39
retroperitoneal fibrosis	224	rhomboid fossa	502
retroperitoneal lymph node dissection	226	rhomboid major muscle	500
		rhomboid minor muscle	500
retroperitoneum	12	rhombus	39
retropubic space	488	rhonchi	158
retroversion of the uterus	239	rhythmical nystagmus	129
retroverted uterus	239	rib	492
return to clinic	594	ribavirin	211
reverse transcriptase-polymerase chain reaction	81	ribonucleic acid	511
		ribonucleoprotein	511
reverse transcription	510	ribosomal RNA	511
reversed occlusion	149	ribosome	508
reversed passive hemagglutination	81	ribostamycin	427
		rickets	337
reversible ischemic neurological deficit	306	rifabutin	427
		rifampicin	168, 427
review of systems	70	Rift Valley fever	108
Revised European-American Lymphoma classification	263	right atrial enlargement	179
		right atrium	470
revolutions per min	439	right bundle branch block	179
Rh blood group	267	right colic artery	474
rhabdomyolysis	285	right coronary artery	471
rhabdomyosarcoma	288	right flexure of colon	482
rhachis	7	right gastric artery	474
rhenium	435	right gastroepiploic artery	474
rhesus factor	592	right hepatic artery	472
rheumatic fever	110, 340	right hypochondriac region	450
rheumatic heart disease	184	right inguinal region	452
rheumatism	278	right lobe	484
rheumatoid arthritis	110, 286	right lower lobe	466, 468
rheumatoid arthritis hemagglutination test	283	right lower quadrant	452
		right (left) lower quadrant pain	120
rheumatoid factor	283	right lung	466
rheumatoid nodule	281	right lymphatic duct	478
rheumatoid vasculitis	114	right middle lobe	466, 468
rheumatologist	60	right sternal border	175
rheumatology	65	right upper lobe	466, 468
rhinencephalon	502	right upper quadrant	452

right (left) upper quadrant pain	120	roundworm	199
right ventricle	470	route of infection	106
right ventricular assist device	192	roxithromycin	427
right ventricular failure	186	-rrhaphy	18
right ventricular hypertrophy	175	-rrhea	18
right ventricular pressure	181	-rrhexis	18
right-angled triangle	39	RS (respiratory syncytial) virus infection	109
right-handedness	294	rubber gloves	77
right-sided heart failure	186	rubella	27, 109, 325, 330
rigor	105	rubeola	109, 330
riluzole	315	rubeosis iridis	129
ring	40	rubidium	434
ring finger	444	rule	46
ringed sideroblast	267	rule of nines	320
ringing in the ears	28	rule out	593
ringworm	28, 318, 325	ruler	78
ringworm of the feet	318	rumbling	196
risperidone	316	rupture	26, 198
rituximab	433	rusty	39
Rocky Mountain spotted fever	109	ruthenium	435
rod neutrophil	264	rutherfordium	436
roentgen	439		
roentgen diagnosis	84		
roentgenium	436		

S

rokitamycin	427	sabot heart	180
rolandic fissure	502	saccule	460
Rolfing	119	sacral anesthesia	87
roll over	330	sacral cord	504
root	2	sacral nodes	479
root canal	464	sacral plexus	506
root canal filling	152	sacral region	452
root canal treatment	152	sacral vertebra	492
root of the nose	460	sacralization	284
root pain	121	sacroiliac joint	495
root planing	152	sacroiliitis	286
ropinirole hydrochloride	315	sacrum	494
rosacea	141	saddle nose	141
roseola	110	saddle-back nose	141
roseola infantum	339	safety glasses	135
rotablation	191	safety pin	78
rotation test	143	sagittal plane	448
rotational atherectomy	191	salazosulfapyridine	211, 288
rotator cuff injury	284	saliva	147, 512
rough endoplasmic reticulum	508	salivary calculus	148
rouleau formation	264	salivary gland	464
round ligament of femur	496	salivary gland scintigraphy	150
round ligament of liver	484	salivary stone	148
round window	459	salivation	147
rounds	66	salmeterol	169

Salmonella	202
salmonellosis	206
salpingitis	27, 143, 238
salpingocyesis	237
salpingography	9
salpingo-oophorectomy	243
salpingoscopy	143, 236
salpinx	9
salt-free diet	90
samarium	435
sanatorium	52
sanguine	6
sanguis	6
saphenous nerve	506
sarco-	16
sarcoid	16, 18
sarcoidosis	113, 165
sarcoma	16, 83
sartorius muscle	500
satanophobia	296
sauna	118
sawtooth	40
scab	318, 320
scabies	27, 325
scala tympani	459
scala vestibuli	459
scald head	318
scale	78, 320
scalene triangle	39
scaling	152
scalp	442
scalpel	88
scandium	434
scanning electron microscope	79
scanning laser ophthalmoscope	131
scanty menstruation	228
scapha	458
scaphocephalus	332
scaphocephaly	332
scaphoid	197
scaphoid bone	492
scapula	492
scapular region	452
scapulohumeral periarthritis	278, 284
scar	83
scarlatina	330
scarlet	39
scarlet fever	330
sceletus	6
Schedule for Affective Disorders and Schizophrenia	304
schistocytosis	264
Schistosoma	199
schizophrenia	312
school doctor	57
School Health Law	46
school of dentistry	62
school of medicine	62
school of nursing	62
school of pharmacy	62
school of veterinary medicine	62
school physician	57
school refusal	343
schoolchild	330
schooling	74
schwannoma	313
sciatic nerve	506
sciatic pain	121
sciatica	121
scintigraphy	80
scintillating scotoma	126
scintiscan	80
scirrhous	37
scirrhous gastric carcinoma	205
scirrhus	37
scissors	88
scissors gait	298
sclera	456
scleral buckling	137
scleritis	133
sclero-	16
scleroderma	16, 17, 111, 114
scleroderma renal crisis	328
scleroiritis	16
-sclerosis	18
scoliosis	281
-scope	18
scotoma	132
scratch	319
scratch test	323
scrotal mass	217
scrotal swelling	217
scrotal tongue	148
scrotum	488
scrub nurse	59
scrub typhus	108
scurf	318
seaborgium	436

sealant	152	seminiferous tubule	488
seamen's insurance	49	seminoma	224
seasonal affective disorder	595	semis	24
seasonal influenza	155	semitendinosus muscle	500
sebaceous glands	462	senile	244, 295
seborrhea	325	senile dementia	295
seborrheic dermatitis	324	senility	244
seborrheic keratosis	324	sennoside	211
sebum palpebrale	127	sensitive	295
second	439	sensorineural hearing loss	142
secondary fracture	282	sensory area	503
secondary glaucoma	134	sensory nerve action potential	304
secondary hypertension	184	sensory nerve ending	462
secondary infection	106	sensory speech center	503
secondary sex characteristics	245	sensus luminis	127
second-degree burn	320	sentence completion test	304
secrete	407	sentinel hospitals	110
secretin test	202	sentinel lymph node biopsy	236
secundum artem	24	separation	74
sedate	407	separation of pharmacy from medical practice	42
sedative	314	sepsis	107
segmental bronchus	466	septal deviation	141
segmental diagnosis	85	septic arthritis	286
segmented neutrophil	264	septicemia	27
seizure	293	septum pellucidum	502
selective aldosterone blocker	188	sequence of events	96
selective celiac angiography	203	sequestration	284
selective estrogen receptor modulator	241, 289	sequestrum	284
selective serotonin reuptake inhibitor	314	serine protease inhibitor	275
selective vagotomy	214	serious condition	76
selegiline hydrochloride	315	serious illness	73
selenium	434	sero-	16
self-care unit	55	serologic test	78
self-limited	92	serologic test for syphilis	236
self-monitoring of blood glucose	257	serology	63
self-rating depression scale	596	seronegative	16
sella turcica	251	serosa	480
semen bank	242	serositis	16
semi-	12	serotonin	250
semicircle	40	serotonin receptor agonist	122
semicircular canal	460	serotonin-dopamine antagonist	316
semicoma	12	serotonin-noradrenaline reuptake inhibitor	314
semilunar	12	serous fluid	512
semilunar bone	492	serous layer	480
semilunar cartilage	496	serrated	40
seminal vesicle	488	serratus anterior muscle	498
seminal vesiculitis	236	serratus posterior inferior muscle	

	500	short stature	245, 331
serratus posterior superior muscle		short tandem repeat	510
	500	short-acting inhaled β_2-agonist	169
serum amyloid A protein	595	short-acting insulin	258
serum creatinine	219	shortness of breath	154, 172, 261
serum diagnosis	84	short-stay facility for the elderly	55
serum iron	268	shot	26
serum protein electrophoresis	599	shoulder	444
serum prothrombin conversion accelerator	599	shoulder blade	444
		shoulder girdle	492
sesquipedalian words	20	shoulder joint	495
severe	121	shuffle	294
severe acute pancreatitis	114	shuffling gait	298
severe acute respiratory syndrome	107, 166	si opus sit	24
		sialadenitis	151
severe combined immunodeficiency	596	sialidase	575
		sialoadenitis	151
severe erythema exudativum multiforme	116	sialography	150
		sialolith	148
sex	71	sialolithiasis	151
sex chromatin	508	sialolithotomy	152
sex chromosome	508	sib	73
sex gland	488	sibling	73
sex hormone-binding globulin	234	sick sinus syndrome	183
sex-linked inheritance	74	sickle cell anemia	269
sexual desire	228	sickness	72
sexual intercourse	228	sideburns	442
sexual precocity	244	sideroblast	267
sexually transmitted disease	237	sideroblastic anemia	269
shaggy	319	siemens	439
shagreen skin	319	sievert	439
shaking chills	105	sigh	154
shaking palsy	27	sight	37, 125
shape	39	sigmoid artery	474
shared care	43	sigmoid colon	482
sharp	121	sigmoidoscopy	204
shelf operation	292	sign language interpreter	58
shift to the left	264	signet ring	40
shifting dullness	197	signet ring cell	82
shin	446	signetur	24
shinbone	27	sildenafil citrate	242
shingles	26	silent myocardial ischemia	185
short gastric artery	474	silent thyroiditis	251
short increment sensitivity index	142	silicon	434
		silicosis	165
short leg brace	290	silver	435
short leg cast	289	silver filling	152
short lingual frenulum	332	simple sequence length polymorphism	510
short PR interval	178		

simulated patient	68	skipped pulse	172
simulator	68	skodaic resonance	157
simultaneous perception	132	skull	442
sine	22	skull radiography	251
singer's nodes	140	skull traction	291
single fiber electromyogram	283	sky blue	39
single nephron glomerular filtration rate	219	slang	2
single nucleotide polymorphism	509	sleep	74, 104
single radial immunodiffusion	80	sleep apnea	140
single-photon emission computed tomography	80	sleep apnea syndrome	167
		sleep-disordered breathing	167
singultus	27, 155	sleepiness	297
sinoatrial conduction time	181	sleeplessness	104
sinoatrial node	470	sleeptalking	104
sinobronchial syndrome	163	sleepwalker	104
sinus arrhythmia	174	sleepwalking	104
sinus bradycardia	174	sleeve gastrectomy	260
sinus nodal reentrant tachycardia	174	slim	105
		sling	289
sinus nodal reentry tachycardia	174	slipped capital femoral epiphysis	287
sinus node recovery time	181	slipped disc	26
sinus rhythm	173	slit-lamp biomicroscopy	131
sinus tachycardia	174	slough	318
sinus trouble	27	slow heartbeat	172
sinuses of dura mater	476	slow pulse	172
sinusitis	27, 144	slow reacting substance of anaphylaxis	159
sinusoid	484		
sisomicin	428	slow wave sleep	304, 600
sister	73	small bowel	480
sitafloxacin	428	small cell lung carcinoma	166
sitagliptin	258	small child	330
site	37	small intestine	480
sitology	35	small saphenous vein	478
sitz bath	89	small-for-dates infant	331
six-pack	277	small-for-gestational-age infant	331
sixth disease	339	smallpox	107
sizofiran	431	smarting	121
skeletal	6	smegma	231
skeletal muscle	498	smell	140
skeletal traction	291	smoking	74
skeleton	6	smoking cessation clinic	169
skiascopy	131	smoldering leukemia	271
skin	75, 318, 462	smooth endoplasmic reticulum	508
skin biopsy	324	smooth muscle	498
skin graft	329	smooth muscle antibody	597
skin grafting	329	snapping finger	285
skin traction	291	sneeze	139
skin-associated lymphoid tissue	595	sneezing	139, 154
		sniffles	155

Term	Page
snivel	139
snore	140
snoring	140
snout reflex	301
snow	25
snuffles	155
SOAP format	96
SOAPIE format	96
soapsuds enema	90
sociable	296
social history	70
social insurance	48
Social Insurance Agency	49
social medicine	64
social security	49
social skills training	316
socialized medicine	43
society-managed health insurance	48
sodium	434
sodium channel blocker	189
sodium nitroprusside	189
sodium picosulfate	211
soft chancre	237
soft contact lens	136
soft diet	90
soft exudate	130
soft palate	464
soft pulse	173
soft x-ray	329
solar keratosis	324
sole	37, 446, 453
soleus muscle	500
solid diet	90
solid food	194
sōma	5
somatic chromosome	508
somatic pain	120
somato-	16
somatoform disorder	312
somatomedin	249
somatomedin C	249
somatosensory	16
somatosensory evoked potential	304
somatotropin	249, 344
somatotype	5, 16
somnambulism	104
somnambulist	104
somniloquism	104
somnolence	297
son	73
sorafenib	433
sorafenib tosilate	224
sore	28, 318
sore ears	120
sore eyes	120
sore throat	28, 120, 140
sore tongue	147, 261
soreness	120
soul	37
source of information	70
source-oriented medical record	95
source-skin distance	599
South American hemorrhagic fever	107
space-occupying lesion	598
sparfloxacin	428
spasm	293
spasmodic	293
spasmodic croup	340
spastic diplegia	306
spastic gait	298
spastic paralysis	298
special nursing home for the elderly	55
specialist	57, 59
specialized function hospital	52
specialty board system	67
specific behavioral objective	67
specific dynamic action	105
specific gravity	598
spectacles	126
spectinomicin	428
spectrum	37
speculum	37
speculum examination	231
speech and hearing therapist	58
speech audiometry	142
speech discrimination test	142
speech reception threshold test	142
speech therapist	600
speech therapy	145, 316
sperm	235
sperm bank	242
sperm function test	235
spermatozoon	235
sphenoid bone	492
sphenoid sinus	460
sphenoid sinusitis	144

sphenoidal sinus	460	splitting	121
sphenoiditis	144	splitting of heart sounds	175
sphere	40	spondylo-	16
spherocyte	264	spondylodesis	291
spherocytosis	264	spondylolisthesis	8, 16, 288
sphygmomanometer	77	spondylolysis	16, 288
spider angioma	197	spondylolytic spondylolisthesis	288
spider telangiectasia	197	spondylos	8
spina	7	spondylosis deformans	288
spina bifida	342	sponge bath	89
spinal	7	spontaneous bacterial peritonitis	210
spinal anesthesia	87	spontaneous occlusion of the circle of Willis	307
spinal canal	455		
spinal canal stenosis	288	spontaneously hypertensive rat	597
spinal column	278	spoon nail	262, 321
spinal cord	504	sporotrichin test	323
spinal cord injury	288	sports medicine	64
spinal cord stimulation	123	spotting	28
spinal deformity	278	spouse	73
spinal extrapyramidal tract	504	sprain	37, 278
spinal fusion	291	sprained finger	279
spinal muscular atrophy	341	spray	328
spinal nerves	505	spur cell	264
spinal pyramidal tract	504	spurting bleeding	261
spinalis muscle	500	sputum	155
spindle	40	sputum culture	159
spine	40, 278, 492	squamocolumnar junction	480
spinobulbar muscular atrophy	112, 309	squamous cell carcinoma	84, 166
spinocerebellar degeneration	111, 309	squamous intraepithelial lesion	239
spinous layer	462	square	39
spiral	40	squaric acid dibutylester	329
spiral CT	79	squeeze dynamometer	283
spiramycin	428	squint	27, 125
spirometer	18, 162	ST depression	179
spirometry	162	ST elevation	179
spironolactone	188	stab neutrophil	264
splashing sound	198	stabbing	121
spleen	485	stable angina	185
splēn	8	staccato speech	302
splenectomy	215, 276	staff doctor	59
splenic	8	staff nurse	59
splenic artery	474	stagger	294
splenic flexure	482	staggers	28
splenic pulp	485	staghorn calculus	219
splenic vein	478	stalk	40
splenomegaly	8, 18, 198, 262	stammer	294
splicing	510	standard language test of aphasia	304
splint	279	standardization	3

standardized mortality rate	44, 93
standardized patient	68
standing posture	76
stapedectomy	145
stapedial reflex	141
stapedioplasty	145
stapes	459
stapes fenestration	145
staphylitis	150
staphylococcal scalded skin syndrome	600
staphylococcus	17
Staphylococcus aureus	202
Staphylococcus saprophyticus	219
stapler	89
star	40
-stasis	19
State Children's Health Insurance Program	50
state medicine	43
state-run hospital	52
static exercise	290
statim	24
statins	259
stationary	38
statoconium	460
statue	38
stature	38
status convulsivus	331
steato-	16
steatohepatitis	16
steatorrhea	16, 197
steeple sign	334
ST-elevation myocardial infarction	185
stella	40
stellate	40
stellate ganglion block	123, 190
stem cell transplantation	276
stenosis	198
steppage gait	298
stereognosis	302
stereognostic perception	302
stereopsis	132
stereotactic irradiation	600
stereotactic radiosurgery	317
stereotactic radiotherapy	117
sterile	229
sterile technique	87
sterility	229
sternal	5
sternal line	454
sternal region	450
sternal-occipital-mandibular immobilizer	290
sternoclavicular joint	495
sternocleidomastoid muscle	498
sternocleidomastoid region	450
sternon	5
sternotomy	5
sternum	5, 492
stethoscope	77
stiff shoulder	278
stimulant	27
Stimulants Control Law	46
stinging	121
stirrup	459
stoma	6
stoma care	212
stomach	444, 480
stomach trouble	194
stomachus	5
stomal ulcer	205
stomatitis	6, 150
stomatodysodia	148
stomatology	64
-stomy	19
stone dissolvent	211
stool	196, 215
stool extraction	90
stopwatch	77
strabismus	27, 125
strain	37
strained back	279
straining to void	216
stratum basale	462
stratum corneum	462
stratum granulosum	462
stratum papillare	462
stratum reticulare	462
stratum spinosum	462
strawberry tongue	148
strep throat	27
streptococcal pharyngitis	27
streptococcal pyrogenic exotoxin	322
Streptococcus pneumoniae	160
streptokinase-streptodornase	597
streptomycin	428

Term	Page
streptomycin sulfate	168
stress echocardiography	181
stress fracture	282
stress incontinence	217
stretcher	90
striae distensae	245
striae gravidarum	231
striated muscle	498
striatonigral degeneration	112, 308
stridor	154, 157
stripping of varicose veins	192
stripping of varicose veins and subfascial ligation of perforator	192
stroke	25, 294
Stroke Impairment Assessment Set	298
stroke rehabilitation nursing	61
stroke volume	181
strong pulse	173
strontium	435
structural gene	510
struvite calculus	218
stumble	294
stump	88
stupor	297
stuporous	297
stutter	294
sty	127
stye	26, 127
sub-	12
subacute	91
subacute bacterial endocarditis	186
subacute combined degeneration of spinal cord	308
subacute hepatitis	207
subacute myelo-optico-neuropathy	116, 309
subacute necrotizing encephalomyelopathy	307
subacute sclerosing panencephalitis	112, 307
subacute thyroiditis	251
subarachnoid anesthesia	87
subarachnoid block	123
subarachnoid hemorrhage	307
subarachnoid space	504
subclavian artery	472
subclavian muscle	498
subclavian vein	476
subclinical infection	106
subconjunctival hemorrhage	128
subcostal	12
subcutaneous	12
subcutaneous emphysema	156
subcutaneous fat	245
subcutaneous fatty tissue	462
subcutaneous injection	86
subcutaneous nodules	280
subcutaneous tissue	462
subdural hematoma	307
subdural space	504
subendocardial myocardial infarction	185
subglottic laryngitis	144
subjective data	96
sublingual cyst	148
sublingual gland	464
sublingual tablet	86
submandibular duct	464
submandibular gland	464
submandibular nodes	478
submaxillary gland	464
submental nodes	478
submerged tooth	149
submucosa	480
submucous layer	480
submucous resection of inferior nasal concha	146
submucous resection of nasal septum	146
subsegmental atelectasis	161
substance dependence	312
substance withdrawal syndrome	303
substantia nigra	504
substernal pain	120
substitution therapy	117
subthalamic nucleus	503
subtotal gastrectomy	214
subungual hematoma	321
subzonal insemination	242
succussion sound	198
succussion splash	198
sucralfate hydrate	210
sudamina	27
sudden cardiac death	176
sudden deafness	113, 143
sudden death	93

Term	Page
sudden infant death syndrome	339
sudden unexplained death	176
sudor	512
sudoriferous glands	462
suffix	2, 17
suffocation	154
suicidal behavior	296
suicidal ideation	296
suicidal thought	296
suicide	74
suicide attempt	296
sulbactam/cefoperazone	427
sulcus of cerebrum	502
sulfa	38
sulfamethoxazole/trimethoprim	428
sulfonylurea	600
sulfonylurea compound	258
sulfur	38, 434
sultamicillin	427
sumatriptan succinate	122
summary	70, 93
summary of the hospital course	93
sun protection factor	318
sunburn	318
sunglasses	126
sunnitinib	433
sunstroke	105
super-	12
supercilium	442, 456
superconducting quantum interference device	599
superego	38
superficial cervical nodes	478
superficial circumflex iliac artery	476
superficial epigastric artery	476
superficial femoral artery	474
superficial pain	120
superficial palmar arterial arch	472
superficial palmar venous arch	476
superficial peroneal nerve	506
superficial punctate keratitis	133
superficial reflex	301
superficial temporal artery	472
superficial temporal artery-middle cerebral artery anastomosis	316
superficial temporal vein	476
superinfection	12
superior	448
superior cerebellar artery	472
superior extensor retinaculum	500
superior limbic keratoconjunctivitis	133
superior lingular segment (S^4)	468
superior mediastinum	468
superior mesenteric artery	474
superior mesenteric vein	478
superior nasal meatus	460
superior oblique muscle	458
superior phrenic artery	472
superior rectal artery	474
superior rectus muscle	458
superior sagittal sinus	476
superior segment (S^6)	468
superior thyroid artery	472
superior turbinate	460
superior vena cava	476
superior vena cava syndrome	166
supernumerary tooth	149
superoxide dismutase	598
supersecretion	12
supination	279
supinator muscle	498
supine hypotensive syndrome	231
supine position	76
support hospital for regional medical care	52
supporting tissue	512
supportive center for long-term care for the elderly	55
supportive therapy	118
suppository	86
suppurate	319
suppurative arthritis	286
supra-	12
supraclavicular	12
supraclavicular fossa	450
supraclavicular nerve	505
supraclavicular nodes	478
supranuclear	38
supraorbital region	450
suprapubic	12
suprapubic lithotomy	226
suprapubic pain	216
suprarenal gland	490
suprascapular nerve	505
suprascapular region	452
supraventricular tachycardia	174

sural region	453
surface anesthesia	87
surface electrode	283
surface lines	454
surfactant protein A	159
surfactant protein D	159
surgeon	59
surgery	64, 86
surgical clipping	317
surgical hand scrub	87
surgical instruments	88
surgical site infection	599
surgical treatment	118
survival rate	92
suspected diagnosis	84, 85
suspended traction	291
suspension of medical practice	42
suspicion	85
sustained virological response	201
Sutton's law	171
suture	88
swallowing	195
swan-neck deformity	281
sway-back nose	141
swaying gait	298
sweat	512
sweat glands	462
sweating	105
swelling	173, 216
swine-origin influenza A virus	160
swollen and indurated prostate	217
sycosis	37, 325
sycosis vulgaris	27
syllabus	67
sylvian aqueduct	502
sylvian fissure	502
sympathectomy	123
sympathetic block	123
sympathetic nerve	506
symptom	72
symptomatic therapy	118
symptoms of the digestive tract	194
syn-	12
synchronized intermittent mandatory ventilation	170
syncopal	293
syncope	293
syndactyly	333
syndesmophyte	284
syndrome	12
syndrome of inappropriate secretion of antidiuretic hormone	253
synesthesia	301
synovectomy	291
synovial bursa	501
synovial fluid	513
synovial fluid analysis	284
synthesis	12
synthetic graft	192
syphilis	27, 109, 237
syringe	86
syringomyelia	112, 342
syrup	86
syrupus	24
system of medical services	42
system review	70, 95
Systematized Nomenclature of Medicine	3
Systematized Nomenclature of Pathology	4
systemic disease	106
systemic inflammatory response syndrome	107
systemic lupus erythematosus	110, 114, 327
systemic vascular resistance	600
systolic anterior motion	181
systolic blood pressure	75
systolic murmur	175
systolic time intervals	182

T

tabes dorsalis	308
tablet	86
tachy-	16
tachycardia	16, 172, 245
tachypnea	16, 154
tacrolimus hydrate	288, 328
tactile fremitus	156
taenia coli	482
Taenia saginata	199
Taenia solium	199
tai chi	118
tail of the pancreas	484
tailor-made medicine	118
talampicillin	428
talaporfirin sodium	170
talipes calcaneus	280

talipes cavus	280	telephone number	71
talipes equinovarus	280, 340	telithromycin	428
talipes equinus	280	tellurium	435
tall stature	245	telomerase	511
talus	494	telomere	511
tamoxifen	431	temper	295
tamoxifen citrate	241	temperament	295
tampon	241	temperature	75
tamsulosin hydrochloride	224	temperature sensation	301
tandem gait	298	temperature sense	301
tangent screen	132	temple	442
tantalum	435	temporal arteritis	111, 114, 187
tape measure	78	temporal bone	492
taping	289	temporal lobe	502
target cell	264	temporal muscle	498
tarry stool	195, 196	temporal region	450
tarsal bone	494	temporary problem	96
tarsal gland	456	temporary threshold decay test	142
tarsal scaphoid bone	494	temporary threshold shift	142
tarsal triquetrum	494	temporomandibular joint	495
tarsometatarsal joint	495	temporomandibular joint disorder	
tarsus	38, 456		152
tartar	147	temsirolimus	433
taste	147	tenacious	155
tattoo	321	tender	121, 197
tautology	371	tenderness	121, 197
taxonomy of educational objectives		tendo	6
	66	tendon	501
tazobactam/piperacillin	428	tendon reflex	300
T-cell growth factor	602	tendon sheath	501
teaching hospital	52	tendovaginitis	6, 285
team nursing	89	tenesmus	196
tear film breakup time	129	tenia	38
tearing	121	tennis elbow	279
tears	126	tenodesis	6
tebipenem pivoxil	428	tenofovir disoproxil fumarate	275
technetium	435	tenōn	6
technical terminology	2	tenosynovectomy	291
technical terms	2	tenosynovitis	285
tectorial membrane	459	tense	295
teethe	330	Tensilon test	305
tegafur	430, 431	tension headache	120
tegafur-gimeracil-oteracil	431	tension-free vaginal mesh	243
tegafur-uracil	431	tentative diagnosis	84
tegmentum mesencephali	504	ter in die	24
teicoplanin	428	tera-	20
tela subcutanea	462	teratology	63
teleangiectasis	17	teratoma	83
telemedicine	43	terbinafine hydrochloride	329

terbium	435	therapeutic drug monitoring	86
terebrating	121	therapeutic exercise	290
teres major muscle	498	therapeutic plan	96
teres minor muscle	498	thermanesthesia	301
terminal bronchiole	466	thermesthesia	301
terminal care	118	thermo-	16
terminal deoxynucleotidyl transferase	267	thermography	182, 322
terminal stage	91	thermometer	16, 77
terminology of medical education	66	thermoregulation	16
tesla	439	thiamazole	258
test for tubal patency	236	thiamphenicol	428
Test of English as a Foreign Language	66	thiazides	188
Test of English for International Communication	67	thiazolidinedione derivative	258
		thigh	446
testicle	488	thin	105
testicular	7	thin blood	25
testicular pain	228	thin-layer chromatography	81
testicular sperm extraction	242	thinly-haired	319
testicular tumor	223	thiotepa	431
testis	7, 488, 490	third molar tooth	147, 464
testosterone	234	third ventricle	502
test-tube baby	25	third-degree burn	320
tetanus	27, 109	thirst	244
tetanus immune globulin	603	thirsty	244
tetany	246	thirsty fever	105
tetracycline	428	thoracentesis	17, 163
tetrahydrocannabinol	124, 603	thoracic	5
tetraiodothyronine	247	thoracic aorta	472
thalamic pain	294	thoracic aortic aneurysm	187
thalamus	503	thoracic cavity	455
thalassemia	269	thoracic cord	504
thalidomide	274	thoracic duct	478
Thalidomide Education and Risk Management System	274	thoracic endovascular aortic repair	192
thallium	436	thoracic nerve	505
thallium treadmill stress test	181	thoracic outlet syndrome	284
thallium-201 myocardial perfusion scanning	181	thoracic respiration	154
		thoracic surgeon	59
thanato-	94	thoracic surgery	64
thanatology	94	thoracic vertebra	492
thanatophobia	94	thoraco-	16
thanatopsis	94	thoracocentesis	163
thanatosis	94	thoracolumbar fascia	501
theca	35	thoracoplasty	5, 170
thecal	35	thoracoscopic biopsy	163
thenar eminence	446	thoracoscopic bullectomy	170
therapeutic abortion	242	thoracoscopic pneumonectomy	170
		thoracoscopy	16, 163
		thoracostomy tube	169

thoracotomy	16, 170	thyroid carcinoma	252
thorax	5, 156, 444	thyroid cartilage	495
thorium	436	thyroid function test	247
threatened abortion	238	thyroid gland	490
three-day measles	330	thyroid hormone resistance	115
three-dimensional conformal radiotherapy	117	thyroid nodules	246
three-dimensional echocardiography	181	thyroid stimulating immunoglobulin	248
thrill	175	thyroidectomy	259
thrix	6	thyroid-stimulating hormone	248
throat	442	thyroid-stimulating hormone receptor antibody	248
throbbing	121	thyrotoxicosis	251
thrombectomy	191	thyrotropin	248
thrombin time	265	thyrotropin human alfa	248
thrombin-antithrombin III complex	266	thyrotropin-binding inhibitory immunoglobulin	248
thrombo-	16	thyrotropin-releasing hormone	604
thromboangiitis obliterans	114, 187	thyroxine	247
thrombocyte count	263	thyroxine-binding globulin	248
thrombocytopenia	18, 265	tibia	6, 27, 494
thrombocytosis	265	tibial	6, 448
thromboelastogram	602	tibial nerve	506
thromboembolism	16	tibialgia	6
thromboendarterectomy	191	tibialis anterior muscle	500
thrombolysis	16, 17	tibiofibular joint	495
thrombolytic agent	189	tic	38, 300
thrombomodulin	266, 275	tic douloureux	121
thrombophlebitis	187	tick	38
thrombotest	265	tick-borne encephalitis	108
thrombotic microangiopathy	273	ticlopidine hydrochloride	190, 315
thrombotic thrombocytopenic purpura	115, 273	tidal volume	162
throw up	28	tight pain	172
thrush	27, 150	tin	435
thulium	435	tine test	158
thumb	444	tinea	38, 325
thumb forceps	89	tinea capitis	325
thumb-sucking	330	tinea corporis	325
thymectomy	259, 317	tinea cruris	27, 325
thymine	511	tinea manus	325
thymus	490	tinea manuum	325
thymus and activation-regulated chemokine	323	tinea pedis	28, 325
thymus and activation-regulated chemokine	601	tinea unguinum	325
		tinea versicolor	318, 325
		tingle	295
thyrocervical trunk	472	tinnitus	28, 139
thyroglobulin	248	tinnitus retraining therapy	145
thyroid antagonist	258	tinnitus test	142
		tip of the nose	460

tip of tongue	464
tiredness	104
tissue	512
tissue fluid	512
tissue plasminogen activator	189, 315
tissue polypeptide antigen	604
titanium	434
TNF-receptor-associated periodic syndrome	604
TNM Classification of Malignant Tumors	85
to-and-fro murmur	175
tobramycin	428
tocilizumab	289
tocodynamometer	235
tocolysis	230
tocolytic agent	241
toddle	330
toes	446
tokodynamometer	235
toluene diisocyanate	602
tomography	79, 161
-tomy	19
tongue	464
tongue blade	77
tongue depressor	77
tongue deviated	148
tonic neck reflex	333
tonometry	131
tonsil	465
tonsilla	465
tonsillar fossa	465
tonsillar swelling	141
tonsillectomy	146
tonsillectomy and adenoidectomy	146
tonsillitis	28, 144
tooth	147, 442, 464
tooth cavity	147
tooth extraction	152
tooth mobility	149
tooth replantation	153
tooth socket	465
tooth transplantation	153
toothache	120, 147
toothbrush	147
toothed forceps	89
toothless	149
top of the head	442
tophus	140, 246
topical	38
topical beta blocker	136
topiramate	316
topo-	68
topography	68
topology	68
TORCH syndrome	338
toremifene	431
tormenting	121
torricelli	439
torsade de pointes	179
torso	444
torticollis	28, 285, 332
tortuosity	40
tortuous	38
torture	38
torus	40
torus palatinus	150
tosufloxacin	428
total abdominal hysterectomy	243
total anomalous pulmonary venous return	183
total artificial heart	192
total bile acid	200
total bilirubin	199
total blood volume	602
total body irradiation	276
total cholesterol	250
total elbow arthroplasty	292
total elbow replacement	292
total gastrectomy	214
total hip arthroplasty	291
total hip replacement	291
total iron-binding capacity	268
total knee arthroplasty	291
total knee replacement	291
total lung capacity	162
total lymphocyte count	265
total nodal irradiation	276
total parenteral nutrition	91
total peripheral resistance	182
total pneumonectomy	171
total vaginal hysterectomy	243
touchy	295
toxemia of pregnancy	238
toxic epidermal necrolysis	326
toxic megacolon	206
toxic shock syndrome	326
toxic shock syndrome toxin	322

Term	Page
toxic shock-like syndrome	326
trabeculectomy	137
trabeculotomy	137
trachea	5, 28
tracheal	5
tracheal cartilage	495
tracheal deviation	156
tracheal sounds	157
tracheal suctioning	168
tracheal tube	168
tracheia	5
tracheoesophageal fistula	338
tracheostomy	5, 170
tracheotomy	19, 170
trachoma	133
trachoma-inclusion conjunctivitis	133
traction	87
traction therapy	290
traditional Chinese medicine	119
trafermin	329
tragus	458
tranquilizer	314
trans-	12
transactional analysis	316
transbronchial aspiration biopsy	163
transbronchial biopsy	163
transbronchial lung biopsy	163
transcatheter arterial chemoembolization	213
transcatheter arterial embolization	213
transcellular fluid	512
transcranial Doppler ultrasonography	305
transcription	511
transcriptome	511
transcutaneous electrical nerve stimulation	123
transcutaneous pacing	190
transdermal patch	189
transection	88
transepidermal water loss	322
transesophageal echocardiography	181
transfemoral amputation	292
transfer RNA	511
transferrin	268
transferrin receptor	268
transfixion	87
transforming growth factor	603
transfusion reaction	274
transfusion-related acute lung injury	166
transhepatic arterial infusion	213
transhumeral amputation	292
transient abnormal myelopoiesis	336
transient global amnesia	302
transient ischemic attack	294, 306
transient tachypnea of the newborn	334
transitional stage	91
transjugular intrahepatic portosystemic shunt	213
translation	511
translocation	12, 511
transmural myocardial infarction	185
transplant coordinator	57
transplant surgery	63
transplantation	12
transposition of great vessels	183
transposon	511
transpupillary thermotherapy	136
transradial amputation	292
transrectal ultrasonography	220
transsphenoidal surgery	317
transtibial amputation	292
transtracheal aspiration biopsy	163
transudation	84
transurethral biopsy	221
transurethral laser-induced prostatectomy	226
transurethral lithotripsy	225
transurethral microwave thermotherapy	226
transurethral needle ablation	226
transurethral prostatectomy	226
transurethral resection	226
transurethral resection of bladder tumor	226
transurethral resection of the prostate	226
transurethral ureterolithotripsy	226
transurethral vaporization of the prostate	226
transverse	448
transverse colon	482
transverse incision	88
transverse pancreatic artery	474

Term	Page
transverse presentation	232, 233
transverse sinus	476
transverse tarsal joint	495
transversus abdominis muscle	500
trapezium	39
trapezium bone	492
trapezius muscle	498
trapezoid	39
trapezoid bone	492
trastuzumab	241, 433
trauma	73
traumatic brain injury	306
traumatic perforation of the tympanic membrane	143
travel medicine	65
treadmill stress test	180
treadmill test	180
treatment	85
treatment room	54
trembling	294
tremor	245, 294
trench mouth	151
trephination	88
Treponema pallidum	235
Treponema pallidum hemagglutination test	236
Treponema pallidum immobilization test	236
tretinoin	429, 525
tri-	12
triage	44
triage tag	44
triangle	39
triangular bone	492
triangular fibrocartilage complex	280
triangular fossa	458
triangular prism	40
triazolam	314
tricarboxylic acid cycle	602
triceps brachii muscle	498
triceps muscle of arm	498
triceps muscle of calf	500
triceps reflex	300
triceps skinfold	605
triceps skinfold thickness	245
triceps surae muscle	500
triceps surae reflex	300
trichiasis	127
trichlormethiazide	188
trichobezoar	209
Trichomonas vaginalis	235
trichophagia	6
trichophytia	325
trichophytosis	28
trichothiodystrophy	326
Trichuris	199
tricuspid	12
tricuspid atresia	183
tricuspid regurgitation	184
tricuspid stenosis	184
tricuspid valve	470
tricuspid valve insufficiency	184
tricuspid valve stenosis	184
tricyclic antidepressant	314
trifascicular block	179
trifocal glasses	135
trigeminal ganglion	505
trigeminal nerve	505
trigeminal neuralgia	121
trigeminy	12, 173
trigger	72
trigger finger	285
triglyceride	250
trigone of the bladder	486
trigonum vesicae	486
triiodothyronine	247
triiodothyronine resin uptake	248
triple vaccine	343
triplets	229
-tripsy	19
triquetrum	492
trismus	148
trochanter major	494
trochanter minor	494
trochanteric region	452
troche	86
trochlear nerve	505
-trophy	19
tropical	38
tropical medicine	65
tropicamide	136
trouble	72
trouble in ~	71
truncal obesity	245
trunk	444
trunk incurvation	333
TSH receptor anomaly	115
tsutsugamushi disease	108

tuba uterina	9
tubal ligation	242
tubal obstruction	144
tubal pregnancy	9, 237
tubal stenosis	143
tube feeding	212
tubercular	38
tuberculin test	158
tuberculosis	18, 28, 107
tuberculosis hospital	52
Tuberculosis Prevention Law	46
tuberculous	38
tuberculous spondylitis	287
tuberosity of tibia	494
tuberous sclerosis	116, 326
tubulointerstitial nephritis	222
tularemia	108
tumor	83
tumor marker	201
tumor necrosis factor	604
tumor suppressor gene	510
tumor-associated antigen	601
tumor-induced osteomalacia	255
tumor-infiltrating lymphocyte	603
tumor-specific antigen	605
tumor-specific transplantation antigen	605
tungsten	435
tunica mucosa	480
tunica serosa	480
tunica submucosa	480
tuning fork	78
tuning fork test	142
turbidimetric immunoassay	82
turbinate	460
turbinectomy	146
tutorial system	67
twang	140
twins	229
twin-twin transfusion syndrome	232
twitching	127
tyloma	320
tympanic	38
tympanic cavity	458
tympanic insufflation	143
tympanic membrane	139, 458
tympanic membrane perforation	140
tympanites	197
tympanitic	38, 197
tympanometry	142
tympanoplasty	145
tympanosclerosis	143
tympanostomy	145
type 1 diabetes mellitus	255
type 2 diabetes mellitus	255
type and cross-match	602
typhoid fever	107
typhus	108
tyrosinuria	333

U

ubenimex	429
ulcer	28, 320
ulcerative colitis	113, 206
ulcus duodeni	205
ulcus ventriculi	205
ulna	492
ulnar	448
ulnar artery	472
ulnar nerve	505
ulnar vein	476
ultra-	12
ultrafiltration	12, 225
ultrafiltration rate	606
ultrasonography	12, 80
ultrasound biomicroscopy	131
ultraviolet	607
ultraviolet B	329
ultraviolet keratitis	133
ultraviolet spectrophotometry	81
umbilical	6
umbilical artery	474
umbilical cord	232
umbilical hernia	210, 339
umbilical region	450
umbilicus	6, 444
un-	12
unbalanced diet	194, 261
unconcerned	295
unconjugated bilirubin	199
unconjugated hyperbilirubinemia	268
unconscious	12, 76
unconsciousness	28, 293
uncorrected visual acuity	131
uncountable noun	329
underarm hairs	444
undergraduate medical education	66
undernourishment	244

undersurface of foot	453	ununseptium	437
underwater exercise	290	ununtrium	436
undescended testis	236	upper arm	444
undifferentiated	12	upper esophageal sphincter	480
undifferentiation	84	upper extremity	444
unemployment	74	upper eyelid	456
unemployment insurance	48	upper gastrointestinal bleeding	204
unerupted tooth	149	upper gastrointestinal series	203
uneven bite	149	upper gastrointestinal tract	480
ungual	8	upper jaw	442
unguentum	24	upper limb	444
unguis	8, 462	upper lip	442
uni-	12	upper motor neuron	606
unidentified clinical syndrome	104	upper respiratory tract	466
unidentified complaint	104	upper respiratory tract infection	163
Unified Medical Language System	3	upset stomach	194
unilateral	12	upside-down stomach	25
unilateral renal mass	217	uranium	436
unilocular	12	uranoschisis	332
uninhibited contraction	223	urate calculus	218
Unio Internationalis Contra Cancrum	606	urate crystal	284
		urea breath test	201
unipolar depression	312	uremia	223
United States Medical Licensing Examination	68	uremic acidosis	219
		uremic breath	217
United States Pharmacopeia	85	uremic fetor	217
universal health insurance	48	ureter	38, 486
university	62	ureterectomy	226
university hospital	52	ureteritis	223
university of health sciences	62	ureteropelvic junction	486
university of medical science	62	ureterovesical junction	486
university of medical welfare	62	urethra	38, 488
university of nursing and welfare	62	urethral catheterization	224
university of pharmacy	62	urethral discharge	217
university of social welfare	62	urethral stent	224
university of welfare	62	urethralgia	216
unlicenced medical practice	44	urethritis	223
unmarried	74	urethroplasty	226
unnatural death	93	urethroscopy	221
unpadded cast	289	urge incontinence	217
unresolved problem	96	-uria	19
unsaturated iron-binding capacity	268	uric acid	606
		uricaciduria	218
unstable	295	uridine diphosphate	606
unstable angina	185	uridine monophosphate	606
ununhexium	437	uridine triphosphate	607
ununoctium	437	urinal	38, 90
ununpentium	436	urinalysis	78, 217
ununquadium	436	urinary	38

urinary bladder	486
urinary flow rate	220
urinary frequency	216
urinary homovanillic acid	333
urinary incontinence	216
urinary lithiasis	223
urinary organ	486
urinary output	216
urinary retention	216
urinary sediment	218
urinary stream	216
urinary system	486
urinary tract	486
urinary tract infection	223
urinary urgency	216
urinary vanillylmandelic acid	333
urination	216
urine	513
urine ardor	216
urine culture	219
urine cytology	219
urine odor	148
urinometry	219
uro-	16
urobilinogenuria	218
urodynamic study	220
urodynamics	220
urodynia	216
uroflometer	220
uroflowmeter	220
uroflowmetry	220
urogenital	16
urogenital region	452
urogenital system	75
urokinase	189
urolithiasis	16, 223
urologist	60
urology	65
ursodeoxycholic acid	211
urticaria	28, 318, 320
urticaria pigmentosa	324
urtication	320
usual interstitial pneumonia	164
ut dictum	24
uterine	6
uterine appendages	489
uterine bleeding	229
uterine cancer	239
uterine cervix cancer	239
uterine corpus carcinoma	239
uterine muscle relaxant	241
uterine muscle stimulant	241
uterine myoma	239
uterine myomectomy	243
uterine prolapse	239
uterine tube	488
uteroplacental insufficiency	237
uterus	6, 28, 488
utricle	460
uvea	456
uveitis	134
uvula	464
uvulitis	150
uvulopalatopharyngoplasty	146

V

vaccinate	407
vaccination	343
vaccine-associated paralytic poliomyelitis	607
vaccinia immune globulin	608
vagal nerve stimulation	316
vagina	489
vagina tendinis	501
vaginal birth after cesarean section	243
vaginal bleeding	28, 229
vaginal discharge	228
vaginal introitus	489
vaginal orifice	489
vaginal speculum	37, 78
vaginal spotting	229
vaginal vault	231
vaginismus	229
vaginitis	238
vaginoscopy	236
vagus nerve	505
valacyclovir hydrochloride	329
vallate papilla	464
valproic acid	316
valvular disease of the heart	28
valvular heart disease	183
vanadium	434
vancomycin	428
vancomycin-resistant enterococcus infection	109
vancomycin-resistant staphylococcus aureus infection	109

vanillylmandelic acid	333, 609	veno-arterial bypass	192
variable number tandem repeats		veno-occlusive disease	208
	510	venous	7
variant angina pectoris	185	venous hum	176
varicella	28, 110, 325, 330	ventilation-perfusion scan	161
varicella vaccine	344	ventilator-associated pneumonia	164
varicella-zoster immune globulin	328	ventilatory receptor	162
varicella-zoster virus	322	ventral	16, 448
varicose veins of lower extremities		ventral decubitus	76
	187	ventral hernia	210
variegate porphyria	257	ventricle	470
vas	6	ventricular activation time	607
vas deferens	488	ventricular aneurysm	185
vascular dementia	311	ventricular assist device	192
vascular murmur	198	ventricular assist system	192
vascular permeability factor	609	ventricular drainage	317
vascular spider	197	ventricular extrasystole	174
vascular surgeon	59	ventricular fibrillation	174
vascular surgery	64	ventricular premature complex	
vasectomy	242	(contraction)	174
vaseline	328	ventricular puncture	317
vaso-	16	ventricular septal defect	183
vasoconstriction	16	ventricular tachycardia	174
vasoconstrictor	189	ventriculo-	16
vasodilation	6	ventriculoatrial shunt	317
vasodilator	189	ventriculography	16, 305
vasomotor	16	ventriculometry	16
vasopressin	249, 259	ventriculoperitoneal shunt	317
vasopressor	189	ventriculoperitoneostomy	317
vasospastic angina	185	ventriculopuncture	317
vasovagal reflex	176	ventriculoscopy	305
vastus intermedius muscle	500	ventro-	16
vastus lateralis muscle	500	ventrolateral	16
vastus medialis muscle	500	verbal order	609
vectorcardiogram	180	vermifuge	211
vegan	261	vernacular	2
veganism	261	vernal conjunctivitis	133
vegetarian	261	verotoxin	609
vegetarianism	261	verotoxin-producing *Escherichia*	
vegetation	176	*coli*	334
vegetative state	297	verruca	28, 320
vein	476	versus	22
vena	7	vertebra	8
venereal disease	237	vertebral	8
Venereal Disease Research Laboratory test	236	vertebral angiography	305
		vertebral artery	472
venereal wart	25	vertebral canal	455
venereologist	60	vertebral column	492
Venezuelan equine encephalitis	108	vertebral region	452

Term	Page
vertebrobasilar insufficiency	306
verteporfin	136
vertex	442
vertical	448
vertical banded gastroplasty	260
vertical infection	106
vertical plane	448
vertiginous	139
vertigo	28, 139, 172, 293
very low birth weight infant	331
very low calorie diet	90
very-high-density lipopretein	608
very-low-density lipopretein	609
vesica	8
vesical	8, 38
vesicle	28, 38, 320
vesicoureteral reflux	223
vesicular sounds	157
vestibular nerve	460, 505
vestibular neuronitis	144
vestibule	459
vestibule of vagina	489
vestibulocochlear nerve	460
vestibulum nasi	460
veterinarian	57
vibration sense	302
Vibrio cholerae	202
Vibrio parahaemolyticus	202
vibro-acoustic stimulation test	235
vice president	62
vice-director	59
vidarabine	329
vide	22
videlicet	22
video display terminal	126
video-assisted thoracoscopic surgery	170
vilirization	244
villous	38
villus	38, 40
vinblastine	431
vincristine	431
vincristine sulfate	274
vindesine	431
vinorelbine	431
violent; excruciating	121
VIPoma	255
viral capsid antigen	608
viral hepatitis	109, 207
viral infection	106
virilism	240, 244
virus	28
virus-associated hemophagocytic syndrome	607
visceral fat	245
visceral pain	120
visceral pleura	468
visceral sensation	302
visceral sense	302
viscid	155
viscous	38
viscus	38
visible peristalsis	197
vision	125
visiting nursing	61
visual acuity	125
visual analog scale	122
visual display terminal	126
visual evoked potential	133
visual field	132
visual field defect	132
visual impairment	125
visual laser ablation of the prostate	226
visual organ	456
visual sense	125
vital capacity	162
vital signs	75
vitamin B_{12}	268, 274
vitamin B_6	274
vitamin D	289
vitamin D receptor anomaly	115
vitamin D-dependent rickets	337
vitiligo	319
vitiligo vulgaris	326
vitrectomy	137
vitreous body	456
vitreous clouding	129
vitreous floater	129
vitreous fluorophotometry	132
vitreous hemorrhage	129
vitreous opacity	129
vitreous surgery	137
vocal cord	466
vocal cord paralysis	141
vocal cord polyp	144
vocal fremitus	158
voice disturbance	140

voice training	145
voiding cystourethrography	221
volar	444, 446
volt	439
volvulus	338
vomit	28, 195
vomiting	195
vomitus	195
voriconazole	428
vulva	489
vulvar pruritus	229
vulvitis	238

W

waist	38, 444
waiting room	55
wale	318
walk unaided	330
walker	90, 290
walking stick	279
wandering pacemaker	179
ward	55
warfarin potassium	189
wart	28, 318, 320
washed red blood cells	276
waste	38
water deprivation test	250
water-hammer pulse	173
watery stool	196
watt	439
waxy cast	218
WDHA syndrome	255
weak pulse	173
weakness	104
weaning	343
weaning food	343
weariness	104
webbed neck	332
weber	439
wedging vertebra	284
weep	26, 319
weight	75, 105
weight gain	105
weight loss	105
weight-bearing joint	278
welfare	49
welfare center for the elderly	55
Welfare Law for the Elderly	47
well leg raising test	281
well-developed	76
well-nourished	76
welt	318
West Nile fever	108
Western blotting	610
Western equine encephalitis	108
wet dream	27, 228
wet-bulb globe temperature index	610
wheal	318, 320
wheelchair	90
wheeze	154, 158
wheezing	154
whiplash	279
whiplash-associated disorders	285
whipworm	199
whispered bronchophony	157
whispered pectoriloquy	157
white	39
white blood cell cast	218
white blood cell count	263
white clot syndrome	273
white flow	229
white mouth	27
white-coat hypertension	173
whites	27, 228
whitish	39
whitlow	326
WHO classification of lymphoid neoplasms	263
WHO's pain relief ladder	122
whole blood	275
whooping cough	27, 330
wind	26
windpipe	28
wing	55
wing of the nose	460
wisdom tooth	147, 464
withdrawal bleeding	234
withdrawal syndrome	196
WMA Declaration of Lisbon on the Rights of the Patient	44
WMA International Code of Medical Ethics	44
womb	28
women's health nursing	60
wooden spatula	77
wooden-shoe heart	180
word structure	2

word-formation	2
workmen's accident compensation insurance	49
World Medical Association	44
worries	71
worsening	91
wound	61, 73
wound dehiscence	88
wrist	444
wrist cock-up splint	290
wrist joint	495
wristdrop	298
wrist-hand orthosis	290
writer's cramp	293
wrong diagnosis	85
wryneck	28, 285, 332

X

xanthelasma	245
xanthine derivatives	167
xanthochromia	305
xanthoma	245
xanthomatosis	256
xenon	435
xenophobia	296
xeroderma	321
xeroderma pigmentosum	116, 325
xerosis	35, 321
xerostomia	151
xiphoid process	450
X-linked dominant	74
X-linked gene	509
X-linked inheritance	74
X-linked lymphoproliferative syndrome	271
X-linked recessive	74
x-ray diagnosis	84
x-ray examination	78
x-ray film	79
X-ray room	54

Y

yard	439
yellow	39
yellow fever	108
yellow jaundice	26
yellow ligaments	496
yellowish	39
Y-linked gene	509
yoga	119
young adult mean	283
ytterbium	435
yttrium	435

Z

zalcitabine	275
zanamivir hydrate	168
zidovudine	275
zinc	434
zinc oxide ointment	328
zirconium	435
zona fasciculata	490
zona glomerulosa	490
zona reticularis	490
zonisamide	315, 316
zoonosis	106
zoophobia	297
zoster immune globulin	328
zygoma	492
zygomatic bone	492
zygomatic region	450
zygote intrafallopian transfer	242

冠名用語索引

A

Achard-Thiers syndrome	254
Achilles reflex	300
Achilles tendon	501
Achilles tendon reflex	300
Achilles tendon rupture	285
Adam's apple	442
Adams-Stokes syndrome	176
Addison disease	115, 254
Adie syndrome	129
Adson test	282
Albert suture	88
Albright hereditary osteodystrophy	252
Allen test	176
Alport syndrome	222
Alzheimer disease	308
(dementia of the) Alzheimer type	311
Amsler chart	132
Andersen disease	257
Apert syndrome	341
Apgar score	317, 331
Argyll Robertson pupil	129
Arnold-Chiari malformation	306
Arthus reaction	323
Ascher syndrome	150
Aschoff-Tawara node	470
Asherman syndrome	239
Asperger syndrome	313
Auerbach plexus	483
Auspitz sign	321
Austin Flint murmur	175
Ayerza syndrome	186

B

Babinski reflex	301
Bainbridge reflex	177
Baker cyst	280
Balint syndrome	301
Ballet sign	246
Banti syndrome	270
Bárány pointing test	143
Bárány test	143
Barr body	508
Barré-Liéou syndrome	285
Barrett esophagus	205
Barthel index	92
Bartholin gland	489
bartholinitis	238
Bartter syndrome	254
Basedow disease	251
Bassen-Kornzweig syndrome	256
Battle sign	141
Bauhin valve	482
Bazin disease	325
Beau lines	321
Beck triad	176
Becker muscular dystrophy	309
Beckwith-Wiedeman syndrome	339
Bednar aphtha	332
Behçet disease	111, 114, 150
Bell palsy	299
Bence Jones proteins	263
Benedikt syndrome	299
Berger disease	221
Bernard-Soulier syndrome	273
Bertin columns	486
Besnier prurigo	324
Bezold triad	142
Billroth I	214
Billroth II	214
Binet intelligence test	334
Binswanger disease	311
Biot respiration	157
Bitot spots	128
Blalock-Taussig operation	191
Bloom syndrome	336
Blount disease	287
Blumberg sign	197
Bochdalek hernia	338
Boerhaave syndrome	205
Böhler angle	280
Borg scale	156
Borrmann classification	199
(patent) Botallo duct	183
Bouchard nodes	280
Bourneville disease	326
Bowen disease	327

Bowman capsule	486
braille	125
Brenner tumor	239
Bright disease	26
Brinkman index	156
Broadbent sign	176
Broca aphasia	302
Broca center	503
Brown-Séquard syndrome	299
Brudzinsky sign	298
Brugada syndrome	174
Brunner gland	483
Brushfield spots	128
Bruton disease	335
Budd-Chiari syndrome	113, 208
Buerger disease	114, 187
Burkitt lymphoma	272
Byler disease	208

C

Caffey disease	340
Calot triangle	484
Camurati-Engelmann syndrome	341
Caplan syndrome	165
Carney complex	188
Caroli disease	209
Carpenter syndrome	341
Castleman disease	272
Chaddock reflex	301
Chadwick sign	231
Chagas disease	340
Charcot joint	280
Charcot triad	196, 298
Charcot-Marie-Tooth disease	310
Chédiak-Higashi syndrome	272
Cheyne-Stokes respiration	157
Chiari-Frommel syndrome	253
Child classification	199
Chopart joint	495
Christmas disease	274
Churg-Strauss syndrome	165
Chvostek sign	246
Coats disease	134
Cockcroft-Gault formula	220
Codman exercise	290
Cogan syndrome	141
Colles fracture	282
Conn syndrome	253
Cooley anemia	269
Coombs test	267
Coopernail sign	233
Cope sign	197
Cori disease	257
Corrigan pulse	173
(organ of) Corti	459
Costen syndrome	141
Coulter counter	263
Courvoisier sign	198
Cowden disease	207
Cowper gland	488
Creutzfeldt-Jakob disease	109, 112, 311
Crigler-Najjar syndrome	335
Crohn disease	113, 206
Cronkhite-Canada syndrome	207
Crow-Fukase syndrome	112, 273
Cruveilhier-Baumgarten syndrome	198
Cullen sign	198
Curling ulcer	205
Curschmann spiral	159
Cushing disease	116, 252
Cushing syndrome	253
Cushing triad	298
Cushing ulcer	205

D

Da Costa syndrome	188
Darier disease	324
Darier sign	320
Darwin tubercle	140
de Musset sign	177
de Quervain disease	285
de Toni-Fanconi syndrome	337
DeBakey classification	182
Dercum disease	245
Descemet membrane	456
Devic disease	308
Diamond-Blackfan anemia	335
Dick test	323, 334
Dieulafoy ulcer	205
DiGeorge syndrome	336
Disse space	484
Döhle inclusion body	264
Donath-Landsteiner test	268
Doppler echocardiography	181
Doppler ultrasonography	80, 305
Douglas cul-de-sac	231, 489

Douglas pouch	489
Down syndrome	336
Dressler syndrome	186
Dubin-Johnson syndrome	208
Duchenne muscular dystrophy	308
Duhring disease	324
Dukes classification	199
Duncan disease	271
Dupuytren contracture	281
Duroziez sign	177

E

Ebstein anomaly	183
Edwards syndrome	336
Ehlers-Danlos syndrome	337
Eisenmenger complex	183
Ellsworth-Howard test	250
Epley maneuver	145
Epstein pearls	332
Epstein-Barr virus	267
Epstein-Barr virus associated nuclear antigen	544
Erb-Duchenne paralysis	335
eustachian salpingitis	143
eustachian tube	459
Evans syndrome	273
Ewart sign	176
Ewing sarcoma	288

F

Fabry disease	113, 336
fallopian pregnancy	237
fallopian tube	488
(tetralogy of) Fallot	183
Fanconi anemia	336
Felty syndrome	111, 286
Fishberg concentration test	220
Fisher syndrome	112, 310
Fitz-Hugh and Curtis syndrome	232
Fogarty catheter	191
Foley catheter	225
Fontan operation	191
Fordyce spots	149
Forestier disease	287
Forrester classification	182
Foster Kennedy syndrome	130
Fournier gangrene	237
Foville syndrome	299
Fowler position	77

Frei test	323
Frenzel glasses	132
Frey syndrome	151
Friedreich ataxia	310
Fröhlich syndrome	253
Froment sign	303

G

Gaenslen sign	281
Gaffky scale	160
Gaisböck syndrome	271
Gardner syndrome	207
Garland triangle	157
gasserian ganglion	505
Gaucher disease	257
Gerota fascia	501
Gerstmann syndrome	302
Gerstmann-Sträussler-Scheinker disease	112, 311
Gianotti-Crosti syndrome	339
Gilbert syndrome	208
Gilles de la Tourette syndrome	310
Girdlestone operation	292
Gitelman syndrome	254
Glanzmann disease	273
Gleason score	221
Goldmann perimeter	132
Golgi apparatus	508
Goodpasture syndrome	221
Gordon reflex	301
Gordon syndrome	254
Gorlin syndrome	327
Gottron sign	321
Gowers sign	299
Gradenigo syndrome	143
Graefe sign	246
Graham Steell murmur	176
Graves disease	251
Grawitz tumor	223
Grey Turner sign	198
Grocco triangle	157
Guillain-Barré syndrome	112, 310
Günther disease	335
Guthrie test	333

H

Hageman factor	556
Hallpike maneuver	141
Halsted operation	243

Ham test	268	Hurler syndrome		337
Hamilton depression rating scale	303	Hutchinson teeth		149
Hamman sign	158	Hutchinson triad		237
Hamman-Rich syndrome	164			
Hand-Schüller-Christian disease	342			

J

Hansen disease	328	
Harrison groove	156	jacksonian epilepsy	297
Hartmann operation	214	Jaeger test type	131
Hashimoto disease	251	Jendrassik maneuver	300
Hashimoto thyroiditis	251	Joffroy sign	246

K

Hassall corpuscle	490		
haversian system	494		
Heberden nodes	280	Kallmann syndrome	240
Heerfoldt syndrome	165	Kanner syndrome	343
Hegar sign	231	Kaplan-Meier survival curve	92
Heimlich maneuver	168	Kaposi sarcoma	272
Heinz body	264	Karnofsky scale	92
Heller operation	214	Kartagener syndrome	183
Henle loop	486	Kasabach-Merritt syndrome	326
Henoch-Schönlein purpura	340	Kaufmann therapy	241
Hertel exophthalmometer	131	Kaup index	331
Herxheimer reaction	233	Kawasaki disease	111, 340
Hesselbach triangle	452	Kayser-Fleischer ring	197
Highmore antrum	460	Kearns-Sayer syndrome	342
Hill sign	173	Kehr sign	262
Hill-Sachs lesion	284	Keith-Wagener classification	131
hippocratic face	76	Kelman phacoemulsification	136
Hippocratic Oath	45	Kent bundle	179
Hirschsprung disease	338	Kerckring folds	482
His bundle	470	Kerley B lines	180
His bundle electrogram	180	Kernig sign	298
Hodgkin disease	272	Kienböck disease	285
Hodgkin lymphoma	272	Kiesselbach area	141, 460
Hoffmann sign	301	Killian operation	146
Holmes phenomenon	300	Killip classification	177
Holter electrocardiograph	180	Kimmelstiel-Wilson syndrome	222
Holter monitor	180	Klatskin tumor	209
Homans sign	177	Kleine-Levin syndrome	312
Horner syndrome	158	Klinefelter syndrome	240
Hounsfield unit	79	Klippel-Feil syndrome	341
Houston valves	482	Klumpke paralysis	335
Howell-Jolly body	264	Klüver-Bucy syndrome	312
Hubbard tank	290	Kocher forceps	89
Huhner test	235	Kocher incision	88
Hunt syndrome	299	Koebner phenomenon	321
Hunter glossitis	151, 262	Koplik spots	148
Hunter syndrome	337	Korotkoff sounds	75
Huntington chorea	310	Korsakoff syndrome	302
Huntington disease	112, 310	kosher food	91
		Krabbe disease	337

Krukenberg tumor	233
Kugelberg-Welander disease	342
Kupffer cells	484
Kussmaul respiration	246
Kveim test	323

L

Ladd syndrome	338
Lamaze method	230
Lambert-Eaton myasthenic syndrome	158
Landolt ring	131
(islets of) Langerhans	490
Langerhans cell histiocytosis	114, 342
Lasègue sign	281
Laurence-Moon-Biedle syndrome	253
Leber hereditary optic neuropathy	135
Legg-Calvé-Perthes disease	286
Leigh disease	307
Lembert suture	88
Lennox-Gastaut syndrome	332
Leopold maneuvers	232
Leriche syndrome	177
Lesch-Nyhan syndrome	337
Leser-Trélat sign	321
Letterer-Siwe disease	342
Levin tube	211
(dementia with) Lewy bodies	312
Lewy body	305
Leydig cells	490
Lhermitte sign	298
Libman-Sacks endocarditis	186
Liddle syndrome	254
Lieberkühn gland	483
Lisfranc joint	495
Little disease	306
Löffler endocarditis	186
Löffler syndrome	164
Löfgren syndrome	161
Löwenberg sign	177
Lown-Ganong-Levine syndrome	178
Lucas sign	332
Ludloff sign	282
Ludwig angina	151
Luys body	503
Lyell syndrome	326
Lynch syndrome	207

M

Macewen sign	333
Mallory body	204
Mallory-Weiss syndrome	204
malpighian corpuscle	486
Mantoux test	158
Marcus Gunn pupil	129
Marfan syndrome	337
Marie-Strümpell disease	287
Mariotte spot	132
Marshall-Marchetti-Krantz operation	226
Master two-step test	180
McArdle disease	257
McBurney incision	88
McBurney sign	197
McCune-Albright syndrome	252
Meckel diverticulum	206
Medusa head	197
Mees lines	321
meibomian gland	456
Meige syndrome	311
Meigs syndrome	233
Meissner plexus	483
Mendelson syndrome	163
Ménétrier disease	205
Meniere disease	113, 144
Merkel cell	462
Merseburg triad	246
Mikulicz syndrome	151
Miles operation	214
Millard-Gubler syndrome	299
Miller-Abbott tube	212
Millon test	333
Milroy disease	177
Minamata disease	309
Mirizzi syndrome	198
Moebius sign	246
Mondor disease	177
Monteggia fracture	282
Morgagni foramen	466
Morgagni hernia	338
Morison pouch	483
Moro embrace reflex	333
Moro reflex	333
Morton disease	285
Muir-Torre syndrome	207
Munchausen syndrome	313

Munchausen syndrome by proxy 343
Murphy sign 197

N

nabothian cyst 231
Nägele rule 230
Negri bodies 305
Nélaton catheter 224
Nelson syndrome 253
Netherton syndrome 325
Niemann-Pick disease 257
Nightingale Pledge 44
Nikolsky sign 321
Nissen fundoplication 214
Nissl body 504
non-Hodgkin lymphoma 272
Noonan syndrome 240

O

(sphincter of) Oddi 484
Ogilvie syndrome 199
Oguchi disease 135
Oliver sign 177
Ollier disease 288
Oppenheim reflex 301
Ortolani sign 333
Osgood-Schlatter disease 287
Osler node 177
Osler-Weber-Rendu disease 274
(nevus of) Ota 326

P

pacchionian body 504
pacinian corpuscle 462
Paget disease of bone 286
Paget disease of breast 240
Pancoast syndrome 158
Paneth cell 483
Papanicolaou smear test 235
Parinaud syndrome 301
Parkinson disease 27, 112, 308, 317
Paul-Bunnell test 267
Pel-Ebstein fever 262
Pelger-Huët nuclear anomaly 264
Perez reflex 333
Perry syndrome 308
Peutz-Jeghers syndrome 207
Peyer patches 483

Peyronie disease 237
Pfannenstiel incision 88
Phalen test 282
Pick disease 308
pickwickian syndrome 156
Pierre Robin syndrome 332
Plummer disease 251
Plummer-Vinson syndrome 262
Pompe disease 257
Pott disease 287
Pott fracture 282
Poupart ligament 496
Prader-Willi syndrome 338
Pringle disease 116, 326
Prinzmetal angina 185
Puestow procedure 215
Purkinje fibers 470

Q

Queckenstedt test 305
Quincke edema 320

R

Ramsay Hunt syndrome 299
Ranson criteria 204
Raynaud phenomenon 321
Recklinghausen disease 116
Reed-Sternberg cell 269
Refsum disease 311
Reifenstein syndrome 240
(insula of) Reil 502
Reinke edema 141
Reiter syndrome 286
Rett syndrome 313
Retzius space 488
Reye syndrome 339
Reynolds pentad 196
Richter hernia 210
Richter syndrome 271
Riedel thyroiditis 252
Riga-Fede disease 332
Rinne test 142
Röhrer index 331
Rokitansky-Aschoff sinus 484
rolandic fissure 502
Romano-Ward syndrome 183
Romberg test 300
Rorschach test 304
Roth spots 130

Roux-en-Y anastomosis	214	sylvian fissure	502
Rovsing sign	197	Syme amputation	292
Rumpel-Leede phenomenon	262		

S

T

Salmonella	202	Takayasu arteritis	111, 187
salmonellosis	206	Takayasu disease	114, 187
Santorini duct	484	Tay syndrome	337
Scarpa triangle	452	Tay-Sachs disease	257
Schamberg disease	327	Tenon capsule	458
Schatzki ring	203	Terson syndrome	130
Scheuermann disease	287	Thomas test	281
Schilling test	268	Tietze syndrome	156
Schiötz tonometer	131	Tinel sign	303
Schirmer test	128	Todd paralysis	297
Schlemm canal	456	Tolosa-Hunt syndrome	307
Schmidt syndrome	255	Traube semilunar space	157
Schmorl nodule	284	Treacher Collins syndrome	341
Schwann sheath	506	Treitz ligament	482
schwannoma	313	Trendelenburg position	77
Sengstaken-Blakemore tube	212	Trendelenburg test	333
Sertoli cells	488	Trousseau sign	246
Sézary syndrome	327	Trousseau syndrome	177
Sheehan syndrome	252	Turner syndrome	240
Shulman syndrome	285	Tzanck test	324
Shy-Drager syndrome	111, 310		
Sims position	77	## V	
Sipple syndrome	255		
Sjögren syndrome	111, 114, 151	Valsalva method	190
skodaic resonance	157	Vater papilla	482
Smith fracture	282	Venturi mask	168
Snellen chart	131	Verner-Morrison syndrome	255
Somogyi phenomenon	247	(lichen) Vidal	325
Stauffer syndrome	223	Vincent angina	151
Steele-Richardson-Olszewski syndrome	308	Virchow node	198
		Virchow triad	177
Stein-Leventhal syndrome	238	Vogt-Koyanagi-Harada syndrome	134
Stellwag sign	246	Volkmann contracture	281
Stensen duct	464	von Gierke disease	257
Stevens-Johnson syndrome	326	von Hippel-Lindau disease	313
Stickler syndrome	341	von Recklinghausen disease	313
Still disease	111, 286	von Willebrand disease	273
struvite calculus	218	von Willebrand factor	266
Sturge-Weber syndrome	342		
Swan-Ganz catheter	181	## W	
Sweet disease	327		
Swyer-James syndrome	161	Waardenburg syndrome	337
Sydenham chorea	310	Waldenström macroglobulinemia	273
sylvian aqueduct	502	Waldeyer tonsillar ring	465
		Wallenberg syndrome	306
		Waterhouse-Friderichsen syndrome	340

Waters projection	150
Watson-Schwartz test	250
Weber syndrome	299
Weber test	142
Wechsler Adult Intelligence Scale	303
Wechsler Intelligence Scale for Children	334
Wegener granulomatosis	111, 114, 165
Weil disease	208
Weil-Felix reaction	322
Wenckebach block	179
Werdnig-Hoffmann disease	341
Wermer syndrome	255
Wernicke aphasia	302
Wernicke center	503
Wernicke encephalopathy	311
West syndrome	332
Westermark sign	180
Westphal sign	300
Wharton duct	464
Whipple disease	206
Whipple operation	215
Whipple triad	246
Whitmore disease	108
Wickham striae	320
Williamson sign	158
(circle of) Willis	471
Wilms tumor	342
Wilson disease	209
(foramen of) Winslow	482
Wirsung duct	484
Wiskott-Aldrich syndrome	339
Wolff-Parkinson-White syndrome	179
Wolfram syndrome	336
Wolman disease	256
Wood lamp	322

Y

Yatabe-Guilford Personality Inventory	303
Young syndrome	235

Z

Zenker diverticulum	204
Zieve syndrome	208
Zollinger-Ellison syndrome	255

薬剤商品名索引

ア

アイエーコール	429
アイソボリン	430
アイトロール	189
アキネトン	315
アクアチム軟膏・クリーム・ローション	426
アクチバシン	189
アクテムラ	289
アクトス	258
アクプラ	429
アクラシノン	429
アクロマイシン	428
アクロマイシン軟膏	428
アザクタム	422
アザルフィジン EN	288
アズノール	153
アスピリン	122
アセオシリン	428
アセチルスピラマイシン	428
アダラート	188
アドエア	169
アトニン-O	241
アドリアシン	429, 430
アバスチン	433
アパプロ	188
アービタックス	433
アピドラ	258
アプレゾリン	189
アベロックス	426
アポルブ	224
アーマイ	428
アマージ	122
アマスリン	424
アマリール	258
アミサリン	189
アムビゾーム	422
アムロジン	188
アモリン	422
アラセナ-A	329
アラバ	288
アリセプト	315
アリミデックス	429
アリムタ	168
アルケラン	430
アルサルミン	210
アルダクトンA	188
アルツ	289
アルドメット	189
アルファロール	289
アレビアチン	315
アログリセム	258
アンカロン	189
アンコチル	425

イ

イスコチン	168, 425
イセパシン	425
イソジンガーグル	153
イダマイシン	430
イトリゾール	329, 426
イノバン	189
イホマイド	430
イミグラン	122
イムノマックス-γ	430
イリノテカン	429
イリボー	211
イレッサ	168, 433
インダシン	122
インタール	167
インデラル	188
イントロンA	430

ウ

ヴァイデックス	275
ウイントマイロン	426
ウリトス	224
ウルソ	211
ウロキナーゼ	189

エ

MSコンチン	122
エクサシン	425
エクザール	431
エクジェイド	274
エクセグラン	316
エサンブトール	425
エストラサイト	430
エストラダーム	241

エスポー	274	カナマイシン軟膏	426
エバステル	145	カネンドマイシン	422
エパデール	259	カバサール	315
エビスタ	289	ガバペン	316
エビリファイ	316	カフェルゴット	122
エピルビシン	430	カプトリル	188
エピレオプチマル	316	カルセド	429
エフトール	168, 425	カルベニン	427
エフビー	315	カルボプラチン	429
エポジン	274	カロナール	122
エポセリン坐剤	424	カンプト	429
エムトリバ	275		
エリスロシン	425	キ	
エリスロシン軟膏	425	キシロカイン	123, 189
エリスロマイシン	425	キネダック	258
エルシトニン	289	ギャバロン	315
エルプラット	430	キュバール	169
塩酸コカイン	122	キロサイド	429
塩酸バンコマイシン	428		
塩酸プロカルバジン	431	ク	
塩酸モルヒネ	122	クエストラン	259
エンドキサン	429	グラクティブ	258
エンブレル	288	クラバモックス	422
		クラビット	426
オ		クラビット点眼液	426
オイグルコン	258	クラフォラン	424
オーガンマ	430	クラリシッド	422
オキシコンチン	122	クラリス	422
オキシテトラコーン	427	グラン	274
オーグメンチン	422	グリコラン	258
オゼックス	428	グリベック	274, 433
オゼックス点眼液	428	グルコバイ	258
オノン	167	グルトパ	315
オピアル	122	クレスチン	431
オピスタン	122	グレースビット	428
オメガシン	422	クロザリル	316
オメプラゾン	211	クロミッド	241
オラスポア	424	クロラムフェニコール点眼液	423
オラセフ	424	クロロマイセチン	423
オラペネム小児用細粒	428	クロロマイセチンサクシネート	423
オルガラン	275	クロロマイセチン耳科用液	423
オンコビン	274, 431		
		ケ	
カ		ケイテン	424
カイトリル	211	ケイペラゾン	422
カソデックス	224	ケテック	428
ガチフロ	425	ケニセフ	423
ガチフロ点眼液	425	ケフラール	422
カナマイシン	426	ケフレックス	423

薬剤商品名索引

コ

ゲンタシン	425
ゲンタシン点眼液・軟膏	425
コアキシン	423
コスメゲン	429
コホリン	429
コムタン	315
コリマイシンS	423
コルヒチン	259
コレキサミン	259
コロネル	211
コンサータ	314

サ

サイクロセリン	168, 424
サイトテック	210
ザイボックス	426
サイメリン	430
サイモグロブリン	276
ザイロリック	259
サガミシン	426
ザジテン	145
サーバリックス	242
サマセフ	423
サラゾピリン	211
サレド	274
サワシリン	422
サンセファール	424
サンテマイシン点眼液	426
サンドスタチン	258
サンピロ	136
サンラビン	429

シ

ジェニナック	425
ジェムザール	168, 430
シオマリン	426
ジオン	212
ジギトキシン	189
ジゴキシン	189
ジスロマック	422
シセプチン点眼液	428
シナジス	344
シナシッド	427
ジフルカン	425
シプロキサン	424
ジメリン	258
ジャヌビア	258
ジュリナ	241
ジョサマイシン	426
シンビット	189
シンメトレル	168, 315
シンレスタール	259

ス

スオード	427
スタラシド	431
スーテント	433
ストックリン	275
スパラ	428
スプリセル	433
スミフェロン	211, 430
スルペラゾン	427

セ

セイブル	258
ゼヴァリン	433
ゼチーア	259
セパトレン	424
セファメジン α	423
ゼフィックス	211
セフォタックス	424
セフォビッド	424
セフォペラジン	424
セフスパン	423
セフゾン	423
セフテム	423
セフメタゾン	423
セフラコール	423
セララ	188
セルシン	314
セレベント	169
センセファリン	423

ソ

ゾシン	428
ソセゴン	123
ソニフィラン	431
ゾビラックス	329
ソフラチュール	425
ゾラデックス	224
ソルシリン	422
ゾレア	167

タ

ダイアモックス	136, 188
タイケルブ	433

タイセファコール	423	トブラシン	428
ダウノマイシン	274, 429	トブラシン点眼液	428
タガメット	210	トフラニール	314
ダカルバジン	429	トポテシン	429
タキソテール	429, 431	トミポラン	422
タキソール	431	トミロン	423
タケスリン	423	ドラール	314
タゴシッド	428	ドルコール	427
タシグナ	433	トレドミン	314
タツレキシン	423	トレリーフ	315
タミフル	168	トロビシン	428
ダラシン	423		
ダラシン S	423	**ナ**	
ダラシン T ゲル	423	ナイキサン	122
タリビッド	427	ナイスタチン	427
タリビッド点眼液・耳科用液	427	ナウゼリン	211
タルセバ	168, 433	ナベルビン	431
ダントリウム	316		
タンナルビン	211	**ニ**	
チ		ニゾラール	329, 426
チウラジール	258	ニッパスカルシウム	427
チエナム	425	ニトプロ	189
チオデロン	431	ニドラン	429
チノ	211	ニトログリセリン	189
チラーヂン	258	ニトロール	189
チラーヂン S	258	ニューモバックス NP	168
ツ		**ネ**	
ツベラクチン	425	ネオイスコチン	425
ツベルミン	168, 425	ネオフィリン	167
		ネクサバール	224, 433
テ		ネスプ	274
ティーエスワン	431		
ディフェリン	329	**ノ**	
テグレトール	315	ノイアート	275
テスパミン	431	ノイセフ	423
デスモプレシン	259, 540	ノバミン	211
デパケン	316	ノバントロン	430
デュロテップ MT パッチ	122	ノルバデックス	241, 431
テラルビシン	431		
		ハ	
ト		バイアグラ	242
ドイル	422	バイアスピリン	190
ドキシル	429, 430	ハイカムチン	431
トスキサシン	428	バイシリン G	424
ドパストン	315	ハイドレア	430
トピナ	316	ハイビッド	275
ドプス	315	パオスクレー	212
		パキシル	314

薬剤名索引

バクシダール	426	ビレスパ	168
バクシダール点眼液	426		
バクタ	428	**フ**	
バクトラミン	428	5-FU	430
バクトロバン鼻腔用軟膏	426	ファスティック	258
パクリタキセル	431	ファーストシン	424
パシル	427	ファムビル	329
パズクロス	427	ファルモルビシン	430
バストシリン	422	ファロム	425
パセトシン	422	ファンガード	426
ハーセプチン	241, 433	ファンギゾン	422
パナシッド	427	フィニバックス	424
パナルジン	190, 315	ブイフェンド	428
バナン	424	フィブラスト	329
パニマイシン	424	フィルデシン	431
パニマイシン点眼液	424	フェアストン	431
ハベカシン	422	フェノバール	315
バラクルード	211	フエロン	211, 430
バラシリン	426	フェンタニル	122
パラプラチン	429	フォサマック	289
パラマイシン軟膏	422	フォーチミシン	422
パラミヂン	259	フォトフリン	170
ハルシオン	314	フサン	275
バルトレックス	329	フシジンレオ軟膏	425
ハルナール	224	ブスルフェクス	429
パルミコート	169	フトラフール	430, 431
バレオン	426	フラグミン	275
パーロデル	241, 259, 315	フラジオマイシン	425
パンスポリン	424	プラビックス	315
パンスポリンT	424	プリバス	224
ヒ		ブリプラチン	429
		プリミドン	316
ビクシリン	422	フルイトラン	188
ビクシリンS	422	プルゼニド	211
ビクリン	422	フルタイド	169
ピシバニール	431	フルダラ	430
ビスダイン	136	フルツロン	429
ビスタマイシン	427	フルナーゼ	145
ヒスロン	241	ブルフェン	122
ヒスロンH	431	フルマーク	425
ヒドラ	425	フルマリン	425
ヒドラジット	425	ブレオ	429
ピトレシン	259	プレタール	315
ピノルビン	431	プレベナー	344
ビブラマイシン	424	プロアクト	424
ピマリシン点眼液・眼軟膏	427	プログラフ	288
ヒュミラ	289	プロゲホルモン	241
ピラマイド	168, 427	プロジフ	425
ビリアード	275	プロスタルモン	241

プロスタンディン	189
プロトピック	328
プロプレス	188
プロベラ	431
フロモックス	423
フロリード	426
フロリードF	329
フロリードゲル・腟坐剤	426

ヘ

ペガシス	211
ベガモックス点眼液	426
ベザトールSR	259
ベサノイド	429
ベスタチン	429
ベストコール	423
ベストロン点眼液・耳科用液	423
ペニシリンGカリウム	427
ベネシッド	259
ペプシド	430, 432
ヘプセラ	211
ペプレオ	431
ベルケイド	274, 433
ペルマックス	315
ペングッド	422
ペンタサ	211
ペントシリン	427

ホ

ホスミシン	425
ホスミシンS	425
ホスミシンS点耳液	425
ボスミン	189
ボトックス	315
ボノテオ	289
ポララミン	145
ボルタレン	122
ボンシルFP	329, 425
ボンゾール	241
ホンバン	429

マ

マイトマイシン	431
マイロターグ	433
マキシピーム	423
マクジェン	136
マブリン	429

ミ

ミオカマイシン	426
ミケラン	136
ミコブテイン	427
ミドリン	136
ミニプレス	188
ミノマイシン	426
ミフロール	430

ム

ムコフィリン	167

メ

メイアクトMS	423
メイセリン	423
メガキサシン	425
メキシチール	189
メジコン	167
メソトレキセート	431
メタコリマイシン	423
メデマイシン	426
メバロチン	259
メリシン	427
メルカゾール	258
メロペン	426

モ

モダシン	422
モービック	122

ユ

ユーエフティ	431
ユーゼル	430
ユナシン	427
ユナシンS	422
ユリノーム	259

ラ

ラキソベロン	211
ラジカット	315
ラシックス	188
ラステット	430, 432
ラピアクタ	168
ラミクタール	316
ラミシール	329
ランダ	429
ランタス	258
ランドセン	316

リ

リウマトレックス	288
リカマイシン	427
リコモジュリン	275
リスパダール	316
リタリン	314
リツキサン	433
リファジン	427
リフレックス	314
リマクタン	168, 427
リマチル	288
硫酸アミカシン	422
硫酸キニジン	189
硫酸ストレプトマイシン	168, 428
硫酸ポリミキシン	427
リルテック	315
リレンザ	168
リンコシン	426
リン酸コデイン	122

ル

ルセンティス	136
ルリッド	427

レ

レキップ	315
レクシヴァ	275
レザフィリン	170
レスタミン	145
レダマイシン	424
レトロビル	275
レバチオ	189
レペタン	123
レベトール	211
レミケード	211, 289
レメロン	314
レリフェン	122

ロ

ロイケリン	431
ロイコプロール	274
ロイコボリン	430
ロイスタチン	429
ロイナーゼ	430
ロセフィン	424
ロペミン	211
ロメバクト	426
ロメフロン点眼液・耳科用液	426

ワ

ワーファリン	189

著者略歴：1960年，京都大学医学部卒業．横須賀米国海軍病院，Genesee Hospital, Rochester, NY, Lahey Clinic, Boston にて臨床研修．天理よろづ相談所病院消化器内科医員，近畿大学医学部内科講師・助教授，天理よろづ相談所病院消化器内科部長・副院長歴任．
日本消化器病学会功労会員，日本消化器内視鏡学会功労会員，日本POS医療学会評議員，日本医学英語教育学会名誉会員

著　書：肝・胆道・膵疾患へのアプローチ（医学書院）
POSのカルテ：POMRの正しい書き方（金芳堂）
整形外科医のための医学英語論文の書き方（メジカルビュー社）
臨床英文の正しい書き方（金芳堂）

分担執筆：消化器内視鏡治療（朝倉書店）
内科学診断基準マニュアル（中外医学社）
今日の内科学（医歯薬出版）
薬と病気の本（保健同人社）
上手い！といわれる診療録の書き方（金原出版）

訳　書：医の倫理：医師・看護婦のジレンマ（紀伊国屋書店）
難しい患者さんとのコミュニケーションスキル（金芳堂）
医学冠名用語辞典（朝倉書店）

プラクティカル医学英語辞典

2010年5月1日　第1版第1刷発行〈検印省略〉

著　　者	羽白　清	HAJIRO, Kiyoshi
発 行 者	市井輝和	
発 行 所	株式会社金芳堂	
	〒606-8425 京都市左京区鹿ケ谷西寺ノ前町34番地	
	振　替　01030-1-15605	
	電　話　075-751-1111（代）	
	http://www.kinpodo-pub.co.jp	
印　　刷	共同印刷工業株式会社	
製　　本	株式会社兼文堂	

©羽白清，金芳堂，2010
落丁・乱丁本は直接小社へお送りください．お取り替え致します．

Printed in Japan
ISBN978-4-7653-1423-7

・**JCOPY** <（社）出版者著作権管理機構　委託出版物>
本書の無断複写は著作権法上での例外を除き禁じられています．複写される場合は，その都度事前に，（社）出版者著作権管理機構（電話03-3513-6969, FAX 03-3513-6979, e-mail：info@jcopy.or.jp）の許諾を得てください．